Stockley's Herbal Medicines Interactions

Stockley's Herbal Medicines Interactions

A guide to the interactions of herbal medicines

Second Edition

Editors

Elizabeth Williamson BSc, PhD, MRPharmS, FLS
Samuel Driver BSc
Karen Baxter BSc, MSc, MRPharmS

Expert Contributor

C Rhoda Lee BPharm, PhD, MRPharmS

Editorial Staff

Elizabeth S Foan BA (Cantab)
Rebecca E Garner BSc
Claire L Preston BPharm, PGDipMedMan, MRPharmS
Julia Sawyer BPharm, DipPharmPrac, MRPharmS
Jennifer M Sharp BPharm, DipClinPharm, MRPharmS
Nilufer Virani BSc, MPharm, MRPharmS

Published by Pharmaceutical Press

I Lambeth High Street, London SE1 7JN, UK

© Pharmaceutical Press 2013

(**PP**) is a trade mark of Pharmaceutical Press

Pharmaceutical Press is the publishing division of the Royal Pharmaceutical Society

First edition published 2009
Second edition 2013

Typeset by Laserwords Private Limited, Chennai, India

Printed in Great Britain by TJ International, Padstow, UK

ISBN 978 0 85711 026 8

Contents

Preface

This second edition of *Stockley's Herbal Medicines Interactions* continues in the same vein as the first edition, in providing expertly assessed, constructive, practical advice on the potential interactions of herbal medicines (which for the purposes of this publication are also taken to include nutritional supplements and some items of food) with conventional drugs. As with the first edition, the group behind *Stockley's Herbal Medicines Interactions* remains a seemingly unique collaboration between those with in-depth knowledge of herbal medicines and the team that writes *Stockley's Drug Interactions,* who are experienced in assessing the literature on drug interactions and providing advice on their management.

The main development for this edition is an extension of the range of herbal medicines covered, with around 40 further monographs added, an increase of almost a third. Inevitably, much of the literature published since the last edition pertains to those herbs already covered, and we have additionally revised and revalidated much of the standing text. The interaction monographs for St John's wort alone now stand at over 50, with a total of nearly 800 across the publication.

The interactions of herbal medicines continue to attract much interest and, healthcare professionals still freely admit their lack of knowledge in this area. However, recent research suggests that patients expect those selling complementary and alternative medicines to have an understanding of their safe use, with 90% of respondents expecting that interactions with conventional drugs would be checked for, with a similar number in another survey stating that they expected doctors to learn about CAM in order to provide advice to their patients. This publication therefore continues to serve an important purpose, and our aim, as ever, has been to critically evaluate the published literature and present it in a familiar, easy-to-handle format, so that the busy healthcare professional can quickly access the information and apply it to their clinical situation.

This publication attempts to answer the same questions we address in *Stockley's Drug Interactions,* namely:

- Are the drugs and substances in question known to interact or is the interaction only theoretical and speculative?

- If they do interact, how serious is it?

- Has it been described many times or only once?

- Are all patients affected or only a few?

- Is it best to avoid these two substances altogether or can the interaction be accommodated in some way?

- And what alternative and safer drugs can be used instead?

Stockley's Herbal Medicines Interactions follows the same easy-to-read format as our other publications, with the text organised into a series of individual monographs, all with a common format. In addition, we have included sections on nomenclature, to help users identify herbal medicines that they or their patients may be familiar with under a different name; uses, so that those less familiar with herbal medicines can put their use into context; and constituents, to allow us to address interactions that occur as a result of a substance common to several plants. A pharmacopoeia section is also included for those herbal medicines, dietary supplements and nutraceuticals that have entries in the latest editions (at time of press) of the *British Pharmacopoeia,* the *European Pharmacopoeia* and the *United States Pharmacopoeia*. An indication of the constituents that the herbal medicine may be standardised for is also provided where necessary, but note that this does not necessarily mean that all marketed products are standardised in this way. In addition, we have added the simple, intuitive ratings system that users of *Stockley's Interaction Alerts* and *Stockley's Drug Interactions Pocket Companion* will already be familiar with.

As with all Stockley products, the text is written for a worldwide audience. Terminology has been carefully considered and international terms have been added where it was thought helpful to do so. This and the inclusion of the synonyms and pharmacopoeia sections will, we hope, cater for the needs of healthcare professionals around the world.

As always, the Editorial team have had assistance from many other people in developing this publication, and the Editors gratefully acknowledge the help and guidance that they have provided. The continued support of the Technology and Production teams, particularly Karl Parsons and Linda Paulus, who are instrumental in transforming our data into a useable output. We are also grateful for the support of Alina Lourie and of course, Ivan Stockley, whose foundation work in evaluating and assessing drug interactions underpins this current work.

We are always interested in hearing feedback from users of our publications, and have in the past received many useful comments, which help us to develop the product to best meet the needs of the end-user. Anyone who wishes to contact us can do so at the following address: stockley@rpharms.com

Sam Driver, Karen Baxter, and
Elizabeth Williamson
London, October 2012

Structure of the Publication

The basic issues involved in assessing the importance of interactions between herbal medicines (which for the purposes of this publication are also taken to include nutritional supplements and some items of food) and drugs are similar to those for interactions between conventional drugs, but for herbal medicines the picture is complicated by their very nature: they are complex mixtures themselves and there is also a lack of reliable information about their occurrence and relevance. Before using this publication it is advisable to read this short explanatory section so that you know how the drug interaction data have been set out here, and why, as well as the basic philosophy that has been followed in presenting it.

This publication includes almost 200 herbal medicines, nutraceuticals or dietary supplements. For each of these products there is an introductory section, which includes the following sections where appropriate:

- Synonyms and related species or types, sources and related compounds

- Pharmacopoeias

- Constituents

- Uses and indications

- Pharmacokinetics

- Interactions overview

The synonyms, constituents and uses have largely been compiled with reference to a number of standard sources. These include:

- Sweetman SC (ed), *Martindale: The Complete Drug Reference 37*. [online] London: Pharmaceutical Press http://www.medicinescomplete.com/

- Williamson EM, ed. Potter's Herbal Cyclopaedia. Saffron Walden: The C.W. Daniel Company Limited; 2003.

- Barnes J, Anderson LA, Phillipson JD (eds), *Herbal Medicines 3*. [online] London: Pharmaceutical Press http://www.medicinescomplete.com/

- Williamson EM, ed. Major Herbs of Ayurveda. 1st ed. London: Elsevier; 2002.

- USDA, ARS, National Genetic Resources Program. *Germplasm Resources Information Network - (GRIN)* [Online Database]. National Germplasm Resources Laboratory, Beltsville, Maryland. URL: http://www.ars-grin.gov/cgi-bin/npgs/html/taxecon.pl

- Tropicos.org. Missouri Botanical Garden http://www.tropicos.org/

Where the information regarding the nomenclature, constituents and uses of a herb, dietary supplement or nutraceutical is scarce enough not to appear in any of our standard sources, we have used data that has been published in peer-reviewed journals, and in some cases these may be limited to foreign-language articles where only the abstract is translated into English. In these situations we have included the reference so the end-user can see what the information is based on.

Almost 800 interactions monographs are included, each with a common format. These are subdivided into the following sections:

- Abstract or summary for quick reading.

- Clinical evidence, detailing the interaction and citing the clinical evidence currently available.

- Experimental evidence. Due to the nature of interactions with herbal medicines much of the data currently available comes from *animal* and *in vitro* studies. Although this data doesn't always extrapolate to the clinical situation it can be used to provide some idea of the likelihood and potential severity of an interaction. It has been deliberately kept separate from the clinical data, because this type of data is a better guide to predicting outcomes in practice.

- Mechanism, to allow an understanding as to why the interaction may occur.

- Importance and management. As with all Stockley products, providing guidance on how to manage an interaction is our key aim. The short discussion is designed to aid rapid clinical decision making.

- References, a list of all of the relevant references.

Some of the monographs have been compressed into fewer subsections instead of the more usual five, simply where information is limited or where there is little need to be more expansive.

The monographs also carry an adapted form of the drug interaction Hazard/Severity ratings as used in the electronic *Stockley Interactions Alerts,* and *Stockley's Drug Interactions Pocket Companion.* Where difficulties arise in applying ratings to monographs that cover multiple pairs of drug-herb interactions, we have chosen to illustrate the worst-case scenario. Reading the *Importance and Management* section will explain which members of the groups are most likely to represent a problem.

The interactions are rated using three separate categories:

- Action: This describes whether or not any action needs to be taken to accommodate the interaction. This category ranges from 'avoid' to 'no action needed'.

- Severity: This describes the likely effect of an unmanaged interaction on the patient. This category ranges from 'severe' to 'nothing expected'.

- Evidence: This describes the weight of evidence behind the interaction. This category ranges from 'extensive' to 'theoretical, weak'.

These ratings are combined to produce one of five symbols:

 For interactions that have a life-threatening outcome, or where concurrent use is considered to be best avoided.

 For interactions where concurrent use may result in a significant hazard to the patient and so dosage adjustment or close monitoring is needed.

 For interactions where there is a potentially hazardous outcome, but where, perhaps, the data is poor and conclusions about the interaction are difficult to draw.

 For interactions where there is doubt about the outcome of concurrent use, and therefore it may be necessary to give patients some guidance about possible adverse effects, and/or consider some monitoring.

 For interactions that are not considered to be of clinical significance, or where no interaction occurs.

We put a lot of thought in to the original design of these symbols, and have deliberately avoided a numerical or colour-coding system as we did not want to imply any relationship between the symbols or colours. Instead we chose internationally recognisable symbols, which in testing were intuitively understood by our target audience of healthcare professionals.

There are also several 'family monographs' included. These are for constituents that have been demonstrated to interact in their own right, but which are prevalent in a number of herbal medicines, the most common example of this is the flavonoids. This structure allows us to assess the relevant data in one place, and cross reference the reader as appropriate. Because so many herbs contain a multitude of these constituents it would not be possible to cover them in each plant monograph.

Data Selection

This publication has been produced by the team that writes *Stockley's Drug Interactions,* with the help and guidance of an expert in the herbal medicines field. The same rigorous approach that is used to produce *Stockley's Drug Interactions* has been applied here, although with some notable differences, particularly in the selection of data for inclusion. The data on interactions are of widely varying quality and reliability, and this is even more the case when considering interactions between herbal medicines and conventional drugs. The best information comes from clinical studies carried out on large numbers of patients under scrupulously controlled conditions; however, with herbal medicines these are sparse. Indeed those that there are, have already been included in *Stockley's Drug Interactions*. What this publication attempts to do is assess the wealth of data from *animal* and *in vitro* studies, which would not normally be considered for inclusion in *Stockley's Drug Interactions*.

As with all our publications we undertake extensive literature searching, we consider guidance published by regulatory bodies and we aim to avoid citing secondary literature wherever possible. Some of the studies cited in herb-drug interaction articles or publications are of doubtful quality and some are merely speculation. We have included them because they appear in other reference sources for interactions, but we have attempted to put their results and recommendations in perspective.

The herbal medicines, dietary supplements and nutraceuticals selected for inclusion have been chosen on the basis of their popularity and/or because they have interaction reports associated with them.

Nomenclature

Every care has been taken to correctly identify the herbal medicine involved in interactions. The botanical nomenclature and the vast number of colloquial names used for the plants can be very confusing. We have therefore adopted one name for each herbal medicine that is used consistently throughout the monograph, and indeed across the publication. However, we are aware that we will not always have selected the most appropriate name for some countries and have therefore included a synonyms field to aid users who know the plant by different names. The synonyms come from several well-respected sources and, where botanical names are used, have been cross-checked against the extremely useful database constructed by Kew (Royal Botanic Gardens, Kew) electronic Plant Information Centre. Available at http://epic.kew.org/epic/). Occasionally the same synonym has been used for more than one herbal medicine, and where we are aware of this, we have been careful to highlight the potential for confusion.

We should also point out that we have chosen the phrase 'conventional medicines' to distinguish those products that are licensed and commonly used in Western medicine. This nomenclature is not meant to imply any preference, it is just simply a way of being clear about which preparation we are discussing.

Similarly, there is the potential for confusion between the synthetic coumarins used as anticoagulants (e.g. warfarin, acenocoumarol) and those coumarins that occur naturally within plants. We have therefore chosen to use the term 'coumarins' for those of synthetic origin, and 'natural coumarins' to distinguish those of plant origin.

Abbreviations

The table below represents the standard abbreviations that may be used without further definition in Stockley's Herbal Medicines Interactions.

ACE	angiotensin-converting enzyme	L	litre(s)
ADP	adenosine diphosphate	LDL	low-density lipoprotein
AIDS	acquired immunodeficiency syndrome	LFT	liver function test
ALT	alanine aminotransferase	LH	luteinising hormone
aPTT	activated partial thromboplastin time	LMWH	low-molecular-weight heparin
AST	aspartate aminotransferase	MAC	minimum alveolar concentration
ATP	adenosine triphosphate	MAO	monoamine oxidase
AUC	area under the time-concentration curve	MAOI	monoamine oxidase inhibitor
AUC_{0-12}	area under the time-concentration curve measured over 0 to 12-hours	MHRA	Medicines and Healthcare products Regulatory Agency (UK)
AV	atrioventricular	MIC	minimum inhibitory concentration
BCRP	breast cancer resistance protein	mEq	milliequivalent(s)
BP	blood pressure	mg	milligram(s)
BP	British Pharmacopoeia	mL	millilitre(s)
bpm	beats per minute	mmHg	millimetre(s) of mercury
CNS	central nervous system	mmol	millimole
COX	cyclo-oxygenase	mol	mole
CSF	cerebrospinal fluid	nmol	nanomole
CSM	Committee on Safety of Medicines (UK) (now subsumed within the Commission on Human Medicines)	NNRTI	non-nucleoside reverse transcriptase inhibitor
		NRTI	nucleoside reverse transcriptase inhibitor
		NSAID	non-steroidal anti-inflammatory drug
ECG	electrocardiogram	OATP	organic anion transporting polypeptide
ECT	electroconvulsive therapy	PCP	pneumocystis pneumonia
e.g.	exempli gratia (for example)	pH	the negative logarithm of the hydrogen ion concentration
EMEA	The European Agency for the Evaluation of Medicinal Products	Ph Eur	European Pharmacopoeia
FDA	Food and Drug Administration (USA)	PPI	proton pump inhibitor
FSH	follicle stimulating hormone	ppm	parts per million
g	gram(s)	PTT	partial thromboplastin time
HAART	highly active antiretroviral therapy	*sic*	written exactly as it appears in the original
HIV	human immunodeficiency virus	SNRI	serotonin and noradrenaline reuptake inhibitor
HRT	hormone replacement therapy		
ibid	*ibidem*, in the same place (journal or book)	SSRI	selective serotonin reuptake inhibitor
		TSH	thyroid-stimulating hormone
i.e.	id est (that is)	UK	United Kingdom
INR	international normalised ratio	USP	The United States Pharmacopeia
IU	international units	US and	United States of America
IUD	intra-uterine device	USA	
kg	kilogram(s)	WHO	World Health Organization

General Considerations

Incidence of herbal medicines interactions

The incidence of interactions between herbal medicines and nutritional supplements with conventional drugs is not yet fully known, and there is no body of reliable information currently available to draw upon when assessing the scale of any possible problem, or predicting clinical outcomes. Even in the case of St John's wort, which is now commonly known to interact with a number of drugs, the clinical significance of some reported cases cannot be accurately evaluated due to the variation in the nature of the herb itself and products made from it. In general, the lack of evidence may be due to under-reporting or unrecognised interactions, but there is also the possibility that many herbal medicines have a generally safe profile and do not interact significantly with drugs. Given the poor quality of information available it can be difficult to put the problem into perspective and in the absence of good evidence, speculation has taken its place. Ivan Stockley, a pioneer in the field of drug-interaction investigation, has often maintained that data on interactions are of widely varying quality and reliability, and stated that 'sometimes they are no more than speculative and theoretical scaremongering guesswork, hallowed by repeated quotation until they become virtually set in stone'. Although these remarks were made in the context of drug interactions, they are even more apposite when applied to herb-drug interactions where anecdotal reports, uncontrolled studies, or data based solely on *animal* studies are the main form of evidence available. These have to be evaluated very carefully before advising patients as to the safety (or not) of combining herbal medicines with either other supplements or with conventional drugs. While many publications uncritically use theoretical evidence to advise on his issue, it risks the danger that patients (and their friends and families) who have already taken supplements and drugs together with no problems, will no longer believe even good advice – and subsequently take incompatible combinations to ill effect. It is also noticeable that whilst anecdotal or theoretical evidence is quite rightly considered unacceptable as evidence of efficacy for herbal products, it seems to be given undue credibility when demonstrating toxicity, and consumers of natural medicines have observed this double standard. Obviously the best answer to this problem is for good and reliable evidence to become available, and for the importance of reports to be based on the nature of the evidence they provide. In the first instance, it would be most useful to know the extent of the problem and the risk or likelihood of a herb-drug interaction arising. However even numbers of people taking supplements is not accurately known, although over the past 10 years several studies have been carried out to try to assess this. Some knowledge of not only who, but how and why people are taking herbal medicines can help to identify potential problems or warn of them before they arise.

Who uses herbal medicines?

The use of herbal medicines and nutritional supplements is increasing dramatically in many parts of the world, especially in Europe, the US and Australasia, as part of the popularity of complementary and alternative medicine (CAM). It is difficult to measure the extent of the use of herbal products by consumers and patients in a largely unregulated market, especially with so many herbal products being sold over the internet, and survey studies that have attempted to do so have often been criticised for flawed methodology. However, there is no doubt that the issue of people taking herbal and nutritional products at the same time as conventional medicines is significant, and the purpose of this publication is to provide information so that this practice can be carried out as safely as possible.

Some idea of the size of the market and its recent growth can be seen from a series of studies carried out over the past few years in the United States. In 1997, the results of a national survey[1] indicated that approximately 12% of the adult responders had taken a herbal remedy in the past year, which was an increase of 380% from 1990, and almost 1 in 5 of those taking prescription drugs were also taking a herbal or vitamin supplement. In 1998 and 1999, a survey of over 2500 adults estimated that 14% of the general population were regularly taking herbal products, and of patients taking prescription drugs, 16% also took a herbal supplement.[2] Data obtained from a separate 1999 survey estimated that 9.6% of US adults used herbal medicines,[3] which was lower than would be expected from the previous study, and illustrates the problems of assessing consumer behaviour accurately, but it is still a significant increase from the 1990 figures. By 2002, figures showed that the annual use of dietary supplements had risen to 18.8%.[4] Although the accuracy of these figures can be questioned, what is also noteworthy is that the studies were carried out in the general population, so it is logical to assume that in the patient population usage could be even higher.

A survey undertaken in the UK in 1994 suggests that the prevalence of alternative medicine use (which included herbal medicines) was 8.5% of the population, whereas in

Germany, in 1996, it was much higher, at 65%. The low figure for the UK could be because of national differences, because different types of use were assessed (1-year versus lifetime) or because at the time, the UK was undergoing a difficult economic period and usually CAM is paid for privately.[5] Useful information about herbal medicinal use can also be obtained from the monetary value of the market. In 2002, French health insurance paid $91 million in partial reimbursements for ginkgo, saw palmetto, and pygeum prescriptions, with a total value of $196 million, and in 2003, German health insurance paid $283 million in reimbursements for prescribed herbal products including ginkgo, St. John's wort, saw palmetto, hawthorn, stinging nettle root and pumpkin seed. These figures do not include non-prescription purchase of herbal remedies, but it is known that in 2003, European countries spent almost $5 billion (at manufacturers' prices) on non-prescription herbal medicines,[6] and of course the cost at consumer level would be very much higher.

1. Eisenberg DM, Davis RB, Ettner SL, Appel S, Wilkey S, Van Rompay M, Kessler RC. Trends in alternative medicine use in the United States, 1990- 1997: results of a follow-up national survey. *JAMA* (1998) 280, 1569–75.
2. Kaufman DW, Kelly JP, Rosenberg L, Anderson TE, Mitchell AA. Recent patterns of medication use in the ambulatory adult population of the United States. The Slone Survey. *JAMA* (2002) 287, 337–44.
3. Ni H, Simile C, Hardy AM. Utilization of complementary and alternative medicine by United States adults: results from the 1999 national health interview survey. *Med Care* (2002) 40, 353–8.
4. Kelly JP, Kaufman DW, Kelley K, Rosenberg L, Anderson TE, Mitchell AA. Recent trends in use of herbal and other natural products. *Arch Intern Med* (2005) 165, 281–6.
5. Ernst E. Prevalence of use of complementary/alternative medicine: – a systematic review. *Bull WHO* (2000) 78, 252–7.
6. De Smet PAGM. Herbal Medicine in Europe – Relaxing Regulatory Standards. *N Engl J Med* (2005) 352, 1176–8.

Herbal medicine use in specific patient groups

(a) Patients with cancer

Certain groups of patients are known, or thought to have, a higher incidence of supplement usage than others. It is generally thought that cancer patients, for example, have an exceptionally high intake of herbal and nutritional supplements. One of the first studies to collate the information available on CAM use in cancer patients was from 1998, when a systematic review of 26 surveys from 13 countries was published. CAM use in adults ranged from 7 to 64%, with an average use of 31.4%.[1] The high degree of variability was thought to be most likely due to different understandings of the term CAM on the part of both investigators and patients, but also illustrates that the results of such surveys must be interpreted very carefully. A subsequent study showed that CAM use (both self-medication and visits to CAM practitioners) had increased significantly from 1998 to 2005 in cancer patients, and it was estimated that more than 80% of all women with breast cancer use CAM, 41% in a specific attempt to manage their breast cancer. The most commonly used herbal products for this purpose in 2005 were flaxseed, green tea, and vitamins (C and E).[2] A US survey of outpatients with cancer found that 83.3% had used at least one CAM. Vitamins and herbal medicines were used by 62.6% of patients, and use was greater in women and those of a younger age.[3] These findings were reflected in a 2005 study which confirmed that of the chemotherapy patients surveyed, 91% reported using at least one form of CAM (most frequently diets, massage, and herbal medicine). Of these patients only 57% discussed the use of at least one of these therapies with their healthcare provider.[4] A report from 2010, exploring CAM use

by patients with cancer, similarly found a high use of such therapies, with 80% of users believing that there were health benefits despite the lack of evidence. Furthermore, 90% of patients believed that doctors should learn about CAM in order to provide advice to their patients.[5]

Herbal medicine use by cancer patients seems to be high in many parts of the world: in New Zealand 49% of cancer patients at a regional centre used CAM (most commonly vitamins, antioxidants, alternative diets, and herbal medicines), to improve the quality of life and in the hope of a cure (47% and 30% of CAM users, respectively). CAM was deemed helpful in the management of their cancer by 71% of patients, and 89% felt that CAM was safe. Younger patients tended to use CAM more.[6] The different patterns of herbal use between cancer patients undergoing palliative or curative chemotherapy has also been studied, and the results confirmed that both groups frequently use herbal remedies concurrently with chemotherapy (37% and 38%, respectively), but with a slightly different intent. Palliative patients tended to show more frequent herbal use than curative patients (78% versus 67%), whereas curative patients used herbal remedies much more often to relieve adverse effects (31% versus 3%).[7]

(b) Patients with HIV infection

The use of CAM is said to be prevalent among patients with HIV infection. A 2008 review analysed the results from 40 different studies in an attempt to establish the impact of CAM use on HIV care. On average, 60% of HIV-positive patients use CAM, with usage seeming to be higher in white Caucasians, those with a higher level of education, and those with greater financial resources. CAM was most commonly used to alleviate the symptoms of HIV, the adverse effects related to antiviral use and to improve quality of life. As with other patient groups, not all patients disclosed the use of CAM, with 38 to 90% stating that their healthcare provider was aware of their use of CAM.[8] A subsequent study similarly found that 36% of patients disclosed CAM use to their healthcare provider, and interestingly, CAM disclosure was associated with a greater adherence to their prescribed antiretroviral regimen.[9]

(c) Patients on weight-loss programmes

Other groups of patients known to use supplements regularly are those on weight loss programmes and most of the weight-loss supplements taken (73.8%) contained stimulants such as ephedra, caffeine, and/or bitter orange. An estimated 15.2% of American adults (women 20.6%, men 9.7%) had used a weight-loss supplement at some time: 8.7% within the past year (women 11.3%, men 6%). Women aged 18 to 34 years used weight-loss supplements the most (16.7%), and use was equally prevalent among ethnic groups and education levels. More worryingly, many adults were long-term users and most did not discuss this practice with their doctor.[10]

(d) Hospital inpatients

A study of herbal medicine use during peri-operative care identified the most commonly used medications and assessed their potential for causing adverse events or drug interactions in patients who were having surgical procedures. Their conclusions were that certain herbal medicines posed a potential danger in peri-operative care (such as St John's wort because of its enzyme-inducing effects, and valerian, because of its sedative effects), but no attempt was made to ascertain the incidence of such events.[11] However, in 2007, a study of 299 patients on the medical wards of two hospitals in Israel found that 26.8% of participants took herbal medicines or dietary supplements, and of these, potential interactions were noted in 7.1%. The authors suggested that most patients are not asked specifically about herbal consumption by their medical team.[12]

(e) Children

Several surveys indicate that herbal use in children is increasing and it has been estimated that 28 to 40% of children might be exposed to herbal preparations for the management of asthma, anxiety, attention deficit hyperactivity disorders, insomnia and respiratory infections.[13,14] A survey of 503 children attending the Royal Children's Hospital, Melbourne, similarly found that the use of CAM by children is common. Herbal products were used by 12% of the group surveyed and a further 8% were taking echinacea products. Sixty-three percent of those reporting CAM use had not discussed this with their treating doctor. The authors concluded that given the potential risk of adverse events associated with the use of CAM or interactions with conventional management, doctors should ask about their use as a part of routine history taking.[15]

1. Ernst E, Cassileth BR. The prevalence of complementary/alternative medicine in cancer: a systematic review. *Cancer* (1998) 83, 777–82.
2. Boon HS, Olatunde F, Zick SM. Trends in complementary/alternative medicine use by breast cancer survivors: comparing survey data from 1998 and 2005. *BMC Womens Health* (2007) 7, 4.
3. Richardson MA, Sanders T, Palmer JL, Greisinger A, Singletary SE. Complementary/alternative medicine use in a comprehensive cancer center and the implications for oncology. *J Clin Oncol* (2000) 18, 2505–14.
4. Yates JS, Mustian KM, Morrow GR, Gillies LJ, Padmanaban D, Atkins JN, Issell B, Kirshner JJ, Colman LK. Prevalence of complementary and alternative medicine use in cancer patients during treatment. *Support Care Cancer* (2005) 13, 806–11.
5. Oh B, Butow P, Mullan B, Beale P, Pavlakis N, Rosenthal D, Clarke S. The use and perceived benefits resulting from the use of complementary and alternative medicine by cancer patients in Australia. *Asia Pac J Clin Oncol* (2010) 6, 342–9.
6. Chrystal K, Allan S, Forgeson G, Isaacs R. The use of complementary/alternative medicine by cancer patients in a New Zealand regional cancer treatment centre. *N Z Med J* (2003) 116, U296.
7. Engdal S, Steinsbekk A, Klepp O, Nilsen OG. Herbal use among cancer patients during palliative or curative chemotherapy treatment in Norway. *Support Care Cancer* (2008) 16, 763–9.
8. Littlewood RA, Vanable PA. Complementary and alternative medicine use among HIV+ people: research synthesis and implications for HIV care. *AIDS Care* (2008) 20, 1002–18.
9. Chenglong C, Yang Y, Gange SJ, Weber K, Sharp GB, Wilson TE, Levine A, Robison E, Goparaju L, Ganhdi M, Merenstein D. Disclosure of complementary and alternative medicine use to health care providers among HIV-infected women. *AIDS Patient Care and STDS* (2009) 23, 965–71.
10. Blanck HM, Serdula MK, Gillespie C, Galuska DA, Sharpe PA, Conway JM, Khan LK, Ainsworth BE. Use of nonprescription dietary supplements for weight loss is common among Americans. *J Am Diet Assoc* (2007) 107, 441–7.
11. Ang-Lee MK, Moss J, Yuan C-S. Herbal medicines and perioperative care. *JAMA* (2001) 286, 208–16.
12. Goldstein LH, Elias M, Ron-Avraham G, Biniaurishvili BZ, Madjar M, Kamargash I, Braunstein R, Berkovitch M, Golik A. Consumption of herbal remedies and dietary supplements amongst patients hospitalized in medical wards. *Br J Clin Pharmacol* (2007) 64, 373–80.
13. Sawini-Sikand A, Schubiner H, Thomas RL. Use of complementary/alternative therapies among children in primary care pediatrics *Ambul Pediatr* (2002) 2, 99–103.
14. Ottolini MC. Complementary and alternative medicine use among children in Washington, DC area *Ambul Pediatr* (2000) 1, 122–5.
15. Lim A, Cranswick N, Skull S, South M. Survey of complementary and alternative medicine use at a tertiary children's hospital *J Paediatr Child Health* (2005) 41, 424–7.

Differences in herbal use in specific population groups

(a) The elderly

CAM use is high in those of 65 years of age and over (27.7% according to one US study), but declines among those aged 75 years and over, and overall, more women than men are CAM users. The highest level of use seems to be among Asians (48.6%), followed by Hispanics (31.6%), Whites (27.7%), and Blacks (20.5%).[1] Data drawn from a 2002 survey that included a supplement on the use of herbal medicines, with the analysis limited to adults aged 65 years and older, showed that herbs were an important component of their own health management. Whereas about 25% of the Asian and Hispanic elderly used herbal medicines, only about 10% of the Black and White elderly used them; the herbs used, and the reasons for doing so, also differed according to ethnicity.[2]

It is also apparent that in the elderly, the use of herbal medicines with conventional medicines, both prescription and non-prescription, is widespread. The risk for adverse interactions was assessed in a Medicare population, using a retrospective analysis of Cardiovascular Health Study interview data from four different years. Of 5052 participants, the median age at the beginning of the study was 75 years, 60.2% were female, 16.6% were African American, and 83.4% were White. From 1994 to 1999 the number using herbal medicines increased from 6.3% to 15.1%, and the number using herbal medicines concurrently with conventional drugs also increased, from 6% to 14.4%. Combinations thought to be potentially risky were noted in 393 separate interviews, with most (379 reports in 281 patients) involving a risk of bleeding due to use of garlic, ginkgo, or ginseng together with aspirin, warfarin, ticlopidine, or pentoxifylline. An additional 786 drug-herb combinations were considered to have some, (again) theoretical or uncertain, risk for an adverse interaction.[3]

The type of products taken obviously reflect the age group taking them, and the most common products used by the elderly are those concerned with ameliorating degenerative or age-related conditions. In a predominantly White (91%) elderly cohort, the use of dietary supplements was surveyed each year from 1994 to 1999 for an average of 359 male (36%) and female (64%) participants aged 60 to 99 years. By 1999, glucosamine emerged as the most frequently used (non-vitamin, non-mineral) supplement followed by ginkgo, chondroitin, and garlic. For women, there was a significant trend of increasing use for black cohosh, starflower oil, evening primrose oil, flaxseed oil, chondroitin, prasterone (dehydroepiandrosterone), garlic, ginkgo, glucosamine, grapeseed extract, hawthorn, and St John's wort. For men, alpha-lipoic acid, ginkgo, and grapeseed extract showed a similar trend.[4]

(b) Children

Surprisingly, herbal medicine and nutritional supplement use in children can also be high, and so is the concurrent use with conventional medicine. A convenience sampling of paediatric emergency department patients in the US was carried out during a 3-month period in 2001, where 153 families participated in the study, with a mean patient age of 5.3 years. Children were given a herbal medicine by 45% of caregivers, and the most common herbal medicines reportedly used were aloe plant or juice (44%), echinacea (33%), and sweet oil (25%).[5]

More recently, 1804 families were interviewed in a study of parents and patients up to 18 years arriving at a large paediatric emergency department in Toronto, Canada. Conventional and herbal medicines or supplements were being used concurrently in 20% of the patients and 15% were receiving more than one herbal medicine simultaneously.

The authors of this study identified possible herb-drug or herb-herb interactions in 16% of children.[6]

(c) Gender

Studies usually show that herbal medicine use is higher in women than men, and this is likely to be true for many reasons, despite the unreliability of figures gained in surveys. Women generally live longer than men, and elderly people take more supplements; women tend to be the primary carers for children and the elderly and also purchase most of the everyday remedies used in the home; and women take more weight-loss products than men. In several studies, it is suggested that women are at least twice as likely to take herbal medicines or supplements as men.[1,7–10]

(d) Educational level and knowledge of herbal products

People of all levels of educational attainment are likely to take herbal and nutritional supplements. Some studies suggest that usage is similar across most education levels,[10] whereas others have found that college graduates appear to have the highest incidence of herbal use.[4,7,11] Despite the generally high levels of education, it is of great concern that consumers do not have a correspondingly high level of knowledge about the products they are consuming. In a study of caregivers who reported giving their child a herbal product, 88% had at least one year of college education. However, 77% of the participants in the study did not believe, or were uncertain, if herbal medicines had any adverse effects; only 27% could name a potential adverse effect, and 66% were unsure, or thought that herbal medicines did not interact with other medications.[5] In a study in Israel of users of 'natural drugs', 56.2% believed they caused no adverse effects.[12] In Australia, the perceptions of emergency department patients towards CAM were assessed by comparing the CAM users (68% of the patients surveyed) with non-users, particularly regarding safety and efficacy. In both cases there was no significant difference between CAM users and non-users, with 44.1% agreeing that CAM is drug-free, and more worryingly, 28.5% agreeing, or strongly agreeing, that CAM is always safe to take with prescription drugs. However, significantly more CAM users agreed that CAM is safe and can prevent people from becoming ill, and furthermore, is more effective than prescription drugs. Moreover, significantly fewer CAM users agreed that prescription drugs are safe to take.[13]

(e) Rural populations

An Australian postal questionnaire survey found that in people living in rural areas of New South Wales the use of CAM is high, with garlic and echinacea being the most used herbal products. Of those responding, 70.3% reported using one or more CAM and 62.7% had visited a complementary practitioner.[14] In Jamaica, concurrent surveys were carried out in Kingston (an urban parish) and Clarendon (a rural parish) in 743 patients who visited health centres and pharmacies. Herbal medicines were taken with conventional medicines by 80% of respondents and 87% of these did not tell their healthcare provider. In the rural community 92% took herbal medicines with conventional medicines, compared with 70% of the urban community.[15]

1. Arcury TA, Suerken CK, Grzywacz JG, Bell RA, Lang W, Quandt SA. Complementary and alternative medicine use among older adults: ethnic variation. *Ethn Dis* (2006) 16, 723–31.
2. Arcury TA, Grzywacz JG, Bell RA, Neiberg RH, Lang W, Quandt SA. Herbal remedy use as health self-management among older adults. *J Gerontol B Psychol Sci Soc Sci* (2007) 62, S142–S149.
3. Elmer GW, Lafferty WE, Tyree PT, Lind BK. Potential interactions between complementary/alternative products and conventional medicines in a Medicare population. *Ann Pharmacother* (2007) 41, 1617–24.
4. Wold RS, Lopez ST, Yau CL, Butler LM, Pareo-Tubbeh SL, Waters DL, Garry PJ, Baumgartner RN. Increasing trends in elderly persons' use of nonvitamin, nonmineral dietary supplements and concurrent use of medications. *J Am Diet Assoc* (2005) 105, 54–63.
5. Lanski SL, Greenwald M, Perkins A, Simon HK. Herbal therapy use in a pediatric emergency department population: expect the unexpected. *Pediatrics* (2003) 111, 981–5.
6. Goldman RD, Rogovik AL, Lai D, Vohra S. Potential interactions of drug-natural health products and natural health products-natural health products among children. *J Pediatr* (2008) 152, 521–6.
7. Schaffer DM, Gordon NP, Jensen CD, Avins AL. Nonvitamin, nonmineral supplement use over a 12-month period by adult members of a large health maintenance organization. *J Am Diet Assoc* (2003) 103, 1500–1505.
8. Richardson MA, Sanders T, Palmer JL, Greisinger A, Singletary SE. Complementary/alternative medicine use in a comprehensive cancer center and the implications for oncology. *J Clin Oncol* (2000) 18, 2505–14.
9. Yates JS, Mustian KM, Morrow GR, Gillies LJ, Padmanaban D, Atkins JN, Issell B, Kirshner JJ, Colman LK. Prevalence of complementary and alternative medicine use in cancer patients during treatment. *Support Care Cancer* (2005) 13, 806–11.
10. Blanck HM, Serdula MK, Gillespie C, Galuska DA, Sharpe PA, Conway JM, Khan LK, Ainsworth BE. Use of nonprescription dietary supplements for weight loss is common among Americans. *J Am Diet Assoc* (2007) 107, 441–7.
11. Kelly JP, Kaufman DW, Kelley K, Rosenberg L, Anderson TE, Mitchell AA. Recent trends in use of herbal and other natural products. *Arch Intern Med* (2005) 165, 281–6.
12. Giveon SM, Liberman N, Klang S, Kahan E. Are people who use "natural drugs" aware of their potentially harmful side effects and reporting to family physician? *Patient Educ Couns* (2004) 53, 5–11.
13. Taylor DMD, Walsham N, Taylor SE, Wong LF. Complementary and alternative medicines versus prescription drugs: perceptions of emergency department patients. *Emerg Med J* (2006) 23, 266–8.
14. Wilkinson JM, Simpson MD. High use of complementary therapies in a New South Wales rural community. *Aust J Rural Health* (2001) 9, 166–71.
15. Delgoda R, Ellington C, Barrett S, Gordon N, Clarke N, Younger N. The practice of polypharmacy involving herbal and prescription medicines in the treatment of diabetes mellitus, hypertension and gastrointestinal disorders in Jamaica. *West Indian Med J* (2004) 53, 400–405.

Attitudes to the use of herbal medicines

People who use herbal medicines and nutritional supplements report their primary source of information as friends or relatives in 80% of cases, and only 45% of those giving their children herbal products report discussing it with either their doctor or pharmacist.[1] In one study, 44.7% never reported herbal usage to their physician, and 11% did so only rarely.[2] Again, this is a general trend found in other studies,[3] sometimes with even higher levels (e.g. up to 70%) of non-reporting seen.[4] In one study in New Zealand only 41% of patients had discussed their CAM use with their oncologist, and almost one-third had started such medicines before being seen at the Cancer Treatment Centre.[5] In a study of hospital inpatients a great cause for concern was that 94% of the patients had not been asked specifically about herbal consumption by the medical team and only 23% of the hospital's medical files of the patients taking herbal medicines or dietary supplements had any record of this fact.[6] In fact, in many studies, even where the question was asked, many patients did not inform their doctor that they were also taking herbal remedies.[7,8]

This serious under-reporting by patients may probably be because they consider herbal medicines safe, even if taken at the same time as prescription drugs.[9] One study found a significant correlation between the belief that herbal medicines can cause adverse effects and the tendency to report their usage to the family physician.[2] Some patients may fear the disapproval of the physician, and since they consider the medicines to be safe, see no reason for inviting problems by disclosing these practices. Unfortunately, even if patients do report their use of herbal medicines to the physician or pharmacist, there is no guarantee that accurate information or advice will be available. Physicians usually underestimate the extent to which their patients use these remedies and often do not ask for information from the patient. Worse still, in one survey 51% of doctors believed that herbal medicines have no or only mild adverse effects and 75% admitted that they had little or no knowledge about what they are.[10] Pharmacists are equally likely to encounter patients taking supplements together with prescription or non-prescription medicines as they may be asked for advice, or they may actually sell or supply the herbal medicine. Many pharmacists (like many doctors) do not feel they have enough basic knowledge themselves, or information readily available, to recommend these safely,[11] although according to a study in an international cohort of pharmacists, 84% have tried CAM at some time in their life, and 81% still felt they had inadequate skills and knowledge to counsel patients.[12] Personal use of dietary supplements was found to correlate with a twofold increase in the likelihood that a pharmacist would recommend them to a patient.[11] A study from 2010, assessing the attitude of pharmacy customers to CAM use found that 92% of customers thought that pharmacies supplying CAM should also provide safety information about their use, with 90% of the opinion that the pharmacist should routinely check for interactions.[13]

1. Lanski SL, Greenwald M, Perkins A, Simon HK. Herbal therapy use in a pediatric emergency department population: expect the unexpected. *Pediatrics* (2003) 111, 981–5.
2. Giveon SM, Liberman N, Klang S, Kahan E. Are people who use "natural drugs" aware of their potentially harmful side effects and reporting to family physician. *Patient Educ Couns* (2004) 53, 5–11.
3. Wold RS, Lopez ST, Yau CL, Butler LM, Pareo-Tubbeh SL, Waters DL, Garry PJ, Baumgartner RN. Increasing trends in elderly persons' use of nonvitamin, nonmineral dietary supplements and concurrent use of medications. *J Am Diet Assoc* (2005) 105, 54–63.
4. Blanck HM, Serdula MK, Gillespie C, Galuska DA, Sharpe PA, Conway JM, Khan LK, Ainsworth BE. Use of nonprescription dietary supplements for weight loss is common among Americans. *J Am Diet Assoc* (2007) 107, 441–7.
5. Chrystal K, Allan S, Forgeson G, Isaacs R. The use of complementary/alternative medicine by cancer patients in a New Zealand regional cancer treatment centre. *N Z Med J* (2003) 116, U296.
6. Goldstein LH, Elias M, Ron-Avraham G, Biniaurishvili BZ, Madjar M, Kamargash I, Braunstein R, Berkovitch M, Golik A. Consumption of herbal remedies and dietary supplements amongst patients hospitalized in medical wards. *Br J Clin Pharmacol* (2007) 64, 373–80.
7. Engdal S, Steinsbekk A, Klepp O, Nilsen OG. Herbal use among cancer patients during palliative or curative chemotherapy treatment in Norway. *Support Care Cancer* (2008) 16, 763–9.
8. Delgoda R, Ellington C, Barrett S, Gordon N, Clarke N, Younger N. The practice of polypharmacy involving herbal and prescription medicines in the treatment of diabetes mellitus, hypertension and gastrointestinal disorders in Jamaica. *West Indian Med J* (2004) 53, 400–405.
9. Taylor DMD, Walsham N, Taylor SE, Wong LF. Complementary and alternative medicines versus prescription drugs: perceptions of emergency department patients. *Emerg Med J* (2006) 23, 266–8.
10. Giveon SM, Liberman N, Klang S, Kahan E. A survey of primary care physicians' perceptions of their patients' use of complementary medicine. *Complement Ther Med* (2003) 11, 254–60.
11. Howard N, Tsourounis C, Kapusnik-Uner J. Dietary supplement survey of pharmacists: personal and professional practices. *J Altern Complement Med* (2001) 7, 667–80.
12. Koh HL, Teo HH, Ng HL. Pharmacists' patterns of use, knowledge, and attitudes toward complementary and alternative medicine. *J Altern Complement Med* (2003) 9, 51–63.
13. Braun LA, Tiralongo E, Wilkinson JM, Spitzer O, Bailey M, Poole S, Dooley M. Perceptions, use and attitudes of pharmacy customers on complementary medicines and pharmacy practice. *BMC Complement Altern Med* (2010) 10, 38.

Interactions between herbal medicines and conventional drugs

An interaction is said to occur when the effects of one drug are changed by the presence of another substance, including herbal medicines, food, drink and environmental chemical agents.

This definition is obviously as true for conventional medicines as it is for herbal medicines. The outcome can be harmful if the interaction causes an increase in the toxicity of the drug. A potential example of this is the experimental increase in toxicity seen when amikacin is given with ginkgo, see Ginkgo + Aminoglycosides, page 240. A reduction in efficacy due to an interaction can sometimes be just as harmful as an increase. For example,

the reduction in ciclosporin levels caused by St John's wort has led to transplant rejection in some cases. See St John's wort + Ciclosporin, page 445.

As with any publication detailing the adverse effects of drug use it would be very easy to conclude after browsing through this publication that it is extremely risky to treat patients with conventional drugs and herbal medicines, but this would be an over-reaction. Patients can apparently tolerate adverse interactions remarkably well, and many interactions can be accommodated for (for example through natural dose titration), so that the effects may not consciously be recognised as the result of an interaction.

One of the reasons it is often difficult to detect an interaction is that, as already mentioned, patient variability is considerable. We now know many of the predisposing and protective factors that determine whether or not an interaction occurs but in practice it is still very difficult to predict what will happen when an individual patient is given two potentially interacting medicines. This effect is compounded when considering the interactions of herbal medicines because they themselves are subject to a degree of variability.

Variability of herbal medicines

Botanical extracts differ from conventional medicines in that they are complicated mixtures of many bioactive compounds. This makes it difficult to assess the contribution of each constituent to the activity of the whole, and this includes evaluating their possible interactions with drugs. Natural products are also liable to a great deal of variation and even when standardised to one of more of their constituents, there can still be differences in the numerous other compounds present, and different constituents will affect different metabolic enzymes. As well as the source material, the method by which an extract is made will also affect its composition, and thus its interaction potential. This is well illustrated by a study looking at echinacea preparations. This study found that a standardised Swiss-registered *Echinacea purpurea* extract mildly inhibited the cytochrome P450 isoenzymes CYP1A2, CYP2C19, and CYP3A4, with CYP3A4 being the most affected. However, when this and a number of other products were screened for their ability to inhibit CYP3A4, the inhibitory potencies of the products were found to vary by a factor of 150.[1]

Sometimes, the overall effect of a herbal extract has a different effect on cytochrome P450 than that of an isolated constituent contained in the extract. For example, a mixture of dietary soya isoflavones containing genistein was found to have no effect on *rat* hepatic CYP1A2 and CYP2E1,[2] whereas isolated genistein was found to inhibit both CYP2E1 and CYP1A2 in experimental studies.[3] Whether this is because of a species difference, a dose-related effect, or due to opposing actions of some constituents within the extract remains to be seen, but it provides another illustration of the dangers of extrapolating results from different types of experiments on individual components to a clinical situation involving a whole mixture.

These brief examples start to illustrate that the mechanisms of drug interactions with herbal medicines bear a great relationship to those of conventional drugs.

1. Modarai M, Gertsch J, Suter A, Heinrich M, Kortenkamp A. Cytochrome P450 inhibitory action of Echinacea preparations differs widely and co-varies with alkylamide content. *J Pharm Pharmacol* (2007) 59, 567–73.

2. Kishida T, Nagamoto M, Ohtsu Y, Watakabe M, Ohshima D, Nashiki K, Mizushige T, Izumi T, Obata A, Ebihara K. Lack of an inducible effect of dietary soy isoflavones on the mRNA abundance of hepatic cytochrome P-450 isozymes in rats. *Biosci Biotechnol Biochem* (2004) 68, 508–15.
3. Helsby NA, Chipman JK, Gescher A, Kerr D. Inhibition of mouse and human CYP 1A- and 2E1-dependent substrate metabolism by the isoflavonoids genistein and equol. *Food Chem Toxicol* (1998) 36, 375–82.

Mechanisms of drug interactions

Some drugs interact together in totally unique ways, but as the many examples in this publication amply illustrate, there are certain mechanisms of interaction that are encountered time and time again. Some of these common mechanisms are discussed here in greater detail than space will allow in the individual monographs, so that only the briefest reference need be made there. This discussion is restricted to those mechanisms that have been extensively investigated with herbal medicines. Readers interested in a more general discussion of mechanisms are referred to *Stockley's Drug Interactions*.

Very many drugs that interact do so, not by a single mechanism, but often by two or more mechanisms acting in concert, although for clarity most of the mechanisms are dealt with here as though they occur in isolation. For convenience, the mechanisms of interactions can be subdivided into those that involve the pharmacokinetics of a drug, and those that are pharmacodynamic.

Pharmacokinetic interactions

Pharmacokinetic interactions are those that can affect the processes by which drugs are absorbed, distributed, metabolised and excreted (the so-called ADME interactions). Although all these mechanisms are undoubtedly relevant to interactions with herbal medicines, this discussion will mainly focus on cytochrome P450 and drug transporter proteins. Other enzymes have been shown to play a role in the interactions of herbal medicines, such as UDP-glucuronyltransferases (UGT), but less is known about their effects.

Cytochrome P450 isoenzymes

Although a few drugs are cleared from the body simply by being excreted unchanged in the urine, most are chemically altered within the body to less lipid-soluble compounds, which are more easily excreted by the kidneys. If this were not so, many drugs would persist in the body and continue to exert their effects for a long time. Some drug metabolism goes on in the serum, the kidneys, the skin and the intestines, but the greatest proportion is carried out by enzymes that are found in the liver, mainly cytochrome P450. Cytochrome P450 is not a single entity, but is in fact a very large family of related isoenzymes, about 30 of which have been found in human liver tissue. However, in practice, only a few specific subfamilies seem to be responsible for most (about 90%) of the metabolism of the commonly used drugs. The most important isoenzymes are: CYP1A2, CYP2C9, CYP2C19, CYP2D6, CYP2E1 and CYP3A4. Some of these isoenzymes are also found in the gut wall.

(a) Enzyme induction

Some herbal medicines can have a marked effect on the extent of first-pass metabolism of conventional drugs by inducing the cytochrome P450 isoenzymes in the gut wall or in the liver. A number of herbs have been studied specifically for their effects on these isoenzymes. Those that appear to cause clinically relevant induction of specific isoenzymes are grouped in a series of tables, along with the conventional drugs that are substrates for this isoenzyme. See the tables Drugs and herbs affecting or metabolised by the cytochrome P450 isoenzyme CYP1A2, page 7, and Drugs and herbs affecting or metabolised by the cytochrome P450 isoenzyme CYP3A4, page 7.

The extent of the enzyme induction depends on the herbal medicine, its dosage, and even the specific extract used (see Variability of herbal medicines, page 5). It may take days or even 2 to 3 weeks to develop fully, and may persist for a similar length of time when the enzyme inducer is stopped. This means that enzyme induction interactions can be delayed in onset and slow to resolve. These effects have been seen with St John's wort, page 437.

If one drug reduces the effects of another by enzyme induction, it may be possible to accommodate the interaction simply by raising the dosage of the drug affected, but this requires good monitoring, and there are obvious hazards if the inducing drug is eventually stopped without remembering to reduce the dosage again. The raised drug dosage may be an overdose when the drug metabolism has returned to normal. This strategy is more complicated with herbal medicines; the intake of a set amount of the herbal medicine would need to be maintained for this approach to work, and this is difficult because the interacting constituent may vary between products, and even between different batches of the same product.

(b) Enzyme inhibition

More common than enzyme induction is the inhibition of enzymes. This results in the reduced metabolism of an affected drug, so that it may begin to accumulate within the body, the effect usually being essentially the same as when the dosage is increased. Unlike enzyme induction, which may take several days or even weeks to develop fully, enzyme inhibition can occur within 2 to 3 days, resulting in the rapid development of toxicity. An example is the effect of grapefruit and grapefruit juice, which seem to inhibit the cytochrome P450 isoenzyme CYP3A4, mainly in the gut, and therefore reduce the metabolism of oral calcium-channel blockers. See Grapefruit + Calcium-channel blockers, page 272.

A number of herbs have been studied specifically for their effects on cytochrome P450 isoenzymes. Those that appear to have clinically relevant effects on specific isoenzymes are grouped in a series of tables, along with the conventional drugs that are substrates for this isoenzyme. See the tables Drugs and herbs affecting or metabolised by the cytochrome P450 isoenzyme CYP1A2, page 7, and Drugs and herbs affecting or metabolised by the cytochrome P450 isoenzyme CYP3A4, page 7.

The clinical significance of many enzyme inhibition interactions depends on the extent to which the serum levels of the drug rise. If the serum levels remain within the therapeutic range the interaction may not be clinically important.

(c) Predicting interactions involving cytochrome P450

It is interesting to know which particular isoenzyme is responsible for the metabolism of drugs because by doing *in vitro* tests with human liver enzymes it is often possible to explain why and how some drugs interact. For example, ciclosporin is metabolised by CYP3A4, and we know that St John's wort is a potent inducer of this isoenzyme, so that it comes as no surprise that St John's wort, page 445, reduces the effects of ciclosporin.

What is very much more important than retrospectively finding out why drugs and herbal medicines interact, is the knowledge such *in vitro* tests can provide about forecasting which other drugs may possibly also interact. This may reduce the numbers of expensive clinical studies in subjects and patients and avoids waiting until significant drug interactions are observed in clinical use. A lot of effort is being put into this area of drug development, and it is particularly important for herbal medicines, where it seems unlikely that expensive clinical studies will be routinely conducted. However, at present such prediction is not always accurate

because all of the many variables that can come into play are not known (such as how much of the enzyme is available, the concentration of the drug at the site of metabolism, and the affinity of the drug for the enzyme). Remember too that some drugs can be metabolised by more than one cytochrome P450 isoenzyme (meaning that this other isoenzyme may be able to 'pick up' more metabolism to compensate for the inhibited pathway); some drugs (and their metabolites) can both induce a particular isoenzyme and be metabolised by it; and some drugs (or their metabolites) can inhibit a particular isoenzyme but not be metabolised by it. With so many factors possibly impinging on the outcome of giving two or more drugs together, it is very easy to lose sight of one of the factors (or not even know about it) so that the sum of 2 plus 2 may not turn out to be the 4 that you have predicted.

Drugs and herbs affecting or metabolised by the cytochrome P450 isoenzyme CYP1A2[†]

Inducers	Substrates*	Inhibitors
Cannabis (modest clinical effects with smoking)	Caffeine	Boswellia (*in vitro* effects with gum resin)
Danshen (*in vitro* effects do not appear to be clinically relevant)	Clomipramine	Chamomile, German (moderate effects with tea given to rats)
Liquorice (glycyrrhizin constituent studied in *mice*, effects may be weaker clinically)	Clozapine	Dandelion (moderate to potent effects with tea given to rats)
St John's wort (*in vitro* induction of only minor clinical relevance)	Duloxetine	Feverfew (*in vitro* evidence only)
	Frovatriptan	Ginkgo (*in vitro* effects do not appear to be clinically relevant)
	Olanzapine	
	Rasagiline	
	Ropinirole	
	Tacrine	
	Theophylline	
	Tizanidine	
	Zolmitriptan	

* shown to be clinically relevant in drug-drug interaction studies
[†] Note that *in vitro* effects are not necessarily replicated *in vivo*; findings *in vivo* often appear weaker than those *in vitro*. The presence of an *in vitro* effect suggests that clinical study is warranted.

Drugs and herbs affecting or metabolised by the cytochrome P450 isoenzyme CYP3A4[†]

Inducers	Substrates*	Inhibitors
Danshen (weak clinical effects)	**Antiarrhythmics** (Amiodarone, Disopyramide, Lidocaine oral, Propafenone, Quinidine)	Bearberry (*in vitro* evidence only, effects vary greatly between products)
Echinacea (*in vitro* studies supported by clinical data, but any effect modest. NB inhibition also reported)	**Anticholinesterases, centrally-acting** (Donepezil, Galantamine)	Bitter orange (juice known to have clinically relevant effects, supplement has no effects; difference possibly due to constituents)
Ginkgo (*in vitro* studies supported by clinical data, but any effect modest. NB inhibition also reported)	**Antihistamines** (Astemizole, Terfenadine)	Black cohosh (effects *in vitro* are probably not clinically relevant)
Liquorice (glycyrrhizin constituent studied in *mice*, effects may be weaker clinically)	**Antimigraine drugs** (Eletriptan, Ergot derivatives)	Cat's claw (*in vitro* studies suggest potent effects)
Rooibos (*in vitro* studies suggest moderate to potent effects)	**Antineoplastics** (Busulfan, Cyclophosphamide, Ifosfamide, Imatinib, Irinotecan, Tamoxifen, Taxanes, Teniposide, Toremifene, Vinblastine, Vincristine)	Cranberry (*in vitro* studies suggest modest effects but studies in humans suggest any effect is not clinically relevant)

table continues

Drugs and herbs affecting or metabolised by the cytochrome P450 isoenzyme CYP3A4[†] (continued)

Inducers	Substrates*	Inhibitors
St John's wort (clinically established, potency appears to vary with hyperforin content)	**Antipsychotics** (Pimozide, Quetiapine)	Echinacea (in vitro studies supported by clinical data, but any effect modest. NB induction also reported)
	Azoles (Itraconazole, Voriconazole)	Feverfew (in vitro evidence only)
	Benzodiazepines and related drugs (Alprazolam, Triazolam, Midazolam; Buspirone, Zolpidem, Zopiclone)	Garlic (effects in vitro are probably not clinically relevant)
	Calcium-channel blockers (Diltiazem, Felodipine, Lercanidipine)	Ginkgo (in vitro studies supported by clinical data, but any effect modest. NB induction also reported)
	Corticosteroids (Budesonide, Dexamethasone, Fluticasone, Hydrocortisone, Methylprednisolone)	Ginseng (ginsenoside constituents studied; in vitro effects are probably not clinically relevant)
	Dopamine agonists (Bromocriptine, Cabergoline)	Goldenseal (in vitro studies suggest potent effects, but studies in humans suggest only modest clinical effects)
	Hormones (Hormonal contraceptives, Oestrogens, Progestogens)	Grapefruit (juice has moderate clinical effects, not known if supplements interact similarly)
	Immunosuppressants (Ciclosporin, Sirolimus, Tacrolimus)	Milk thistle (in vitro studies supported by some clinical data, but any effect modest)
	Opioids (Alfentanil, Buprenorphine, Fentanyl, Methadone)	Pepper (in vitro piperine (a constituent) has some effect, but ethanolic extracts of the fruit had no clinically significant effects)
	Phosphodiesterase type-5 inhibitors (Sildenafil, Tadalafil, Vardenafil)	Resveratrol (in vitro studies suggest modest effects)
	HIV-protease inhibitors (Amprenavir, Atazanavir, Darunavir, Fosamprenavir, Indinavir, Nelfinavir, Ritonavir, Saquinavir, Tipranavir)	Rhodiola (in vitro effects with a root extract)
	Statins (Atorvastatin, Lovastatin, Simvastatin)	Saw palmetto (effects in vitro are not clinically relevant)
	Miscellaneous (Aprepitant, Bosentan, Carbamazepine, Cilostazol, Cisapride, Delavirdine, Dutasteride, Eplerenone, Maraviroc, Reboxetine, Rifabutin, Sibutramine, Solifenacin, Tolterodine)	Schisandra (clinical studies suggest moderate effects)
		Turmeric (curcumin constituent studied; in vitro effects are potent)

* shown to be clinically relevant in drug-drug interaction studies

[†] Note that in vitro effects are not necessarily replicated in vivo; findings in vivo often appear weaker than those in vitro. The presence of an in vitro effect suggests that clinical study is warranted.

Drug transporter proteins

Drugs and endogenous substances are known to cross biological membranes, not just by passive diffusion, but by carrier-mediated processes, often known as transporters. Significant advances in the identification of various transporters have been made, although the contribution of many of these to drug interactions in particular, is still being investigated. The most well known drug transporter protein is P-glycoprotein.

More and more evidence is accumulating to show that some drug interactions occur because they interfere with the activity of P-glycoprotein. This is an efflux pump found in the membranes of certain cells, which can push metabolites and drugs out of the cells and have an impact on the extent of drug absorption (via the intestine), distribution (to the brain, testis, or placenta) and elimination (in the urine and bile). So, for example, the P-glycoprotein in the cells of the gut lining can eject some already-absorbed drug molecules back into the intestine resulting in a reduction in the total amount of drug absorbed. In this way P-glycoprotein acts as a barrier to absorption. The activity of P-glycoprotein in the endothelial cells of the blood-brain barrier can also eject certain drugs from the brain, limiting CNS penetration and effects.

The pumping actions of P-glycoprotein can be experimentally induced or inhibited by some herbal medicines. So for example, the induction (or stimulation) of the activity of P-glycoprotein by capsicum, within the lining cells of the gut, causes digoxin to be ejected into the gut more vigorously. This may result in a fall in the plasma levels of digoxin. See Capsicum + Digoxin, page 126. In contrast, some extracts of danshen appear to inhibit the activity of P-glycoprotein, and may therefore increase digoxin levels. See Danshen + Digoxin, page 185.

There is an overlap between CYP3A4 and P-glycoprotein inhibitors, inducers and substrates. Digoxin is an example of one of the few drugs that is a substrate for P-glycoprotein but not CYP3A4. It is for this reason that it is used as a probe substrate for P-glycoprotein activity, and the effects of herbal medicines on this particular drug have been studied.

Other transporters that are involved in some drug interactions are the organic anion transporters (OATs), organic anion-transporting polypeptides (OATPs) and organic cation transporters (OCTs), which are members of the solute carrier superfamily (SLC) of transporters. The best known example of an OAT inhibitor is probenecid, which affects the renal excretion of a number of drugs. However, the effects of many herbal medicines and drugs on these transporters are less well understood than those of P-glycoprotein, and thus, the role of OAT, OATP and OCT in drug interactions is still being elucidated.

Pharmacodynamic interactions

Pharmacodynamic interactions are those where the effects of one drug are changed by the presence of another drug at its site of action. Sometimes the drugs directly compete for particular receptors but often the reaction is more indirect and involves interference with physiological mechanisms. These interactions are much less easy to classify neatly than those of a pharmacokinetic type.

(a) Additive or synergistic interactions

If two drugs that have the same pharmacological effect are given together the effects can be additive. For example, alcohol depresses the CNS and, if taken in moderate amounts with normal therapeutic doses of herbal medicines (e.g. valerian), may increase drowsiness. See Valerian + Alcohol, page 479.

Sometimes the additive effects are solely toxic (e.g. theoretical additive nephrotoxicity, see Ginkgo + Aminoglycosides, page 240). It is common to use the terms 'additive', 'summation', 'synergy' or 'potentiation' to describe what happens if two or more drugs behave like this. These words have precise pharmacological definitions but they are often used rather loosely as synonyms because in practice it is often very difficult to know the extent of the increased activity, that is to say whether the effects are greater or smaller than the sum of the individual effects.

One particular additive effect is well known to occur between the herbal medicine St John's wort, page 437, and conventional medicines. This is serotonin syndrome. The reasons for this effect are not fully understood, but the serotonin syndrome is thought to occur as a result of overstimulation of the 5-HT$_{1A}$ and 5-HT$_{2A}$ receptors and possibly other serotonin receptors in the central nervous system (in the brain stem and spinal cord in particular) due to the combined effects of two medicines (herbal or conventional). Serotonin syndrome can occur exceptionally after taking only one substance that causes over-stimulation of these 5-HT receptors, but much more usually it develops when two or more drugs (so-called serotonergic or serotomimetic drugs) act in concert. The characteristic symptoms fall into three main areas, namely altered mental status (agitation, confusion, mania), autonomic dysfunction (diaphoresis, diarrhoea, fever, shivering) and neuromuscular abnormalities (hyperreflexia, incoordination, myoclonus, tremor).

The syndrome can develop shortly after one serotonergic drug is added to another, or even if one is replaced by another without allowing a long enough washout period in between, and the problem usually resolves within about 24 hours if both drugs are withdrawn and supportive measures given. Non-specific serotonin antagonists (cyproheptadine, chlorpromazine, methysergide) have also been used for treatment. Most patients recover uneventfully, but there have been a few fatalities.

It is still not at all clear why many patients can take two, or sometimes several serotonergic drugs together without problems, while a very small number develop this serious toxic reaction, but it certainly suggests that there are as yet other factors involved that have yet to be identified. The full story is likely to be much more complex than just the simple additive effects of two drugs.

(b) Antagonistic or opposing interactions

In contrast to additive interactions, there are some pairs of drugs with activities that are opposed to one another. For example the coumarins can prolong the blood clotting time by competitively inhibiting the effects of dietary vitamin K. If the intake of vitamin K is increased, the effects of the oral anticoagulant are opposed and the prothrombin time can return to normal, thereby cancelling out the therapeutic benefits of anticoagulant treatment. It has been proposed that the vitamin K content of herbal medicines may be sufficient to provoke this interaction, but in most cases of normal intake of the herb, this seems unlikely. See Alfalfa + Warfarin and related drugs, page 23, for further discussion of this potential interaction.

Drawing your own conclusions

The human population is a total mixture, unlike selected batches of laboratory animals (same age, weight, sex, and strain etc.). For this reason human beings do not respond uniformly to one or more drugs or even herbal medicines. Our genetic make up, ethnic background, sex, renal and hepatic functions, diseases and nutritional states, ages and other factors (the route of administration, for example) all contribute towards the heterogeneity of our responses. This means that the outcome of giving one or more drugs to any individual for the first time is never totally predictable because it is a new and unique 'experiment'. Even so, some idea of the probable outcome of using a drug or a pair of drugs can be based on what has been seen in other patients: the more extensive the data, the firmer the predictions.

The most difficult decisions concern isolated cases of interaction, many of which only achieved prominence because they were serious. Do you ignore them as 'idiosyncratic' or do you, from that moment onwards, advise against the use of the herbal medicine and conventional drug totally?

There is no simple yes or no answer to these questions, especially as evidence regarding interactions between herbal medicines is often only of an experimental nature. The delicate balance between whether or not to give the drug has then to be set against the actual severity of the reaction reported and weighed up against how essential it is to use the combination in question.

When deciding the possible first-time use of any two drugs in any particular patient, you need to put what is currently known about these drugs against the particular profile of your patient. Read the monograph. Consider the facts and conclusions, and then set the whole against the backdrop of your patients' unique condition (age, disease, general condition, and so forth) so that what you eventually decide to do is well thought out and soundly based. We do not usually have the luxury of knowing absolutely all the facts, so that an initial conservative approach is often the safest.

It is now quite impossible to remember all the known clinically important interactions and how they occur but there are some broad general principles that are worth remembering:

- Be on the alert with any drugs that have a narrow therapeutic window or where it is necessary to keep serum levels at or above a suitable level (e.g. anticoagulants, antidiabetic drugs, antiepileptics, antihypertensives, anti-infectives, antineoplastic cytotoxics, digitalis glycosides, immunosuppressants, etc.).

- Think about the basic pharmacology of the drugs under consideration so that obvious problems (additive CNS depression for example) are not overlooked, and try to think what might happen if drugs that affect the same receptors are used together. And don't forget that many drugs affect more than one type of receptor.

- Keep in mind that the elderly are at risk because of reduced liver and renal function on which drug clearance depends.

Acidophilus

Lactobacillus acidophilus (Lactobacillaceae)

Use and indications

Lactobacillus acidophilus are lactic-acid producing bacterial organisms that are normally present in the human gut. Acidophilus supplements are primarily taken as a probiotic, to restore or maintain healthy microbial flora. Acidophilus has also been used to treat diarrhoea, irritable bowel syndrome, lactose intolerance, urinary tract infections, yeast-based infections (such as those caused by *Candida albicans*) and for general digestive problems. It is available in various forms ranging from capsules to yoghurts.

Pharmacokinetics

No relevant pharmacokinetic data found.

Interactions overview

Acidophilus is a bacterial organism, and therefore it may lead to systemic infection in immunosuppressed patients, although this effect is expected to be rare. Antibacterials and drugs that are dependent on bacterial degradation to release active constituents, namely sulfasalazine, may also be expected to interact with supplemental acidophilus, although the limited evidence available suggests that a clinically relevant interaction is unlikely.

Interactions monographs

- Antibacterials, page 12
- Food, page 12
- Herbal medicines; Soya isoflavones, page 12
- Immunosuppressants, page 12
- Sulfasalazine, page 13

Acidophilus + Antibacterials

The interaction between acidophilus and antibacterials is based on experimental evidence only.

Clinical evidence
No interactions found.

Experimental evidence
Lactobacillus acidophilus are gram-positive, facultative anaerobic bacteria. They can be inhibited or killed by antibacterials that are effective against this bacterial type. **Ampicillin,**[1–3] **ampicillin** with **sulbactam,**[3] **benzylpenicillin,**[2,3] **cefalotin,**[1] **chloramphenicol,**[2,3] **clindamycin,**[1,3,4] **erythromycin,**[2,3] **gentamicin,**[3] **linezolid,**[3] **oxytetracycline,**[3] **penicillin,**[1] **quinupristin/dalfopristin,**[3] **streptomycin,**[3] **tetracycline**[2] and **vancomycin**[3] have been found to inhibit acidophilus populations.

Mechanism
Antibacterials kill or inhibit the growth of bacterial populations through various different mechanisms.

Importance and management
Depending on the particular strain of acidophilus, and the antibacterial dose, the desired therapeutic effect of acidophilus may be significantly reduced or even abolished by these antibacterials.

1. Bayer AS, Chow AW, Concepcion N, Guze LB. Susceptibility of 40 lactobacilli to six antimicrobial agents with broad gram-positive anaerobic spectra. *Antimicrob Agents Chemother* (1978) 14, 720–722.
2. Hummel AS, Hertel C, Holzapfel WH, Franz CMAP. Antibiotic resistances of starter and probiotic strains of lactic acid bacteria. *Appl Environ Microbiol* (2007) 73, 730–739.
3. Klare I, Konstabel C, Werner G, Huys G, Vankerckhoven V, Kahlmeter G, Hildebrandt B, Müller-Bertling S, Witte W, Goossens H. Antimicrobial susceptibilities of *Lactobacillus, Pediococcus* and *Lactococcus* human isolates and cultures intended for probiotic or nutritional use. *J Antimicrob Chemother* (2007) 59, 900–912.
4. Lidbeck A, Edlund C, Gustafsson JÅ, Kager L, Nord CE. Impact of *Lactobacillus acidophilus* administration on the intestinal microflora after clindamycin treatment. *J Chemother* (2005) 1, 630–632.

Acidophilus + Food

No interactions found. Acidophilus is often present in probiotic yoghurt.

Acidophilus + Herbal medicines; Soya isoflavones

Acidophilus does not appear to have a clinically significant affect on the metabolism of soya isoflavones.

Clinical evidence
In a randomised study 20 women who had been successfully treated for breast cancer and 20 women without a history of cancer were given a soya protein isolate containing 640 micrograms/kg of isoflavones daily (34% daidzein, 57% genistein, and 9% glycitein), with three probiotic capsules (*DDS Plus*), containing *Lactobacillus acidophilus* and **Bifidobacterium longum**, daily for 42 days. In general, the probiotics did not affect the plasma isoflavone concentrations, although two of the subjects had altered plasma concentrations of equol, a daidzein metabolite. No adverse effects were reported in the study.[1] In another study, the same probiotic did not alter the cholesterol-lowering effects of the isoflavones.[2]

Experimental evidence
In an experimental study in fermenting soymilk, five isolates of *Lactobacillus* bacteria, including *Lactobacillus acidophilus*, and yeast, increased the bioavailability of the isoflavones, genistein and daidzein.[3]

Mechanism
The gut bacterial flora metabolises daidzein to equol, which is thought to be responsible for reduced breast cancer risk. The authors hypothesised that increasing the populations of bacteria by using probiotics, levels of equol would increase. For more information on the metabolism of isoflavones by bacteria in the gut, see under *pharmacokinetics* in isoflavones, page 300.

Importance and management
Increasing the populations of bacteria in the gut does not appear to have a clinically significant effect on the metabolism of soya isoflavones. Note that the metabolism of isoflavones is variable, due to differences in gut flora between individuals, and so the effects of any interaction between acidophilus and isoflavones are likely to differ between individuals. For more information on the interactions of isoflavones in general, see under isoflavones, page 300.

1. Nettleton JA, Greany KA, Thomas W, Wangen KE, Adlercreutz H, Kurzer MS. Plasma phytoestrogens are not altered by probiotic consumption in postmenopausal women with and without a history of breast cancer. *J Nutr* (2004) 134, 1998–2003.
2. Greany KA, Nettleton JA, Wangen KE, Thomas W, Kurzer MS. Probiotic consumption does not enhance the cholesterol-lowering effect of soy in postmenopausal women. *J Nutr* (2004) 134, 3277–83.
3. Rekha CR, Vijayalakshmi G. Bioconversion of isoflavone glycosides to aglycones, mineral bioavailability and vitamin B complex in fermented soymilk by probiotic bacteria and yeast. *J Appl Microbiol* (2010) 109, 1198–1208.

Acidophilus + Immunosuppressants

An isolated case report describes fatal septicaemia in an immunosuppressed woman taking cyclophosphamide and fludrocortisone who ate live yoghurt containing *Lactobacillus rhamnosus*, which is closely related to acidophilus.

Clinical evidence
A 42-year-old woman taking **cyclophosphamide** and **fludrocortisone** for Sjögren's syndrome, developed pneumonia and secondary *Lactobacillus rhamnosus* septicaemia, which proved to be fatal, after taking a short course of supermarket-own brand live yoghurt for diarrhoea.[1] Note that *Lactobacillus rhamnosus* is a species closely related to *Lactobacillus acidophilus*.

Experimental evidence
No relevant data found.

Mechanism
The immunosuppressed nature of the patient is thought to have provided a more conducive environment for the introduced bacteria to establish a sufficient population to reach a pathogenic threshold.

Importance and management
Although not a drug interaction in the strictest sense, it would be sensible to assume that introducing bacteria in the form of a probiotic to an immunosuppressed patient should be undertaken with great care or perhaps avoided: note that patients who have undergone a transplant and who are immunosuppressed are often advised to avoid foods such as live yoghurts.

Remember that as immunosuppression secondary to corticosteroid use is dependent on numerous factors related to the dose and duration of intake, not all patients taking corticosteroids are likely to be immunosuppressed and therefore they will not necessarily need to avoid acidophilus-containing products.

1. MacGregor G, Smith AJ, Thakker B, Kinsella J. Yoghurt biotherapy: contraindicated in immunosuppressed patients? *Postgrad Med J* (2002) 78, 366–7.

Acidophilus + Sulfasalazine

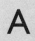

Acidophilus does not appear to affect the pharmacokinetics of sulfasalazine.

Clinical evidence

In a study,[1] twelve patients with rheumatoid arthritis, who had taken sulfasalazine for more than three months, were given a probiotic containing *Lactobacillus acidophilus, Bifidobacterium lactis* and *Streptococcus salivarius* (BLIS BioRestore™) concurrently for seven days. The probiotic did not affect the pharmacokinetics of sulfasalazine to a clinically relevant extent, and although some minor gastrointestinal adverse effects were reported, this is not uncommon with probiotic treatment alone.

Experimental evidence

In an experimental study using cell cultures, about 85 to 95% of sulfasalazine tested was broken down by several different strains of *Lactobacillus acidophilus*.[2]

Mechanism

The azo link of sulfasalazine is split by anaerobic bacteria in the colon to release sulfapyridine and 5-aminosalicylic acid, the latter being the active metabolite that acts locally in the treatment of inflammatory bowel disease. The lipophilic nature of sulfasalazine is thought to enable it to reach the site of azoreductase activity within the bacterial cell by passive diffusion across the cell membrane.

Importance and management

Evidence for an interaction between acidophilus and sulfasalazine is limited. Sulfasalazine is generally thought to be 'activated' by its metabolism to release 5-aminosalicylic acid by bacteria in the colon. By introducing more bacteria, the metabolism could be increased. Metabolism may also occur earlier, in the small intestine, which could be detrimental as one metabolite, sulfapyridine, is rapidly absorbed from the small intestine and can contribute to renal toxicity.

It should be noted, however, that due to differences in gut flora between individuals, the effects of any interaction between acidophilus and sulfasalazine are likely to differ between individuals and the study in patients with rheumatoid arthritis suggests that a clinically relevant interaction is unlikely.

1. Lee HJ, Waller RD, Stebbings S, Highton J, Orlovich DA, Schmierer D, Fawcett JP. The effects of an orally administered probiotic on sulfasalazine metabolism in individuals with rheumatoid arthritis: a preliminary study. *Int J Rheum Dis* (2010) 13, 48–54.
2. Pradhan A, Majumdar MK. Metabolism of some drugs by intestinal lactobacilli and their toxicological considerations. *Acta Pharmacol Toxicol (Copenh)* (1986) 58, 11–15.

African potato

Hypoxis hemerocallidea Fisch.Mey. & Avé-Lall. (Hypoxidaceae)

Synonym(s) and related species

African wild potato, Bantu tulip, *Hypoxis rooperi* T. Moore.

Constituents

The corm or tuber (the 'potato') contains the norlignan diglucoside, hypoxoside. Other constituents include phytosterols, mainly β-sitosterol glycosides and stigmasterol; agglutinins (lectin-like proteins) and various tannins.

Use and indications

African potato is used to treat a wide range of conditions, including cardiovascular diseases, prostrate hypertrophy, urinary tract infections, various types of cancer, epilepsy, and for the prevention of miscarriage. It has also been used as an immunostimulant and has therefore been advocated for AIDS and HIV infection. Clinical evidence for efficacy in these conditions is lacking, but various *in vitro* and *animal* studies have found analgesic, anti-inflammatory, antidiabetic, antioxidant, antiepileptic, antihypertensive and antidiarrhoeal effects.

The constituent hypoxoside has been investigated in phase I studies in cancer patients.

Pharmacokinetics

Hypoxoside is converted by beta-glucosidase in the gut to its aglycone, rooperol. In a pharmacokinetic study in 24 patients with lung cancer who took a single dose of hypoxoside orally as a standardised plant extract, neither free hypoxoside nor rooperol appeared in the serum. Rooperol undergoes complete phase II biotransformation into its major mixed glucuronide-sulphate metabolite, and much smaller quantities of the diglucuronide and disulphate metabolites. Considerable interpatient variation in concentration-time relationships was found, due to an active enterohepatic recirculation in some patients and a distinct lag phase in others.[1]

In various *in vitro* studies, pure rooperol was a potent inhibitor of the cytochrome P450 isoenzymes CYP3A4/5, although an African potato decoction did not affect the pharmacokinetics of the CYP3A4 substrate, efavirenz, in one study, see NNRTIs, page 15. Rooperol may also have some inhibitory effect on CYP2C19. Conversely, pure hypoxoside, stigmasterol and various African potato extracts had more modest inhibitory effects on these isoenzymes.[2] Hypoxoside was a fairly strong inducer of P-glycoprotein, whereas rooperol, stigmasterol and various African potato extracts appeared to have little effect on this drug transporter.[2] However, in another *in vitro* study, African potato extract *inhibited* P-glycoprotein, see *Experimental evidence,* under NNRTIs, page 15. The clinical relevance of these *in vitro* findings remains to be determined; however, as free hypoxoside and rooperol are not present in the systemic circulation[1] the findings may not have any clinical relevance.

Interactions overview

African potato extract had no effect on the pharmacokinetics of a single dose of efavirenz. An *in vitro* study suggests that African potato might increase the uptake of nevirapine, but this is unlikely to be clinically relevant.

Interactions monographs

- Food, page 15
- Herbal medicines, page 15
- NNRTIs, page 15

1. Albrecht CF, Kruger PB, Smit BJ, Freestone M, Gouws L, Miller R, van Jaarsveld PP. The pharmacokinetic behaviour of hypoxoside taken orally by patients with lung cancer in a phase I trial. *S Afr Med J* (1995) 85, 861–5.
2. Nair VD, Foster BC, Thor Arnason J, Mills EJ, Kanfer I. In vitro evaluation of human cytochrome P450 and P-glycoprotein-mediated metabolism of some phytochemicals in extracts and formulations of African potato. *Phytomedicine* (2007) 14, 498–507.

African potato + Food

No interactions found.

African potato + Herbal medicines

No interactions found.

African potato + NNRTIs

African potato had no effect on the pharmacokinetics of a single dose of efavirenz.
An *in vitro* study suggests that African potato increases the uptake of nevirapine.

Clinical evidence

In a pharmacokinetic interaction study in 10 healthy subjects, an African potato aqueous decoction delivering hypoxoside 15 mg/kg daily was given for 14 days with a single 600-mg dose of **efavirenz** given on day 12. There was no difference in the pharmacokinetics of **efavirenz** before and during administration of the African potato decoction.[1]

Experimental evidence

An *in vitro* study into the transport of nevirapine across human intestinal epithelial cells found that a water extract of African potato decreased nevirapine efflux. The extent of this effect was greater than that of verapamil, a known, clinically relevant P-glycoprotein inhibitor, which was used as a positive control.[2]

Mechanism, importance and management

African potato might inhibit the cytochrome P450 isoenzyme CYP3A4 by which efavirenz is metabolised. However, the study suggests that any such effect is not clinically relevant as the pharmacokinetics of efavirenz were not affected by the aqueous African potato extract. Furthermore, efavirenz is an inducer of CYP3A4 and induces its own metabolism on long-term use, and its pharmacokinetics are generally unaffected by potent CYP3A4 inhibitors. No clinically relevant interaction would therefore be expected on concurrent use.

It was suggested that African potato might inhibit P-glycoprotein and increase the uptake of nevirapine, which appears to be a substrate for this transporter protein. However, nevirapine is almost completely absorbed after oral administration, and so it seems unlikely that P-glycoprotein has a clinically relevant effect on its intestinal efflux. As a consequence, P-glycoprotein inhibitors would seem unlikely to affect nevirapine pharmacokinetics.

1. Mogatle S, Skinner M, Mills E, Kanfer I. Effect of African potato (*Hypoxis hemerocallidea*) on the pharmacokinetics of efavirenz. *S Afr Med J* (2008) 98, 945–9.
2. Brown L, Heyneke O, Brown D, van Wyk JPH, Hamman JH. Impact of traditional medicinal plant extracts on antiretroviral drug absorption. *J Ethnopharmacol* (2008) 119, 588–92.

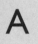
Agnus castus

Vitex agnus-castus L. (Lamiaceae)

Synonym(s) and related species

Agni casti, Chasteberry, Chaste tree, Monk's pepper.

Pharmacopoeias

Agnus Castus Fruit (*BP 2012, PhEur 7.5*); Chaste Tree (*USP35–NF30 S1*).

Constituents

Agnus castus is often standardised to the content of the flavonoid **casticin** and sometimes also the iridoid glycoside **agnuside**. Other major constituents are the **labdane** and **clerodane diterpenes** (including rotundifuran, 6β,7β-diacetoxy-13-hydroxy-labda-8,14-diene, vitexilactone). Other **flavonoids** include orientin, apigenin and penduletin.

Use and indications

Traditional use of the dried ripe fruit of agnus castus focuses on menstrual disorders in women resulting from corpus luteum deficiency, such as amenorrhoea, metrorrhagia and symptoms of premenstrual syndrome, including mastalgia. It has also been used to alleviate some menopausal symptoms and to promote lactation. In men it has been used to suppress libido and treat acne.

Pharmacokinetics

No relevant pharmacokinetic data found. For information on the pharmacokinetics of individual flavonoids present in agnus castus, see under flavonoids, page 213.

Interactions overview

A comprehensive systematic review of data from spontaneous adverse event reporting schemes and published clinical studies, post-marketing surveillance studies, surveys and case reports was carried out in September 2004 to investigate the safety of agnus castus extracts. No drug interactions were identified.[1] Agnus castus extracts used in the data reviewed included *Agnolyt, Agnucaston, Strotan,* and *ZE 440*.

However, agnus castus has dopamine agonist properties, and may therefore interact with drugs with either dopamine agonist or dopamine antagonist actions.

Agnus castus also contains oestrogenic compounds but it is unclear whether the effects of these compounds are additive, or antagonistic, to oestrogen-containing preparations (e.g. hormonal contraceptives and HRT) and oestrogen antagonists (e.g. tamoxifen). Although agnus castus binds with opioid receptors, no serious interaction with opioid analgesics would be expected.

For information on the interactions of flavonoids, see under flavonoids, page 213.

Interactions monographs

- Dopamine agonists or antagonists, page 17
- Food, page 17
- Herbal medicines, page 17
- Oestrogens or Oestrogen antagonists, page 17
- Opioids, page 18

1. Daniele C, Thompson Coon J, Pittler MH, Ernst E. *Vitex agnus castus*: a systematic review of adverse effects. *Drug Safety* (2005) 28, 319–32.

Agnus castus + Dopamine agonists or antagonists

Agnus castus has dopamine agonist properties, and may therefore interact with drugs with either dopamine agonist or dopamine antagonist actions.

Clinical evidence

In a double-blind study in women suffering from mastalgia, agnus castus extracts reduced serum prolactin levels (by about 4 nanograms/mL compared with about 0.6 nanograms/mL for placebo).[1] The agnus castus extracts used in this study were an oral solution, *Mastodynon,* and a tablet, MA 1025 E1.[1]

Experimental evidence

Extracts of agnus castus act as dopamine agonists.[2-5] Some dopaminergic compounds (mainly clerodane diterpenes) isolated from agnus castus have almost identical prolactin-suppressive properties at the D2 receptor to dopamine.[3]

Mechanism

Active compounds of agnus castus and dopaminergics may have additive effects because of their similar pharmacological activity.

Importance and management

While the importance of any potential interaction is difficult to judge, it would be wise to exercise some caution with the concurrent use of agnus castus and dopaminergics that act at the D2 receptor, which is the majority. For dopamine agonists such as **bromocriptine** and **apomorphine**, additive effects and toxicity is a theoretical possibility. Conversely, for dopamine antagonists such as the **antipsychotics** and some antiemetics (such as **metoclopramide** and **prochlorperazine**), antagonistic effects are a theoretical possibility.

1. Wuttke W, Splitt G, Gorkow C, Sieder C. Behandlung zyklusabhängiger Brustschmerzen mit einem Agnus castus-haltigen Arzneimittel. Ergebnisse einer randomisierten, plazebo-kontrollierten Doppelblindstudie. *Geburtshilfe Frauenheilkd* (1997) 57, 569–74.
2. Jarry H, Leonhardt S, Gorkow C, Wuttke W. In vitro prolactin but not LH and FSH release is inhibited by compounds in extracts of Agnus castus: direct evidence for a dopaminergic principle by the dopamine receptor assay. *Exp Clin Endocrinol* (1994) 102, 448–54.
3. Wuttke W, Jarry H, Christoffel V, Spengler B, Seidlová-Wuttke D. Chaste tree (*Vitex agnus-castus*) - Pharmacology and clinical indications. *Phytomedicine* (2003) 10, 348–57.
4. Meier B, Berger D, Hoberg E, Sticher O, Schaffner W. Pharmacological activities of *Vitex agnus-castus* extracts *in vitro. Phytomedicine* (2000) 7, 373–81.
5. Jarry H, Spengler B, Wuttke W, Christoffel V. *In vitro* assays for bioactivity-guided isolation of endocrine active compounds in *Vitex agnus-castus. Maturitas* (2006) 55 (Suppl 1), S26–S36.

Agnus castus + Food

No interactions found.

Agnus castus + Herbal medicines

No interactions found.

Agnus castus + Oestrogens or Oestrogen antagonists

Agnus castus contains oestrogenic compounds. This may result in additive effects with oestrogens or it may oppose the effects of oestrogens. Similarly, agnus castus may have additive effects with oestrogen antagonists or oppose the effects of oestrogen antagonists (e.g. tamoxifen).

Clinical evidence

A 32-year-old woman took a herbal medicine made from agnus castus, on her own initiative, before and in the early follicular phase of her fourth cycle of unstimulated IVF (*in vitro* fertilisation) treatment in order to try to promote ovarian function. In this cycle, she developed 4 follicles, and her serum gonadotrophin and ovarian hormone measurements became disordered. The agnus castus was stopped and she experienced symptoms suggestive of mild ovarian hyperstimulation syndrome in the luteal phase. Two subsequent cycles were endocrinologically normal with single follicles, as were the 3 cycles before she took the herbal preparation.[1]

It has also been suggested that agnus castus may provide relief from menopausal symptoms, see under Chinese angelica, page 146.

Experimental evidence

In receptor-binding studies, extracts of agnus castus were found to contain the flavonoids penduletin, apigenin and vitexin, which are thought to have some oestrogenic effects. Apigenin was identified as the most active, but all were selective for the oestrogen beta receptor.[2,3]

Mechanism

Active compounds of agnus castus may compete for the same oestrogen receptor as hormonal drugs and treatment. The case report suggests that agnus castus has anti-oestrogenic effects (leading to increased FSH and LH). The *in vitro* evidence suggests oestrogenic activity.

Importance and management

Evidence is limited and largely speculative, and it is therefore difficult to predict the outcome of using agnus castus with oestrogens or oestrogen antagonists. The evidence suggests that compounds of agnus castus may compete for the same oestrogen receptor as conventional hormonal drugs, with the outcome of either an overall oestrogenic effect, or an overall oestrogen antagonist effect (see also Chinese angelica, page 146).

The main compounds in agnus castus that have oestrogenic activity are agnuside, apigenin and rotundifuran and they are found, particularly apigenin, ubiquitously in foods and herbs. Phytoestrogens are generally much less potent than endogenous oestrogens and therefore any potential interaction is likely to be modest. However, note that it is probably inappropriate for patients undergoing IVF treatment to take hormonally-active herbal medicines, unless under the advice of an experienced endocrinologist. Similarly, because the possible effect of agnus castus on the efficacy of other oestrogen-containing preparations, such as hormonal contraceptives and HRT is unknown, it would seem sensible to undertake concurrent use with caution, anticipating reduced efficacy or increased oestrogenic adverse effects (e.g. nausea, breast tenderness, headaches). Given the potential consequences of contraceptive failure it may be most prudent to avoid concurrent use. Further study is needed.

1. Cahill DJ, Fox R, Wardle PG, Harlow CR. Multiple follicular development associated with herbal medicine. *Hum Reprod* (1994) 9, 1469–70.
2. Jarry H, Spengler B, Porzel A, Schmidt J, Wuttke W, Christoffel V. Evidence for estrogen receptor beta-selective activity of *Vitex agnus-castus* and isolated flavones. *Planta Med* (2003) 69, 945–7.
3. Jarry H, Spengler B, Wuttke W, Christoffel V. *In vitro* assays for bioactivity-guided isolation of endocrine active compounds in *Vitex agnus-castus. Maturitas* (2006) 55 (Suppl 1), S26–S36.

Agnus castus + Opioids

The interaction between agnus castus and opioids is based on experimental evidence only.

Clinical evidence

No interactions found.

Experimental evidence

Various agnus castus extracts and constituents have been shown to have an affinity to opioid receptors in *in vitro* studies.[1,2] Lipophilic extracts of agnus castus produced an inhibition of binding to μ- and κ-opioid receptors and an aqueous fraction produced an inhibition of binding to δ-opioid receptors in one study.[1] In another study,[2] various extracts were found to bind and activate μ- and δ-opioid receptors, but not κ-opioid receptors.

Another study on *hamster* ovary cells[3] found that extracts of agnus castus acted as agonists at the μ-opioid receptor in a similar way to morphine, another opioid agonist.

Mechanism

Active compounds of agnus castus and opioids may have additive effects because of their similar pharmacological activity.

Importance and management

The importance of this action on opioid receptors is unknown. Agnus castus is not known for any strong analgesic effects or for producing opioid-like dependence, and as no clinical interactions have been reported, it seems unlikely that any important interaction will occur with opioids.

1. Meier B, Berger D, Hoberg E, Sticher O, Schaffner W. Pharmacological activities of *Vitex agnus-castus* extracts *in vitro*. *Phytomedicine* (2000) 7, 373–81.
2. Webster DE, He Y, Chen S-N, Pauli GF, Farnsworth NR, Wang ZJ. Opioidergic mechanisms underlying the actions of *Vitex agnus-castus* L. *Biochem Pharmacol* (2011) 81, 170–177.
3. Webster DE, Lu J, Chen S-N, Farnsworth NR, Wang ZJ. Activation of the μ-opiate receptor by *Vitex agnus-castus* methanol extracts: Implication for its use in PMS. *J Ethnopharmacol* (2006) 106, 216–21.

Agrimony

Agrimonia eupatoria L. (Rosaceae)

Synonym(s) and related species

Agrimonia, Cocklebur, Stickwort.

Pharmacopoeias

Agrimony (*BP 2012, PhEur 7.5*).

Constituents

Agrimony may be standardised to a **tannin** content expressed as **pyrogallol** 2%. Other constituents include **flavonoids**, based on quercetin, kaempferol, apigenin, catechins, epicatechins and procyanidins; various phenolic acids; **triterpenes** including α-amyrin, ursolic and euscapic acids, phytosterols; salicylic and silicic acids.

Use and indications

The dried flowering tops of agrimony are used as a mild astringent and diuretic. They have also been used for diarrhoea in children, mucous colitis, urinary incontinence, cystitis, and as a gargle for sore throats and catarrh.

Pharmacokinetics

No relevant pharmacokinetic data found. For information on the pharmacokinetics of individual flavonoids present in agrimony, see under flavonoids, page 213.

Interactions overview

Experimental studies have found that agrimony has weak blood-glucose-lowering, diuretic, and blood pressure-lowering effects. It therefore has the potential to interact with conventional drugs that have these properties, although there is no clinical evidence for this. For information on the interactions of individual flavonoids present in agrimony, see under flavonoids, page 213, but note that it is unlikely that agrimony would be taken in doses large enough to give the levels of individual flavonoids used in the flavonoid studies (e.g. quercetin 100 mg daily and above).

Interactions monographs

- Antidiabetics, page 20
- Antihypertensives, page 20
- Food, page 20
- Herbal medicines, page 20

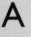

Agrimony + Antidiabetics

The interaction between agrimony and antidiabetics is based on experimental evidence only.

Clinical evidence

No interactions found.

Experimental evidence

In various *in vitro* and *animal* studies, high-dose agrimony has stimulated insulin secretion and reduced hyperglycaemia.[1,2] This suggests that usual doses used as a herbal medicine might have a weak antidiabetic effect, which could be additive with the effects of antidiabetic drugs.

Mechanism

Additive pharmacological effects.

Importance and management

These experimental studies provide limited evidence of a possible blood-glucose-lowering effect of agrimony extracts. Because of the nature of the evidence, applying these results in a clinical setting is extremely difficult. However, if patients taking antidiabetic drugs want to take agrimony it may be prudent to discuss these potential additive effects, and advise an increase in blood-glucose monitoring, should an interaction be suspected.

1. Gray AM, Flatt PR. Actions of the traditional anti-diabetic plant, *Agrimony eupatoria* (agrimony): effects on hyperglycaemia, cellular glucose metabolism and insulin secretion. *Br J Nutr* (1998) 80, 109–14.
2. Swanston-Flatt SK, Day C, Bailey CJ, Flatt PR. Traditional plant treatments for diabetes. Studies in normal and streptozotocin diabetic mice. *Diabetologia* (1990) 33, 462–4.

Agrimony + Antihypertensives

The interaction between agrimony and antihypertensives is based on experimental evidence only.

Clinical evidence

No interactions found.

Experimental evidence

Agrimony has traditionally been used as a diuretic. One study in *rats* found that agrimony had little significant diuretic activity,[1] and another in *cats* found that intravenous agrimony decreased blood pressure over a period of 20 minutes.[2]

Mechanism

It is possible that agrimony has weak antihypertensive effects, and a slight additive reduction in blood pressure could be possible if it is given with antihypertensives.

Importance and management

These experimental studies provide extremely limited evidence of a possible antihypertensive effect of agrimony extracts. Because of the nature of the evidence, applying these results in a clinical setting is extremely difficult, and until more is known, it would be unwise to advise anything other than general caution.

1. Giachetti D, Taddei E, Taddei I. Ricerche sull'attivita' diuretica ed uricosurica di Agrimonia eupatoria L. *Boll Soc Ital Biol Sper* (1986) 62, 705–11.
2. Petkov V. Plants with hypotensive, antiatheromatous and coronarodilatating action. *Am J Chin Med* (1979) 7, 197–236.

Agrimony + Food

No interactions found.

Agrimony + Herbal medicines

No interactions found.

Alfalfa

Medicago sativa L. (Fabaceae)

Synonym(s) and related species

Lucerne, Medicago, Purple medick.

Medicago afghanica Vass, *Medicago grandiflora* (Grossh.) Vass, *Medicago ladak* Vass, *Medicago mesopotamica* Vass, *Medicago orientalis* Vass, *Medicago polia* (Brand) Vass, *Medicago praesativa* Sinsk, *Medicago sogdiana* (Brand) Vass, *Trigonella upendrae* Chowdh. and Rao.

Constituents

The main active constituents of alfalfa are the **isoflavones**, which include **biochanin A**, **formononetin**, **daidzein**, and **genistein**, and the saponins, based on the aglycones hederagenin, medicagenic acid, and soyasapogenols A-E. Other components include the toxic amino acid canavanine; natural coumarins such as coumestrol, lucernol, medicagol, sativol, and daphnoretin; the sterols campestrol and beta-sitosterol; and miscellaneous compounds including vitamins (notably vitamin K), porphyrins, alkaloids (e.g. stachydrine), sugars, minerals and trace elements.

Use and indications

Alfalfa herb is usually used as a source of nutrients, including vitamins. Alfalfa seeds, when germinated, are popular as salad sprouts. Alfalfa has therapeutic properties including lowering blood cholesterol (the saponins) and oestrogenic activity (the isoflavones, page 300).

A possible association between alfalfa and systemic lupus erythematosus has been reported. This has been attributed to the toxic constituent canavanine, which is a structural analogue of arginine and may interfere with arginine functions.[1]

Pharmacokinetics

No relevant data for alfalfa found. For information on the pharmacokinetics of its isoflavone constituents genistein, daidzein, and biochanin A, see isoflavones, page 300.

Interactions overview

Although it has been suggested that alfalfa may interact with antidiabetic medicines and anticoagulants, evidence for this is largely lacking. Alfalfa may interact with immunosuppressants, and has apparently caused transplant rejection in one patient. Potential interactions of specific isoflavone constituents of alfalfa are covered under isoflavones; see antibacterials, page 302, digoxin, page 302, fexofenadine, page 303, nicotine, page 303, paclitaxel, page 303, tamoxifen, page 304, and theophylline, page 305.

Interactions monographs

- Antidiabetics, page 22
- Food, page 22
- Herbal medicines, page 22
- Immunosuppressants, page 22
- Warfarin and related drugs, page 23

1. Akaogi J, Barker T, Kuroda Y, Nacionales DC, Yamasaki Y, Stevens BR, Reeves WH, Satoh M. Role of non-protein amino acid L-canavanine in autoimmunity. *Autoimmun Rev* (2006) 5, 429–35.

A

Alfalfa + Antibacterials

No data for alfalfa found. For the theoretical possibility that broad-spectrum antibacterials might reduce the metabolism of the isoflavone constituents of alfalfa, such as daidzein, by colonic bacteria, and so alter their efficacy, see Isoflavones + Antibacterials, page 302.

Alfalfa + Antidiabetics

An isolated case describes a marked reduction in blood-glucose levels in a diabetic patient who took an alfalfa extract.

Clinical evidence

A case report describes a young man with poorly controlled diabetes (reportedly requiring large doses of insulin for even moderately satisfactory control) who had a marked reduction in blood-glucose levels after taking an oral alfalfa aqueous extract. He also had a reduction in his blood-glucose levels in response to oral manganese chloride, but this effect was not seen in 8 other patients with diabetes.[1]

Experimental evidence

In a study in streptozotocin-induced diabetic *mice,* high levels of alfalfa in the diet (62.5 g/kg) and drinking water (2.5 g/L) resulted in glucose levels that were similar to those in non-diabetic control *mice* and markedly lower than those in streptozotocin-diabetic control *mice.*[2] Insulin-releasing and insulin-like activity was demonstrated for various extracts of alfalfa *in vitro.*[2]

Mechanism

The authors of the case report (from 1962) concluded that the effect of alfalfa was due to the manganese content,[1] but a subsequent *in vitro* study discounted a major role for manganese.[2]

Importance and management

Evidence is very limited, with just one early case report in an atypical patient and an *animal* study using very high doses of alfalfa. There is insufficient data to recommend any action, but it appears unlikely that usual herbal doses of alfalfa will have much, if any, effect on diabetic control.

1. Rubenstein AH, Levin NW, Elliott GA. Hypoglycaemia induced by manganese. *Nature* (1962) 194, 188–9.
2. Gray AM, Flatt PR. Pancreatic and extra-pancreatic effects of the traditional anti-diabetic plant, *Medicago sativa* (lucerne). *Br J Nutr* (1997) 78, 325–34.

Alfalfa + Digoxin

No data for alfalfa found. For the possibility that high-dose biochanin A, an isoflavone present in alfalfa, might increase digoxin levels, see Isoflavones + Digoxin, page 302.

Alfalfa + Fexofenadine

No data for alfalfa found. For the possibility that high-dose biochanin A, an isoflavone present in alfalfa, has been shown to slightly decrease fexofenadine levels in *rats,* see Isoflavones + Fexofenadine, page 303.

Alfalfa + Food

No interactions found.

Alfalfa + Herbal medicines

No interactions found.

Alfalfa + Immunosuppressants

An isolated report describes acute rejection and vasculitis with alfalfa and/or black cohosh in a renal transplant patient taking ciclosporin.

Clinical evidence

A stable kidney transplant patient taking azathioprine 50 mg daily and ciclosporin 75 mg twice daily began to take alfalfa and black cohosh supplements (specific products not stated) on medical advice for severe menopausal symptoms. Her serum creatinine rose from between about 97 to 124 micromol/L up to 168 micromol/L after 4 weeks and, to 256 micromol/L after 6 weeks with no associated change in her ciclosporin levels. Biopsy revealed severe acute rejection with vasculitis and she was treated with corticosteroids and anti-T lymphocyte immunoglobulin with partial improvement in renal function.[1]

Experimental evidence

No relevant data found.

Mechanism

Alfalfa has been reported to cause worsening of systemic lupus erythematosus and immunostimulation, and it was suggested that immunostimulation may have contributed to the acute rejection in this patient.[1]

Importance and management

The evidence of an interaction between alfalfa/black cohosh and immunosuppressants is limited, with the mechanism suggesting that alfalfa is the more likely culprit, although an effect of black cohosh cannot be ruled out. As the effects were so severe in this case it would seem prudent to avoid the use of alfalfa supplements in patients receiving immunosuppressants for serious indications, such as organ transplantation. Similarly, it would seem prudent to avoid the use of alfalfa in those taking immunosuppressants for indications such as eczema, psoriasis or rheumatoid arthritis; however, if these patients particularly wish to take alfalfa a short-term trial of concurrent use is likely to be less hazardous, but patients should be counselled about the possible risks (i.e. loss of disease control).

1. Light TD, Light JA. Acute renal transplant rejection possibly related to herbal medications. *Am J Transplant* (2003) 3, 1608–9.

Alfalfa + Nicotine

For discussion of a study showing that daidzein and genistein present in alfalfa caused a minor decrease in the metabolism of nicotine, see Isoflavones + Nicotine, page 303.

Alfalfa + Paclitaxel

No data for alfalfa found. For the possibility that biochanin A and genistein present in alfalfa might markedly increase paclitaxel levels, see Isoflavones + Paclitaxel, page 303. Note that paclitaxel is used intravenously, and the effect of biochanin A on intravenous paclitaxel does not appear to have been evaluated.

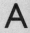

Alfalfa + Tamoxifen

No data for alfalfa found. Data relating to the use of the isoflavone constituents of alfalfa, such as biochanin A, daidzein and genistein, with tamoxifen are covered under Isoflavones + Tamoxifen, page 304.

Alfalfa + Theophylline

No data for alfalfa found. For the possibility that high doses of daidzein present in alfalfa might modestly increase theophylline levels, see Isoflavones + Theophylline, page 305.

Alfalfa + Warfarin and related drugs

Unintentional and unwanted antagonism of warfarin has occurred in patients who ate exceptionally large amounts of some green vegetables, which can contain significant amounts of vitamin K_1. It is predicted that alfalfa may contain sufficient vitamin K to provoke a similar reaction.

Evidence

There is no specific clinical or experimental evidence relating to the use of alfalfa with anticoagulants, but alfalfa is predicted to antagonise coumarin anticoagulants based on its vitamin K content. There are some data on the amount of vitamin K in alfalfa, and lots of data on dietary vitamin K and anticoagulant control.

(a) Vitamin K_1 content of alfalfa

Alfalfa supplements are often promoted on the basis that they contain significant amounts of vitamin K_1, although packaging rarely gives an amount. Alfalfa greens were used in early studies from the 1930s when vitamin K was first identified. In one such study, the amount of vitamin K activity in dried alfalfa was about half that in dried spinach.[1] Green leafy vegetables such as spinach are well known to contain high levels of vitamin K_1, with modern assay techniques giving values of about 500 micrograms/100 g.[2]

Conversely, sprouted alfalfa seeds have been shown to contain far more modest amounts of vitamin K_1 (in the region of 30 micrograms/100 g).[2] It is likely that the seeds themselves would contain even less vitamin K_1. Therefore, the amount of vitamin K_1 in an alfalfa product is likely to depend on the part of the plant used, and would be highest from the green leaf material and lowest from the seeds.

In addition, the way the product is extracted (vitamin K_1 is a fat-soluble vitamin) would affect the vitamin K_1 content. For example, although the leaves of green tea themselves are high in vitamin K_1, the brew prepared from the leaves contains very little vitamin K_1.[3] Therefore an aqueous infusion prepared from alfalfa dried herb would be unlikely to contain much vitamin K_1. Moreover, although the dried herb itself contains high levels of vitamin K_1, it is taken in modest amounts in the form of supplements when compared with, for example, eating spinach as part of a meal. If a capsule containing 500 mg of powdered alfalfa leaf is taken at a dose of 4 capsules three times daily, then the daily intake of alfalfa would be 6 g, which might contain in the region of 15 micrograms of vitamin K daily. This amount seems unlikely to generally affect the response to vitamin K antagonist anticoagulants (such as warfarin), and many products contain less alfalfa than this.

(b) Dietary vitamin K and warfarin activity

There is evidence that the average dietary vitamin K_1 intake is correlated with the efficacy of warfarin. In one study, patients consuming a diet containing more than 250 micrograms daily of vitamin K_1 had a lower INR 5 days after starting warfarin than patients consuming less dietary vitamin K_1 (median INR 1.9 versus 3). Also, the group consuming large amounts of vitamin K_1 needed a higher maintenance warfarin dose (5.7 mg/day versus 3.5 mg/day).[4] In another study, multiple regression analysis indicated that, in patients taking warfarin, the INR was altered by 1, by a weekly change in the intake of vitamin K_1 of 714 micrograms.[5] Similarly, for each increase in daily dietary vitamin K_1 intake of 100 micrograms, the INR decreased by 0.2 in another study.[6]

In a randomised, crossover study in patients taking warfarin or phenprocoumon, increasing the dietary intake of vitamin K_1 by 500% relative to the baseline value (from 118 to 591 micrograms daily) for 4 days only modestly decreased the INR from 3.1 to 2.8 on day 4. Decreasing the dietary intake of vitamin K_1 by 80% (from 118 to 26 micrograms daily) for 4 days increased the INR from 2.6 to 3.3 on day 7.[7]

There is some evidence that patients with a very low dietary vitamin K_1 intake are more sensitive to alterations in intake, and have less stable anticoagulant control. For example, in one study, patients with unstable anticoagulant control were found to have a much lower dietary intake of vitamin K_1, when compared with another group of patients with stable anticoagulant control (29 micrograms daily versus 76 micrograms daily).[8] In another study in 10 patients with poor anticoagulant control taking acenocoumarol, a diet with a low, controlled vitamin K_1 content of 20 to 40 micrograms daily increased the percentage of INR values within the therapeutic range, when compared with a control group of 10 patients not subjected to any dietary restrictions.[9]

Mechanism

The coumarin and indanedione oral anticoagulants are vitamin K antagonists, which inhibit the enzyme vitamin K epoxide reductase so reducing the synthesis of vitamin K-dependent blood clotting factors by the liver. If the intake of dietary vitamin K_1 increases, the synthesis of the blood clotting factors begins to return to normal. As a result the prothrombin time also begins to fall to its normal value. Naturally occurring vitamin K_1 (phytomenadione) is found only in plants.

The natural coumarins present in alfalfa are not considered to be anticoagulants, because they do not have the structural requirements for this activity.

Importance and management

Patients should be counselled on the effects of dietary vitamin K and the need to avoid dramatic dietary alterations while taking warfarin. It would be prudent to avoid large doses of alfalfa leaf supplements as a precaution when taking warfarin or other coumarin anticoagulants. Available evidence suggests that it is unlikely that infusions prepared with water, or alfalfa seeds, would pose any problem, due to the lower vitamin K_1 content.

1. Dam H, Schønheyder F. The occurrence and chemical nature of vitamin K. *Biochem J* (1936) 30, 897–901.
2. USDA National Nutrient Database for Standard Reference, Release 17. Vitamin K (phylloquinone) (µg) Content of selected foods per common measure. http://www.nal.usda.gov/fnic/foodcomp/Data/SR17/wtrank/sr17a430.pdf (accessed 15/03/2012).
3. Booth SL, Madabushi HT, Davidson KW, Sadowski JA. Tea and coffee brews are not dietary sources of vitamin K-1 (phylloquinone). *J Am Diet Assoc* (1995) 95, 82–3.
4. Lubetsky A, Dekel-Stern E, Chetrit A, Lubin F, Halkin H. Vitamin K intake and sensitivity to warfarin in patients consuming regular diets. *Thromb Haemost* (1999) 81, 396–9.
5. Couris R, Tataronis G, McCloskey W, Oertel L, Dallal G, Dwyer J, Blumberg JB. Dietary vitamin K variability affects International normalized ratio (INR) coagulation indices. *Int J Vitam Nutr Res* (2006) 76, 65–74.
6. Khan T, Wynne H, Wood P, Torrance A, Hankey C, Avery P, Kesteven P, Kamali F. Dietary vitamin K influences intra-individual variability in anticoagulant response to warfarin. *Br J Haematol* (2004) 124, 348–54.
7. Franco V, Polanczyk CA, Clausell N, Rohde LE. Role of dietary vitamin K intake in chronic oral anticoagulation: prospective evidence from observational and randomized protocols. *Am J Med* (2004) 116, 651–6.
8. Sconce E, Khan T, Mason J, Noble F, Wynne H, Kamali F. Patients with unstable control have a poorer dietary intake of vitamin K compared to patients with stable control of anticoagulation. *Thromb Haemost* (2005) 93, 872–5.
9. Sorano GG, Biondi G, Conti M, Mameli G, Licheri D, Marongiu F. Controlled vitamin K content diet for improving the management of poorly controlled anticoagulated patients: a clinical practice proposal. *Haemostasis* (1993) 23, 77–82.

Aloe vera

Aloe vera (L.) Burm.f. (Aloaceae)

Synonym(s) and related species

Aloe gel, Barbados aloes, Curacao aloes.

Aloe africana Mill., *Aloe barbadensis* Mill., *Aloe vera* Tourn. ex L., *Aloe vera* (L.) Webb.

Constituents

Aloe vera gel is contained in the mucilaginous tissue that is found in the inner leaf, and should not be confused with aloes, page 27, which is the latex stored in tubules along the leaf margin. Aloe vera gel may be produced by a hand-filleted technique to remove the inner leaf, or by a whole-leaf extraction process where the aloes constituents (anthraquinones) are now usually subsequently removed (e.g. by charcoal filtration).

The principal constituents of the gel are polysaccharides consisting mainly of polymannans, of which **acemannan** is the major one. Other constituents include glycoproteins such as aloctins, and various carboxypeptidases, sterols, saponins, tannins, organic acids, vitamins and minerals. Traces of anthraquinone glycosides may also be present in preparations.

Use and indications

Aloe vera is used topically to aid wound healing from cuts and burns, including sunburn, and is used in many cosmetic preparations such as moisturisers. It is reported to possess anti-inflammatory, antitumour, immunomodulatory and antibacterial properties. Internally, aloe vera is thought to be immunostimulatory and to have mild analgesic, antioxidant and antidiabetic effects.

Pharmacokinetics

No relevant pharmacokinetic data found.

Interactions overview

Aloe vera contains only traces of anthraquinone glycosides, and would therefore not be expected to have any of the interactions of aloes, page 27, or similar herbal medicines, which occur, or are predicted to occur, as a result of their anthraquinone content.

Aloe vera may have blood-glucose-lowering properties and may therefore be expected to interact with conventional drugs that have the same effect. Aloe vera appears to enhance the absorption of some vitamins but the clinical significance of this is not clear.

Interactions monographs

- Antidiabetics, page 25
- Food, page 25
- Herbal medicines, page 25
- Sevoflurane, page 25
- Vitamins, page 25

Aloe vera + Antidiabetics

Aloe vera juice reduces blood-glucose levels in patients with diabetes taking glibenclamide.

Clinical evidence

In placebo-controlled clinical studies, aloe vera juice (80%), one tablespoonful twice daily for 42 days, reduced blood-glucose both in patients with diabetes, either taking **glibenclamide**,[1] or not taking oral antidiabetic drugs,[2] from an average of 14 to 16 mmol/L down to 8 mmol/L over a period of 6 weeks. However, it should be noted that in the study in patients taking **glibenclamide**, there was, unexpectedly, no response to the use of **glibenclamide** alone. In these studies, the aloe vera juice (80%) was prepared from aloe gel and additional flavours and preservatives.

Experimental evidence

There is extensive literature (not cited here) on the possible blood-glucose-lowering effect of various extracts of aloe vera in *animal* models of diabetes, with some studies showing an effect and others not.

Mechanism

Unknown.

Importance and management

It seems possible that some oral preparations of aloe vera might have a clinically important blood-glucose-lowering effect. Indeed, aloe vera has traditionally been used to treat diabetes. It might therefore be prudent to increase the frequency of blood-glucose monitoring if patients taking antidiabetic medication wish to try oral aloe vera preparations.

1. Bunyapraphatsara N, Yongchaiyudha S, Rungpitarangsi V, Chokechaijaroenporn O. Antidiabetic activity of *Aloe vera* L. juice II. Clinical trial in diabetes mellitus patients in combination with glibenclamide. *Phytomedicine* (1996) 3, 245–8.
2. Yongchaiyudha S, Rungpitarangsi V, Bunyapraphatsara N, Chokechaijaroenporn O. Antidiabetic activity of *Aloe vera* L. juice. I. Clinical trial in new cases of diabetes mellitus. *Phytomedicine* (1996) 3, 241–3.

Aloe vera + Food

No interactions found.

Aloe vera + Herbal medicines

No interactions found.

Aloe vera + Sevoflurane

An isolated case report tentatively attributed increased surgical bleeding to the concurrent use of aloe vera and sevoflurane.

Clinical evidence

A 35-year-old woman, who had taken four aloe vera tablets (exact constituents and dose unknown) daily for 2 weeks before undergoing a procedure to excise a haemangioma from her left thigh, lost more than double the amount of blood estimated before surgery.[1] General anaesthesia was induced with propofol 110 mg, fentanyl 100 micrograms and rocuronium 35 mg, followed by tracheal intubation. Sevoflurane 0.5% to 1.3% was used to maintain anaesthesia with nitrous oxide in oxygen, which was supplemented by rocuronium 70 mg and morphine 10.5 mg. The authors suggest a possible interaction between sevoflurane and aloe vera contributed to the excessive bleeding seen.

Experimental evidence

Aloe vera gel extracts inhibited prostaglandin synthesis *in vitro*,[2] and might therefore have antiplatelet activity.

Mechanism

Sevoflurane can inhibit platelet aggregation by inhibiting thromboxane A_2, and aloe vera affects prostaglandin synthesis, which may also impair platelet aggregation. Therefore additive antiplatelet effects may have contributed to the excessive bleeding.[1]

Importance and management

An interaction between aloe vera and sevoflurane is based on a single case report and is by no means proven, especially as the patient's aPTT and INR were not assessed pre-operatively and the authors do state that the vascularity and size of the haemangioma were the most important factors in the blood loss.[1] Because of limited information, the American Society of Anesthesiologists have recommended discontinuation of all herbal medicines 2 weeks before an elective anaesthetic[3,4] and if there is any doubt about the safety of a product, this may be a prudent precaution.[5]

1. Lee A, Chui PT, Aun CST, Gin T, Lau ASC. Possible interaction between sevoflurane and *Aloe vera*. *Ann Pharmacother* (2004) 38, 1651–4.
2. Vázquez B, Avila G, Segura D, Escalante B. Antiinflammatory activity of extracts from *Aloe vera* gel. *J Ethnopharmacol* (1996) 55, 69–75.
3. Larkin M. Surgery patients at risk for herb-anaesthesia interactions. *Lancet* (1999) 354, 1362.
4. Leak JA. Perioperative considerations in the management of the patient taking herbal medicines. *Curr Opin Anaesthesiol* (2000) 13, 321–5.
5. Cheng B, Hung CT, Chiu W. Herbal medicine and anaesthesia. *Hong Kong Med J* (2002) 8, 123–30.

Aloe vera + Vitamins

Aloe vera might delay, and enhance, the absorption of vitamin C and vitamin E.

Clinical evidence

(a) Vitamin C

In a single-dose, randomised study in 8 healthy subjects, aloe vera gel extract 60 mL appeared to enhance the absorption of vitamin C 500 mg. The AUC of ascorbate was increased by about threefold. However, this difference was not statistically significant: it was attributed to the large interindividual differences. There was a second maximum plasma ascorbate level at 8 hours with the gel, and plasma ascorbate was still detectable at 24 hours, suggesting that aloe vera gel might delay, as well as enhance, absorption. Conversely, aloe vera whole leaf extract 60 mL had no significant effect on the absorption of vitamin C.[1]

(b) Vitamin E

In a single-dose, randomised study in 10 healthy subjects, aloe vera gel extract 60 mL increased the AUC of vitamin E 420 mg by 3.7-fold. Aloe vera whole leaf extract 60 mL increased the AUC by about twofold. However, the only statistically significant

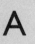

difference was the increase in plasma tocopherol at 8 hours, which occurred with both aloe vera extracts. The time to maximum level was delayed from 4 hours to 8 hours for the gel and to 6 hours for the leaf extract, suggesting that aloe vera might delay, as well as enhance, absorption.[1]

Experimental evidence

No relevant data found.

Mechanism

The authors suggest that the vitamins may be protected from degradation in the intestine by flavonoid antioxidants in the aloe vera extracts and by polysaccharides that may bind to the vitamins, delaying and increasing their absorption.[1]

Importance and management

If confirmed, this appears to be a beneficial interaction, with aloe vera exhibiting the potential to be an adjunct for patients requiring vitamin C and/or E supplementation.

1. Vinson JA, Al Kharrat H, Andreoli L. Effect of *Aloe vera* preparations on the human bioavailability of vitamins C and E. *Phytomedicine* (2005) 12, 760–765.

Aloes

Aloe barbadensis Mill., *Aloe ferox* Mill., *Aloe perryi* Baker (Aloaceae)

Synonym(s) and related species

Aloe barbadensis: Barbados aloes, Curacao aloes, *Aloe vera* Tourn ex L., *Aloe vera* (L.) Webb.

   Aloe ferox: Cape aloes.

   Aloe perryi: Socotrine aloes, Zanzrbar aloes.

   Not to be confused with the gel of Aloe vera, page 24.

Pharmacopoeias

Aloe (*USP35–NF30 S1*); Barbados Aloes (*BP 2012, PhEur 7.5*); Cape Aloes (*BP 2012, PhEur 7.5*); Standardised Aloes Dry Extract (*BP 2012, PhEur 7.5*).

Constituents

Not to be confused with Aloe vera, page 24, which is the gel contained in the mucilaginous tissue that is found in the inner leaf. Aloes is derived from the latex that is stored in tubules along the margin of the leaf. When the outer leaf is cut, latex exudes from the leaf and this exudate, when dried, is aloes. **Anthraquinone glycosides** are major components of aloes and include barbaloin, a glycoside of aloe-emodin to which it may be standardised, and minor glycosides such as aloinosides A and B. Aloe-emodin, chrysophanol, chromones including aloesin, aloeresin E, isoaloeresin D and furoaloesone are also present in small amounts, as are resins.

Use and indications

Aloes has mainly been used internally as a laxative (although, note that this use has generally been superseded) and, in low concentrations, as a flavouring ingredient in food and drink.

Pharmacokinetics

The anthraquinone, emodin, is present in aloes (and similar plants) principally as the inactive glycoside. It travels through the gut, and is then metabolised by microflora to produce the active aglycone emodin, some of which is absorbed. Emodin is genotoxic, and might be metabolised to more toxic metabolites by CYP1A2. However, the relevance of this to the clinical use of drugs (especially CYP1A2 substrates and inducers) is unclear.[1]

Interactions overview

Although aloes have been predicted to interact with a number of drugs that lower potassium levels (such as the corticosteroids and potassium-depleting diuretics), or drugs where the effects become potentially harmful when potassium is lowered (such as digoxin), there appears to be little or no direct evidence that this occurs in practice. A case report describes persistent diarrhoea and raised lopinavir levels when evening primrose oil and a product containing aloes, rhubarb and liquorice were started, see under Evening primrose oil + Lopinavir, page 207.

Interactions monographs

- Corticosteroids, page 28
- Digitalis glycosides, page 28
- Diuretics; Potassium-depleting, page 28
- Food, page 29
- Herbal medicines; Liquorice, page 29
- Quinidine, page 29

1. Mueller ST, Stopper H, Dekant W. Biotransformation of the anthraquinones emodin and chrysophanol by cytochrome P450 enzymes. Bioactivation to genotoxic metabolites. *Drug Metab Dispos* (1998) 26, 540–546.

A

Aloes + Corticosteroids

Theoretically, the risk of hypokalaemia might be increased in patients taking corticosteroids, who also regularly use, or abuse, anthraquinone-containing substances such as aloes.

Clinical evidence

Chronic diarrhoea as a result of long-term use, or abuse, of stimulant laxatives such as aloes can cause excessive water and potassium loss; this has led to metabolic acidosis in one case.[1] Systemic corticosteroids with mineralocorticoid effects can cause water retention and potassium loss. The effect of the over-use of aloes combined with systemic corticosteroids is not known, but, theoretically at least, the risk of hypokalaemia might be increased. Although this is mentioned in some reviews[2] there do not appear to be any reports describing clinical cases of this effect.

Experimental evidence

No relevant data found.

Mechanism

In theory the additive loss of potassium, caused by anthraquinone-containing substances and systemic corticosteroids, may result in hypokalaemia.

Importance and management

The interaction between aloes and corticosteroids is theoretical, but be aware of the potential in patients who regularly use, or abuse, anthraquinone-containing substances such as aloes. However, note that if anthraquinone laxatives are used as recommended (at a dose producing a comfortable soft-formed motion), then this interaction would not be expected to be clinically relevant. See also Senna + Corticosteroids, page 424.

1. Ramirez B, Marieb NJ. Hypokalemic metabolic alkalosis due to Carter's Little Pills. *Conn Med* (1970) 34, 169–70.
2. Hadley SK, Petry JJ. Medicinal herbs: A primer for primary care. *Hosp Pract* (1999) 34, 105–23.

Aloes + Digitalis glycosides

Theoretically, digitalis toxicity could develop if patients regularly use, or abuse, anthraquinone-containing substances such as aloes.

Clinical evidence

Chronic diarrhoea caused by the long-term use, or abuse, of stimulant laxatives such as aloes can cause excessive water and potassium loss, which may cause hypokalaemia that could lead to the development of digitalis toxicity. Although this is often mentioned in reviews[1,2] there do not appear to be any reports describing clinical cases of this effect. However, for mention of a case of **digoxin** toxicity and mild hypokalaemia in a patient stabilised on **digoxin** and furosemide, who started to take a laxative containing *rhubarb* and *liquorice,* see liquorice, page 331.

Experimental evidence

No relevant data found.

Mechanism

Possible pharmacodynamic interaction. The risk of development of digitalis toxicity, including cardiac arrhythmias, is increased by hypokalaemia, which can be induced by the excessive use of anthraquinone laxatives.

Importance and management

This is a theoretical interaction, but it may be prudent to exercise caution in patients who are taking digitalis glycosides and who regularly use, or abuse, anthraquinone-containing substances such as aloes. However, note that if anthraquinone laxatives are used as recommended (at a dose producing a comfortable soft-formed motion), then this interaction would not be expected to be clinically relevant. Consider also Senna + Digitalis glycosides, page 424, for the effects of anthraquinones on digoxin absorption.

1. Boudreau MD, Beland FA. An evaluation of the biological and toxicological properties of *Aloe barbadensis* (Miller), Aloe Vera. *J Environ Sci Health C Environ Carcinog Ecotoxicol Rev* (2006) 24, 103–54.
2. Hadley SK, Petry JJ. Medicinal herbs: a primer for primary care. *Hosp Pract* (1999) 34, 105–23.

Aloes + Diuretics; Potassium-depleting

Theoretically, patients taking potassium-depleting diuretics could experience excessive potassium loss if they also regularly use, or abuse, anthraquinone-containing substances such as aloes.

Clinical evidence

The potassium-depleting diuretics (i.e. **loop diuretics** and **thiazide and related diuretics**) may cause potassium depletion. Chronic diarrhoea caused by long-term use, or abuse, of stimulant laxatives such as aloes, may also lead to excessive water loss and potassium deficiency. This, theoretically, could be increased by concurrent use of these diuretics. This interaction is sometimes mentioned in reviews;[1,2] nevertheless, there is little, if any, direct evidence. There appears to be one case describing a myopathic syndrome related to potassium deficiency (potassium level 1.7 mmol/L) in a patient taking **furosemide** 80 mg daily and with a history of laxative abuse (laxatives not named). However, even this case may not have occurred as a result of an interaction as the patient also had gastroenteritis, causing profuse diarrhoea.[3]

Experimental evidence

No relevant data found.

Mechanism

Possible pharmacodynamic interaction involving additive loss of potassium and water by anthraquinone-containing substances and potassium-depleting diuretics.

Importance and management

This is a theoretical interaction, but be aware of the potential for hypokalaemia in patients who are taking potassium-depleting diuretics and who regularly use, or abuse, anthraquinone-containing substances such as aloes. However, note that if anthraquinone laxatives are used as recommended (at a dose producing a comfortable soft-formed motion), then this interaction is not clinically relevant. See also Senna + Diuretics; Potassium-depleting, page 424, for the effects of anthraquinones on furosemide absorption.

1. Boudreau MD, Beland FA. An evaluation of the biological and toxicological properties of *Aloe barbadensis* (Miller), Aloe Vera. *J Environ Sci Health C Environ Carcinog Ecotoxicol Rev* (2006) 24, 103–54.
2. Hadley SK, Petry JJ. Medicinal herbs: A primer for primary care. *Hosp Pract* (1999) 34, 105–23.
3. Rudolf J, Würker M, Neveling M, Grond M, Haupt WF, Heiss W-D. Dyskaliämische Lähmung bei Furosemidtherapie und gleichzeitigem Laxanzeinabuss. *Med Klin (Munich)* (1999) 94, 391–4.

Aloes + Food

No interactions found. Aloes are used as a flavouring agent in drink.

Aloes + Herbal medicines; Liquorice

Consider Liquorice + Laxatives, page 332, for the potential additive effects of anthraquinone-containing laxatives and liquorice.

Aloes + Lopinavir

For mention of a case of persistent diarrhoea and raised lopinavir levels in an HIV-positive man after starting evening primrose oil and a product containing aloes, rhubarb and liquorice, see Evening primrose oil + Lopinavir, page 207.

Aloes + Quinidine

Consider Senna + Quinidine, page 425 for a potential interaction between anthraquinone-containing laxatives and quinidine.

A

Alpha-lipoic acid

5-(1,2-dithiolan-3-yl)valeric acid

Synonym(s) and related species

Alpha-liponic acid, Lipoic Acid, Thioctic acid.

Pharmacopoeias

Alpha-Lipoic Acid (*USP35–NF30 S1*); Thioctic Acid (*PhEur 7.5*)

Use and indications

Alpha-lipoic acid is a naturally-occurring co-factor, and can be synthesised in humans. As a supplement it is used in the treatment of diabetic neuropathy, and has also been tried in a variety of other conditions such as dementia, glaucoma, liver dysfunction, and vascular disease. It has been used as an antidote in poisoning due to ingestion of the death cap mushroom *Amanita phalloides,* but such use is unproven. Derivatives of alpha-lipoic acid, such as sodium thioctate, ethylenediamine thioctate and thioctamide are used in a similar way. Alpha-lipoic acid has also been used topically as an antioxidant to reduce skin aging.

Pharmacokinetics

Alpha-lipoic acid is absorbed when given orally, with an absolute bioavailability of about 30% for a 200 mg dose.[1] In the body, alpha-lipoic acid is present as the oxidised form, alpha-lipoic acid, and the reduced form dihydrolipoic acid. Its primary metabolic pathways are beta-oxidation and *S*-methylation.[2]

Interactions overview

Alpha-lipoic acid does not appear to interact with acarbose, metformin or glibenclamide (glyburide), and does not appear to alter glycaemic control. Food very slightly decreases the overall absorption of alpha-lipoic acid. Evidence from *animal* studies suggests that alpha-lipoic acid might slightly increase valproate exposure. Theoretically, antioxidants such as alpha-lipoic acid might reduce the efficacy of cytotoxic antineoplastics, such as alkylating agents; however there is limited evidence to suggest that it might improve the efficacy of some of these antineoplastics.

Interactions monographs

- Antidiabetics, page 31
- Antineoplastics, page 31
- Food, page 31
- Herbal medicines, page 32
- Valproate, page 32

1. Teichert J, Kern J, Tritschler HJ, Ulrich H, Preiss R. Investigations on the pharmacokinetics of alpha-lipoic acid in healthy volunteers. *Int J Clin Pharmacol Ther* (1998) 36, 625–8.
2. Teichert J, Hermann R, Ruus P, Preiss R. Plasma kinetics, metabolism, and urinary excretion of alpha-lipoic acid following oral administration in healthy volunteers. *J Clin Pharmacol* (2003) 43, 1257–67.

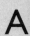

Alpha-lipoic acid + Antidiabetics

Alpha-lipoic acid is reported not to interact with acarbose, metformin or glibenclamide (glyburide). Alpha-lipoic acid appears not to appreciably alter glycaemic control.

Clinical evidence

A study in 24 healthy subjects given tablets containing alpha-lipoic acid 200 mg and **metformin** 500 mg found that the pharmacokinetics of **metformin** were unchanged by the presence of the alpha-lipoic acid, and the authors of the report state that there was also no pharmacodynamic interaction.[1] The report gives very few details. A further single-dose study in 24 healthy subjects found that alpha-lipoic acid 600 mg given with **glibenclamide (glyburide)** 3.5 mg did not result in any clinically relevant pharmacokinetic interaction, and alpha-lipoic acid did not alter the effect of **glibenclamide** on glucose or insulin levels.[2] Similarly, there was no evidence of a change in alpha-lipoic acid pharmacokinetics when it was given with **acarbose** 50 mg. Alpha-lipoic acid alone, and when given with **acarbose**, did not affect glucose or insulin levels.[2]

Alpha-lipoic acid has been widely studied in patients with diabetes for treating diabetic neuropathy. In general, in clinical use, it does not appear to alter glucose control. For example, in one large, well-conducted study in patients with type 2 diabetes, there were no statistically significant differences in HbA$_{1c}$ levels between patients receiving alpha-lipoic acid (intravenously for 3 weeks, followed by oral alpha-lipoic acid or placebo for 6 months) and those receiving placebo. Patients in this study were managed with diet, **oral antidiabetics** and/or **insulin** (just over 60% of patients in each group received insulin).[3]

Experimental evidence

No interactions found.

Mechanism

Alpha-lipoic acid has been shown to improve insulin sensitivity, an effect that might be more apparent with intravenous use rather than oral use.[4] Alpha-lipoic acid can rarely cause an insulin autoimmune syndrome characterised by hypoglycaemia, anti-insulin antibodies, and high insulin levels.[5]

Importance and management

Evidence for an interaction between alpha-lipoic acid and the antidiabetics seems to be limited to the studies cited; nevertheless, some of these studies were large and well designed. The available evidence suggests that no special precautions are necessary if oral alpha-lipoic acid is given to patients taking **acarbose**, **metformin** or **glibenclamide**. No alteration in glycaemic control would generally be expected.

1. Schug BS, Schneider E, Elze M, Fieger-Büschges H, Larsimont V, Popescu G, Molz KH, Blume HH, Hermann R. Study of pharmacokinetic interaction of thioctic acid and metformin. *Eur J Clin Pharmacol* (1997) 52 (Suppl), A140.
2. Gleiter CH, Schreeb KH, Freudenthaler S, Thomas M, Elze M, Fieger-Büschges H, Potthast H, Schneider E, Schug BS, Blume HH, Hermann R. Lack of interaction between thioctic acid, glibenclamide and acarbose. *Br J Clin Pharmacol* (1999) 48, 819–25.
3. Ziegler D, Hanefeld M, Ruhnau KJ, Hasche H, Lobisch M, Schütte K, Kerum G, Malessa R. ALADIN III Study Group. Treatment of symptomatic diabetic polyneuropathy with the antioxidant alpha-lipoic acid: a 7-month multicenter randomized controlled trial (ALADIN III Study). *Diabetes Care* (1999) 22, 1296–1301.
4. Singh U, Jalal I. Alpha-lipoic acid supplementation and diabetes. *Nutr Rev* (2008) 66, 646–57.
5. Takeuchi Y, Miyamoto T, Kakizawa T, Shigematsu S, Hashizume K. Insulin Autoimmune Syndrome possibly caused by alpha lipoic acid. *Intern Med* (2007) 46, 237–9.

Alpha-lipoic acid + Antineoplastics

The interaction between alpha-lipoic acid and cytotoxic antineoplastics is based on experimental evidence only.

Clinical evidence

No interactions found.

Experimental evidence

There are a number of animal studies suggesting that alpha-lipoic acid protects against toxicities of various cytotoxic antineoplastics, for example: cisplatin-induced nephrotoxicity,[1] doxorubicin-induced myocardial toxicity,[2] and cyclophosphamide-induced cardiomyopathy.[3] However, in a leukaemia model in mice, alpha-lipoic acid antagonised the effect of doxorubicin at low concentrations, and was synergistic at high concentrations.[4]

Mechanism

Theoretically, supplements with purported antioxidant activity such as alpha-lipoic acid might reduce the efficacy of cytotoxic antineoplastics that utilise reactive oxygen species for their cytotoxic effect (e.g. alkylating agents, anthracyclines, mitomycin, bleomycin, etoposide, teniposide). This might be apparent in the short term as a reduction in acute toxicity, but longer term it might increase the risk of disease recurrence.[5] Conversely, there is limited evidence that the antioxidant effect of alpha-lipoic acid actually increases cancer cell death at some concentrations.[4]

Importance and management

It has been suggested that antioxidants such as alpha-lipoic acid might reduce the benefits of some cytotoxic chemotherapy drugs (see Mechanism, above). However, it is also possible that they might prove to be useful in attenuating the toxicity of some antineoplastics without altering efficacy, although benefits might be dose and schedule dependent. Note that alpha-lipoic acid is a natural substance synthesised in small amounts by the body, although this does not rule out the possibility of interactions with alpha-lipoic acid supplements. A cautious approach would be to avoid such supplements when undergoing chemotherapy, as has been recommended by some.[5,6] However, others contend this is too cautious.[7] Further study is needed to establish the outcome of using alpha-lipoic acid with specific antineoplastics.

1. Bae EH , Lee J, Ma SK, Kim IJ, Frøkiaer J, Nielsen S, Kim SY, Kim SW. α-Lipoic acid prevents cisplatin-induced acute kidney injury in rats. *Nephrol Dial Transplant* (2009) 24, 2692–2700.
2. Al-Majed AA, Gdo AM, Al-Shabanah OA, Mansour MA. Alpha-lipoic acid ameliorates myocardial toxicity induced by doxorubicin. *Pharmacol Res* (2002) 46, 499–503.
3. Mythili Y, Sudharsan PT, Sudhahar V, Varalakshmi P. Protective effect of DL-alpha-lipoic acid on cyclophosphamide induced hyperlipidemic cardiomyopathy. *Eur J Pharmacol* (2006) 543, 92–6.
4. Dovinová I, Novotný L, Rauko P, Kvasnicka P. Combined effect of lipoic acid and doxorubicin in murine leukemia. *Neoplasma* (1999) 46, 237–41.
5. Labriola D, Livingston R. Possible interactions between dietary antioxidants and chemotherapy. *Oncology (Williston Park)* (1999) 13, 1003–8, 1011–12.
6. CM Jr Bagley. Call for stronger recommendations about supplement use during chemotherapy. *Oncology (Williston Park)* (1999) 13, 1628–31.
7. Reilly P, Gignac M, Chue B, Sardo M . Concerns over antioxidant-chemotherapy interactions overstated. *Oncology (Williston Park)* (1999) 13, 1624, 1627–8.

Alpha-lipoic acid + Food

The absorption of alpha-lipoic acid might be very slightly decreased by a high-fat meal.

Clinical evidence

In a crossover study in 12 healthy subjects, a high-fat breakfast very slightly decreased the AUC of alpha-lipoic acid given as a single 600-mg dose (Thioctacid 600) when compared with the fasted state.[1] The AUC of *R*-alpha-lipoic acid was reduced by 23% and the AUC of *S*-alpha-lipoic acid was reduced by 17%.

Experimental evidence

No interactions found.

Mechanism

Uncertain.

A

Importance and management

The absorption of alpha-lipoic acid appears to be slightly reduced by food. In general, reductions of the extent described in this study are not usually considered to be clinically relevant. However, the authors recommend that to achieve maximal absorption, administration on an empty stomach is preferable.

1. Gleiter CH, Schug BS, Hermann R, Elze M, Blume HH, Gundert-Remy U. Influence of food intake on the bioavailability of thioctic acid enantiomers. *Eur J Clin Pharmacol* (1996) 50, 513–14.

Alpha-lipoic acid + Herbal medicines

No interactions found.

Alpha-lipoic acid + Valproate

The interaction between alpha-lipoic acid and valproate is based on experimental evidence only.

Clinical evidence

No interactions found.

Experimental evidence

In a small study in 3 *rats,* the AUC of valproate was about 30% higher when valproic acid 50 mg/kg and alpha-lipoic acid 50 mg/kg were infused simultaneously compared with valproic acid given alone.[1] In an *in vitro* study in *rat* liver microsomes, the metabolism of valproate to valproyl-CoA was inhibited by alpha-lipoic acid.[1]

Mechanism

It was suggested that alpha-lipoic acid inhibits the metabolism of valproate via mitochondrial beta-oxidation.

Importance and management

These preliminary data from *animals* suggest that alpha-lipioc acid might slightly increase valproate exposure. However, findings from *animals* cannot be directly extrapolated to humans, and these studies require confirmation in humans. Until further information is available, bear the possibility of an interaction in mind in the event of increased valproate levels in patients also taking alpha-lipoic acid.

1. Phua LC, New LS, Goh CW, Neo AH, Browne ER, Chan EC. Investigation of the drug-drug interaction between alpha-lipoic acid and valproate via mitochondrial beta-oxidation. *Pharm Res* (2008) 25, 2639–49.

Androgaphis

Androgaphis paniculata Nees (Acanthaceae)

Synonym(s) and related species

Bhunimba, Green chiretta, Kalmegh.

Not to be confused with Chirata, page 148 (*Swertia chirayita*), which may be referred to as Chiretta.

Constituents

The whole plant contains **diterpene lactone glycosides**, collectively termed **andrographolides**, which are based on the aglycone andrographolide and its derivatives, such as neo-andrographolide, deoxyandrographolide, andrographiside, andropaniside, and others.

Use and indications

Used in Ayurvedic medicine particularly for jaundice as a general liver and digestive system tonic, and as an immune system stimulant for treatment and prevention of infections. It is also used as an anti-inflammatory and antimalarial, and for cardiovascular disorders and diabetes. When used for the common cold, it is commonly combined with *Eleutherococcus senticosus* (Siberian ginseng), page 251, or echinacea, page 191.

Pharmacokinetics

Evidence from *animal* studies suggests that crude extracts of andrographis might induce the cytochrome P450 isoenzymes CYP1A and CYP2B,[1] and might moderately inhibit P-glycoprotein.[2] A further *in vitro* study found that the effect of andrographis extracts varied, with aqueous extracts having less of an inhibitory effect than alcoholic extracts on CYP2C9, CYP2D6 and CYP3A4. In the same study, the constituent andrographolide was found to have inhibitory effects only on CYP3A4.[3] However, there is no certainty that this evidence can be extrapolated to clinical use, and further study is required to assess its clinical application.

Interactions overview

Andrographis may have antidiabetic and antihypertensive effects, and limited evidence suggests that it may interact with conventional drugs with these properties. Andrographis may also have antiplatelet effects, and so it may interact with conventional antiplatelet drugs and anticoagulants, although evidence is sparse.

Interactions monographs

- Anticoagulants, page 34
- Antidiabetics, page 34
- Antihypertensives, page 34
- Antiplatelet drugs, page 34
- Food, page 35
- Herbal medicines, page 35

1. Jarukamjorn K, Don-in K, Makejaruskul C, Laha T, Daodee S, Pearaksa P, Sri-panidkulchai B. Impact of *Androgaphis paniculata* crude extract on mouse hepatic cytochrome P450 enzymes. *J Ethnopharmacol* (2006) 105, 464–7.
2. Junyaprasert VB, Soonthornchareonnon N, Thongpraditchote S, Murakami T, Takano M. Inhibitory effect of Thai plant extracts on P-glycoprotein mediated efflux. *Phytother Res* (2006) 20, 79–81.
3. Pan Y, Abd-Rashid BA, Ismail Z, Ismail R, Mak JW, Pook PCK, Er HM, Ong CE. In vitro determination of the effect of *Androgaphis paniculata* extracts and andrographolide on hepatic cytochrome P450 activities. *J Nat Med* (2100) 65, 440–447.

Andrographis + Anticoagulants

The interaction between andrographis and warfarin is based on experimental evidence only.

Clinical evidence

No interactions found.

Experimental evidence

Kan Jang, (a standardised fixed combination of extracts from *Andrographis paniculata* and *Eleutherococcus senticosus* (Siberian ginseng, see page 251) caused a modest increase in warfarin exposure, but did not alter the effect of warfarin on prothrombin time, in a study in *rats*. One group of *animals* was given an aqueous solution of Kan Jang orally for 5 days, at a dose of 17 mg/kg daily of the active principle **andrographolide** (a dose about 17-fold higher than that recommended for humans). The control group received a similar volume of water only. Sixty minutes after the final daily dose of Kan Jang or water, an aqueous solution of warfarin was given orally, at a dose of 2 mg/kg. The AUC of warfarin was increased by 67%, and its clearance was decreased by 45%, but other pharmacokinetic parameters were similar.[1]

Mechanism

The available evidence suggests that andrographis might have antiplatelet effects (see Andrographis + Antiplatelet drugs, below), which would be expected to prolong bleeding time. This may increase the risk or severity of bleeding if over-anticoagulation with warfarin occurs. It is not clear why high doses of andrographis increase warfarin exposure.

Importance and management

A very high dose of andrographis does not appear to directly affect prothrombin time, but may modestly increase warfarin exposure. As this study suggested that the pharmacodynamic effects of warfarin were not altered, any pharmacokinetic interaction would not be expected to be clinically relevant. However, if the antiplatelet effects of andrographis are confirmed to be clinically important, then an increased risk of bleeding would be anticipated in patients also taking warfarin, as occurs with low-dose aspirin. Therefore, until more is known, some caution is appropriate if andrographis is given in high doses for a long period of time with any anticoagulant.

1. Hovhannisyan AS, Abrahamyan H, Gabrielyan ES, Panossian AG. The effect of Kan Jang extract on the pharmacokinetics and pharmacodynamics of warfarin in rats. *Phytomedicine* (2006) 13, 318–23.

Andrographis + Antidiabetics

The interaction between andrographis and antidiabetics is based on experimental evidence only.

Clinical evidence

No interactions found.

Experimental evidence

Andrographolide[1] and an andrographis decoction[2] lowered blood-glucose levels in *animal* models of diabetes. In one study, the effect was similar to that of Karela (*Momordica charantia*),[2] which has an established antidiabetic effect.

Mechanism

Potentially additive pharmacological effects.

Importance and management

These experimental studies provide limited evidence of the possible blood-glucose-lowering properties of andrographis, but because of the nature of the evidence, applying these results in a clinical setting is extremely difficult. However, if a patient taking antidiabetic drugs wants to take andrographis it may be prudent to discuss these potential additive effects, and advise an increase in blood-glucose monitoring, should an interaction be suspected.

1. Yu B-C, Hung C-R, Chen W-C, Cheng J-T. Antihyperglycemic effect of andrographolide in streptozotocin-induced diabetic rats. *Planta Med* (2003) 69, 1075–9.
2. Reyes BAS, Bautista ND, Tanquilut NC, Anunciado RV, Leung AB, Sanchez GC, Magtoto RL, Castronuevo P, Tsukamura H, Maeda K-I. Anti-diabetic potentials of *Momordica charantia* and *Andrographis paniculata* and their effects on estrous cyclicity of alloxan-induced diabetic rats. *J Ethnopharmacol* (2006) 105, 196–200.

Andrographis + Antihypertensives

Limited evidence suggests that andrographis may have hypotensive properties that may be additive if given with conventional antihypertensives.

Clinical evidence

Anecdotal evidence suggests that some patients have experienced hypotensive effects while taking andrographis.[1]

Experimental evidence

In vitro and *animal* studies found that extracts of andrographis, and various individual diterpenoid constituents have hypotensive effects.[1,2]

Mechanism

Unknown. Andrographis may have antihypertensive effects, and a slight additive reduction in blood pressure is possible if it is given with conventional antihypertensives.

Importance and management

These experimental studies provide limited evidence of the possible hypotensive properties of andrographis. Because of the nature of the evidence, applying these results to a general clinical setting is difficult, and until more is known, it would be unwise to advise anything other than general caution.

1. Yoopan N, Thisoda P, Rangkadilok N, Sahasitiwat S, Pholphana N, Ruchirawat S, Satayavivad J. Cardiovascular effects of 14-deoxy-11,12-didehydroandrographolide and *Andrographis paniculata* extracts. *Planta Med* (2007) 73, 503–11.
2. Zhang CY, Tan BKH. Mechanisms of cardiovascular activity of *Andrographis paniculata* in the anaesthetized rat. *J Ethnopharmacol* (1997) 56, 97–101.

Andrographis + Antiplatelet drugs

The interaction between andrographis and antiplatelet drugs is based on experimental evidence only.

Clinical evidence

No interactions found.

Experimental evidence

In an *in vitro* study, aqueous extracts of andrographis, and two of three individual diterpenoid constituents (all **andrographolides**), inhibited thrombin-induced platelet aggregation.[1] In another study, a preparation of flavones extracted from the root of andrographis, given intravenously, inhibited platelet aggregation and thrombus formation in an experimental model of thrombus production in *dogs*.[2]

Mechanism

Potentially additive pharmacological effects.

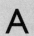

Importance and management

If the antiplatelet effects of andrographis are confirmed to be clinically important, then an increased risk of bleeding would be anticipated in patients taking conventional antiplatelet drugs. Until more is known, this suggests that some caution is appropriate on concurrent use. See also willow, page 485, for more information on herbs that possess antiplatelet properties.

1. Thisoda P, Rangkadilok N, Pholphana N, Worasuttayangkurn L, Ruchirawat S, Satayavivad J. Inhibitory effect of *Andrographis paniculata* extract and its active diterpenoids on platelet aggregation. *Eur J Pharmacol* (2006) 553, 39–45.
2. Zhao H-Y, Fang W-Y. Antithrombotic effects of Andrographis paniculata nees in preventing myocardial infarction. *Chin Med J (Engl)* (1991) 104, 770–775.

Andrographis + Food

No interactions found.

Andrographis + Herbal medicines

No interactions found.

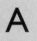

Angel's trumpet

Datura suaveolens Humb. & Bonpl. ex Willd. (Solanaceae)

Synonym(s) and related species

Angel's tears, White angel's trumpet.

Brugmansia suaveolens (Humb. & Bonpl. ex Willd.) Bercht. & C. Presl., *Datura gardneri* Hook.

Not to be confused with Stramonium, which is *Datura stramonium*.

Constituents

The main active constituents of angel's trumpet are the tropane alkaloids **hyoscine** (scopolamine), hyoscyamine and **atropine**. **Flavonoids**, mainly glycosides of kaempferol, and the sterols physalindicanol A and physalindicanol B are also present.

Use and indications

Traditionally, angel's trumpet has been used for the treatment of asthma and for inducing hallucinations in shamanistic rituals. The alkaloid content is very variable and it is known to be toxic (and in some cases fatal) with effects similar to those seen with atropine toxicity.

Pharmacokinetics

No relevant pharmacokinetic data found. For information on the pharmacokinetics of individual flavonoids present in angel's trumpet, see under flavonoids, page 213.

Interactions overview

No interactions with angel's trumpet found. Note that while the alkaloid content may be variable, cases of toxicity have been reported. This suggests that therapeutically equivalent doses of alkaloids may be consumed from herbal preparations containing angel's trumpet and so it might be expected to interact similarly to other antimuscarinics, and in particular, atropine and hyoscine. For information on the interactions of individual flavonoids present in angel's trumpet, see under flavonoids, page 213.

Aniseed

Pimpinella anisum L. (Apiaceae)

Synonym(s) and related species

Anise [Not to be confused with Star anise (*Illicium verum*)], Anisum.

Anisum officinarum Moench., *Anisum vulgare* Gaertn.

Pharmacopoeias

Aniseed (*BP 2012, PhEur 7.5*); Anise Oil (*BP 2012, PhEur 7.5, USP35–NF30 S1*).

Constituents

Aniseed fruit contains 2 to 6% of a volatile oil composed mostly of *trans*-**anethole** (80 to 95%), with smaller amounts of estragole (methyl chavicol), β-caryophyllene and anise ketone (p-methoxyphenylacetone). **Natural coumarins** present include scopoletin, umbelliferone, umbelliprenine and bergapten, and there are numerous **flavonoids** present, including quercetin, apigenin and luteolin.

Use and indications

Aniseed dried fruit, or oil distilled from the fruit, are used mainly for their antispasmodic, carminative and parasiticide effects. Aniseed also is reputed to have mild oestrogenic effects, page 38. In foods, aniseed is used as a spice and flavouring.

Pharmacokinetics

Studies in *rats* suggested that *trans*-anethole did not alter cytochrome P450 activity, but increased UDP-glucuronyltransferase activity (a phase II biotransformation reaction).[1]

In another study in *rats,* aniseed oil enhanced the absorption of glucose from the gut, probably by increasing the activity of the Na+-K+ ATPase and consequently the sodium gradient needed for glucose transport.[2]

For information on the pharmacokinetics of individual flavonoids and natural coumarins present in aniseed, see under flavonoids, page 213 and natural coumarins, page 356, respectively.

Interactions overview

Evidence is very limited. Aniseed appears to have some oestrogenic effects, but the clinical relevance of this is unclear. For information on the interactions of individual flavonoids present in aniseed, see under flavonoids, page 213. Although aniseed contains natural coumarins, the quantity of these constituents is not established, and therefore the propensity of aniseed to interact with other drugs because of their presence is unclear. Consider natural coumarins, page 356, for further discussion of the interactions of natural coumarin-containing herbs.

Interactions monographs

- Food, page 38
- Herbal medicines, page 38
- Oestrogens, page 38

1. Rompelberg CJ, Verhagen H, van Bladeren PJ. Effects of the naturally occurring alkenylbenzenes eugenol and trans-anethole on drug-metabolizing enzymes in the rat liver. *Food Chem Toxicol* (1993) 31, 637–45.
2. Kreydiyyeh SI, Usta J, Knio K, Markossian S, Dagher S. Aniseed oil increases glucose absorption and reduces urine output in the rat. *Life Sci* (2003) 74, 663–73.

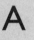

Aniseed + Food

No interactions found.

Aniseed + Herbal medicines

No interactions found.

Aniseed + Oestrogens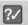

The interaction between aniseed and oestrogens is based on experimental evidence only.

Clinical evidence
No interactions found.

Experimental evidence
In a yeast oestrogen screen assay, the fruit oil from aniseed was oestrogenic.[1] In another study, an aqueous extract from aniseed had selective oestrogen receptor modulator-like properties (i.e. properties like those of drugs such as raloxifene) in various *in vitro* assays (stimulation and differentiation of osteoblasts, antiestrogenic effect on breast cancer cells, and absence of proliferative effects on cervical adenocarcinoma cells).[2]

Mechanism
Active compounds from aniseed appear to have oestrogenic activity and might compete for the same oestrogen receptor as conventional hormonal drugs and treatment.

Importance and management
These experimental studies provide limited evidence of the possible oestrogenic activity of aniseed. Because of the nature of the evidence, applying these results in a clinical setting is extremely difficult, and until more is known, it would be unwise to advise anything other than general caution.

1. Tabanca N, Khan SI, Bedir E, Annavarapu S, Willett K, Khan IA, Kirimer N, Baser KHC. Estrogenic activity of isolated compounds and essential oils of *Pimpinella* species from Turkey, evaluated using a recombinant yeast screen. *Planta Med* (2004) 70, 728–35.
2. Kassi E, Papoutsi Z, Fokialakis N, Messari I, Mitakou S, Moutsatsou P. Greek plant extracts exhibit selective estrogen receptor modulator (SERM)-like properties. *J Agric Food Chem* (2004) 52, 6956–61.

Aristolochia

Aristolochia species (Aristolochiaceae)

Synonym(s) and related species

The nomenclature of these and related plants has given rise to confusion with other, non-toxic plants. This has been exacerbated by the fact that different Chinese names have been used for each species. Great care is needed.

Birthwort has been used as a collective name for the *Aristolochia* species, but it has also been used for one of the species, *Aristolochia clematitis* L. The Chinese name Mu Tong has been used to refer to some of the *Aristolochia* species.

Aristolochia clematitis L. and *Aristolochia fangchi* are the most common species used in herbal medicines, but many others are also used. *Aristolochia fangchi* has been referred to by the Chinese names Fang Chi, Fang Ji, Guang Fang Ji. However, note that *Stephania tetrandra* is also known as Fang Ji.

Aristolochia reticulata NUTT., also known as Serpentary, Snakeroot and Texan snakeroot, has been used as a herbal medicine, although note that the term Snakeroot has also been used to describe other species.

Constituents

All species contain a range of toxic aristolochic acids and aristolactams.

Use and indications

Aristolochic acids and aristolactams are nephrotoxic, carcinogenic and cytotoxic. Numerous deaths have resulted from aristolochic acid nephropathy and associated urothelial cancer, caused by ingestion of aristolochia both medicinally and from contamination of food. All plants of the family Aristolochiaceae are banned in Europe and elsewhere, and should be avoided.

Pharmacokinetics

No relevant pharmacokinetic data found.

Interactions overview

No interactions with aristolochia found.

Arjuna

Terminalia arjuna (Roxb. ex DC.) Wight & Arn. (Combretaceae)

Synonym(s) and related species

Arjun myrobalan.

Terminalia cuneata Roth.

Pharmacopoeias

Terminalia Arjuna Stem Bark (*BP 2012*).

Constituents

The main constituents of the bark are **triterpenoid** saponins including arjunic acid, arjunolic acid, arjungenin and arjunglycosides, and high levels of **flavonoids**, such as arjunone, arjunolone, luteolin, and quercetin. Polyphenols, particularly gallic acid, ellagic acid and oligomeric proanthocyanidins are also present.

Use and indications

Arjuna is widely used in Ayurvedic medicine for the treatment of cardiovascular disorders including coronary artery disease, heart failure, hypertension and hypercholesterolaemia. A number of small clinical studies have supported this use.

Pharmacokinetics

No relevant pharmacokinetic data found. For information on the pharmacokinetics of individual flavonoids present in arjuna, see under flavonoids, page 213.

Interactions overview

Arjuna appears to have some effects on cardiovascular function, which may lead to interactions with conventional drugs used for similar indications. However, if anything, these interactions may be beneficial. Arjuna may also affect thyroid function, which could alter the control of both hyper- and hypothyroidism.

For information on the interactions of individual flavonoids present in arjuna, see under flavonoids, page 213.

Interactions monographs

- Cardiovascular drugs, page 41
- Food, page 41
- Herbal medicines, page 41
- Thyroid and Antithyroid drugs, page 41

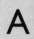

Arjuna + Cardiovascular drugs

Arjuna appears to have some effects on cardiovascular function that may be of benefit when given with conventional cardiovascular drugs.

Clinical evidence

The effect of arjuna on angina pectoris, congestive heart failure, left ventricular mass, and hyperlipidaemia has been investigated in a number of small studies in patients with various cardiovascular disorders (these have been the subject of a review[1]). In some of these studies, patients were also taking conventional drugs. For example, in one double-blind, crossover study in 58 patients with stable angina, the addition of powdered stem bark extract (500 mg every 8 hours) for one week, decreased the number of angina episodes and the need for **nitrate** therapy during episodes of angina (about 5.7 mg/week versus 18.2 mg/week with placebo).[2] In another double-blind crossover study in patients with refractory congestive heart failure, the addition of bark extract 500 mg every 8 hours for 2 weeks to conventional therapy (**digoxin**, maximally tolerated **furosemide** and **spironolactone**, **vasodilators**; **ACE inhibitors**, **nifedipine** or **nitrates**) led to improvements in signs and symptoms of heart failure. This improvement was maintained over long-term evaluation in an open phase, when patients continued the bark extract at the same dosage. The only notable adverse effect was a rise in serum potassium (from about 3.8 to 4.3 mmol/L).[3] Another randomised placebo-controlled study in patients with coronary heart disease found that adding arjuna bark powder 500 mg daily to existing medication decreased lipid peroxide levels (a marker of atherosclerosis) and caused a significant decrease in cholesterol levels.[4]

Experimental evidence

Numerous pharmacological studies in *animals* (which have been the subject of a review[1]) have shown that arjuna has cardiotonic activity, positive or negative inotropic effects (depending on the type of extract), causes bradycardia, has hypotensive effects, antioxidant activity, and lipid-lowering effects.

Mechanism

Unknown. Arjuna is purported to have inotropic and hypotensive effects, as well as lipid-lowering effects. These effects might be additive with those of conventional cardiovascular drugs. See Arjuna + Thyroid and Antithyroid drugs, below, for the possibility that some of the cardiovascular effects of arjuna might occur via an antithyroid action.

Importance and management

Arjuna has been used in small numbers of patients taking a variety of conventional cardiovascular drugs, apparently without particular problems, and with possible additional benefit.

1. Dwivedi S. *Terminalia arjuna* Wight & Arn. – a useful drug for cardiovascular disorders. *J Ethnopharmacol* (2007) 114, 114–29.
2. Bharani A, Ganguli A, Mathur LK, Jamra Y, Raman PG. Efficacy of *Terminalia arjuna* in chronic stable angina: a double-blind, placebo-controlled, crossover study comparing *Terminalia arjuna* with isosorbide mononitrate. *Indian Heart J* (2002) 54, 170–175.
3. Bharani A, Ganguly A, Bhargava KD. Salutary effect of *Terminalia Arjuna* in patients with severe refractory heart failure. *Int J Cardiol* (1995) 49, 191–9.
4. Gupta R, Singhal S, Goyle A, Sharma VN. Antioxidant and hypocholesterolaemic effects of *Terminalia arjuna* tree-bark powder: a randomised placebo-controlled trial. *J Assoc Physicians India* (2001) 49, 231–5.

Arjuna + Food

No interactions found.

Arjuna + Herbal medicines

No interactions found.

Arjuna + Thyroid and Antithyroid drugs

The interaction between arjuna and thyroid or antithyroid drugs is based on experimental evidence only.

Clinical evidence

No interactions found.

Experimental evidence

In a study in *animals,* arjuna bark extract appeared to inhibit thyroid function. Giving **levothyroxine** increased the level of thyroid hormones, increased the heart to body-weight ratio, as well as increasing cardiac and hepatic lipid peroxidation. When the plant extract was given simultaneously, the level of thyroid hormones, and also the cardiac lipid peroxidation, were decreased. These effects were comparable to those of a standard antithyroid drug, **propylthiouracil**. When arjuna bark extract was given to euthyroid *animals,* thyroid hormone levels were decreased, whereas the hepatic lipid peroxidation increased, indicating drug-induced liver toxicity.[1]

Mechanism

Arjuna may deplete thyroid hormones.

Importance and management

Although the evidence is experimental, until more is known, it might be prudent to avoid the use of arjuna in patients requiring levothyroxine (or any thyroid hormone), because of the possibility of reduced efficacy. If patients want to try arjuna, their thyroid function should be monitored more frequently. An additive effect with antithyroid drugs such as propylthiouracil might also occur, and therefore similar caution would seem advisable.

Since in euthyroid *animals,* thyroid hormones were decreased and hepatic lipid peroxidation was increased, the authors suggest that high amounts of this plant extract should not be consumed, as hepatotoxicity as well as hypothyroidism may occur.[1]

1. Parmar HS, Panda S, Jatwa R, Kar A. Cardio-protective role of Terminalia arjuna bark extract is possibly mediated through alterations in thyroid hormones. *Pharmazie* (2006) 61, 793–5.

A

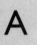

Artichoke

Cynara scolymus L. (Asteraceae)

Synonym(s) and related species

Alcachofa, Bur artichoke, Cynara, Globe artichoke.
Cynara cardunculus Moris.
Not to be confused with Jerusalem artichoke.

Pharmacopoeias

Artichoke Leaf (*BP 2012, PhEur 7.5*); Artichoke Leaf Dry Extract (*BP 2012, PhEur 7.5*).

Constituents

Artichoke leaf is usually standardised to the caffeoylquinic acid derivative, **chlorogenic acid**. Other major constituents are **flavonoid glycosides** based on luteolin, including cynaroside and scolymoside, and sesquiterpene lactones including cynaropicrin.

Use and indications

The leaf extract has been traditionally used for liver and digestive disorders, especially dyspepsia and nausea, and to promote bile secretion. Its use now focuses more on hypercholesterolaemia, hyperlipidaemia and irritable bowel syndrome, and some cardiovascular disorders such as atherosclerosis. Artichoke flowers are also used as food and artichoke extracts are used as flavouring agents.

Pharmacokinetics

No relevant pharmacokinetic data found. For information on the pharmacokinetics of individual flavonoids present in artichoke, see under flavonoids, page 213.

Interactions overview

No interactions with artichoke found. For information on the interactions of individual flavonoids present in artichoke, see under flavonoids, page 213.

Asafoetida

Ferula asafoetida H.Karst. (Apiaceae)

Synonym(s) and related species

Asafetida, Asant, Devil's dung, Gum asafetida.

Asafoetida is obtained from various *Ferula* species, the main sources being *Ferula asafoetida* L. or *Ferula foetida* (Bunge) Regel.

Note that Giant fennel (*Ferula communis* L.), although a species of *Ferula,* contains certain constituents that are distinct from asafoetida and will not be dealt with in this monograph.

Constituents

The gum resin contains ferulic acid esters and free ferulic acid, asaresinotannols, farnesiferols A, B and C, **natural coumarin** derivatives including saradaferin, gummosin, asacoumarins and assafoetidnols, and an essential oil composed of disulfides, polysulfanes, monoterpenes and phenylpropanoids. The sesquiterpene dienones, fetidones A and B, samarcandin and galbanic acid are also present. *Ferula foetida* also contains foetisulfides and foetithiophenes.

Use and indications

Asafoetida is used for its carminative, antispasmodic and expectorant properties in chronic bronchitis, pertussis, and specifically for intestinal flatulent colic.

Pharmacokinetics

Little information is available. Studies in *rats* fed with asafoetida suggest that, it did not stimulate levels of cytochrome P450, and glucuronyl transferase activity remained unaffected.[1]

Interactions overview

In theory the use of asafoetida with conventional antihypertensives may be expected to produce additive hypotensive effects. Although it has been suggested that asafoetida may interact with anticoagulants, the available data does not appear to support this prediction.

Interactions monographs

- Antihypertensives, page 44
- Food, page 44
- Herbal medicines, page 44
- Warfarin and related drugs, page 44

1. Sambaiah K, Srinivasan K. Influence of spices and spice principles on hepatic mixed function oxygenase system in rats. *Indian J Biochem Biophys* (1989) 26, 254–8.

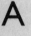

Asafoetida + Antihypertensives

The interaction between asafoetida and antihypertensives is based on experimental evidence only.

Clinical evidence

No interactions found.

Experimental evidence

In a study in *rats,* asafoetida gum extract significantly reduced mean arterial blood pressure.[1]

Mechanism

In theory the use of asafoetida with conventional antihypertensives may be expected to produce additive hypotensive effects.

Importance and management

Because of the nature of the evidence, applying these results in a clinical setting is extremely difficult, and until more is known, it would be unwise to advise anything other than general caution.

1. Fatehi M, Farifteh F, Fatehi-Hassanabad Z. Antispasmodic and hypotensive effects of *Ferula asafoetida* gum extract. *J Ethnopharmacol* (2004) 91, 321–4.

Asafoetida + Food

No interactions found.

Asafoetida + Herbal medicines

No interactions found.

Asafoetida + Warfarin and related drugs

The interaction between asafoetida and warfarin and related drugs is a prediction only.

Clinical evidence

No interactions found.

Experimental evidence

Some reviews[1] and monographs list asafoetida as having the potential to increase the risk of bleeding or potentiate the effects of **warfarin**.

Mechanism

This appears to be based on the fact that asafoetida contains natural coumarins, but these are not thought to have the structural requirements for anticoagulant activity. For more information, see Natural coumarins + Warfarin and related drugs, page 360.

Importance and management

There appears to be no evidence to support the prediction of an interaction between warfarin and asafoetida, and some data to suggest that an interaction is unlikely to occur. No special precautions therefore appear to be needed if patients taking warfarin or related anticoagulants also wish to take asafoetida.

1. Heck AM, DeWitt BA, Lukes AL. Potential interactions between alternative therapies and warfarin. *Am J Health-Syst Pharm* (2000) 57, 1221–7.

Ashwagandha

Withania somnifera (L.) Dunal (Solanaceae)

Synonym(s) and related species

Winter cherry.

Physalis somnifera L.

Note that ashwagandha has also been known as Indian ginseng, which should not be confused with the common ginsengs, page 251.

Pharmacopoeias

Ashwagandha Root (*USP35–NF30 S1*); Powdered Ashwagandha Root (*USP35–NF30 S1*); Powdered Ashwagandha Root Extract (*USP35–NF30 S1*).

Constituents

The major constituents of the root are steroidal lactones, with several series known as the withanolides (designated A-Y to date), glycowithanolides (sitoindosides), the withasomniferols (A-C), withastramonolide and withaferin A. The extract also contains phytosterols and alkaloids such as ashwagandhine, ashwagandhinine, anahygrine, withasomnine, withaninine and others.

Use and indications

Use of ashwagandha root originates in Ayurvedic medicine, and it is used as a tonic for debility and as an adaptogen and immune modulator. It has sedative and anti-inflammatory effects and is used for a wide range of conditions including hypercholesterolaemia.

Pharmacokinetics

No relevant pharmacokinetic data found.

Interactions overview

Although ashwagandha may have blood-glucose-lowering effects, these seem to be mild, and would not generally be expected to affect the control of diabetes with conventional medicines. Ashwagandha may affect the reliability of digoxin assays, and interfere with the control of hypo- and hyperthyroidism.

Interactions monographs

- Antidiabetics, page 46
- Digoxin, page 46
- Food, page 46
- Herbal medicines, page 46
- Laboratory tests, page 46
- Thyroid and Antithyroid drugs, page 46

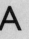

Ashwagandha + Antidiabetics

Limited evidence suggests that ashwagandha has blood-glucose-lowering effects, which may be additive with conventional antidiabetics.

Clinical evidence

In 6 subjects with mild type 2 diabetes, giving powdered root of ashwagandha 1 g three times daily after meals for 30 days reduced blood-glucose levels by 12% (from 11.5 to 10.1 mmol/L – timing of sample in relation to meals not stated).[1] These subjects discontinued any blood-glucose-lowering drugs before the study, and 6 control subjects continued treatment with **glibenclamide**. These control subjects also had a reduction in blood-glucose of 12%. This study is difficult to interpret, because there was no placebo group.

Experimental evidence

No interactions found.

Mechanism

Unknown. Additive blood-glucose-lowering effects might be anticipated with antidiabetics.

Importance and management

The limited evidence suggests that ashwagandha might have blood-glucose-lowering effects. Until further information is available, if a patient taking antidiabetic drugs wants to take ashwagandha it may be prudent to discuss these potential additive effects, and advise an increase in blood-glucose monitoring, should an interaction be suspected. However, bear in mind that, although ashwagandha has been used for a wide number of complaints, it does not appear to be used for diabetes, suggesting that any effects are mild, and probably not clinically relevant.

1. Andallu B, Radhika B. Hypoglycemic, diuretic and hypocholesterolemic effect of winter cherry (*Withania somnifera*, Dunal) root. *Indian J Exp Biol* (2000) 38, 607–9.

Ashwagandha + Digoxin

Ashwagandha has been shown to interfere with some methods of measuring serum digoxin levels, see Ashwagandha + Laboratory tests, below.

Ashwagandha + Food

No interactions found.

Ashwagandha + Herbal medicines

No interactions found.

Ashwagandha + Laboratory tests

Digoxin levels might be spuriously elevated when assayed using a fluorescence polarization immunoassay in patients taking ashwagandha. Ashwagandha does not interfere with *in vitro* assays for carbamazepine, gentamicin, paracetamol, phenytoin, phenobarbital, procainamide, salicylate, theophylline, tobramycin or valproic acid.

Clinical evidence

No interactions found.

Experimental evidence

(a) Digoxin

In a study, *mice* fed two ashwagandha extracts (in quantities that equated to human doses) developed apparent serum digoxin levels of 0.46 nanograms/mL and 0.57 nanograms/mL one hour after feeding, as assessed by a fluorescence polarisation immunoassay (FPIA) of digoxin (Abbott Laboratories). A further ashwagandha extract did not produce detectable digoxin levels by FPIA. No digoxin was detected for any of the three extracts using a monoclonal antibody-based digoxin assay (Beckman) or a microparticle enzyme immunoassay (MEIA, Abbott Laboratories).[1] Similar findings were seen *in vitro*, with interference seen at lower concentrations of ashwagandha extracts with the FPIA assay, than with the MEIA and Beckman assays.[1] In other similar studies by the same research group, an enzyme-linked chemiluminescent immunosorbent assay (ECLIA) for digoxin (Bayer),[2] and the Tina-quant assay (Roche),[3] were not affected by ashwagandha.

(b) Other drugs

In *in vitro* tests, ashwagandha extract had no effect on immunoassays (Roche) for carbamazepine, gentamicin, paracetamol, phenytoin, phenobarbital, procainamide, salicylate, theophylline, tobramycin or valproic acid.[1]

Mechanism

Some withanolides (major constituents of ashwagandha) are structurally similar to digoxin, and might therefore interfere with the digoxin immunoassay.[1]

Importance and management

The *animal* data available suggest that in patients taking digoxin and ashwagandha, digoxin levels might be spuriously elevated when assayed using a fluorescence polarization immunoassay. Further clinical study is needed.

1. Dasgupta A, Peterson A, Wells A, Actor JK. Effect of Indian Ayurvedic medicine ashwagandha on measurement of serum digoxin and 11 commonly monitored drugs using immunoassays: study of protein binding and interaction with Digibind. *Arch Pathol Lab Med* (2007) 131, 1298–1303.
2. Dasgupta A, Kang E, Olsen M, Actor JK, Datta P. Interference of Asian, American, and Indian (Ashwagandha) ginsengs in serum digoxin measurements by a fluorescence polarization immunoassay can be minimized by using a new enzyme-linked chemiluminescent immunosorbent or turbidimetric assay. *Arch Pathol Lab Med* (2007) 131, 619–21.
3. Dasgupta A, Reyes MA. Effect of Brazilian, Indian, Siberian, Asian, and North American ginseng on serum digoxin measurement by immunoassays and binding of digoxin-like immunoreactive components of ginseng with Fab fragment of antidigoxin antibody (Digibind). *Am J Clin Pathol* (2005) 124, 229–36.

Ashwagandha + Thyroid and Antithyroid drugs

Limited evidence suggests that ashwagandha increases thyroid hormone levels and therefore interfere with the control of hypo- and hyperthyroidism.

Clinical evidence

A 32-year-old healthy woman developed clinical symptoms of thyrotoxicosis, and was found to have elevated levels of thyroid hormones when she increased the dose of capsules containing ashwagandha herbal extract she had been taking for chronic fatigue. The symptoms and raised thyroid hormone levels resolved on stopping the product.[1]

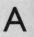

Experimental evidence

In a study in *mice,* ashwagandha root extract 1.4 g/kg given daily for 20 days by gastric intubation increased serum levels of thyroid hormones, triiodothyronine and thyroxine, by 18% and 111%, respectively.[2]

Mechanism

Unknown. Additive effects with thyroid hormones might be anticipated.

Importance and management

Although the evidence is limited, until more is known, it might be prudent to advise caution if patients taking **levothyroxine** (or other thyroid hormones) want to take ashwagandha because of the possibility of an increase in effects. Furthermore, on the basis of this evidence, ashwagandha may be expected to antagonise the effects of antithyroid drugs, such as **propylthiouracil**. In both cases it may be prudent to consider monitoring thyroid function tests if symptoms of hypo- or hyperthyroidism begin to emerge.

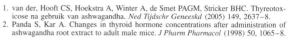

1. van der, Hooft CS, Hoekstra A, Winter A, de Smet PAGM, Stricker BHC. Thyreotoxicose na gebruik van ashwagandha. *Ned Tijdschr Geneeskd* (2005) 149, 2637–8.
2. Panda S, Kar A. Changes in thyroid hormone concentrations after administration of ashwagandha root extract to adult male mice. *J Pharm Pharmacol* (1998) 50, 1065–8.

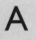

Asparagus

Asparagus officinalis L. (Asparagaceae)

Synonym(s) and related species

Sparrowgrass.

Not to be confused with Shatavari, page 427, which is *Asparagus racemosus*.

Constituents

Asparagus contains **saponins** called asparagosides, steroidal glycosides, asparagusic acid and its derivatives, **flavonoids** (including rutin, kaempferol and quercetin) and various amino acids and polysaccharides. Asparagus is also a source of folic acid, vitamin K_1 and other vitamins.

Use and indications

The root and green parts of asparagus have been used as a diuretic, laxative, cardiac tonic and sedative. The young shoots are eaten as a foodstuff. Asparagusic acid may be nematocidal.

Pharmacokinetics

No relevant pharmacokinetic data for asparagus found. For information on the pharmacokinetics of individual flavonoids present in asparagus, see flavonoids, page 213.

Interactions overview

No interactions with asparagus found; however, note that asparagus contains a moderate amount of vitamin K and may therefore reduce the effectiveness of warfarin and other similar anticoagulants if eaten in large quantities. For information on the interactions of individual flavonoids present in asparagus, see under flavonoids, page 213.

Interactions monographs

- Food, page 49
- Herbal medicines, page 49
- Warfarin and related drugs, page 49

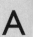

Asparagus + Food

No interactions found, but note that asparagus is extensively used as a foodstuff.

Asparagus + Herbal medicines

No interactions found.

Asparagus + Warfarin and related drugs

Patients taking coumarins and indanediones should avoid taking excessive amounts of asparagus because of its vitamin K_1 content.

Evidence, mechanism, importance and management

Asparagus[1] contains a moderate amount of vitamin K_1, which reduces the effect of coumarin and indanedione anticoagulants, which are vitamin K antagonists. Patients taking these anticoagulants are advised to maintain a regular amount of vitamin K from the diet. They should therefore avoid taking excessive amounts of asparagus.

1. USDA National Nutrient Database for Standard Reference, Release 17. Vitamin K (phylloquinone) (μg) Content of selected foods per common measure. http://www.nal.usda.gov/fnic/foodcomp/Data/SR17/wtrank/sr17a430.pdf (accessed 11/04/2008).

Astragalus

Astragalus membranaceus Bunge (Fabaceae)

Synonym(s) and related species

Huang qi.

Astragalus membranaceus (Fisch.) Bunge var *mongholicus* (Bunge.) P.K.Hsaio.

Not to be confused with the pharmaceutical excipient, tragacanth (*Astragalus gummifer*).

Pharmacopoeias

Astragalus Root (*BP 2009*); Processed Astragalus Root (*BP 2009*).

Constituents

The key constituents are **triterpene saponins**, which include the astragalosides I-VIII and their acetyl derivatives, the agroastragalosides I-IV, the astramembranins I and II and others. **Isoflavones** are also present, mainly glycosides of calycosin and formononetin, with astrapterocarpan, kumatakenin and numerous hydroxyl and methoxyl derivatives of pterocarpan and isoflavan; and a series of polysaccharides known as astragaloglucans.

Use and indications

Astragalus is traditionally used in Chinese medicine as a tonic to strengthen the immune system, for viral infections, fatigue and loss of blood. It is now used as a liver protectant, an adjunct in chemotherapy and impaired immunity, and for a variety of other conditions such as cardiovascular disease and diabetic complications. Some indications are supported by pharmacological and clinical studies.

Pharmacokinetics

Little data is available, but in a study in one healthy subject, who was given astragalus root decoction orally twice daily before meals of bread and honey for 5 days, urine samples were found to contain calycosin and formononetin and various isoflavonoid glucuronide metabolites. These data, and data from *in vitro* studies, demonstrate that the isoflavones in astragalus could be absorbed and metabolised by the intestine.[1] For more information about the pharmacokinetics of isoflavones, see under isoflavones, page 300.

Interactions overview

Astragalus appears to alter the immune response, but the effect this has on treatment with interleukins, interferons, antiretrovirals, and antineoplastics does not appear to be established. For information about the interactions of individual isoflavones present in astragalus, see under isoflavones, page 300.

Interactions monographs

- Antineoplastics, page 51
- Antiretrovirals, page 51
- Cytokines, page 51
- Food, page 52
- Herbal medicines, page 52

1. Xu F, Zhang Y, Xiao S, Lu X, Yang D, Yang X, Li C, Shang M, Tu P, Cai S. Absorption and metabolism of Astragali radix decoction: in silico, in vitro, and a case study in vivo. *Drug Metab Dispos* (2006) 34, 913–24.

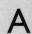

Astragalus + Antineoplastics

Astragalus improved the response to chemotherapy with mitomycin, a vinca alkaloid and cisplatin in one study. Limited experimental data suggests that astragalus may diminish the immunosuppressant effects of cyclophosphamide.

Clinical evidence

In one small randomised clinical study in Chinese patients with non-small cell lung cancer, the addition of an infusion of astragalus to a chemotherapy regimen of **mitomycin**, **vinca alkaloid** and **cisplatin** (MVP) improved response rate (40% versus 36.7%) and median survival (11 months versus 7 months), when compared with a control group receiving MVP alone.[1]

Experimental evidence

In a study in **cyclophosphamide**-primed *rats,* giving a partially purified fraction of astragalus before mononuclear cell grafting markedly enhanced the ability of the *rats* to reject the graft. This suggests that astragalus reversed the immunosuppressant effect of **cyclophosphamide**.[2] Conversely, in a similar study, astragalus appeared to prolong the life of bone marrow cells transplanted into *mice* pretreated with **cyclophosphamide**, as well as promoting blood cell production.[3] Furthermore, in another study in *rats,* pretreatment with astragalus and *Ligustrum lucidium* (glossy privet) for 12 days had no effect on the degree or duration of myelosuppression (neutrophil and platelet counts) seen after a single dose of **cyclophosphamide**.[4]

Mechanism

Unknown, although many *in vitro* studies have shown that astragalus has immunostimulating effects.

Importance and management

The preclinical and preliminary clinical evidence suggests that astragalus might have immunomodulating activity and effects on blood cell production, and might therefore have beneficial effects if it is given with antineoplastics. Some have interpreted the preclinical data showing increased rejection of a xenograft[2] as suggesting that astragalus might decrease the effects of immunosuppressive therapy, and recommend caution with the combination. The evidence is extremely limited, and apparently conflicting, nevertheless it may be prudent to consider the risk-benefit ratio of using the herb, especially in those given immunosuppressant treatment for life-threatening conditions.

1. Zou YH, Liu XM. [Effect of astragalus injection combined with chemotherapy on quality of life in patients with advanced non-small cell lung cancer]. *Zhongguo Zhong Xi Yi Jie He Za Zhi* (2003) 23, 733–5.
2. Chu DT, Wong WL, Mavligit GM. Immunotherapy with Chinese medicinal herbs. II. Reversal of cyclophosphamide-induced immune suppression by administration of fractionated *Astragalus membranaceus in vivo. J Clin Lab Immunol* (1988) 25, 125–9.
3. Zhu X-L, Zhu B-D. Mechanisms by which *Astragalus membranaceus* injection regulates hematopoiesis in myelosuppressed mice. *Phytother Res* (2007) 21, 663–7.
4. Khoo KS, Ang PT. Extract of astragalus membranaceus and ligustrum lucidum does not prevent cyclophosphamide-induced myelosuppression. *Singapore Med J* (1995) 36, 387–90.

Astragalus + Antiretrovirals

Long-term astragalus use does not appear to reduce the efficacy of zidovudine or zalcitabine.

Clinical evidence

A randomised, placebo-controlled study, found that a combination of five herbs containing astragalus, *Glycyrrhiza glaba* L. (Liquorice), *Artemisia capillaris* Thunb., *Morus alba* L. (Mulberry), and *Carthamus tinctorius* L. (Safflower) may enhance the activity of antiretrovirals in patients with HIV. Over a period of 24 weeks antiretroviral-naive subjects received a combination of **zidovudine** 200 mg three times daily and **zalcitabine** 750 micrograms three times daily plus either the combined herbs 2.5 g three times daily or placebo. Forty patients receiving the herbs had a significantly greater decline in viral load than 20 patients receiving placebo. In addition, the CD4 cell count in the herbal group was significantly increased from the baseline value from week 12 onwards. No serious adverse events were reported in either of the two groups.[1]

Experimental evidence

No relevant data found.

Mechanism

Unknown, although many *in vitro* studies have shown that astragalus has immunostimulating effects.

Importance and management

Although not an interactions study, the findings provide some evidence that if patients take astragalus concurrently with the NRTIs zidovudine or zalcitabine no major adverse interaction would be expected, and efficacy should not be compromised. Because the herbal product used contained three different herbs, a beneficial effect for a combination of astragalus and antiretroviral drugs is still far from proven.

1. Sangkitporn S, Shide L, Klinbuayaem V, Leenasirimakul P, Wirayutwatthana NA, Leechanachai P, Dettrairat S, Kunachiwa W, Thamlikitkul V. Efficacy and safety of zidovudine and zalcitabine combined with a combination of herbs in the treatment of HIV-infected Thai patients. *Southeast Asian J Trop Med Public Health* (2005) 36, 704–8.

Astragalus + Cytokines

Preliminary evidence suggests that astragalus may be beneficial when given with interferon alfa or interleukin-2.

Clinical evidence

In a controlled study in 235 patients, astragalus appeared to act synergistically with **interferon alfa** for the topical treatment of chronic cervicitis associated with viral infection. Local application of astragalus extract plus **interferon** was similar in efficacy to twice the dose of **interferon** alone, and more effective than astragalus alone.[1]

Experimental evidence

Various *in vitro* studies have found that astragalus extract potentiates the cytotoxic effect of **interleukin-2** against renal cell carcinoma by about tenfold.[2,3]

Mechanism

Unknown, although many *in vitro* studies have found that astragalus has immunostimulating effects.

A

Importance and management

The above preliminary evidence suggests that astragalus might have immunomodulating activity and might therefore be beneficial when given with interferons or interleukin-2.

1. Qian Z-W, Mao S-J, Cai X-C, Zhang X-L, Gao F-X, Lu M-F, Shao X-S, Li Y-Y, Yang X-K, Zhuo Y, Shi L-Y, Duan S-M, Hou Y-D. Viral etiology of chronic cervicitis and its therapeutic response to a recombinant interferon. *Chin Med J (Engl)* (1990) 103, 647–51.
2. Wang Y, Qian X-J, Hadley HR, Lau BHS. Phytochemicals potentiate interleukin-2 generated lymphokine-activated killer cell cytotoxicity against murine renal cell carcinoma. *Mol Biother* (1992) 4, 143–6.
3. Chu D-T, Lepe-Zuniga J, Wong WL, LaPushin R, Mavligit GM. Fractionated extract of Astragalus membranaceus, a Chinese medicinal herb, potentiates LAK cell cytotoxicity generated by a low dose of recombinant interleukin-2. *J Clin Lab Immunol* (1988) 26, 183–7.

Astragalus + Food

No interactions found.

Astragalus + Herbal medicines

No interactions found.

Avens

Geum urbanum L. (Rosaceae)

Synonym(s) and related species

Benedict's herb, Colewort, Geum, Herb bennet, Wood avens.

Constituents

The main actives found in the whole plant are the tannins, gallotannins and ellagitannins, including sanguiin H6, casuarictin, pedunculagin, potentillin and tellimagrandin. Other polyphenols include gallic, caffeic and chlorogenic acids, gein (a phenolic glycoside of eugenol), **flavonoids** and volatile oil containing eugenol.

Use and indications

Avens has been used as an astringent in diarrhoea, a haemostatic, and an anti-inflammatory.

Pharmacokinetics

No relevant pharmacokinetic data found.

Interactions overview

No interactions with avens found.

Bacopa

Bacopa monnieri (L.) Wettst. (Scrophulariaceae)

Synonym(s) and related species

Brahmi, Thyme leaved gratiola.

Gratiola monnieria L., *Herpestis monniera* Kunth., *Lysimachia monnieri* L., *Moniera cuneifolia* Michx.

Pharmacopoeias

Bacopa (*USP35–NF30 S1*); Bacopa Monnieri (*BP2012*); Powdered Bacopa (*USP35–NF30 S1*); Powdered Bacopa Extract (*USP35–NF30 S1*).

Constituents

Bacopa contains a wide range of triterpene glycosides, including the bacopa saponins, known as bacosides and bacopasaponins. Cucurbitacins, known as bacobitacins and cucurbitacin E, the alkaloids brahmine and herpestine, phenylethanoid glycosides (including the monnierasides and plantioside B), and the **flavonoids** apigenin and luteolin have also been isolated.

Use and indications

Bacopa is an important herb in Ayurvedic medicine, which is increasingly being used in the West. The bacosides have been found, in a number of studies, to enhance the memory and cognitive processes. Bacopa has also been used as an anti-inflammatory, analgesic, antipyretic, sedative, and for the treatment of asthma and bronchitis. Recent toxicological studies suggest that the herb is relatively safe in normal use.

Pharmacokinetics

No relevant pharmacokinetic data found. For information on the pharmacokinetics of individual flavonoids present in bacopa, see under flavonoids, page 213.

Interactions overview

No interactions with bacopa found. For information on the interactions of individual flavonoids present in bacopa, see under flavonoids, page 213.

Baical skullcap

Scutellaria baicalensis Georgi (Lamiaceae)

Synonym(s) and related species

Huang qin.

Scutellaria lanceolaria Miq., *Scutellaria macrantha* Fisch.

Pharmacopoeias

Baical Skullcap Root (*PhEur 7.5*); Scutellariae Baicalensis Root (*BP2012*).

Constituents

The major active components of the root are the **flavonoids** baicalein, baicalin (the glucuronide of baicalein), chrysin, oroxylin A, tenaxin I, skullcapflavones I and II, wogonin, wogonoside, and many other hydroxylated methoxyflavones.

Use and indications

Baical skullcap root has been used traditionally, especially in Chinese medicine, as a remedy for inflammation, infections, dermatitis, allergic diseases, hyperlipidaemia, atherosclerosis and stress-related disorders.

Pharmacokinetics

No relevant pharmacokinetic data found specifically for baical skullcap, but see flavonoids, page 213, for information on individual flavonoids present in baical skullcap.

Interactions overview

Baical skullcap is the constituent of a number of Chinese medicines, such as sho-saiko-to, saiko-ka-ryukotsu-borei-to and sairei-to; these interactions are covered under bupleurum, page 98. For information on the interactions of individual flavonoids present in the herb, see under flavonoids, page 213, particularly the monograph Flavonoids + Ciclosporin, page 217, where baical skullcap was given as a source of flavonoids.

Interactions monographs

- Food, page 56
- Herbal medicines, page 56

B

Baical skullcap + Caffeine

For mention that sho-saiko-to (of which baical skullcap is one of 7 constituents) slightly reduces the metabolism of caffeine, see Bupleurum + Caffeine, page 99.

Baical skullcap + Carbamazepine

For mention that saiko-ka-ryukotsu-borei-to and sho-saiko-to (of which baical skullcap is one of a number of constituents) do not affect the pharmacokinetics of carbamazepine in *animal* studies, see Bupleurum + Carbamazepine, page 99.

Baical skullcap + Ciclosporin

For mention that baical skullcap, given as a specific source of flavonoids, may affect the pharmacokinetics of ciclosporin, see Flavonoids + Ciclosporin, page 217.

Baical skullcap + Food

No interactions found.

Baical skullcap + Herbal medicines

No interactions found.

Baical skullcap + Ofloxacin

For mention that sairei-to and sho-saiko-to (of which baical skullcap is one of a number of constituents) do not affect the pharmacokinetics of ofloxacin, see Bupleurum + Ofloxacin, page 99.

Baical skullcap + Tolbutamide

For conflicting evidence from *animal* studies that sho-saiko-to (of which baical skullcap is one of 7 constituents) might increase or decrease the rate of absorption of tolbutamide, see Bupleurum + Tolbutamide, page 99.

Balm of Gilead

Populus × *gileadensis* Rouleau and other *Populus* species (Salicaceae)

Synonym(s) and related species

Balsam Poplar, Gileadensis, Poplar buds

Populus candicans Ait., *Populus tacamahacca* Mill., *Populus balsamifera* L., *Populus nigra* L., and others.

Note that Canada Balsam from the fir tree *Abies balsamea* (L.) Mill. is sometimes known as Balm of Gilead. Mecca balsam, a resin from *Commiphora opobalsamum* Engl. (Burseraceae) has also been used as a synonym for Balm of Gilead.

Not to be confused with Poplar bark, which is also from *Populus* species.

Constituents

The leaf buds, collected before they open, contain phenolic glycosides including **salicin** (a **salicylate**) , and populin, and a volatile oil consisting of α-caryophyllene as the major component with cineole, bisabolene, farnesene and actophenone. **Flavonoids** present include apigenin, chrysin and others, and some *Populus* species may have constituents which differ slightly.

Use and indications

Balm of Gilead has expectorant, stimulant, antipyretic and analgesic activity, and is used mainly in cough mixtures.

Pharmacokinetics

No relevant pharmacokinetic data found for Balm of Gilead, but note that salicin, a constituent of Balm of Gilead, is metabolised to salicylic acid in the body. For more information, see willow, page 485. See also flavonoids, page 213 for information on the flavonoid components of Balm of Gilead.

Interactions overview

No specific interactions found. Balm of Gilead contains salicin, a precursor of salicylic acid, and clinically relevant levels of this have been achieved by taking some herbs, although this does not necessarily equate to the antiplatelet effect of the herb. For a discussion about the use of herbs with antiplatelet effects in conjunction with antiplatelet drugs and anticoagulants, see willow, page 485.

See also flavonoids, page 213 for information on the interactions of individual flavonoid components of Balm of Gilead.

Bayberry

Myrica cerifera L. (Myricaceae)

Synonym(s) and related species

Candleberry, Myrica, Southern bayberry, Southern wax myrtle, Waxberry, Wax myrtle.

Constituents

The root bark, which is used therapeutically, contains **triterpenes** including myriceric acid A, myrica acid, myricadiol, myriceron caffeoyl ester, taraxerol and taraxerone, and the **flavonoid**, myricitrin.

Use and indications

Bayberry bark is used for coughs and colds, and for diarrhoea and other gastrointestinal disorders. It is also used topically for wounds and as a douche for vaginal discharge.

Pharmacokinetics

No relevant pharmacokinetic data found.

Interactions overview

No interactions with bayberry found.

Bearberry

Arctostaphylos uva-ursi (L.) Spreng (Ericaceae)

Synonym(s) and related species

Uva-ursi.

Pharmacopoeias

Bearberry Leaf (*BP 2012, Ph Eur 7.5*).

Constituents

The major active constituent is **arbutin (hydroquinone beta-glucoside)**, with methylarbutin, 4-hydroxyacetophenone glucoside and galloyl arbutin. Whole or cut dried bearberry leaves may contain not less than 7% anhydrous **arbutin** (*BP 2009, Ph Eur 6.4*). Iridoids (such as monotropein), **flavonoids** (such as myricetin and quercetin), and tannins (including corilagin) are also present.

Use and indications

Bearberry leaves and preparations are traditionally used for urinary tract infections. The use of arbutin and hydroquinone as skin-whitening agents has been investigated.

Pharmacokinetics

After oral ingestion, arbutin is hydrolysed in the urine to hydroquinone,[1–3] which has antiseptic properties, but in large doses is irritant and cytotoxic. However, it is rapidly conjugated in the urine, mainly as hydroquinone glucuronide and hydroquinone sulfate.[2] The presence of *Escherichia coli* in an infected urinary tract may enhance hydroquinone levels, by reversing the conjugation process and metabolising them back into free, active hydroquinone.[3] Alkalinisation of the urine seems to be unnecessary for improving the antiseptic properties of hydroquinone or arbutin.[3]

In vitro studies[4,5] suggest that aqueous and ethanol extracts of commercially available bearberry leaf products, markedly inhibit CYP3A4 and CYP2C19, whereas methanol extracts appear to have low to moderate activity against these isoenzymes. However, the effect on CYP3A4 varied greatly between products.[4] Bearberry alcoholic extracts were also found to inhibit CYP3A4, and interfere with the activity of P-glycoprotein *in vitro,* causing inhibition after 1 hour of exposure, and induction after 18 hours.[4] The clinical significance of these effects is unknown.

Interactions overview

An isolated case of lithium toxicity has been reported in a patient who took a herbal diuretic containing bearberry among other ingredients, see under Parsley + Lithium, page 364. For information on the interactions of individual flavonoid constituents of bearberry, see under flavonoids, page 213.

Interactions monographs

- Food, page 60
- Herbal medicines, page 60
- Lithium, page 60

1. Schindler G, Patzak U, Brinkhaus B, von Niecieck A, Wittig J, Krähmer N, Glöckl I, Veit M. Urinary excretion and metabolism of arbutin after oral administration of *Arctostaphylos uvae ursi* extract as film-coated tablets and aqueous solution in healthy humans. *J Clin Pharmacol* (2002) 42, 920–927.
2. Quintus J, Kovar K-A, Link P, Hamacher H. Urinary excretion of arbutin metabolites after oral administration of bearberry leaf extracts. *Planta Med* (2005) 71, 147–52.
3. Siegers C, Bodinet C, Ali SS, Siegers C-P. Bacterial deconjugation of arbutin by *Escherichia coli*. *Phytomedicine* (2003) 10 (Suppl 4), 58–60.
4. Chauhan B, Yu C, Krantis A, Scott I, Arnason JT, Marles RJ, Foster BC. In vitro activity of uva-ursi against cytochrome P450 isoenzymes and P-glycoprotein. *Can J Physiol Pharmacol* (2007) 85, 1099–1107.
5. Scott IM, Leduc RI, Burt AJ, Marles RJ, Arnason JT, Foster BC. The inhibition of human cytochrome P450 by ethanol extracts of North American botanicals. *Pharm Biol* (2006) 44, 315–27.

B

Bearberry + Food

No interactions found.

Bearberry + Herbal medicines

No interactions found.

Bearberry + Lithium

For mention of a case of lithium toxicity in a woman who had been taking a non-prescription herbal diuretic containing corn silk, *Equisetum hyemale,* juniper, buchu, parsley and bearberry, all of which are believed to have diuretic actions, see under Parsley + Lithium, page 364.

Bee pollen

Arctostaphylos uva-ursi (L.) Spreng (Ericaceae)

Synonym(s) and related species

Honeybee pollen.

Bee pollen consists of flower pollen and nectar from male seed flowers, which is mixed with secretions from a worker honey bee. Note that there are products made from pollen alone, such as *Cernilton* (Rye grass pollen), which will not be dealt with in this monograph.

Constituents

The constituents of bee pollen depend to some extent on the flower species from which it has been harvested. It usually contains phytosterols, essential fatty acids including linoleic and alpha-linolenic acids, **flavonoids** and other polyphenols, minerals, and small amounts of B vitamins and vitamin C. Coumaroyl spermine and spermidine derivatives have been isolated from Brazilian bee pollen.

Use and indications

Bee pollen has been taken for prostate enlargement and to reduce the risk of atherosclerosis, hypertension and to improve cognition. Bee pollen from *Brassica campestris* is widely used in China as a natural food supplement to strengthen the body's resistance against diseases, including cancer. There is little supporting evidence for any of these uses. It should be avoided by people allergic to bee stings and to pollen because of the risk of a hypersensitivity reaction.

Pharmacokinetics

No relevant pharmacokinetic data found.

Interactions overview

A case report suggests that bee pollen might interact with warfarin. No other interactions appear to have been reported.

Interactions monographs

- Food, page 62
- Herbal medicines, page 62
- Warfarin, page 62

B

Bee pollen + Food

No interactions found.

Bee pollen + Herbal medicines

No interactions found.

Bee pollen + Warfarin

A case report describes an increased INR when a patient taking warfarin started to take bee pollen.

Clinical evidence

A 71-year-old man, who had been taking warfarin for 3 years, was noted to have an INR of 7.1 at a routine monitoring appointment. Although he was taking a number of potentially interacting drugs, and a vitamin and herbal supplement, his INR had been stable for the previous 9 months; however, one month earlier the patient had starting taking bee pollen granules 5 g twice daily. Warfarin was withheld until the INR returned to within the therapeutic range, and the patient was restabilised on a dose of warfarin that was 5 mg per week lower, while continuing to take the bee pollen. Over the next 7 months his INR was successfully maintained within the therapeutic range.[1]

Experimental evidence

No relevant data found.

Mechanism

The authors suggested that the flavonoid content of bee pollen might have inhibited the cytochrome P450 isoenzymes involved in the metabolism of warfarin, particularly CYP2C9. However, consider also *Pharmacokinetics,* under Flavonoids, page 213.

Importance and management

Evidence for an interaction between bee pollen and warfarin appears to be restricted to this case report and as such the general relevance of this case is unknown. Because of the many other factors influencing anticoagulant control, it is not possible to reliably ascribe a change in INR specifically to a drug interaction in a single case report without other supporting evidence. It may be better to advise patients taking warfarin to discuss the use of any herbal products they wish to try, and to increase monitoring if this is thought advisable. Cases of uneventful use should be reported, as they are as useful as possible cases of adverse effects.

1. Hurren KM, Lewis CL. Probable interaction between warfarin and bee pollen. *Am J Health-Syst Pharm* (2010) 67, 2034–7.

Berberine

Types, sources and related compounds

Berberine is an isoquinoline alkaloid found in many plants, particularly berberis, page 66, bloodroot, page 84, coptis, page 168, goldenseal, page 265, and greater celandine, page 277.

Use and indications

Berberine is bactericidal, amoebicidal and fungicidal. It has been used for many conditions, such as amoebic dysentery and diarrhoea, inflammation and liver disease. Berberine is also said to possess some antiepileptic, uterine stimulant and hypotensive effects, and is slightly sedative.

Pharmacokinetics

Berberine appears to undergo significant hepatobiliary excretion, including metabolism by cytochrome P450. Its metabolism in *rats* was partially affected by a known experimental inhibitor of cytochrome P450 isoenzymes.[1] In one *in vitro* study,[2] berberine appeared to increase CYP3A4 levels. In other *in vitro* studies,[3–5] it showed modest inhibition of CYP3A4 activity (see ciclosporin, page 64). It also appears to inhibit CYP2D6,[4,5] CYP2C8,[5] and CYP2E1,[5] but it does not significantly inhibit CYP2C9,[4,5] CYP2C19 and CYP1A2.[5]

Berberine also appears to be a substrate of P-glycoprotein, as the biliary excretion of berberine in the *rat* was inhibited by the P-glycoprotein inhibitor ciclosporin, page 64, and both ciclosporin, and verapamil, another P-glycoprotein inhibitor, improved berberine absorption.[1] Berberine may also be a substrate of organic cation transporters, as its biliary excretion was inhibited by the organic cation transporter inhibitor quinidine.

Interactions overview

Although a number of studies have used conventional drugs to study berberine metabolism, data on potentially clinically relevant interactions is sparse: the most significant interaction of berberine appears to be its potential to increase ciclosporin levels.

Interactions monographs

- Anxiolytics, page 64
- Ciclosporin, page 64
- Food, page 64
- Herbal medicines, page 64
- Hyoscine (Scopolamine), page 64
- Paclitaxel, page 65

1. Tsai P-L, Tsai T-H. Hepatobiliary excretion of berberine. *Drug Metab Dispos* (2004) 32, 405–12.
2. Budzinski JW, Trudeau VL, Drouin CE, Panahi M, Arnason JT, Foster BC. Modulation of human cytochrome P450 3A4 (CYP3A4) and P-glycoprotein (P-gp) in Caco-2 cell monolayers by selected commercial-source milk thistle and goldenseal products. *Can J Physiol Pharmacol* (2007) 85, 966–78.
3. Budzinski JW, Foster BC, Vandenhoek S, Arnason JT. An *in vitro* evaluation of human cytochrome P450 3A4 inhibition by selected commercial herbal extracts and tinctures. *Phytomedicine* (2000) 7, 273–82.
4. Chatterjee P, Franklin MR. Human cytochrome P450 inhibition and metabolic-intermediate complex formation by goldenseal extract and its methylenedioxyphenyl components. *Drug Metab Dispos* (2003) 31, 1391–7.
5. Etheridge AS, Black SR, Patel PR, So J, Mathews JM. An *in vitro* evaluation of cytochrome P450 inhibition and p-glycoprotein interaction with goldenseal, *Ginkgo biloba*, grape seed, milk thistle, and ginseng extracts and their constituents. *Planta Med* (2007) 73, 731–41.

Berberine + Anxiolytics

The interaction between berberine and anxiolytics is based on experimental evidence only.

Clinical evidence
No interactions found.

Experimental evidence
The effect of berberine was investigated using two experimental anxiety models in the *mouse*. Berberine showed anxiolytic effects in these models at a dose of 100 mg/kg, and sedative effects at a dose of 500 mg/kg. Berberine was found to enhance the anxiolytic effects of **buspirone** in the elevated plus-maze test, whereas the anxiolytic effects of berberine were not affected by **diazepam**.[1]

Mechanism
Berberine may have effects on brain monamines.

Importance and management
The doses of berberine given in this study were extremely large, compared with those used in clinical studies in humans. Any interactions seem unlikely to be clinically significant.

1. Peng W-H, Wu C-R, Chen C-S, Chen C-F, Leu Z-C, Hsieh M-T. Anxiolytic effect of berberine on exploratory activity of the mouse in two experimental anxiety models: interaction with drugs acting at 5-HT receptors. *Life Sci* (2004) 75, 2451–62.

Berberine + Ciclosporin ⚠

Berberine appears to increase the bioavailability and trough blood levels of ciclosporin. *Animal* **studies suggest that ciclosporin may affect the intestinal absorption and elimination of berberine possibly by inhibiting P-glycoprotein.**

Clinical evidence
A study in 6 kidney transplant patients looked at the effects of berberine on the pharmacokinetics of ciclosporin. The patients were taking ciclosporin 3 mg/kg twice daily for an average of 12 days before berberine 200 mg three times daily for 12 days was added. The AUC and trough blood levels of ciclosporin were increased by about 35% and 88%, respectively. The peak ciclosporin level was decreased but this was not statistically significant.[1] A clinical study by the same authors in 52 stable kidney transplant patients taking ciclosporin and given berberine 200 mg three times daily for 3 months found that the ciclosporin trough levels were increased by about 24% when the berberine-treated group was compared with 52 similar patients taking ciclosporin without berberine. The ciclosporin levels in 8 patients fell after berberine was stopped. Creatinine clearance was not significantly altered, and no serious adverse effects were reported.[1]

A single-dose study in healthy subjects found conflicting results. Six subjects given a single 6-mg/kg dose of ciclosporin daily found that berberine 300 mg twice daily, taken for 10 days before the dose of ciclosporin, had no significant effects on the pharmacokinetics of ciclosporin. However, a separate study in another 6 subjects given a single 3-mg/kg dose of ciclosporin found that a single 300 mg dose of berberine increased the AUC of ciclosporin by 19.2%. No adverse events were reported in this study.[2]

Experimental evidence
A study in *rats* found that intravenous ciclosporin 20 mg/kg did not significantly affect the AUC of intravenous berberine 10 to 20 mg/kg in the blood, but ciclosporin did decrease the AUC of berberine in the liver and the bile.[3] Another study in *rats* also found that ciclosporin increased the intestinal absorption of berberine.[4]

Mechanism
The mechanism for the increase in ciclosporin levels seen in the clinical studies is unclear, although it has been suggested that it may be due to inhibition of CYP3A by berberine.

Animal studies suggest that ciclosporin may also affect the handling of berberine possibly by inhibiting P-glycoprotein, therefore affecting its intestinal absorption and its distribution into the bile and liver.

Importance and management
Although the increase in ciclosporin levels is not sufficiently severe to suggest that the concurrent use of berberine should be avoided, it may make ciclosporin levels less stable. If concurrent use is undertaken, ciclosporin levels should be well monitored, and the dose of ciclosporin adjusted accordingly.

1. Wu X, Li Q, Xin H, Yu A, Zhong M. Effects of berberine on the blood concentration of cyclosporin A in renal transplanted recipients: clinical and pharmacokinetic study. *Eur J Clin Pharmacol* (2005) 61, 567–72.
2. Xin H-W, Wu X-C, Li Q, Yu A-R, Zhong M-Y, Liu Y-Y. The effects of berberine on the pharmacokinetics of ciclosporin A in healthy volunteers. *Methods Find Exp Clin Pharmacol* (2006) 28, 25–9.
3. Tsai P-L, Tsai T-H. Hepatobiliary excretion of berberine. *Drug Metab Dispos* (2004) 32, 405–12.
4. Pan G-Y, Wang G-J, Liu X-D, Fawcett JP, Xie Y-Y. The involvement of P-glycoprotein in berberine absorption. *Pharmacol Toxicol* (2002) 91, 193–7.

Berberine + Food

No interactions found.

Berberine + Herbal medicines

No interactions found.

Berberine + Hyoscine (Scopolamine)

The interaction between berberine and hyoscine (scopolamine) is based on experimental evidence only.

Clinical evidence
No interactions found.

Experimental evidence
Berberine 100 and 500 mg/kg, given orally for 7 to 14 days significantly improved hyoscine-induced amnesia in *rats,* measured using a step-through passive avoidance task. This antiamnesic effect of berberine was completely reversed by hyoscine methobromide, implying that the antiamnesic action of berberine may be through the peripheral rather than central nervous system.[1]

Mechanism
The authors suggest that the mechanism may partially be through alpha$_2$-adrenoceptor blockade by berberine, leading to an increase in the release of adrenaline (epinephrine) and a subsequent increase in glucose supply to the brain.

Importance and management
The experimental evidence for this interaction is very limited and there appears to be no data to suggest that berberine may improve memory or reverse the effects of drugs that affect memory, such as hyoscine, in humans. This is unlikely to be a clinically significant

interaction, especially as the doses used in the study were many times those used in human studies of berberine.

1. Peng W-H, Hsieh M-T, Wu C-R. Effect of long-term administration of berberine on scopolamine-induced amnesia in rats. *Jpn J Pharmacol* (1997) 74, 261–6.

Berberine + Paclitaxel

The interaction between berberine and paclitaxel is based on experimental evidence only.

Clinical evidence

No interactions found.

Experimental evidence

An *in vitro* study found that pre-treatment with berberine blocked the anticancer effects of paclitaxel in six cancer cell line cultures (oral cancer, gastric cancer and colon cancer).[1]

Mechanism

Unknown.

Importance and management

This appears to be the only published study of an antagonistic effect between berberine and paclitaxel. Further study is required to confirm these *in vitro* results, and to explore their clinical relevance.

1. Lin H-L, Liu T-Y, Wu C-W, Chi C-W. Berberine modulates expression of *mdr*1 gene product and the responses of digestive track cancer cells to paclitaxel. *Br J Cancer* (1999) 81, 416–22.

B

Berberis

Berberis vulgaris L. and *Berberis aristata* DC. (Berberidaceae)

Synonym(s) and related species

Barberry, Berberidis, Pipperidge bush.

Berberis chitria Lindl., *Berberis dumetorum* Gouan, *Berberis floribunda* Wall.

Constituents

The root and stem of all species contain isoquinoline alkaloids such as **berberine**, berbamine, jatrorrhizine, oxyberberine, palmatine, magnoflorine, oxyacanthine and others.

Use and indications

Used for many conditions, especially infective, such as amoebic dysentery and diarrhoea; inflammation and liver disease. The main constituent berberine is bactericidal, amoebicidal and fungicidal. It has some antiepileptic, uterine stimulant and hypotensive effects and is slightly sedative, as are jatrorrhizine and palmatine.

Pharmacokinetics

No relevant pharmacokinetic data found specifically for berberis, but see berberine, page 63, for information on this constituent of berberis.

Interactions overview

No interactions with berberis found. For information on the interactions of one of its constituents, berberine, see under berberine, page 63.

Bergamot oil

Citrus bergamia Risso (Rutaceae)

Synonym(s) and related species

Bergamot essence, Bergamot orange.

Citrus aurantium subsp. bergamia Wight & Arn., is also used and is closely related to Bitter orange, page 75, which is *Citrus aurantium* var *amara*.

Constituents

Bergamot essential oil is obtained by expression from the fruit peel and contains a volatile fraction consisting of monoterpene and sesquiterpene hydrocarbons and their oxygenated derivatives, including linalyl acetate, limonene and linalool, and some **natural coumarins**, particularly the **furanocoumarins**, bergamottin and **5-methoxypsoralen** (bergapten).

Use and indications

Bergamot oil is included in some preparations for upper respiratory-tract disorders. It has photosensitising properties due to the presence of furanocoumarins and has been used topically with UV light for the treatment of psoriasis. Berg-amot oil is also used in perfumery, as a flavouring in foods such as Earl Grey and Lady Grey tea, and in aromatherapy.

Pharmacokinetics

No relevant pharmacokinetic data found. For information on the pharmacokinetics of individual furanocoumarins present in bergamot oil, see under natural coumarins, page 356.

Interactions overview

Theoretically, bergamot oil might increase the photosen-sitising effect of psoralens as it contains the psoralen, 5-methoxysporalen. For information on the interactions of individual furanocoumarins present in bergamot oil, see under natural coumarins, page 356.

Interactions monographs

- Food, page 68
- Herbal medicines, page 68
- Psoralens, page 68

Bergamot oil + Food

No interactions found. Note that bergamot oil is used as a citrus flavouring agent in foods.

Bergamot oil + Herbal medicines

No interactions found. Theoretically, the photosensitising effect of bergamot oil might be additive with that of other herbs with photosensitising properties, although whether this is clinically relevant is uncertain.

Bergamot oil + Psoralens

The interaction between bergamot oil and psoralens is based on a prediction only.

Clinical evidence

No interactions found. However, note that bergamot oil has been used topically with phototherapy (UV light) for treating psoriasis in order to reduce the dose of UV required[1] and cases of phototoxic skin reactions have been reported after exposure to topical or aerosolised bergamot oil and subsequent sun exposure or UVA exposure on a sunbed.[2] Therefore it is possible that the phototoxic effects of bergamot oil might be additive with those of photosensitising drugs such as the psoralens.

Experimental evidence

No relevant data found.

Mechanism

Furanocoumarins such as 5-methoxypsoralen in bergamot oil are known photosensitisers.

Importance and management

Although the interaction between bergamot oil and the psoralens is only a prediction, it might be prudent to be cautious with the use of bergamot oil (particularly when applied topically) in patients undergoing treatment with psoralens or other photosensitising drugs. Warn patients that phototoxic reactions have been reported with bergamot oil aromatherapy products.

1. Valkova S. UVB phototherapeutic modalities. Comparison of two treatments for chronic plaque psoriasis. *Acta Dermatovenerol Alp Panonica Adriat* (2007) 16, 26–30.
2. Kaddu S, Kerl H, Wolf P. Accidental bullous phototoxic reactions to bergamot aromatherapy oil. *J Am Acad Dermatol* (2001) 45, 458–61.

B

Betacarotene

Types, sources and related compounds

Provitamin A.

Pharmacopoeias

Betacarotene (*BP 2012, PhEur 7.5*); Beta Carotene (*USP35–NF30 S1*); Beta Carotene Capsules (*USP35–NF30 S1*).

Use and indications

Betacarotene is a **carotenoid** precursor to vitamin A (retinol). It is a natural pigment found in many plants including fruit and vegetables (such as carrots) and is therefore eaten as part of a healthy diet, and is also used as a food colouring. Betacarotene supplements are usually taken for the prevention of vitamin A deficiency and for reducing photosensitivities in patients with erythropoietic protoporphyria. It is also used for age-related macular degeneration and has been investigated for possible use in cardiovascular disease and cancer prevention.

Pharmacokinetics

Betacarotene is the most studied carotenoid of the hundreds that exist in nature. It is a fat soluble precursor of vitamin A (retinol) and a large part of the metabolism to vitamin A takes place in the gastrointestinal mucosa where its absorption may be sensitive to changes in gastric pH, see proton pump inhibitors, page 72. This could be a contributing factor to the large interindividual variation seen in betacarotene absorption. As betacarotene intake increases, vitamin A production from the carotenoid is reduced.[1]

Betacarotene potentiated the induction of the cytochrome P450 isoenzyme CYP2E1 by alcohol in *rats*;[2] however, it did not significantly affect CYP1A1/2.

Interactions overview

Orlistat reduces betacarotene absorption, heavy long-term alcohol intake may interfere with the conversion of betacarotene to vitamin A, and the desired effect of betacarotene supplementation may be reduced by colchicine and omeprazole. Betacarotene reduces the benefits that combined simvastatin and nicotinic acid have on cholesterol, and reduces ciclosporin levels. Combined use with colestyramine or probucol modestly reduces dietary betacarotene absorption. Clinically relevant interactions are unlikely between betacarotene and tobacco, but note that smokers are advised against taking betacarotene. For the interactions of betacarotene with food or lycopene, see Lycopene + Food, page 337, and Lycopene + Herbal medicines; Betacarotene, page 337.

Interactions monographs

- Alcohol, page 70
- Ciclosporin, page 70
- Cimetidine, page 70
- Colchicine, page 70
- Lipid regulating drugs, page 71
- Orlistat, page 71
- Proton pump inhibitors, page 72
- Tobacco, page 72

1. Patrick L. Beta-carotene: The controversy continues. *Altern Med Rev* (2000) 5, 530–545.
2. Kessova IG, Leo MA, Lieber CS. Effect of β-carotene on hepatic cytochrome P-450 in ethanol-fed rats. *Alcohol Clin Exp Res* (2001) 25, 1368–72.

B

Betacarotene + Alcohol

Heavy consumption of alcohol may interfere with the conversion of betacarotene to vitamin A.

Clinical evidence

In the Alpha-Tocopherol, Beta-Carotene Cancer Prevention Study (ATBC), an almost 7-year long large randomised placebo-controlled study in men, an alcohol intake of more than 12.9 g daily by 109 heavy drinkers reduced the serum concentrations of betacarotene 20 mg daily by up to 13%. These findings were independent of dietary carotenoid intake.[1]

Experimental evidence

In an experimental study in *baboons* fed alcohol for 2 to 5 years and given 30 mg/L and then 45 mg/L doses of betacarotene (*Solatene* capsules) daily for 33 days and 29 days respectively, the serum levels of betacarotene were higher in those fed alcohol than those that were not fed alcohol. When betacarotene was stopped, its clearance was delayed in the *baboons* fed alcohol. Betacarotene was also found to potentiate the hepatotoxicity of alcohol.[2]

Mechanism

This interaction is complex. Betacarotene and alcohol may share similar biochemical pathways; one experimental study in *rats* found that betacarotene potentiated the induction of the cytochrome P450 isoenzyme CYP2E1 by alcohol.[3] Alcohol also reduces the levels of **vitamin A**, of which betacarotene is the precursor. It has therefore been suggested that alcohol interferes with the conversion of betacarotene to **vitamin A**.[4]

Importance and management

Information about an interaction between betacarotene and alcohol is limited, and the effects in *animals* and humans are conflicting. It appears that the long-term intake of alcohol causes some changes in betacarotene disposition, and it would therefore seem sensible to try to limit alcohol intake if betacarotene supplementation is necessary.

1. Albanes D, Virtamo J, Taylor PR, Rautalahti M, Pietinen P, Heinonen OP. Effects of supplemental β-carotene, cigarette smoking, and alcohol consumption on serum carotenoids in the Alpha-Tocopherol, Beta-Carotene Cancer Prevention Study. *Am J Clin Nutr* (1997) 66, 366–72.
2. Leo MA, Kim C-I, Lowe N, Lieber CS. Interaction of ethanol with β-carotene: delayed blood clearance and enhanced hepatotoxicity. *Hepatology* (1992) 15, 883–91.
3. Kessova IG, Leo MA, Lieber CS. Effect of β-carotene on hepatic cytochrome P-450 in ethanol-fed rats. *Alcohol Clin Exp Res* (2001) 25, 1368–72.
4. Leo MA, Lieber CS. Alcohol, vitamin A, and β-carotene: adverse interactions, including hepatotoxicity and carcinogenicity. *Am J Clin Nutr* (1999) 69, 1071–85.

Betacarotene + Ciclosporin

A study in 10 kidney transplant patients found that an antioxidant vitamin supplement containing betacarotene modestly reduced ciclosporin blood levels.

Clinical evidence

A randomised placebo-controlled study, in 10 kidney transplant patients taking ciclosporin, found that the addition of an antioxidant vitamin supplement for 6 months containing vitamin C 500 mg, vitamin E 400 units and betacarotene 6 mg daily reduced the ciclosporin blood level by 24%. An associated improvement in renal function, indicated by an increase in glomerular filtration rate of 17%, was also seen and may have been associated with reduced ciclosporin levels.[1]

Experimental evidence

No relevant data found.

Mechanism

Unknown.

Importance and management

The clinical significance of this study is unclear as there appear to be no published case reports of any adverse effects due to this interaction. Furthermore, a decrease in ciclosporin levels of 24% is fairly modest, and other studies have found that vitamin C 1 g daily and vitamin E 300 mg daily may slightly decrease ciclosporin levels, so the potential for a clinically significant interaction with betacarotene alone is unclear. However, until more is known it may be prudent to consider an interaction with betacarotene if a sudden or unexplained reduction in stable ciclosporin levels occurs. More study is needed, particularly with regard to the concurrent use of standard, commercially available multivitamin preparations.

1. Blackhall ML, Fassett RG, Sharman JE, Geraghty DP, Coombes JS. Effects of antioxidant supplementation on blood cyclosporin A and glomerular filtration rate in renal transplant recipients. *Nephrol Dial Transplant* (2005) 20, 1970–1975.

Betacarotene + Cimetidine

An interaction between betacarotene and cimetidine is based on experimental evidence only.

Clinical evidence

No interactions found.

Experimental evidence

In an *animal* study, *rats* were given intragastric alcohol to induce mucosal damage. When the *rats* were pretreated with betacarotene 1 mg/kg, the number of mucosal lesions was decreased by 63%. However, when cimetidine 50 mg/kg was given with the betacarotene, 30 minutes before the alcohol, the damaging effects of the alcohol appeared to be enhanced.[1]

Mechanism

The exact mechanism is unclear.

Importance and management

This is a relatively old study and there do not appear to be any clinical reports in the literature. Furthermore the dose of betacarotene used is roughly 10-fold greater than the recommended daily intake of betacarotene. Therefore a clinically relevant interaction with cimetidine seems unlikely.

1. Garamszegi M, Jávor T, Sütő G, Vincze Á, Tóth G, Mózsik G. Effect of atropine, PGF$_{2\alpha}$ and cimetidine on the β-carotene induced cytoprotection in ethanol-treated rats. *Acta Physiol Hung* (1989) 73, 221–4.

Betacarotene + Colchicine

The desired effect of betacarotene supplementation may be reduced in those taking colchicine.

Clinical evidence

Divided doses of colchicine 1.9 mg to 3.9 mg daily reduced the serum levels of betacarotene 10 000 units daily (about 6 mg) in 5 obese subjects. Levels returned to normal when colchicine was stopped.[1] However, in another study, long-term use of colchicine 1 mg to 2 mg daily for 3 years had no effect on the serum levels of diet-derived carotene in 12 patients with familial Mediterranean fever.[2]

B

Experimental evidence

No relevant data found.

Mechanism

The mechanism is unclear. Colchicine causes reversible malabsorption in the gastrointestinal tract by disturbing epithelial cell function and inhibiting cell proliferation. It also lowered the serum levels of cholesterol in the first study. All these factors could have an effect on the absorption of betacarotene, which largely takes place in the gastrointestinal mucosa and whose distribution is dependent on the presence of lipoproteins.

Importance and management

The evidence for a possible interaction between betacarotene and colchicine is limited to two relatively old studies. While supplemental betacarotene absorption appears to be reduced, betacarotene ingested as part of the normal diet appears to be unaffected. Based on these two findings, and the fact that there is large interindividual variation in betacarotene absorption, it is difficult to recommend a clinical course of action other than to be aware that the desired effect of betacarotene supplementation may be reduced in those taking colchicine.

1. Race TF, Paes IC, Faloon WW. Intestinal malabsorption induced by oral colchicine. Comparison with neomycin and cathartic agents. *Am J Med Sci* (1970) 259, 32–41.
2. Ehrenfeld M, Levy M, Sharon P, Rachmilewitz D, Eliakim M. Gastrointestinal effects of long-term colchicine therapy in patients with recurrent polyserositis (familial Mediterranean fever). *Dig Dis Sci* (1982) 27, 723–7.

Betacarotene + Food

See under Lycopene + Food, page 337.

Betacarotene + Herbal medicines; Lycopene

Betacarotene may alter the absorption of lycopene, see Lycopene + Herbal medicines; Betacarotene, page 337.

Betacarotene + Lipid regulating drugs

Betacarotene reduces the benefits that combined simvastatin and nicotinic acid have on HDL-cholesterol. Colestyramine and probucol reduce the serum levels of betacarotene eaten as part of a normal diet.

Clinical evidence

In a 3-year study in 146 patients with clinical coronary disease, an antioxidant regimen consisting of betacarotene 25 mg, vitamin E 800 units, vitamin C 1 g and selenium 100 micrograms daily, halved the beneficial rise of high-density lipoprotein-cholesterol (HDL2) caused by combined treatment with **simvastatin** 10 to 20 mg and **nicotinic acid** (**niacin**) 2 to 4 g daily.[1]

There do not appear to be any studies on the effect of lipid regulating drugs on the absorption of betacarotene from supplements; however, a 3-year study of 303 hypercholesterolemic subjects given **colestyramine** in doses of 8 g to 16 g daily, according to tolerance, found that the serum levels of *dietary*-derived betacarotene were reduced by about 40% after 2 months. **Probucol** 500 mg twice daily was then added, and 2 months later the serum levels of betacarotene were reduced by an additional 39% (representing an overall decrease of 65%).[2]

Experimental evidence

No relevant data found.

Mechanism

Unknown. Betacarotene is a fat-soluble substance, and therefore its absorption and distribution is dependent on the presence of lipoproteins, which might be reduced by colestyramine.

Importance and management

There appears to be only one study investigating the effects of betacarotene on treatment with lipid lowering drugs; however, the study was well-designed, long-term, and large. Antioxidant supplementation including betacarotene appears to suppress the beneficial effects of the combined treatment of simvastatin and nicotinic acid on high-density lipoprotein-cholesterol, higher levels of which reduce the risk of major cardiovascular events. The authors suggest that their results indicate that the use of antioxidants to prevent cardiovascular events should be questioned. What this means for patients taking lower therapeutic doses of betacarotene (recommended daily intake is about 6 mg daily, about one-quarter of the dose used in the study) is unclear. However, there is potential for a severe detrimental effect on concurrent use. Therefore, until more is known it would seem prudent to avoid concurrent use, unless there is a clear defined clinical need for betacarotene supplementation.

The use of colestyramine and probucol appears to lower betacarotene levels, but the clinical importance of this does not appear to have been established.

1. Brown BG, Zhao X-Q, Chait A, Fisher LD, Cheung MC, Morse JS, Dowdy AA, Marino EK, Bolson EL, Alaupovic P, Frohlich J, Albers JJ. Simvastatin and niacin, antioxidant vitamins, or the combination for the prevention of coronary disease. *N Engl J Med* (2001) 345, 1583–92.
2. Elinder LS, Hådell K, Johansson J, Mølgaard J, Holme I, Olsson AG, Walldius G. Probucol treatment decreases serum concentrations of diet-derived antioxidants. *Arterioscler Thromb Vasc Biol* (1995) 15, 1057–63.

Betacarotene + Orlistat

Orlistat decreases the absorption of supplemental betacarotene.

Clinical evidence

A randomised study in healthy subjects found that about two-thirds of a supplemental dose of betacarotene was absorbed in the presence of orlistat. The study included 48 patients in 4 groups, given placebo, or betacarotene in doses of 30 mg, 60 mg, or 120 mg. The betacarotene was given within about 30 minutes of the orlistat.[1]

Experimental evidence

No relevant data found.

Mechanism

Orlistat reduces dietary fat absorption by inhibiting gastrointestinal lipase. Consequently, it reduces the absorption of fat-soluble vitamins.

Importance and management

Evidence is limited to one study, but what is known suggests that orlistat decreases the absorption of supplemental betacarotene. To maximise vitamin absorption, the manufacturers recommend that any multivitamin preparations should be taken at least 2 hours before or after orlistat, such as at bedtime.[2,3] The US manufacturers suggest that patients taking orlistat should be advised to take multivitamins, because of the possibility of reduced vitamin levels.[3]

1. Zhi J, Melia AT, Koss-Twardy SG, Arora S, Patel IH. The effect of orlistat, an inhibitor of dietary fat absorption, on the pharmacokinetics of β-carotene in healthy volunteers. *J Clin Pharmacol* (1996) 36, 152–9.
2. Xenical (Orlistat). Roche Products Ltd. UK Summary of product characteristics, June 2008.
3. Xenical (Orlistat). Roche Pharmaceuticals. US Prescribing information, July 2008.

Betacarotene + Proton pump inhibitors

The desired effect of betacarotene supplementation may be reduced in those taking proton pump inhibitors.

Clinical evidence

In a study in 10 healthy subjects the AUC of a single 120-mg dose of betacarotene was halved by pretreatment with **omeprazole** 20 mg twice daily for 7 days.[1]

Experimental evidence

No relevant data found.

Mechanism

The exact mechanism is unclear. Betacarotene is absorbed in the small intestine by a simple passive-diffusion process. It has been suggested that omeprazole may retard this diffusion,[1] and that delayed gastric emptying may also contribute.[2]

Importance and management

Evidence for an interaction between betacarotene and omeprazole is limited, and as there is large interindividual variability in betacarotene absorption, the true bioavailability of the carotenoid can vary greatly even before omeprazole is taken. Coupled with the fact that betacarotene is a normal part of the healthy diet, it is very difficult to assess the true clinical importance of this interaction. Be aware that the desired effect of betacarotene supplements may be reduced or abolished by the concurrent use of omeprazole. If the suggested mechanism is correct, other proton pump inhibitors are likely to affect betacarotene absorption similarly.

1. Tang G, Serfaty-Lacrosniere C, Ermelinda Camilo M, Russell RM. Gastric acidity influences the blood response to a β-carotene dose in humans. *Am J Clin Nutr* (1996) 64, 622–6.
2. Øster-Jørgensen E, Rasmussen L. Blood response to a β-carotene dose. *Am J Clin Nutr* (1998) 67, 349–53.

Betacarotene + Tobacco

There is a slight increased risk of lung cancer in smokers taking betacarotene supplements.

Clinical evidence

In the Alpha-Tocopherol, Beta-Carotene Cancer Prevention Study (ATBC), an almost 7-year long large randomised placebo-controlled study in men, tobacco smoking did not significantly affect the serum concentrations of betacarotene 20 mg daily. These findings were independent of dietary carotenoid intake.[1] However, in this study, the risk of lung cancer was slightly, but significantly, increased in those patients receiving betacarotene supplements (18% increase).[2]

Experimental evidence

No relevant data found.

Mechanism

Unknown.

Importance and management

Evidence for an interaction between tobacco smoking and betacarotene is limited, but a clinically significant effect of tobacco smoking on absorption of betacarotene supplementation seems unlikely. However, unexpectedly, well-designed studies have found a slight increased risk of lung cancer in smokers taking betacarotene supplements. There is no clear explanation for this, and there is much debate about whether this is a true effect. Until more is known it may be prudent for smokers to avoid betacarotene supplements, and to counsel the patient on smoking cessation and the health benefits of consuming five portions of fruit and vegetables daily as part of a balanced diet. Note that the Food Standards Agency in the UK advises people who smoke not to take betacarotene supplements because of an increased risk of lung cancer.[3]

1. Albanes D, Virtamo J, Taylor PR, Rautalahti M, Pietinen P, Heinonen OP. Effects of supplemental carotene, cigarette smoking, and alcohol consumption on serum carotenoids in the Alpha-Tocopherol, Beta-Carotene Cancer Prevention Study. *Am J Clin Nutr* (1997) 66, 366–72.
2. Anon . The effect of vitamin E and beta carotene on the incidence of lung cancer and other cancers in male smokers: the Alpha-Tocopherol, Beta Carotene Cancer Prevention Study Group. *N Engl J Med* (1994) 330, 1029–35.
3. Food Standards Agency Betacarotene http://www.eatwell.gov.uk/healthydiet/nutritionessentials/vitaminsandminerals/betacarotene/ (accessed 14/10/2008).

B

Bilberry

Vaccinium myrtillus L. (Ericaceae)

Synonym(s) and related species

Blaeberry, Bogberry, Huckleberry, Hurtleberry, Myrtillus, Whortleberry.

Note that the synonym Blueberry has also been used, but the name Blueberry is the more commonly accepted name for the North American native plants such as *Vaccinium angustifolium* Aiton (Lowbush Blueberry) and *Vaccinium corymbosum* L. (Northern Highbush Blueberry).

Pharmacopoeias

Dried Bilberry (*BP 2012, PhEur 7.5*); Fresh Bilberry (*BP 2012, PhEur 7.5*); Fresh Bilberry Fruit Dry Extract, Refined and Standardised (*BP 2012, PhEur 7.5*); Powdered Bilberry Extract (*USP35–NF30 S1*).

Constituents

The berries contain **anthocyanins**, mainly glucosides of cyanidin, delphinidin, malvidin, petunidin and peonidin. Standardised extracts containing not less than 0.3% of **anthocyanins** expressed as cyanidin-3-glucoside chloride (dried drug), or not less than 1% tannins, expressed as pyrogallol (dried drug), are often used (*BP 2009, Ph Eur 6.4*). Bilberry berries also contain **flavonoids** (including catechins, quercetin-3-glucuronide and hyperoside), and vitamin C.

Use and indications

Traditionally bilberry has been used to treat diarrhoea, haemorrhoids and venous insufficiency, gastrointestinal inflammation and urinary complaints. It has now found a more specific use in improving visual acuity, by improving blood flow to the retina, and for its vasoprotective properties as an anti-atherosclerotic.

Pharmacokinetics

For general information about the pharmacokinetics of anthocyanins, see under flavonoids, page 213.

An *in vitro* study investigated the effects of bilberry extract (at a concentration likely to be attainable in the human intestine) on the uptake of estrone-3-sulfate by the transporter protein OATP-B. Estrone-3-sulfate was used as it is known to be an OATP-B substrate. The bilberry extract inhibited estrone-3-sulfate uptake by about 75%, which was considered to be a potent effect.[1] OATP-B is known to have a role in the absorption of drugs such as fexofenadine, glibenclamide and pravastatin, and therefore this study suggests that bilberry extract may decrease the absorption of these drugs, which could result in a reduction in their effects. However, no clinical reports of an interaction between bilberry and these or other drugs appear to have been published.

Interactions overview

No interactions with bilberry found. For information on the interactions of individual flavonoids found in bilberry, see under flavonoids, page 213.

1. Fuchikami H, Satoh H, Tsujimoto M, Ohdo S, Ohtani H, Sawada Y. Effects of herbal extracts on the function of human organic anion-transporting polypeptide OATP-B. *Drug Metab Dispos* (2006) 34, 577–82.

Bistort

Persicaria bistorta (L.) Sampaio (Polygonaceae)

Synonym(s) and related species

Adderwort, Dragonwort, English Serpentary, Osterick, Snakeweed.

Polygonum bistorta L., , *Polygonum bistortoides* Pursh, *Bistorta major* S.F. Gray.

Pharmacopoeias

Bistort rhizome (*BP 2012, PhEur 7.5*).

Constituents

The bistort root and rhizome contain polyphenolic compounds, mainly **flavonoids** (e.g. catechins and quercetin), ellagic acid, and the **triterpenes**, friedelanol and 5-glutinen-3-one.

Use and indications

Bistort is traditionally used as an astringent and anti-inflammatory agent.

Pharmacokinetics

No relevant pharmacokinetic data found. For information on the pharmacokinetics of individual flavonoids found in bistort, see under flavonoids, page 213.

Interactions overview

No interactions with bistort found. For information on the interactions of individual flavonoids found in bistort, see under flavonoids, page 213.

Bitter orange

Citrus aurantium var amara L. (Rutaceae)

Synonym(s) and related species

Bigaradier, Pomeranze, Seville orange.

Note that Bitter orange is closely related to Bergamot, page 67, which has been known as *Citrus aurantium* subsp. bergamia Wight & Arn.

Pharmacopoeias

Bitter-orange Epicarp and Mesocarp (*PhEur 7.5*); Bitter-orange Epicarp and Mesocarp Tincture (*BP 2012 PhEur 7.5*); Bitter-orange Flower (*BP 2012, PhEur 7.5*); Dried Bitter-orange Peel (*BP 2012*); Neroli Oil (*PhEur 7.5*).

Constituents

Bitter orange contains the sympathomimetic alkaloid **oxedrine** (**synephrine**), **flavonoids** (hesperidin, narin-genin, tangeretin and others; often referred to as citrus bioflavonoids), and natural coumarins (umbelliferone, 6,7-dimethoxycoumarin, and the furanocoumarins 6,7-dihydroxybergamottin and bergapten). The volatile oil is mostly composed of limonene. Some sources standardise the flowers to **flavonoid** content, expressed as naringin, and the peel to essential oil content.

Use and indications

Bitter orange is traditionally used as a carminative and for other digestive disorders. It is also said to possess antihypertensive, anti-inflammatory, analgesic and antibac-terial properties. Bitter-orange extract is included in some herbal anorectic preparations as it contains oxedrine, which is claimed to increase metabolism; however cardiovas-cular adverse effects are associated with this constituent (see under Caffeine + Herbal medicines; Bitter orange, page 111). Interestingly bitter orange has also been pro-moted as an appetite stimulant. The flowers have been used as a sedative, and the peel and the oils are used widely as flavourings in foods and conventional medicines. Bitter orange is used to make marmalade. The juice of bitter orange has been used in studies of drug metabolism as a comparator to grapefruit juice, but it is not used as a medicine or beverage.

Pharmacokinetics

A bitter orange supplement (containing oxedrine but no 6,7-dihydroxybergamottin) did not inhibit the cytochrome P450 isoenzymes CYP1A2 (see caffeine, page 111), CYP2E1 (see chlorzoxazone, page 76), or CYP2D6 (as assessed with debrisoquine[1]) in clinical studies.

The effects of bitter orange on CYP3A4 are uncertain. A bitter orange supplement (containing oxedrine but no 6,7-dihydroxybergamottin) did not inhibit CYP3A4

(see midazolam, page 77). However, the juice of bitter orange (containing the furanocoumarins bergapten and 6,7-dihydroxybergamottin) inhibited intestinal CYP3A4 (see felodipine, page 77), but probably has no effect on hepatic CYP3A4 (see indinavir, page 77). The juice may also inhibit P-glycoprotein transport (see dextromethorphan, page 76). Differences in active constituents might be part of the explanation for the differences in effects seen on CYP3A4.

For information on the pharmacokinetics of individual flavonoids present in bitter orange, see flavonoids, page 213, and for the pharmacokinetics of individual furanocoumarins, see under natural coumarins, page 356.

Interactions overview

The juice of bitter orange has been used in some drug interaction studies (as a comparator to grapefruit juice, page 270). Information from these studies has been included here, but note that it should not be directly extrapolated to herbal medicines containing bitter orange, because some differences in interaction potential have been seen.

A bitter orange decoction increased ciclosporin levels in *animals,* whereas the juice of bitter orange does not appear to interact clinically. A bitter orange supplement does not appear to affect the pharmacokinetics of chlor-zoxazone, debrisoquine or midazolam, suggesting a lack of interaction with substrates of the cytochrome P450 isoen-zymes CYP2E1, CYP2D6 and CYP3A4, respectively. The juice of bitter orange does not appear to affect the pharma-cokinetics of indinavir, but it may raise dextromethorphan and felodipine levels.

For a possible interaction of supplements containing bitter orange with caffeine, resulting in adverse cardiac effects, see Caffeine + Herbal medicines; Bitter orange, page 111.

For specific interactions of citrus flavonoids such as naringenin, see flavonoids, page 213, and for citrus furanocoumarins such as bergapten, see natural coumarins, page 356.

Interactions monographs

- Chlorzoxazone, page 76
- Ciclosporin, page 76
- Dextromethorphan, page 76
- Felodipine, page 77
- Food, page 77
- Indinavir, page 77
- Midazolam, page 77

1. Gurley BJ, Gardner SF, Hubbard MA, Williams DK, Gentry WB, Carrier J, Khan IA, Edwards DJ, Shah A. In vivo assessment of botanical supplementation on human cytochrome P450 phenotypes: *Citrus aurantium, Echinacea purpurea,* milk thistle, and saw palmetto. *Clin Pharmacol Ther* (2004) 76, 428–40.

B

Bitter orange + Chlorzoxazone

A bitter orange supplement did not alter the metabolism of chlorzoxazone in one study and is therefore unlikely to alter the pharmacokinetics of drugs that are metabolised by CYP2E1.

Clinical evidence

In a study in 12 healthy subjects, a bitter orange supplement, standardised to synephrine 4%, was given at a dose of 350 mg twice daily for 28 days with a single 250-mg dose of chlorzoxazone given before and at the end of the treatment with bitter orange. The metabolism of chlorzoxazone was not affected by the concurrent use of bitter orange. The supplement was analysed and found to contain the stated amount of synephrine (equivalent to a daily dose of about 30 mg), and none of the furanocoumarin, 6,7-dihydrobergamottin.[1]

Experimental evidence

No relevant data found.

Mechanism

No mechanism expected.

Importance and management

Chlorzoxazone is used as a probe drug for CYP1E2 activity, and therefore these results also suggest that a pharmacokinetic interaction between this bitter orange supplement and other CYP1E2 substrates is unlikely.

1. Gurley BJ, Gardner SF, Hubbard MA, Williams DK, Gentry WB, Carrier J, Khan IA, Edwards DJ, Shah A. In vivo assessment of botanical supplementation on human cytochrome P450 phenotypes: *Citrus aurantium, Echinacea purpurea,* milk thistle, and saw palmetto. *Clin Pharmacol Ther* (2004) 76, 428–40.

Bitter orange + Ciclosporin

Bitter orange juice does not appear to affect the pharmacokinetics of ciclosporin in humans. However, a bitter orange decoction increased ciclosporin levels in *animals*.

Clinical evidence

In a randomised, crossover study, 7 healthy subjects were given a single 7.5-mg/kg dose of ciclosporin 30 minutes after consuming about 240 mL of bitter orange juice. Bitter orange juice did not affect the AUC or the maximum serum levels of ciclosporin, although it appeared to delay the absorption of ciclosporin in some subjects. This was in contrast to the effects of grapefruit juice.[1] The bitter orange juice was prepared by squeezing fresh fruit and freezing it until needed (up to 6 weeks). It was determined to contain 6,7-dihydroxybergamottin at a concentration of about 30 micromol/L.

Experimental evidence

In a study in *pigs,* 200 mL of a decoction of bitter orange increased the maximum levels and AUC of ciclosporin 10 mg/kg by 64% and 46%, respectively. One of the 5 *animals* used in the study developed ciclosporin toxicity. The decoction was prepared by boiling the crude drug with water for about 2 hours. Each 200 mL dose was prepared from the equivalent of 20 g of crude drug, and was determined to contain 1.12 mmoL of flavonoids, mostly naringin. It was not assayed for furanocoumarin content.[2]

Mechanism

The results of an *animal* study[2] suggested that bitter orange alters the absorption of ciclosporin, possibly by affecting intestinal P-glycoprotein. It is possible that the differing findings in humans represents differing absorption characteristics between species, but it also seems likely that they could be related to the different preparations of bitter orange (juice and a decoction) used in the studies. Note that, in the clinical study, the furanocoumarin 6,7-dihydroxybergamottin did not interact.[1] In the *animal* study, the extent of the interaction was not related to the flavonoid content.[2]

Importance and management

There only appear to be two studies investigating an interaction between bitter orange and ciclosporin, one of them using the juice in humans and another using a decoction in *animals*. What is known suggests that the juice of bitter orange is unlikely to affect the pharmacokinetics of ciclosporin. However, the *animal* study suggests that a decoction of bitter orange may increase ciclosporin levels and therefore some caution may be warranted if patients taking ciclosporin wish to take bitter orange supplements. Careful consideration should be given to the risks of using the supplement; in patients receiving ciclosporin for severe indications, such as transplantation, it seems unlikely that the benefits will outweigh the risks. If concurrent use is undertaken then close monitoring of ciclosporin levels seems warranted.

1. Edwards DJ, Fitzsimmons ME, Schuetz EG, Yasuda K, Ducharme MP, Warbasse LH, Woster PM, Schuetz JD, Watkins P. 6',7'-dihydroxybergamottin in grapefruit juice and Seville orange juice: effects on cyclosporine disposition, enterocyte CYP3A4, and P-glycoprotein. *Clin Pharmacol Ther* (1999) 65, 237–44.
2. Hou Y-C, Hsui S-L, Tsao C-W, Wang Y-H, Chao P-DL. Acute intoxication of cyclosporin caused by coadministration of decoctions of the fruits of *Citrus aurantium* and the pericarps of *Citrus grandis*. *Planta Med* (2000) 66, 653–5.

Bitter orange + Dextromethorphan

Bitter orange juice increases the absorption of dextromethorphan.

Clinical evidence

In a study, 11 healthy subjects were given a single 30-mg dose of dextromethorphan hydrobromide at bedtime, followed by 200 mL of water or freshly-squeezed bitter orange juice. Measurement of the amount of dextromethorphan and its metabolites in the urine indicated that the bioavailability of dextromethorphan was increased by more than fourfold by bitter orange juice. Dextromethorphan levels were still raised 3 days later, indicating a sustained effect of the juice. The effects were similar to those of grapefruit juice.[1]

Experimental evidence

No relevant data found.

Mechanism

It was suggested that these fruit juices increased the absorption of dextromethorphan by inhibiting the cytochrome P450 isoenzyme CYP3A and P-glycoprotein in the gut wall, although the authors note that other transporter proteins may be involved. Note that dextromethorphan is commonly used as a probe substrate for CYP2D6; however, in this study, analysis of the metabolites demonstrated that the metabolism of dextromethorphan by CYP2D6 in the liver was not affected.[1] Similarly, a bitter orange supplement did not alter CYP2D6 activity as assessed by debrisoquine metabolism.[2]

Importance and management

While the study discussed shows a clear pharmacokinetic interaction, it has no direct clinical relevance to bitter orange supplements (it was used in the study as a comparator to assess the likely mechanisms of the effect of *grapefruit juice*). How the effects of the juice of bitter orange relate to the peel of bitter orange, which is one of the parts used medicinally, is unclear. However, note that the effects of *grapefruit juice* are thought to be in part related to 'contamination' with constituents of the peel, so some interaction might occur. Further study is needed.

Note that it is important not to extrapolate the interaction seen with the juice to other CYP2D6 substrates since inhibition of CYP2D6 was not thought to be the mechanism.

1. Di Marco MP, Edwards DJ, Wainer IW, Ducharme MP. The effect of grapefruit juice and seville orange juice on the pharmacokinetics of dextromethorphan: the role of gut CYP3A and P-glycoprotein. *Life Sci* (2002) 71, 1149–60.
2. Gurley BJ, Gardner SF, Hubbard MA, Williams DK, Gentry WB, Carrier J, Khan IA, Edwards DJ, Shah A. In vivo assessment of botanical supplementation on human cytochrome P450 phenotypes: *Citrus aurantium, Echinacea purpurea,* milk thistle, and saw palmetto. *Clin Pharmacol Ther* (2004) 76, 428–40.

Bitter orange + Felodipine

Bitter orange juice increased the exposure to felodipine in one study.

Clinical evidence

In a randomised study, 10 healthy subjects were given a single 10-mg dose of felodipine with 240 mL of bitter orange juice or orange juice (as a control). The AUC and maximum serum levels of felodipine were increased by 76% and 61%, respectively, when compared with orange juice. The effects were similar in magnitude to those of grapefruit juice.[1] The bitter orange juice was prepared by squeezing fresh fruit and freezing it until needed. It was analysed and found to contain the furanocoumarins bergapten, 6,7-dihydrobergamottin and bergamottin.

Experimental evidence

No relevant data found.

Mechanism

It was suggested that bitter orange juice inhibited the metabolism of felodipine (a drug that undergoes high first-pass metabolism) by the cytochrome P450 isoenzyme CYP3A4 in the intestine. This is similar to the effect seen with grapefruit juice, for which the furanocoumarins are known to be required for an interaction to occur.

Importance and management

There appears to be only one study investigating the effect of bitter orange on the pharmacokinetics of felodipine, and it relates to the juice, so has no direct clinical relevance to bitter orange supplements. The effects seen in the study were similar, although slightly smaller, than those seen with *grapefruit juice*. Felodipine should not be given with the juice or peel of *grapefruit juice* because of the increased effects on blood pressure that may result, and some extend this advice to other grapefruit products. See Grapefruit + Calcium-channel blockers, page 272. Extrapolating these suggestions to bitter orange implies that it may be prudent to be cautious if patients taking felodipine wish to take bitter orange products made from the peel. Conversely, a bitter orange supplement did not alter the metabolism of midazolam by CYP3A4, see below, so it is by no means clear that the effects of the juice can be extrapolated to the herbal products.

1. Malhotra S, Bailey DG, Paine MF, Watkins PB. Seville orange juice-felodipine interaction: comparison with dilute grapefruit juice and involvement of furocoumarins. *Clin Pharmacol Ther* (2001) 69, 14–23.

Bitter orange + Food

No interactions found. Note that bitter orange is commonly used as a flavouring, and in marmalade, but this is not expected to result in a high dietary intake.

Bitter orange + Herbal medicines; Caffeine-containing

For an interaction between bitter orange and the caffeine content of some herbs resulting in adverse cardiac effects, see Caffeine + Herbal medicines; Bitter orange, page 111.

B

Bitter orange + Indinavir

Bitter orange juice did not alter indinavir pharmacokinetics in one study.

Clinical evidence

In a study in 13 healthy subjects, about 200 mL of freshly-squeezed bitter orange juice had no effect on the pharmacokinetics of indinavir. In this study indinavir 800 mg was given every 8 hours for 4 doses; with water or bitter orange juice given with the last 2 doses. Grapefruit juice also had no effect.[1] The juices were determined to contain 6,7-dihydroxybergamottin at a concentration of about 40 micromol/L.[1]

Experimental evidence

No relevant data found.

Mechanism

No mechanism expected. The authors suggest that bitter orange juice does not affect the metabolism of indinavir by the cytochrome P450 isoenzyme CYP3A4 in the intestine, as has been seen with other drugs. See felodipine, page 77. This may be because the first-pass metabolism of indinavir is low.

Importance and management

Evidence regarding an interaction between indinavir and bitter orange comes from one study, which used the juice rather than the peel or flowers of bitter orange, which are the parts used medicinally. However, this information, and what is known about midazolam, page 77, suggests that bitter orange supplements are unlikely to affect the metabolism of indinavir.

1. Penzak SR, Acosta EP, Turner M, Edwards DJ, Hon YY, Desai HD, Jann MW. Effect of Seville orange juice and grapefruit juice on indinavir pharmacokinetics. *J Clin Pharmacol* (2002) 42, 1165–70.

Bitter orange + Midazolam

A bitter orange supplement did not alter the metabolism of midazolam in one study.

Clinical evidence

In a study[1] in 12 healthy subjects, bitter orange (*Citrus aurantium*) 350 mg, standardised to 4% synephrine, was given twice daily for 28 days with a single 8-mg oral dose of midazolam before and at the end of this period. The metabolism of midazolam was not affected by the concurrent use of bitter orange. The supplement was analysed and found to contain the stated amount of synephrine (equivalent to a daily dose of about 30 mg), and none of the furanocoumarin, 6,7-dihydroxybergamottin.

Experimental evidence

No relevant data found.

B

Mechanism

No mechanism expected. The bitter orange supplement used here may not have interacted because of a lack of furanocoumarins.[1] In the study here, the bitter orange supplement used did not contain the one furanocoumarin tested for, 6,7-dihydroxybergamottin.

Importance and management

Direct evidence about an interaction between midazolam and bitter orange appears to be limited to one clinical study. However, its findings suggest that this bitter orange supplement is unlikely to affect the metabolism of midazolam. Midazolam is used as a probe drug for CYP3A4 activity, and therefore these results also suggest that a pharmacokinetic interaction between bitter orange supplements and other substrates of CYP3A4 is unlikely. Bearing in mind the proposed mechanisms, it is possible that this applies only to supplements that do not contain furanocoumarins.

1. Gurley BJ, Gardner SF, Hubbard MA, Williams DK, Gentry WB, Carrier J, Khan IA, Edwards DJ, Shah A. In vivo assessment of botanical supplementation on human cytochrome P450 phenotypes: Citrus aurantium, Echinacea purpurea, milk thistle, and saw palmetto. *Clin Pharmacol Ther* (2004) 76, 428–40.

Black cohosh

Actaea racemosa L. (Ranunculaceae)

Synonym(s) and related species

Black snakeroot, Bugbane, Cimicifuga, Macrotys actaea, Rattleroot, Rattleweed.

Actaea monogyna Walter, *Cimicifuga racemosa* (L.) Nutt., *Macrotrys actaeoides* Rafin.

Note that the synonym Squaw root has been used for both Black cohosh and the unrelated Blue cohosh, page 85 (*Caulophyllum thalictroides*), and care should be taken to avoid any confusion between the two.

Pharmacopoeias

Black Cohosh (*PhEur 7.5, USP35–NF30 S1*); Black Cohosh Fluidextract (*USP35–NF30 S1*); Black Cohosh Tablets (*USP35–NF30 S1*); Powdered Black Cohosh (*USP35–NF30 S1*); Powdered Black Cohosh Extract (*USP35–NF30 S1*).

Constituents

The main active constituents are **triterpene glycosides** (to which it may be standardised) including actein, and several series of related compounds such as the cimicifugosides, the cimiracemosides, cimigenol and its derivatives, 26-deoxyactein and many others. Phenylpropanoid esters such as the cimiracemates A-D, isoferulic and ferulic acids and methylcaffeate are present, as are the quinolizidine alkaloids including cytisine and *N*-methylcytisine. The presence of the oestrogenic isoflavone formononetin is disputed.

Use and indications

Black cohosh is widely used to treat peri- and postmenopausal symptoms. It is also used as an antirheumatic, antitussive and sedative, and for the treatment of dysmenorrhoea and premenstrual disorders.

Pharmacokinetics

An *in vitro* study isolated six triterpene glycosides with inhibitory activity against the cytochrome P450 isoenzyme CYP3A4 from a powdered preparation of black cohosh.

However, the CYP3A4-inhibitory activity of these compounds was very weak,[1] and the clinical data using midazolam, page 81, as a probe drug for CYP3A4 suggests that this activity is not clinically relevant. Similarly, two clinical studies using debrisoquine as a probe substrate of CYP2D6 suggested that black cohosh (standardised to 0.2% or 2.5% triterpene glycosides) has no clinically relevant effect on this isoenzyme.[2,3]

Black cohosh root extract had no clinically relevant effects on the activity of CYP1A2 or CYP2E1, see caffeine, page 80, and chlorzoxazone, page 80, respectively.

Studies with digoxin, page 80, suggest that black cohosh does not affect P-glycoprotein activity.

Interactions overview

Black cohosh does not appear to interact with caffeine, chlorzoxazone, digoxin or midazolam. Limited data suggests that black cohosh may antagonise the activity of cisplatin. For a case report describing transplant rejection in a patient taking a supplement containing alfalfa and black cohosh, see Alfalfa + Immunosuppressants, page 22.

Interactions monographs

- Antineoplastics, page 80
- Caffeine, page 80
- Chlorzoxazone, page 80
- Digoxin, page 80
- Food, page 80
- Herbal medicines, page 81
- Midazolam, page 81
- Oestrogens or Oestrogen antagonists, page 81

1. Tsukamoto S, Aburatani M, Ohta T. Isolation of CYP3A4 Inhibitors from the Black Cohosh (*Cimicifuga racemosa*). *Evid Based Complement Alternat Med* (2005) 2, 223–6.
2. Gurley BJ, Gardner SF, Hubbard MA, Williams DK, Gentry WB, Khan IA, Shah A. In vivo effects of goldenseal, kava kava, black cohosh, and valerian on human cytochrome P450 1A2, 2D6, 2E1, and 3A4/5 phenotypes. *Clin Pharmacol Ther* (2005) 77, 415–26.
3. Gurley BJ, Swain A, Hubbard MA, Williams DK, Barone G, Hartsfield F, Tong Y, Carrier DJ, Cheboyina S, Battu SK. Clinical assessment of CYP2D6-mediated herb-drug interactions in humans: effects of milk thistle, black cohosh, goldenseal, kava kava, St. Johns wort, and *Echinacea*. *Mol Nutr Food Res* (2008) 52, 755–63.

B

Black cohosh + Antineoplastics

The interaction between black cohosh and antineoplastics is based on experimental evidence only.

Clinical evidence

No interactions found.

Experimental evidence

An *in vitro* study using mouse mammary tumour cells found that liquid extracts of black cohosh caused a small reduction in the cytotoxicity of **cisplatin**. The extracts were standardised to 3% triterpene glycosides and were given in doses of 100 times the expected human dose.[1]

Mechanism

Unknown.

Importance and management

Evidence is extremely limited. This data cannot reasonably be extrapolated to patients being treated with an antineoplastic regimen for breast cancer, because the dose of black cohosh used was much higher than the usual human dose, and the same study found that black cohosh may have *potentiated* the effects of other antineoplastics (such as **docetaxel** and **doxorubicin**).

Probably of more clinical relevance are the potential oestrogenic effects of black cohosh. Although these effects are not fully understood, they may have an important impact on the outcome of treatment for oestrogen-dependent breast cancer (see also Oestrogens or Oestrogen antagonists, page 81).

1. Rockwell S, Liu Y, Higgins SA. Alteration of the effects of cancer therapy agents on breast cancer cells by the herbal medicine black cohosh. *Breast Cancer Res Treat* (2005) 90, 233–9.

Black cohosh + Caffeine

Black cohosh does not significantly affect the pharmacokinetics of caffeine.

Clinical evidence

In a study in 12 healthy subjects, black cohosh root extract 1.09 g twice daily (standardised to 0.2% triterpene glycosides) for 28 days, did not significantly affect the pharmacokinetics of caffeine 100 mg.[1]

Experimental evidence

No relevant data found.

Mechanism

These studies investigated whether black cohosh had any effect on the cytochrome P450 isoenzyme CYP1A2 by which caffeine is metabolised.

Importance and management

Evidence appears to be limited to this one study, which suggests that black cohosh does not raise caffeine levels.

Caffeine is used as a probe drug for CYP1A2 activity, and therefore these results also suggest that a pharmacokinetic interaction between black cohosh and other CYP1A2 substrates is unlikely.

1. Gurley BJ, Gardner SF, Hubbard MA, Williams DK, Gentry WB, Khan IA, Shah A. In vivo effects of goldenseal, kava kava, black cohosh, and valerian on human cytochrome P450 1A2, 2D6, 2E1, and 3A4/5 phenotypes. *Clin Pharmacol Ther* (2005) 77, 415–26.

Black cohosh + Chlorzoxazone

Black cohosh does not significantly affect the pharmacokinetics of chlorzoxazone.

Clinical evidence

In a study in 12 healthy subjects, black cohosh root extract 1.09 g twice daily (standardised to 0.2% triterpene glycosides) for 28 days, did not significantly affect the pharmacokinetics of chlorzoxazone 250 mg.[1]

Experimental evidence

No relevant data found.

Mechanism

These studies investigated whether black cohosh had any effect on the cytochrome P450 isoenzyme CYP2E1 by which chlorzoxazone is metabolised.

Importance and management

Evidence appears to be limited to this one study, which suggests that black cohosh does not raise chlorzoxazone levels.

Chlorzoxazone is used as a probe drug for CYP2E1 activity, and therefore these results also suggest that a pharmacokinetic interaction between black cohosh and other CYP2E1 substrates is unlikely.

1. Gurley BJ, Gardner SF, Hubbard MA, Williams DK, Gentry WB, Khan IA, Shah A. In vivo effects of goldenseal, kava kava, black cohosh, and valerian on human cytochrome P450 1A2, 2D6, 2E1, and 3A4/5 phenotypes. *Clin Pharmacol Ther* (2005) 77, 415–26.

Black cohosh + Digoxin

A standardised black cohosh extract did not alter the pharmacokinetics of digoxin in one study.

Clinical evidence

In a randomised study, 16 healthy subjects were given a black cohosh extract 20 mg twice daily (standardised to 2.5% triterpene glycosides) for 14 days with a single 400-microgram oral dose of digoxin on day 14. There were no significant changes in the pharmacokinetics of digoxin, and no serious adverse effects were reported.[1]

Experimental evidence

No relevant data found.

Mechanism

Digoxin is used as a probe drug to assess the effects of other substances on P-glycoprotein.

Importance and management

This study suggests that black cohosh does not interact with digoxin, and is unlikely to interact with other drugs that are transported by P-glycoprotein.

1. Gurley BJ, Barone GW, Williams DK, Carrier J, Breen P, Yates CR, Song P-f, Hubbard MA, Tong Y, Cheboyina S. Effect of milk thistle (*Silybum marianum*) and black cohosh (*Cimicifuga racemosa*) supplementation on digoxin pharmacokinetics in humans. *Drug Metab Dispos* (2006) 34, 69–74.

Black cohosh + Food

No interactions found.

Black cohosh + Herbal medicines

No interactions found.

Black cohosh + Immunosuppressants

For a case report describing transplant rejection in a patient taking a supplement containing alfalfa and black cohosh, see Alfalfa + Immunosuppressants, page 22.

Black cohosh + Midazolam

Black cohosh does not affect the pharmacokinetics of midazolam.

Clinical evidence
In a study in 19 healthy subjects given black cohosh extract (standardised to triterpene glycosides 2.5%) 40 mg twice daily for 28 days with a single 8-mg oral dose of **midazolam** on day 28, there was no change in the pharmacokinetics of **midazolam**. In addition, black cohosh had no effect on the duration of **midazolam**-induced sleep.[1] Similarly, in another study in 12 non-smoking healthy subjects given black cohosh root extract (standardised to triterpene glycosides 0.2%) 1090 mg twice daily for 28 days, there was no significant change in the pharmacokinetics of a single 8-mg oral dose of **midazolam**.[2]

Experimental evidence
No relevant data found.

Mechanism
These studies investigated whether black cohosh had any effect on the cytochrome P450 isoenzyme CYP3A4 by which midazolam is metabolised.

Importance and management
Black cohosh is unlikely to interact with midazolam, and as midazolam is used as a probe drug for CYP3A4 activity, black cohosh is also unlikely to induce or inhibit the metabolism of other CYP3A4 substrates.

1. Gurley B, Hubbard MA, Williams DK, Thaden J, Tong Y, Gentry WB, Breen P, Carrier DJ, Cheboyina S. Assessing the clinical significance of botanical supplementation on human cytochrome P450 3A activity: comparison of a milk thistle and black cohosh product to rifampin and clarithromycin. *J Clin Pharmacol* (2006) 46, 201–13.
2. Gurley BJ, Gardner SF, Hubbard MA, Williams DK, Gentry WB, Khan IA, Shah A. *In vivo* effects of goldenseal, kava kava, black cohosh, and valerian on human cytochrome P450 1A2, 2D6, 2E1, and 3A4/5 phenotypes. *Clin Pharmacol Ther* (2005) 77, 415–26.

Black cohosh + Oestrogens or Oestrogen antagonists

Black cohosh contains oestrogenic compounds. This may result in additive effects with oestrogens or it may oppose the effects of oestrogens. Similarly, black cohosh may have additive effects with oestrogen antagonists or oppose the effects of oestrogen antagonists (e.g. tamoxifen). See Chinese angelica + Oestrogens or Oestrogen antagonists, page 146, for more information.

B

Black haw

Viburnum prunifolium L. (Caprifoliaceae)

Synonym(s) and related species

American sloe, Nanny bush, Stagbush.

Constituents

The stem and root bark of black haw contain **iridoid glycosides** based on penstemide, with patrinoside and others. They also contain **natural coumarins**, such as scopoletin and aesculetin, and **triterpenes**, including oleanolic and ursolic acids.

Use and indications

Traditionally black haw has been used as a uterine tonic, for preventing miscarriage in the latter stages of pregnancy, to reduce pain and bleeding after childbirth, and for dysmenorrhoea.

Pharmacokinetics

No relevant pharmacokinetic data found. For information on the pharmacokinetics of individual natural coumarins present in black haw, see under coumarins, page 356.

Interactions overview

No interactions with black haw found. Although black haw contains natural coumarins, the quantity of these constituents is not established, and therefore the propensity of black haw to interact with other drugs because of their presence is unclear. Consider coumarins, page 356, for further discussion of the interactions of coumarin-containing herbs.

Blessed thistle

Cnicus benedictus L. (Asteraceae)

Synonym(s) and related species

Cnicus, Holy thistle.

Carbeni benedicta (L.) Benth., *Carbenia benedicta* Adans., *Carduus benedictus* (L.) Thell., *Centaurea benedicta* (L.) L.

Not to be confused with Milk thistle, page 349, which is *Silybum marianum*.

Constituents

The major constituents of blessed thistle are lignans including arctigenin, trachelogenin, nortracheloside and their derivatives; and the sesquiterpene lactones cnicin and salonitenolide. There is also a small amount of essential oil composed of cinnamaldehyde, cuminaldehyde, citronellol and fenchone.

Use and indications

Traditionally, blessed thistle is used orally for digestive complaints and anorexia, and as an expectorant in catarrh. It is also applied topically as an anti-haemorrhagic and to aid wound healing.

Pharmacokinetics

No relevant pharmacokinetic data found.

Interactions overview

No interactions with blessed thistle found.

Bloodroot

Sanguinaria canadensis L. (Papaveraceae)

Synonym(s) and related species

Red Indian paint, Red puccoon, Red root, Sanguinaria.

Tetterwort has been used for both bloodroot and the unrelated Greater celandine, page 277 (*Chelidonium majus*), and care should be taken to avoid any confusion between the two.

Note that *Sanguinaria australis* Greene, *Sanguinaria canadensis* var. *rotundifolia* (Greene) Fedde and *Sanguinaria dilleniana* Greene have also been referred to as bloodroot.

Constituents

The rhizome contains isoquinoline alkaloids including **sanguinarine**, chelerythrine, sanguidaridine, oxysanguinaridine, **berberine**, coptisine, protopine and others.

Use and indications

Bloodroot is found in cough preparations and topical preparations used to treat skin infections and burns. Bloodroot extracts are also used as an antiplaque agent in some toothpastes and mouthwashes.

Pharmacokinetics

No relevant pharmacokinetic data found specifically for bloodroot, but see berberine, page 63, for more details on this constituent.

Interactions overview

No interactions with bloodroot found. However, for the interactions of one of its constituents, berberine, see under berberine, page 63.

Blue cohosh

Caulophyllum thalictroides (L.) Michx. (Berberidaceae)

Synonym(s) and related species

Caulophyllum, Papoose root.

Leontice thalictroides L.

Note that the synonym Squaw root has been used for both Blue cohosh and the unrelated Black cohosh, page 79 (*Cimicifuga racemosa*), and care should be taken to avoid any confusion between the two.

A sub-species, *Caulophyllum thalictroides* subsp. robustum (Maxim.) M.Hiroe. (*Caulophyllum robustum* Maxim.) contains similar constituents.

Constituents

Blue cohosh root contains alkaloids including anagyrine, baptifoline, methylcytisine (caullophylline), magnoflorine, thalictroidine, taspine, lupanine, *O*-acetylbaptifolin, caulophyllumine B, sparteine and others. Triterpene saponins based on hederagenin, including the caulosaponins and caulosides are also present.

Use and indications

Traditionally blue cohosh has been used specifically for menstrual disorders such as amenorrhoea, threatened miscarriage, and to facilitate childbirth, although there is no evidence of safety or efficacy during pregnancy. Of particular concern is the finding that some constituents of blue cohosh may have abortifacient, teratogenic and embryotoxic effects and therefore its use in pregnancy cannot be recommended. Blue cohosh has also been used traditionally to treat rheumatism, and to expel worms.

Pharmacokinetics

In an *in vitro* study, a methanolic extract of blue cohosh root did not inhibit the cytochrome P450 isoenzymes CYP3A4, CYP2D6, CYP1A2 or CYP2C19; however, an alkaloid fraction obtained from the methanolic extract did inhibit these isoenzymes. When the alkaloids were tested individually, methylcytisine had little effect, but caulophyllumine B, *O*-acetylbaptifolin, anagyrine and lupanine all had some inhibitory effect, particularly against CYP2C19, and there was greater inhibition when tested together.[1] The clinical relevance of these *in vitro* findings remains to be determined.

Interactions overview

No interactions with blue cohosh found.

1. Madgula VLM, Ali Z, Smillie T, Khan IA, Walker LA, Khan SI. Alkaloids and saponins as cytochrome P450 inhibitors from blue cohosh (*Caulophyllum thalictroides*) in an *in vitro* assay. *Planta Med* (2009) 75, 329–32.

Bogbean

Menyanthes trifoliata L. (Menyanthaceae)

Synonym(s) and related species

Buckbean, Marsh trefoil, Menyanthes.

The name Bog myrtle, most commonly used for *Myrica gale* (Myricaceae), has also been used for *Menyanthes trifoliata*.

Pharmacopoeias

Bogbean leaf (*BP 2012, PhEur 7.5*).

Constituents

Bogbean leaf contains the iridoids foliamenthin, 7′,8′-dihydrofoliamenthin, loganin, menthiafolin and sweroside; polyphenolics such as caffeic, chlorogenic, protocatechuic and ferulic acids, and **flavonoids**, including hyperin, kaempferol, quercetin, rutin and trifolioside. Other constituents include the pyridine alkaloids gentianine and gentianidine; triterpenes including lupeol, betulin, and betulinic acid; carotenoids, such as carotene and loliolide; and the **natural coumarins**, scopoletin and braylin.

Use and indications

Bogbean has been used for rheumatism, rheumatoid arthritis and other inflammatory diseases, and as a bitter tonic.

Pharmacokinetics

No relevant pharmacokinetic data for bogbean found, but see under flavonoids, page 213, for information on individual flavonoids present in bogbean.

Interactions overview

No interactions with bogbean found. Some have suggested that bogbean may interact with anticoagulants, presumably based on its natural coumarin content, but the coumarins present are not known to possess the structural requirements necessary for anticoagulant activity. For more information, see Natural coumarins + Warfarin and related drugs, page 360. For information on the interactions of individual flavonoids present in bogbean, see under flavonoids, page 213.

Boldo

Peumus boldus Molina (Monimiaceae)

Synonym(s) and related species

Boldus, Boldi folium, Peumus.

Boldea fragrans Gay, *Boldu boldus* Lyons.

Pharmacopoeias

Boldo leaf (*BP 2012, PhEur 7.5*); Boldo leaf dry extract (*BP 2012, PhEur 7.5*).

Constituents

Alkaloids are the main constituents of boldo leaf and these include **boldine**, isoboldine and dehydroboldine among others. Extracts may be standardised to contain a minimum of 0.1% of total alkaloids (dried extracts), or 0.5% of total alkaloids (aqueous extracts), expressed as **boldine** (*BP 2009, Ph Eur 6.4*). Boldo also contains **coumarin**. Volatile oils present include low levels of ascaridole, which is toxic: it is this constituent that has led to the suggestion the dose and duration of treatment with boldo should be restricted.

Use and indications

Boldo is used as an aid to slimming, although there is little or no evidence to support this use. It is also traditionally used for dyspepsia, digestive disturbances, constipation, gallstones, liver disorders, cystitis, and rheumatism. Recent research has shown boldine to be a potent antioxidant.

Pharmacokinetics

No relevant pharmacokinetic data found.

Interactions overview

There is little data regarding boldo. One case report suggests that it may interact with warfarin.

Interactions monographs

- Food, page 88
- Herbal medicines, page 88
- Warfarin and related drugs, page 88

Boldo + Food

No interactions found.

Boldo + Herbal medicines

No interactions found.

Boldo + Warfarin and related drugs

A report describes a woman taking warfarin whose INR rose modestly when she began to take boldo and fenugreek.

Clinical evidence

A woman taking **warfarin** for atrial fibrillation whose INR was normally within the range 2 to 3 had a modest rise in her INR to 3.4, apparently due to the use of 10 drops of boldo after meals and one capsule of **fenugreek** before meals. A week after stopping these two herbal medicines her INR had fallen to 2.6. When she restarted them, her INR rose to 3.1 after a week, and to 3.4 after 2 weeks. Her INR was later restabilised in her normal range, while continuing to take these two herbs, by reducing the **warfarin** dosage by 15%.[1] The patient had no undesirable reactions (e.g. bruising or bleeding).

Experimental evidence

No relevant data found.

Mechanism

The mechanism of this apparent interaction remains unknown, and it is not known whether both herbs or just one was responsible for what happened. Both boldo and fenugreek have been reported to contain natural coumarins, but it is unclear whether they have any anticoagulant activity. See natural coumarins, page 356 for more information on the interactions of coumarin-containing herbs.

Importance and management

Evidence is limited to one isolated case. Because of the many other factors influencing anticoagulant control, it is not possible to reliably ascribe a change in INR specifically to a drug interaction in a single case report without other supporting evidence. It may be better to advise patients to discuss the use of any herbal products they wish to try, and to increase monitoring if this is thought advisable. Cases of uneventful use should be reported, as they are as useful as possible cases of adverse effects.

1. Lambert JP, Cormier J. Potential interaction between warfarin and boldo-fenugreek. *Pharmacotherapy* (2001) 21, 509–12.

Boneset

Eupatorium perfoliatum L. (Asteraceae)

Synonym(s) and related species

Common boneset, Feverwort, Thoroughwort.

Eupatorium chapmanii Small.

Note that the name Boneset has also been used for *Symphytum officinale* (Boraginaceae) and the synonym Feverwort has also been used for Centaury (*Centaurium erythraea*), and it should also not be confused with Feverfew (*Tanacetum parthenium*).

Constituents

Sesquiterpene lactones present in boneset include helenalin, euperfolin, euperfolitin, eufoliatin, eufoliatorin and euperfolide. **Diterpenes** such as dendroidinic acid and hebeclinolide have been reported, as well as the phytosterols sitosterol and stigmasterol, and the **flavonoids** kaempferol, quercetin, and rutin. A series of immunostimulatory polysaccharides (mainly 4-*O*-methylglucuroxylans) have also been found.

Use and indications

Boneset is traditionally used for influenza, acute bronchitis, and nasopharyngeal catarrh.

Pharmacokinetics

No relevant pharmacokinetic data found. For information on the pharmacokinetics of individual flavonoids present in boneset, see under flavonoids, page 213.

Interactions overview

No interactions with boneset found. For information on the interactions of individual flavonoids present in boneset, see under flavonoids, page 213.

Boswellia

Boswellia serrata Roxb. (Burseraceae)

Synonym(s) and related species

The gum resin obtained from *Boswellia serrata* is known as Indian frankincense, Indian olibanum, or Salai guggul.

Not to be confused with other types of frankincense, which are extracted from other *Boswellia* species and used for their aromatic properties.

Pharmacopoeias

Indian Frankincense (*BP 2012, PhEur 7.5*).

Constituents

The main active constituents are the **boswellic acids**, which are lipophilic pentacyclic **triterpene** acids. The keto derivatives, 11-keto-beta-boswellic acid and acetyl-11-keto-beta-boswellic acid, are thought to be particularly potent anti-inflammatory agents. The volatile oils of *Boswellia serrata* characteristically contain the diterpenes isoincensole and isoincensole acetate.

Use and indications

Boswellia serrata is used for inflammatory disorders including collagenous colitis (a cause of chronic diarrhoea), peritumoural oedema, rheumatoid arthritis and other chronic conditions. There is mounting clinical evidence to support its use. The boswellic acids have immunomodulatory effects and are anti-inflammatory via a number of mechanisms.

Pharmacokinetics

In an *in vitro* study, aqueous extracts of *Boswellia serrata* did not inhibit common cytochrome P450 drug metabolising enzymes. However, the gum resin was found to have some inhibitory effects on the cytochrome P450 isoenzymes CYP1A2 and CYP2D6, and more potent inhibitory effects on CYP2C8, CYP2C9, CYP2C19 and CYP3A4, although the clinical relevance of these effects is not clear. It was established that cytochrome P450 inhibition occurs irrespective of boswellic acid content, and the constituents responsible for this effect are not removed during the manufacturing of a commercially available product tested in the study (*Boswellia serrata* extract, *H15*).[1] Another *in vitro* study found that keto derivatives of boswellic acids (from a *Boswellia serrata* extract, *H15*) inhibited P-glycoprotein in a dose-dependent manner. It was suggested that the low bioavailability of some of the boswellic acid derivatives means that boswellia is unlikely to have a clinically significant effect on P-glycoprotein at the blood-brain barrier, but that it may inhibit gastrointestinal P-glycoprotein at clinically relevant doses.[2]

Interactions overview

Some evidence suggests that food may beneficially increase the bioavailability of boswellic acids, but other interaction data is generally lacking. It seems possible that boswellia may interact with conventional drugs by inhibiting P-glycoprotein and/or cytochrome P450 isoenzymes (see *pharmacokinetics,* above), but the data is too sparse to make any meaningful predictions.

Interactions monographs

- Conventional drugs, page 91
- Food, page 91
- Herbal medicines, page 91

1. Frank A, Unger M. Analysis of frankincense from various *Boswellia* species with inhibitory activity on human drug metabolising cytochrome P450 enzymes using liquid chromatography mass spectrometry after automated on-line extraction. *J Chromatogr A* (2006) 1112, 255–62.
2. Weber C-C, Reising K, Müller WE, Schubert-Zsilavecz M, Abdel-Tawab M. Modulation of Pgp function by boswellic acids. *Planta Med* (2006) 72, 507–13.

Boswellia + Conventional drugs

No interactions found.

Boswellia + Food

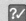

Food appears to beneficially increase the bioavailability of boswellic acids.

Clinical evidence
In a crossover study, 12 healthy subjects, after fasting for 10 hours, were given a single 786-mg dose of dry extract (gum resin) of *Boswellia serrata* (standardised to 55% boswellic acids) with a high-fat meal. The plasma AUCs of the boswellic acids were increased by between about 1.8- to 5-fold by the high-fat meal, and the maximum plasma levels were increased by up to 6-fold. No serious adverse events were noted.[1]

Experimental evidence
No relevant data found.

Mechanism
Unknown.

Importance and management
These data show that food intake can significantly increase the bioavailability of boswellic acids, and suggest that *Boswellia serrata* extracts should be taken with meals, as therapeutic levels may not be achieved when taken on an empty stomach.

1. Sterk V, Büchele B, Simmet T. Effect of food intake on the bioavailability of boswellic acids from a herbal preparation in healthy volunteers. *Planta Med* (2004) 70, 1155–60.

Boswellia + Herbal medicines

No interactions found.

B

Bromelain

Ananas comosus (L.) Merr. (Bromeliaceae)

Synonym(s) and related species

Ananase, Pineapple.

Pharmacopoeias

Bromelains (*BP 2012, PhEur 7.5*).

Constituents

Bromelain is a crude, aqueous extract obtained from the pineapple plant, containing a number of proteolytic enzymes. The most common type is stem bromelain, which is extracted from the stem of the pineapple.

Use and indications

There is some clinical evidence for anti-arthritic and anti-inflammatory effects of bromelain, and it is sometimes used as an alternative to NSAIDs. It is also used to treat bruising, swollen and painful joints, as an analgesic and wound-healing agent, and as a skin debrider for the treatment of burns. It possesses anti-oedematous, antithrombotic, fibrinolytic and immunomodulatory activities. It also has *in vivo* antitumoral activity. Bromelain can cause allergies in susceptible individuals.

Pharmacokinetics

No relevant pharmacokinetic data found.

Interactions overview

Although bromelain appears to increase the levels of some antibacterials, the clinical relevance of this is unknown.

Interactions monographs

- Amoxicillin, page 93
- Food, page 93
- Herbal medicines, page 93
- Tetracycline, page 93

Bromelain + Amoxicillin

Bromelain appears to moderately increase amoxicillin levels.

Clinical evidence

In a placebo-controlled study, subjects undergoing surgery were given a single 500-mg dose of amoxicillin and a single 80-mg dose of bromelain 3 hours before surgery. When compared with placebo, bromelain appeared to increase intra-operative amoxicillin levels in tissue, serum and skin samples. Amoxicillin levels were still higher in the bromelain group 3 hours after surgery.[1]

Experimental evidence

No relevant data found.

Mechanism

The reason for this interaction is unclear, but it is possible that bromelain increases the uptake of amoxicillin into tissues.

Importance and management

The clinical relevance of these increased levels is unclear, but as the increases were only moderate (serum concentration increased by 62%) it seems likely to be small.

1. Tinozzi S, Venegoni A. Effect of bromelain on serum and tissue levels of amoxycillin. *Drugs Exp Clin Res* (1978) 4, 39–44.

Bromelain + Food

No interactions found.

Bromelain + Herbal medicines

No interactions found.

Bromelain + Tetracycline

Bromelain appears to moderately increase tetracycline levels.

Clinical evidence

In a crossover study, 10 subjects were given tetracycline 500 mg, either alone, or with bromelain 80 mg. Bromelain appeared to increase the serum levels of tetracycline by up to about fourfold. Higher serum and urine levels were also found when the study was repeated using multiple doses of the two preparations.[1]

Experimental evidence

No relevant data found.

Mechanism

Unknown.

Importance and management

The clinical significance of this interaction is unclear but higher levels of tetracycline may result in an improved outcome, but also an increased risk of adverse effects.

1. Renzini VG, Varengo M. Die Resorption von Tetracycline in Gegenwart von Bromelinen bei oraler Application. *Arzneimittelforschung* (1972) 22, 410–412.

Broom

Cytisus scoparius (L.) Link. (Fabaceae)

Synonym(s) and related species

Besom, Broomtops, Hogweed, Irish broom, Scoparium, Scoparius, Scotch broom.

Sarothamnus scoparius (L.) Koch., *Sarothamnus vulgaris* Wim., *Spartium scoparium* L.

Not to be confused with Butcher's broom, page 104, which is *Ruscus aculeatus* L.

Constituents

The flowering tops contain **flavonoids** including scoparin (scoparoside), and the quinolizidine alkaloid sparteine. There is also a small amount of volatile oil present.

Use and indications

Broom is used traditionally for cardiac disorders including arrhythmias, and may also have diuretic and peripheral vasoconstrictor activity. Sparteine may have strong oxytocic activity.

Pharmacokinetics

No relevant pharmacokinetic data found. For information on the pharmacokinetics of individual flavonoids present in broom, see under flavonoids, page 213.

Interactions overview

No interactions with broom found. For information on the interactions of individual flavonoids present in broom, see under flavonoids, page 213.

Buchu

Agathosma betulina (P.J.Bergius) Pillans (Rutaceae)

Synonym(s) and related species

Bucco, Diosma, Round buchu, Short buchu.

Hartogia betulina Berg.

The use of *Agathosma crenulata* (L.) Pillans (commonly known as Oval buchu), and *Agathosma serratifolia* (Curt.) Spreeth (commonly known as Long buchu), is also allowed. *Agathosma* species were formerly known as *Barosma*.

Constituents

Buchu leaf contains a volatile oil composed of diosphenol (buchu camphor), pulegone, isopulegone, 8-mercapto-*p*-methan-3-one, menthone, isomenthone and others, and the **flavonoids** diosmin, hesperidin, rutin and others.

Use and indications

Buchu preparations are used as diuretics, for bladder and kidney infections, stomach aches, rheumatism, and coughs and colds.

Pharmacokinetics

No relevant pharmacokinetic data found. For information on the pharmacokinetics of individual flavonoids present in buchu, see under flavonoids, page 213.

Interactions overview

An isolated case of lithium toxicity has been reported in a patient who took a herbal diuretic containing buchu among other ingredients, see under Parsley + Lithium, page 364. For information on the interactions of individual flavonoids present in buchu, see under flavonoids, page 213.

Interactions monographs

- Food, page 96
- Herbal medicines, page 96

B

Buchu + Food

No interactions found.

Buchu + Herbal medicines

No interactions found.

Buchu + Lithium

For mention of a case of lithium toxicity in a woman who had been taking a non-prescription herbal diuretic containing corn silk, *Equisetum hyemale,* juniper, buchu, parsley and bearberry, all of which are believed to have diuretic actions, see under Parsley + Lithium, page 364.

Bugleweed

Lycopus virginicus Michx., and *Lycopus europaeus* L. (Lamiaceae)

Synonym(s) and related species

Sweet bugle, Water bugle.

Lycopus europaeus (European bugleweed) is known more commonly as Gypsywort, and both species are used interchangeably for medicinal purposes.

Constituents

Neither species has been exhaustively investigated chemically. The main constituents of *Lycopus virginicus* are polyphenolics, such as **flavonoids** based on apigenin and luteolin. Caffeic, chlorogenic, ellagic and rosmarinic acids, and isopimarane **diterpenoids** are also present. *Lycopus europaeus* contains similar **flavonoids** and **diterpenoids**.

Use and indications

Both species of *Lycopus* are used to treat mild hyperthyroidism and its associated symptoms, and there is some supporting experimental and clinical evidence for this. They are also used as sedatives and cough remedies.

Pharmacokinetics

No relevant pharmacokinetic data found specifically for bugleweed, but see flavonoids, page 213, for more detail on individual flavonoids present in the herb.

Interactions overview

No interactions with bugleweed found, but see flavonoids, page 213, for the interactions of individual flavonoids present in bugleweed.

Bupleurum

Bupleurum falcatum L. (Apiaceae)

Synonym(s) and related species

Chai hui, Hare's ear, Saiko.

Bupleurum chinense DC., *Bupleurum fruticosum* L., and *Bupleurum scorzonerifolium* Willd., are also used medicinally, but *Bupleurum longiradiatum* Turcz. is toxic and should be avoided.

Constituents

Bupleurum root contains a range of triterpene saponins, the **saikosaponins** and saikogenins. There are also polysaccharides known as bupleurans, and phytosterols present.

Use and indications

Bupleurum is used for chills, fevers, as an anti-inflammatory and general tonic. It is also used for liver disorders and menstrual and uterine problems. Anti-inflammatory and immune-modulatory activities have been demonstrated in laboratory tests. Bupleurum root is an ingredient of a number of traditional Chinese and Japanese herbal medicines such as Sho-saiko-to (Xiao Chai Hu Tang) and Sairei-to, see the table Constituents of some Chinese herbal medicines containing bupleurum, see below. These Chinese medicines are used for similar reasons as bupleurum.

Pharmacokinetics

Saikosaponin a, and its monoglycoside and aglycones, were detectable in the plasma of *rats* when saikosaponin a was given orally. Absorption of other derivatives, structural isomers and their monoglycosides and aglycones, which were formed in the gastrointestinal tract, depended on food intake. The pharmacological effects of saikosaponin a given orally may therefore differ depending on conditions of the gastrointestinal tract.[1]

Saikosaponins a, c and d are metabolised extensively in the *mouse* gut to at least 27 metabolites in a complex manner. A study in *rats* to determine which of these metabolites are active, based on their corticosterone-secreting activity, found that saikosaponin a, saikosaponin d and their intestinal metabolites prosaikogenin F and prosaikogenin G showed strong activity. Other compounds and metabolites showed varying degrees of biological activity so the degree to which metabolism occurs is likely to affect pharmacological and clinical effects.[2]

Interactions overview

No interactions with bupleurum alone found. Bupleurum is the main constituent of a number of Chinese herbal medicines, such as sho-saiko-to, saiko-ka-ryukotsu-borei-to and sairei-to. Sho-saiko-to slightly inhibits caffeine metabolism. Neither sho-saiko-to nor sairei-to appear to alter the pharmacokinetics of ofloxacin. Sho-saiko-to may modestly affect the absorption of tolbutamide but blood-glucose levels appear to be minimally affected.

Constituents of some Chinese herbal medicines containing bupleurum

	Proportion of herbs in the medicines (parts)		
	Sho-saiko-to[1]	Sairei-to[2]	Saiko-ka-ryukotsu-borei-to[3]
Alismatis (rhizome)		4	
Atractylodes lancea (rhizome)		3	
Bupleuri (root)	7	7	5
Cinnamomi (cortex), see *Cassia*, page 133		1.5	3
Fossilia Ossis Mastodi			2.5
Ginseng (root), see *Ginseng*, page 251	3	3	2.5
Glycyrrhizae (root), see *Liquorice*, page 329	2	2	
Hoelen		3	3
Ostreae testa			2.5
Pinelliae (tuber)	5	5	4
Polyporus		3	
Scutellariae (root), see *Baical skullcap*, page 55	3	3	2.5
Zizyphi (fruit)	3	3	2.5
Zingiberis (rhizome), see *Ginger*, page 235	1	1	1

1. Ohnishi N, Okada K, Yoshioka M, Kuroda K, Nagasawa K, Takara K, Yokoyama T. Studies on interactions between traditional herbal and western medicines. V. Effects of Sho-saiko-to (Xiao-Cai-hu-Tang) on the pharmacokinetics of carbamazepine in rats. *Biol Pharm Bull* (2002) 25, 1461–6.
2. Fujitsuka N, Goto K, Takeda S, Aburada M. The diuretic effect of Sairei-to is mediated by nitric oxide production in pentobarbital-anesthetized rats. *J Pharmacol Sci* (2004) 94, 185–91.
3. Ohnishi N, Nakasako S, Okada K, Umehara S, Takara K, Nagasawa K, Yoshioka M, Kuroda K, Yokoyama T. Studies on interactions between traditional herbal and western medicines. IV: lack of pharmacokinetic interactions between Saiko-ka-ryukotsu-borei-to and carbamazepine in rats. *Eur J Drug Metab Pharmacokinet* (2001) 26, 129–35.

Interactions monographs

- Caffeine, page 99
- Carbamazepine, page 99
- Food, page 99
- Herbal medicines, page 99
- Ofloxacin, page 99
- Tolbutamide, page 99

1. Fujiwara K, Ogihara Y. Pharmacological effects of oral saikosaponin a may differ depending on conditions of the gastrointestinal tract. *Life Sci* (1986) 39, 297–301.
2. Nose M, Amagaya S, Ogihara Y. Corticosterone secretion-inducing activity of saikosaponin metabolites formed in the alimentary tract. *Chem Pharm Bull (Tokyo)* (1989) 37, 2736–40.

Bupleurum + Caffeine

Sho-saiko-to slightly reduces the metabolism of caffeine, but this is not expected to be clinically important.

Evidence, mechanism, importance and management

In a study, 26 healthy subjects were given **sho-saiko-to** 2.5 g twice daily for 5 days, with a single 150-mg dose of caffeine on days 1 and 5. By assessing the metabolites of caffeine, it was estimated that **sho-saiko-to** caused a 16% inhibition of the cytochrome P450 isoenzyme CYP1A2.[1]

Note that **sho-saiko-to** is a Chinese herbal medicine of which bupleurum is one of 7 constituents. Any modest effect is therefore not directly attributable to bupleurum alone. See the table Constituents of some Chinese herbal medicines containing bupleurum, page 98.

The clinical significance of this finding is unclear, but is likely to be small, although further studies would help to clarify this.

1. Saruwatari J, Nakagawa K, Shindo J, Nachi S, Echizen H, Ishizaki T. The in-vivo effects of sho-saiko-to, a traditional Chinese herbal medicine, on two cytochrome P450 enzymes (1A2 and 3A) and xanthine oxidase in man. *J Pharm Pharmacol* (2003) 55, 1553–9.

Bupleurum + Carbamazepine

Any interaction between sho-saiko-to and saiko-ka-ryukotsu-borei-to and carbamazepine is based on experimental evidence only.

Clinical evidence

No interactions found.

Experimental evidence

A study in *rats* found that the simultaneous administration of single doses of carbamazepine and **sho-saiko-to**, of which bupleurum is one of 7 constituents, delayed and lowered (by 45%) the maximum plasma concentrations of carbamazepine. The AUC of carbamazepine-epoxide was also modestly reduced by 32%, but there was no change in elimination rate. In a related study *rats* were pretreated with **sho-saiko-to** daily for 2 weeks, and then 24 hours later, given a single dose of carbamazepine. Although this tended to reduce the maximum carbamazepine level, there was no significant effect on the pharmacokinetics of carbamazepine.[1]

In a further study, *rats* treated with **saiko-ka-ryukotsu-borei-to** (of which bupleurum is one of 10 constituents) either as a single dose or as a daily dose for one week, experienced no change in the pharmacokinetics of a single dose of carbamazepine given 3 hours after the Chinese herbal medicine.[2]

Mechanism

It was found that sho-saiko-to delayed gastric emptying, and so it could delay absorption of carbamazepine when given at the same time. It is unlikely that sho-saiko-to or saiko-ka-ryukotsu-borei-to affect the metabolism of carbamazepine.[1]

Importance and management

While information regarding an interaction between bupleurum and carbamazepine is limited to experimental data using Chinese herbal medicines of which bupleurum is only one constituent, they provide some reassurance that these products are unlikely to affect the metabolism of carbamazepine. The first product, sho-saiko-to, slightly delayed the absorption of carbamazepine, especially when given simultaneously, but since the extent of absorption was not significantly altered, this is unlikely to be clinically relevant. Other main constituents of the products also seem unlikely to interact. See

the table, Constituents of some Chinese herbal medicines containing bupleurum, page 98, for a list of the constituents.

1. Ohnishi N, Okada K, Yoshioka M, Kuroda K, Nagasawa K, Takara K, Yokoyama T. Studies on interactions between traditional herbal and western medicines. V. Effects of Sho-saiko-to (Xiao-Cai-hu-Tang) on the pharmacokinetics of carbamazepine in rats. *Biol Pharm Bull* (2002) 25, 1461–6.
2. Ohnishi N, Nakagawa S, Okada K, Umehara S, Takara K, Nagasawa K, Yoshioka M, Kuroda K, Yokoyama T. Studies on interactions between traditional herbal and western medicines. IV: lack of pharmacokinetic interactions between Saiko-ka-ryukotsu-borei-to and carbamazepine in rats. *Eur J Drug Metab Pharmacokinet* (2001) 26, 129–35.

Bupleurum + Food

There is limited experimental evidence from *animal* studies that the absorption of saikosaponins (the main constituents of bupleurum) might differ when taken with food as opposed to the fasting state, see pharmacokinetics, page 98.

Bupleurum + Herbal medicines

No interactions found.

Bupleurum + Ofloxacin

Sho-saiko-to and Sairei-to do not appear to affect the pharmacokinetics of ofloxacin.

Evidence, mechanism, importance and management

The bioavailability and urinary recovery of a single 200-mg oral dose of ofloxacin were not significantly altered in 7 healthy subjects by two Chinese herbal medicines, **Sho-saiko-to** and **Sairei-to**, which contain bupleurum as the main ingredient.[1] There would therefore seem to be no reason for avoiding concurrent use. Information about other quinolones is lacking. Other main constituents of these products also seem unlikely to interact with ofloxacin. See the table Constituents of some Chinese herbal medicines containing bupleurum, page 98, for a list of the constituents.

1. Hasegawa T, Yamaki K, Nadai M, Muraoka I, Wang L, Takagi K, Nabeshima T. Lack of effect of Chinese medicines on bioavailability of ofloxacin in healthy volunteers. *Int J Clin Pharmacol Ther* (1994) 32, 57–61.

Bupleurum + Tolbutamide

The interaction between sho-saiko-to and tolbutamide is based on experimental evidence only.

Clinical evidence

No interactions found.

Experimental evidence

In a single-dose study in *rats,* the initial rate of gastrointestinal absorption of tolbutamide 50 mg/kg given as a suspension was modestly increased when given simultaneously with **sho-saiko-to**, of which bupleurum is one of 7 constituents. The maximum tolbutamide level was slightly increased, by 21%; however, there was no difference in tolbutamide AUC, clearance or elimination half-life. The decrease in plasma glucose levels was greater during the first hour and less in the period 5 to 8 hours after both drugs were given, when compared with tolbutamide alone. However, at a maximum, **sho-saiko-to** increased the blood-glucose-lowering effects of tolbutamide by about 11%, which was not statistically significant.[1]

In contrast, in a similar study, the absorption of tolbutamide was delayed when tolbutamide was given 1 hour after the **sho-saiko-to**.[2]

Mechanism

In vitro studies have shown that sho-saiko-to increases the permeability of jejunal epithelial cells to tolbutamide, which could explain the increased absorption in the first study.[1] Conversely, the second study found that sho-saiko-to decreases gastric emptying rate (see also Bupleurum + Carbamazepine, page 99), which could explain the finding of delayed absorption.

Importance and management

These preliminary studies provide some evidence that sho-saiko-to might alter the absorption of tolbutamide, but because of their contrasting findings (one showed an increased rate of absorption and one showed delayed absorption), no conclusions can be drawn. The rate of absorption of tolbutamide is probably unlikely to alter clinical efficacy. This suggestion is supported by the finding of minimal changes in blood-glucose levels in one of the studies. Note that any interaction cannot be directly attributed to bupleurum as sho-saiko-to contains a number of constituents, any one of which may be responsible for the effects seen. See the table, Constituents of some Chinese herbal medicines containing bupleurum, page 98, for a list of the constituents.

1. Nishimura N, Naora K, Hirano H, Iwamoto K. Effects of Sho-saiko-to on the pharmacokinetics and pharmacodynamics of tolbutamide in rats. *J Pharm Pharmacol* (1998) 50, 231–6.
2. Nishimura N, Naora K, Hirano H, Iwamoto K. Effects of *Sho-saiko-to* (*Xiao Chai Hu Tang*), a Chinese traditional medicine, on the gastric function and absorption of tolbutamide in rats. *Yakugaku Zasshi* (2001) 121, 153–9.

Burdock

Arctium lappa L. (Asteraceae)

Synonym(s) and related species

Bardane, Beggar's buttons, Great burr, Greater burdock, Lappa, Thorny burr.

Arctium majus Bernh.

Constituents

Burdock leaves and root contain lignans including arctigenin, arctiin and matairesinol, and various sesquiterpenes including arctiol, β-eudesmol, petasitolone, fukinanolide, and fukinone are also found in the leaves. The seeds contain a series of lappaols.

Use and indications

Burdock is usually taken for skin conditions and as an anti-inflammatory and antiseptic agent. The lignans have anti-proliferative effects *in vitro* and arctiin has oestrogenic effects.

Pharmacokinetics

An *in vitro* study suggests that ethanol extracts of burdock root were only weak inhibitors of the cytochrome P450 isoenzymes CYP3A4 and CYP2C19.[1]

Interactions overview

No interactions with burdock found.

1. Scott IM, Leduc RI, Burt AJ, Marles RJ, Arnason JT, Foster BC. The inhibition of human cytochrome P450 by ethanol extracts of North American botanicals. *Pharm Biol* (2006) 44, 315–27.

Burnet

Sanguisorba officinalis L. (Rosaceae)

Synonym(s) and related species

Garden burnet, Greater burnet, Sanguisorba.

Sanguisorba polygama F. Nyl.

Formerly known as *Poterium officinale* A. Gray.

Not to be confused with Burnet saxifrage (Lesser burnet).

Pharmacopoeias

Greater Burnet Root (*BP 2012*); Sanguisorba Root (*PhEur 7.5*).

Constituents

The root and rhizome contain the sanguisorbins A-E, which are **triterpene glycosides** based on ursolic acid. Burnet also contains ziyu glycosides I and II and related compounds, and numerous polyphenolics, including a series of ellagitannins known as sanguiins H1 to H6, and tannins.

Use and indications

Burnet has antimicrobial, antihaemorrhagic and astringent properties, which have been demonstrated experimentally but not clinically. Burnet is used to treat infections, ulcerative colitis and diarrhoea, burns and inflammatory conditions, and to stem excessive bleeding.

Pharmacokinetics

No relevant pharmacokinetic data found.

Interactions overview

Evidence of any interactions with burnet is sparse, but one *animal* study suggests that it may reduce the bioavailability of ciprofloxacin.

Interactions monographs

- Food, page 103
- Herbal medicines, page 103
- Quinolones, page 103

Burnet + Food

No interactions found.

Burnet + Herbal medicines

No interactions found.

Burnet + Quinolones

The interaction between burnet and quinolones is based on experimental evidence only.

Clinical evidence
No interactions found.

Experimental evidence
In an *animal* study, *rats* were given a burnet powdered extract 2 g/kg and **ciprofloxacin**, both orally. The maximum levels and AUC of **ciprofloxacin** were found to be reduced by 94% and 78%, respectively, by the herb.[1]

Mechanism
It is possible that the metal cations present in the extract may have formed chelates with ciprofloxacin thereby reducing its bioavailability.[1]

Importance and management
Evidence is limited, but it appears that burnet may reduce the bioavailability of ciprofloxacin. Burnet was given in a clinically relevant dose, and the reduction in levels seen would therefore be expected to result in a clinically relevant reduction in the efficacy of ciprofloxacin. With other chelation interactions with ciprofloxacin, separating administration to reduce the admixture of the two drugs in the gut minimises any interaction. In general, ciprofloxacin should be taken at least 2 hours before, and not less than 4 to 6 hours after, drugs that it may chelate with, such as those containing polyvalent cations; this would appear to include burnet. The majority of the quinolone antibacterials are known to interact with polyvalent cations in the same way as ciprofloxacin, and it would therefore seem prudent to extend this caution to all of them.

1. Zhu M, Wong PYK, Li RC. Influence of *Sanguisorba officinalis*, a mineral-rich plant drug, on the pharmacokinetics of ciprofloxacin in the rat. *J Antimicrob Chemother* (1999) 44, 125–8.

B

Butcher's broom

Ruscus aculeatus L. (Ruscaceae)

Synonym(s) and related species

Box holly, Kneeholm, Kneeholy, Pettigree, Sweet broom.

Not to be confused with Broom, page 94, which is *Cystisus scoparius* (L.) Link.

Pharmacopoeias

Butcher's broom (*BP 2012, PhEur 7.5*).

Constituents

Butcher's broom contains a range of saponins, including ruscine and ruscoside, which are based on **ruscogenin** (1-beta-hydroxydiosgenin) and neoruscogenin. The related glycosides aculeosides A and B are present in the root. Extracts are often standardised to contain a minimum of 1% of total sapogenins, expressed as **ruscogenins** (*BP 2012, Ph Eur 7.5*).

Use and indications

Butcher's broom is used mainly for chronic venous insufficiency, in varicose veins and haemorrhoids, for example. It is also reported to be anti-inflammatory and to reduce vascular permeability. There are a number of studies in support of these uses.

Pharmacokinetics

No relevant pharmacokinetic data found.

Interactions overview

No interactions with Butcher's broom found.

Butterbur

Petasites hybridus (L.) G.Gaertn., B.Mey. & Scherb. (Asteraceae)

Synonym(s) and related species

Blatterdock, Bog rhubarb, Bogshorns, Butterdock, Butterfly dock, Capdockin, Flapperdock, Umbrella plant.

Petasites officinalis Moench, *Petasites ovatus* Hill, *Petasites sabaudus* Beauv., *Petasites vulgaris* Desf., *Tussilago petasites*.

Constituents

All parts of the plant contain sesquiterpenes and unsaturated pyrrolizidine alkaloids. During storage, some of the constituents undergo transformation, thus the final composition of herbal preparations may vary depending on storage conditions.

Use and indications

Butterbur is used for the prophylaxis of migraines, and as an anti-spasmodic agent for chronic cough or asthma. It has also been used successfully for the prevention of gastric ulcers, and to treat patients with irritable bladder and urinary tract spasms. It has also been used as a diuretic and cardiotonic. The pyrrolizidine alkaloids are hepatotoxic, and have been shown to be carcinogenic and mutagenic in pre-clinical studies.

Pharmacokinetics

No relevant pharmacokinetic data found.

Interactions overview

Many theoretical interactions have been proposed, including the suggestion that butterbur may interact through effects on histamine H_1 receptors. A post-marketing surveillance study identified over 50 patients taking antihistamines and a butterbur extract (Ze 339), without evidence of either a beneficial or an adverse effect.[1]

1. Käufeler R, Polasek W, Brattström A, Koetter U. Efficacy and safety of butterbur herbal extract Ze 339 in seasonal allergic rhinitis: postmarketing surveillance study. *Adv Therapy* (2006) 23, 373–84.

Caffeine

The information in this monograph relates specifically to caffeine. A number of herbs contain significant amounts of caffeine, to which many of their pharmacological effects may be attributed. Their caffeine content also means that they have the potential to interact in the same way as caffeine itself, although note that the levels of caffeine are likely to vary widely between different herbal medicines and products. Also, remember that the herbs often contain active constituents other than caffeine, and the reader should refer to the relevant herb for other potential interactions.

Types, sources and related compounds

Caffeine (1,3,7-trimethylxanthine, coffeinum, guaranine, koffein, methyltheobromine, théine) is found in significant quantities, in approximate order of highest to lowest levels: in the seeds of guarana, page 279, the leaves of tea, page 463, the nuts of cola, page 165, the beans of coffee, page 162, the leaves of maté, page 339, and the beans of cocoa, page 156. Cocoa contains significant amounts of the xanthine theobromine. Note that rooibos, page 409, and honeybush, page 291, which are commonly used as a tea-like beverage, do not contain caffeine.

Pharmacopoeias

Caffeine (*BP 2012, PhEur 7.5, USP35−NF30 S1*); Caffeine Hydrate (*BP 2012*); Caffeine Monohydrate (*PhEur 7.5*); Caffeine Citrate Injection (*USP35−NF30 S1*); Caffeine Citrate Oral Solution (*USP35−NF30 S1*).

Conventional drugs that are known inhibitors of the metabolism of caffeine[1]

Drug	Reduction in clearance	Prolongation of half-life	Recommendation
Potent inhibitors (clearance reduced by two-thirds or more)			
Clinafloxacin	84%		An increase in the stimulant and adverse effects of caffeine
Enoxacin	78 to 83%		(headache, jitteriness, restlessness, insomnia) may be
Fluvoxamine	80%	6- to 10-fold	possible in susceptible patients if they continue to consume
Idrocilamide	90%	8.4-fold (from 7 hours to 59 hours)	large amounts of caffeine. They should be warned to reduce their caffeine intake if problems develop.
Oral psoralens	69%	10.2-fold (from 5.6 hours to 57 hours)	
Moderate inhibitors (clearance reduced by one- to two-thirds)			
Artemisinin	35%		Unlikely to be clinically important in most patients, but
Cimetidine	31 to 42%	45 to 96%	bear this interaction in mind if the adverse effects of
Ciprofloxacin	33 to 53%		caffeine (headache, jitteriness, restlessness, insomnia)
Disulfiram	30 to 50%		become troublesome.
Mexiletine	48 to 57%	75% (from 4 hours to 7 hours)	
Norfloxacin	35%		
Pefloxacin	47%		
Pipemidic acid	63%		
Propafenone	35%	54% (from 3.82 hours to 5.9 hours)	
Tiabendazole	66%	140%	
Minor inhibitors (clearance reduced by 20 to 30%)			
Combined oral contraceptives		from 4 to 6 hours up to 8 to 11 hours	No action necessary.
Fluconazole	25%		Increases of this magnitude are very unlikely to cause any
Grapefruit juice (1.2 litres)	23%	31%	clinically relevant effects.
HRT	29%		
Terbinafine	21%	31%	
Verapamil	25%	26% (from 4.6 hours to 5.8 hours)	

1. Compiled from Baxter K (ed), Stockley's Drug Interactions. [online] London: Pharmaceutical Press <http://www.medicinescomplete.com> (accessed on 15/09/10).

Uses and administration

Extracts of caffeine-containing herbs have been used medicinally for their stimulant and diuretic effects, and may be promoted as slimming aids and for boosting energy. As foods, caffeine and caffeine-containing herbs are very widely consumed as beverages and, on regular consumption, partial tolerance develops to many of the pharmacological effects of caffeine. Caffeine may induce dependence, and stopping intake abruptly can cause withdrawal. Consumption of excess caffeine can cause anxiety, sleeplessness, tremor, palpitations and headache.

Caffeine-containing beverages have been associated with various health benefits in epidemiological studies, which have been attributed to other constituents such as the flavonoids.

Pharmacokinetics

Caffeine is predominantly metabolised via N3-demethylation to paraxanthine by the cytochrome P450 isoenzyme CYP1A2, and is often used as a probe substrate to study the effect of medicines and other substances on this isoenzyme.[1,2] The elimination half-life of caffeine is about 3 to 6 hours in adults, and is about twofold longer in people who do not regularly consume caffeine.[2]

In one study, the pharmacokinetics and subjective effects of caffeine were similar whether consumed as coffee or cola.[3]

(a) Inhibitors of caffeine metabolism

There are a number of medicines that are known inhibitors of the cytochrome P450 isoenzyme CYP1A2, by which caffeine is metabolised, and these are listed in the table Drugs and herbs affecting or metabolised by the cytochrome P450 isoenzyme CYP1A2, page 7. Very few of these actually have warnings regarding their use with caffeine-containing beverages, so warnings are unlikely to be needed with concurrent use of caffeine, including that from caffeine-containing herbs. Nevertheless, if an increase in the stimulant and adverse effects of caffeine is seen in patients taking these drugs (most likely with those drugs that are potent inhibitors of caffeine metabolism), then the intake of caffeine should be reduced.

(b) Inducers of caffeine metabolism

Barbiturates and phenytoin induce CYP1A2, by which caffeine is metabolised, and they would therefore be expected to reduce the effects of caffeine, including that from caffeine-containing herbs.

Interactions overview

Caffeine is a vasopressor and stimulant and it therefore may antagonise the effects of antihypertensive drugs and benzodiazepines. It may also cause serious adverse effects if used with other drugs or herbs with similar effects, such as phenylpropanolamine, bitter orange and ephedra, page 202. Caffeine may interfere with the dexamethasone suppression test, and the efficacy of adenosine and dipyridamole used during cardiac imaging. Caffeine may raise clozapine levels, and has modest effects on the absorption of some analgesics, but probably does not significantly affect lithium levels.

Note that caffeine is known to have diuretic effects. Therefore caffeine-containing herbs may produce a degree of additive diuresis with other diuretics.

The inhibitory effects of conventional drugs on caffeine metabolism, and management recommendations, are summarised in the table Conventional drugs that are known inhibitors of the metabolism of caffeine, page 106.

Interactions monographs

- Adenosine, page 108
- Antihypertensives, page 108
- Aspirin or Diclofenac, page 108
- Benzodiazepines and related drugs, page 109
- Clozapine, page 109
- Dexamethasone, page 110
- Dipyridamole, page 110
- Food; Caffeine-containing, page 110
- Herbal medicines; Bitter orange, page 111
- Lithium, page 111
- Nicotine, page 112
- Paracetamol (Acetaminophen), page 112
- Phenylpropanolamine, page 113
- Theophylline, page 113

1. Sharma A, Pilote S, Bélanger PM, Arsenault M, Hamelin BA. A convenient five-drug cocktail for the assessment of major drug metabolizing enzymes: a pilot study. *Br J Clin Pharmacol* (2004) 58, 288–97.
2. Carrillo JA, Benitez J. Clinically significant pharmacokinetic interactions between dietary caffeine and medications. *Clin Pharmacokinet* (2000) 39, 127–53.
3. Liguori A, Hughes JR, Grass JA. Absorption and subjective effects of caffeine from coffee, cola and capsules. *Pharmacol Biochem Behav* (1997) 58, 721–6.

Caffeine + Adenosine

Caffeine can inhibit the effects of adenosine infusions used in conjunction with radionuclide myocardial imaging.

Clinical evidence

Studies in healthy subjects, on the way xanthine drugs such as caffeine possibly interact with adenosine, have shown that caffeine reduces the increased heart rate and the changes in blood pressure caused by infusions of adenosine,[1,2] and attenuates adenosine-induced vasodilatation.[3]

Experimental evidence

Because of the quality of the clinical evidence (controlled pharmacokinetic studies), experimental data have not been sought.

Mechanism

Caffeine has an antagonistic effect on adenosine receptors.[4] It appears to have opposite effects on the circulatory system: caffeine causes vasoconstriction whereas adenosine infusions generally cause vasodilatation.[1] Consequently their concurrent use is likely to result in opposing effects.

Importance and management

Caffeine can inhibit the effects of adenosine infusions used in conjunction with radionuclide myocardial imaging. The manufacturers of adenosine state that xanthine-containing drinks (tea, coffee, chocolate, cola drinks, etc.) should be avoided for at least 12 hours before imaging,[5] and this should be taken to include caffeine-containing herbs or supplements. In a recent study in 70 patients, measurable caffeine serum levels were found in 74% of patients after 12 hours of self-reported abstention from caffeine-containing products. Patients with caffeine serum levels of at least 2.9 mg/L had significantly fewer stress symptoms (chest tightness, chest pain, headache, dyspnoea, nausea, dizziness) than those with lower serum levels. The authors suggest that a 12-hour abstention from caffeine-containing products may be insufficient, and could result in false-negative results.[6]

There appears to be no direct evidence regarding the effects of caffeine on the use of adenosine boluses to revert supraventricular tachycardias.

1. Smits P, Schouten J, Thien T. Cardiovascular effects of two xanthines and the relation to adenosine antagonism. *Clin Pharmacol Ther* (1989) 45, 593–9.
2. Smits P, Boekema P, De Abreu R, Thien T, van't Laar A. Evidence for an antagonism between caffeine and adenosine in the human cardiovascular system. *J Cardiovasc Pharmacol* (1987) 10, 136–43.
3. Smits P, Lenders JWM, Thien T. Caffeine and theophylline attenuate adenosine-induced vasodilation in humans. *Clin Pharmacol Ther* (1990) 48, 410–418.
4. Fredholm BB. On the mechanism of action of theophylline and caffeine. *Acta Med Scand* (1985) 217, 149–53.
5. Adenoscan (Adenosine). Sanofi-Aventis. UK Summary of product characteristics, September 2005.
6. Majd-Ardekani J, Clowes P, Menash-Bonsu V, Nunan TO. Time for abstention from caffeine before an adenosine myocardial perfusion scan. *Nucl Med Commun* (2000) 21, 361–4.

Caffeine + Antihypertensives

Caffeine can cause a modest increase in blood pressure, which may be relevant to patients with hypertension.

Clinical evidence

In a number of studies, acute caffeine intake, comparable to the usual population intake, was found to cause an increase of about 5 to 15 mmHg in systolic blood pressure and 5 to 10 mmHg in diastolic blood pressure.[1] However, studies of repeated intake generally showed more modest increases. For example, in one meta-analysis of 7 caffeine studies (median daily dose 410 mg), the increase in blood pressure was about 4/2 mmHg.[2]

It is unclear whether the form caffeine is taken in makes a difference. For example, one meta-analysis found that blood pressure increases after coffee intake were lower than that from pure caffeine.[2] See also Coffee + Antihypertensives, page 163.

There appears to be very little evidence on the effect of caffeine intake on blood pressure in treated hypertensive patients. One single-dose study suggested that coffee attenuated the effects of beta blockers. See Coffee + Antihypertensives, page 163.

Experimental evidence

Because of the extensive clinical evidence available, experimental data have not been sought.

Mechanism

Caffeine is an antagonist of endogenous adenosine, and as a result of this, it causes vasoconstriction, which raises blood pressure. It has been suggested that tolerance develops to this effect. However, it is possible that near complete sensitivity to caffeine is restored each day after an "overnight fast", and that during the day the increase in blood pressure seen with each caffeine intake is proportionally less than the previous intake, until a plateau is reached (available adenosine receptors are saturated).[1] This is possible with moderate intake of caffeine (3 to 4 drinks of caffeine-containing beverages).[1]

Importance and management

An extensively studied interaction. Some consider that the modest increase in blood pressure of about 4/2 mmHg with caffeine intake has little relevance, whereas others consider it important.[1] Bear in mind the possibility that caffeine intake from herbal supplements might modestly increase blood pressure, and that this might not be advisable in patients with poorly controlled hypertension.

Interactions of antihypertensive drugs and specific caffeine-containing herbal medicines are discussed in the individual monographs. Consider also Cocoa + Antihypertensives, page 157, Coffee + Antihypertensives, page 163, Cola + Antihypertensives, page 166, and Tea + Antihypertensives, page 464.

1. James JE. Critical review of dietary caffeine and blood pressure: a relationship that should be taken more seriously. *Psychosom Med* (2004) 66, 63–71.
2. Noordzij M, Uiterwaal CS, Arends LR, Kok FJ, Grobbee DE, Geleijnse JM. Blood pressure response to chronic intake of coffee and caffeine: a meta-analysis of randomized controlled trials. *J Hypertens* (2005) 23, 921–8.

Caffeine + Aspirin or Diclofenac

Caffeine modestly increases the bioavailability, rate of absorption and plasma levels of aspirin. Adding caffeine to diclofenac may improve its efficacy in the treatment of migraine.

Evidence, mechanism, importance and management

In a study in healthy subjects, caffeine citrate 120 mg given with a single 650-mg dose of aspirin increased the AUC of aspirin by 36%, increased its maximum plasma levels by 15%, and increased its rate of absorption by 30%.[1] This confirms the results of previous studies.[2,3] These studies suggest that caffeine could modestly potentiate the efficacy of aspirin by a pharmacokinetic mechanism. However, a meta analysis of randomised, controlled studies concluded that there was no therapeutic advantage in adding caffeine to analgesic doses of aspirin in patients experiencing postoperative pain.[4]

In a placebo-controlled study in patients with migraine, there was a non-significant trend towards improved analgesic effect in patients receiving diclofenac softgel capsules 100 mg and caffeine 100 mg, when compared with diclofenac alone, although the sample size was too small to provide meaningful results.[5]

Caffeine is commonly included in aspirin preparations as an analgesic adjuvant, but its overall value still remains unclear. It seems unlikely that caffeine-containing herbs will have any detrimental effect as a result of their caffeine content if they are given with these analgesics. However, note that if aspirin or diclofenac formulated with caffeine is given there is the potential for caffeine adverse effects (such as headache, jitteriness, restlessness, and insomnia). Caffeine intake should be reduced if this occurs.

1. Thithapandha A. Effect of caffeine on the bioavailability and pharmacokinetics of aspirin. *J Med Assoc Thai* (1989) 72, 562–6.
2. Yoovathaworn KC, Sriwatanakul K, Thithapandha A. Influence of caffeine on aspirin pharmacokinetics. *Eur J Drug Metab Pharmacokinet* (1986) 11, 71–6.
3. Dahanukar SA, Pohujani S, Sheth UK. Bioavailability of aspirin and interacting influence of caffeine. *Indian J Med Res* (1978) 68, 844–8.
4. Zhang WY, Po ALW. Do codeine and caffeine enhance the analgesic effect of aspirin?– A systematic overview. *J Clin Pharm Ther* (1997) 22, 79–97.
5. Peroutka SJ, Lyon JA, Swarbrick J, Lipton RB, Kolodner K, Goldstein J. Efficacy of diclofenac sodium softgel 100 mg with or without caffeine 100 mg in migraine without aura: a randomized, double-blind, crossover study. *Headache* (2004) 44, 136–41.

Caffeine + Benzodiazepines and related drugs

Caffeine appears to antagonise the effects of the benzodiazepines (mainly sedative effects, but possibly also anxiolytic effects). The effects of zopiclone might be similarly antagonised.

Clinical evidence

(a) Benzodiazepines

In a study in healthy subjects, a single 250-mg or 500-mg dose of caffeine (added to decaffeinated coffee) counteracted the drowsiness and mental slowness induced by a single 10- to 20-mg dose of **diazepam**.[1] The same or a similar study has been reported elsewhere.[2] Conversely, in a study in 6 healthy subjects, the concurrent use of caffeine 6 mg/kg and **diazepam** 300 micrograms/kg did not antagonise the effects of either drug; however, caffeine caused a minor 22% reduction in **diazepam** levels.[3] In one study the sedative effects of **midazolam**[4] were moderately antagonised by caffeine 250 mg but not 125 mg, and there is also some evidence to suggest that caffeine and **clonazepam**[5] or **triazolam**[6] have mutually opposing effects.

No pharmacokinetic interaction appears to occur between caffeine and **midazolam**[7] or **alprazolam**.[8]

(b) Non-benzodiazepine hypnotics

Zopiclone 7.5 mg appears to counter the stimulant effects of caffeine 300 mg more easily than caffeine counters the sedative effects of **zopiclone**.[6] In one study, no pharmacokinetic interaction occurred between **zolpidem** 10 mg and caffeine 300 mg (added to decaffeinated coffee), and the hypnotic effects of **zolpidem** were unchanged.[9] However, a placebo-controlled, crossover study in 12 healthy subjects found that caffeine 250 mg and 500 mg reversed the pharmacodynamic effects (such as sedation, reduced tapping speed, reaction time) caused by **zolpidem** 7.5 mg. Even though the pharmacodynamic effects of **zolpidem** were reduced by caffeine, the AUC of **zolpidem** was increased by 41% by caffeine 500 mg, when compared with placebo.[10]

Experimental evidence

Because of the extensive clinical evidence available, experimental data have not been sought.

Mechanism

Uncertain. One suggestion is that caffeine can block adenosine receptors, leading to CNS stimulation, which would antagonise the CNS depressant effects of the benzodiazepines.[11] Another suggestion is that the stimulant effects of caffeine and the sedative effects of benzodiazepines are simply antagonistic.

Importance and management

The evidence suggests that caffeine, particularly at higher doses, at least partially reduces the sedative and performance-impairing effects of benzodiazepines and related hypnotics. This would appear

to be a disadvantage at night, but may possibly be useful the next morning, although caffeine should not be considered an antidote to the residual effects of these hypnotics. The extent to which caffeine reduces the anxiolytic effects of the benzodiazepines remains uncertain (it needs assessment), but be alert for reduced benzodiazepine effects if both are used.

1. Mattila MJ, Nuotto E. Caffeine and theophylline counteract diazepam effects in man. *Med Biol* (1983) 61, 337–43.
2. Mattila MJ, Palva E, Savolainen K. Caffeine antagonizes diazepam effects in man. *Med Biol* (1982) 60, 121–3.
3. Ghoneim MM, Hinrichs JV, Chiang C-K, Loke WH. Pharmacokinetic and pharmacodynamic interactions between caffeine and diazepam. *J Clin Psychopharmacol* (1986) 6, 75–80.
4. Mattila MJ, Vainio P, Nurminen M-L, Vanakoski J, Seppälä T. Midazolam 12 mg is moderately counteracted by 250 mg caffeine in man. *Int J Clin Pharmacol Ther* (2000) 38, 581–7.
5. Gaillard J-M, Sovilla J-Y, Blois R. The effects of clonazepam, caffeine and the combination of the two drugs on human sleep. In: Koella WP, Rüther E, Schulz H, eds. Sleep '84 New York: Gustav Fischer Verlag; 1985. p. 314–15.
6. Mattila ME, Mattila MJ, Nuotto E. Caffeine moderately antagonizes the effects of triazolam and zopiclone on the psychomotor performance of healthy subjects. *Pharmacol Toxicol* (1992) 70, 286–9.
7. Blakey GE, Lockton JA, Perrett J, Norwood P, Russell M, Aherne Z, Plume J. Pharmacokinetic and pharmacodynamic assessment of a five-probe metabolic cocktail for CYPs 1A2, 3A4, 2C9, 2D6 and 2E1. *Br J Clin Pharmacol* (2004) 57, 162–9.
8. Schmider J, Brockmöller J, Arold G, Bauer S, Roots I. Simultaneous assessment of CYP3A4 and CYP1A2 activity in vivo with alprazolam and caffeine. *Pharmacogenetics* (1999) 9, 725–34.
9. Mattila MJ, Nurminen M-L, Vainio P, Vanakoski J. Zolpidem 10 mg given at daytime is not antagonized by 300 mg caffeine in man. *Eur J Clin Pharmacol* (1998) 54, 421–5.
10. Cysneiros RM, Farkas D, Harmatz JS, von Moltke LL, Greenblatt DJ. Pharmacokinetic and pharmacodynamic interactions between zolpidem and caffeine. *Clin Pharmacol Ther* (2007) 82, 54–62.
11. Niemand D, Martinell S, Arvidsson S, Svedmyr N, Ekström-Jodal B. Aminophylline inhibition of diazepam sedation: is adenosine blockade of GABA-receptors the mechanism? *Lancet* (1984) i, 463–4.

Caffeine + Clozapine

Caffeine minimally increases clozapine exposure, but greater increases in clozapine concentrations and adverse effects have been reported in individual cases.

Clinical evidence

In a controlled study in 12 healthy subjects,[1] caffeine 400 mg to 1 g daily increased the AUC and decreased the clearance of a single 12.5-mg dose of clozapine by 19% and 14%, respectively. In a crossover study, 6 coffee-drinking patients taking clozapine were given decaffeinated or caffeine-containing instant coffee for 7 days. The plasma levels of clozapine were 26% higher while the patients were taking caffeine-containing coffee.[2] However, a greater interaction was reported in a previous study in 7 patients, which found that clozapine concentrations *decreased* by 47% when the subjects *avoided* caffeine for 5 days, and increased again when caffeine consumption was resumed.[3]

A patient taking clozapine for schizophrenia had an exacerbation of his psychotic symptoms, which was attributed to caffeinated **coffee** (5 to 10 cups daily). The problem resolved when the patient stopped drinking caffeine-containing beverages. He had previously not had any problems when consuming caffeine coffee while taking haloperidol 30 mg and procyclidine 30 mg daily.[4]

A 31-year-old woman taking clozapine 550 mg daily developed increased daytime sleepiness, sialorrhoea and withdrawn behaviour after taking caffeine (about 1.2 g daily, as drinks and tablets). Her plasma clozapine concentrations fell from 1.5 micrograms/mL to 0.63 micrograms/mL when her caffeine intake was stopped.[5]

A 66-year-old woman taking clozapine 300 mg daily developed supraventricular tachycardia (180 bpm) when she was given 500 mg of intravenous caffeine sodium benzoate to increase seizure length during an ECT session. Verapamil was needed to correct the arrhythmia. Before taking clozapine she had received caffeine sodium benzoate in doses of up to 1 g during ECT sessions without problems.[6]

Experimental evidence

Because of the quality of the clinical evidence (controlled pharmacokinetic studies), experimental data have not been sought.

Mechanism

Unknown. Both caffeine and clozapine are sensitive substrates of CYP1A2, but neither are known to be inhibitors of this isoenzyme. In the best designed study, the effects were negligible.

Importance and management

The pharmacokinetic interaction between caffeine and clozapine would appear to be established. Based on the data from one of the studies[3] the UK manufacturer of clozapine states that clozapine dose adjustments might be necessary if patients change their intake of caffeine-containing beverages.[7] However, the data from the controlled studies[2,1] suggests that the effect of caffeine on clozapine pharmacokinetics is negligible to slight at most, and is unlikely to be of clinical relevance in most patients, particularly if clozapine serum concentrations are established and well monitored, and if caffeine intake remains fairly stable and moderate. Possible exceptions are if large doses of caffeine are given during ECT treatment or if for some other reason the caffeine intake suddenly increases or decreases markedly. Patients taking clozapine should probably avoid taking large doses of caffeine-containing herbal preparations.

1. Hägg S, Spigset O, Mjörndal T, Dahlqvist R. Effect of caffeine on clozapine pharmacokinetics in healthy volunteers. *Br J Clin Pharmacol* (2000) 49, 59–63.
2. Raaska K, Raitasuo V, Laitila J, Neuvonen PJ. Effect of caffeine-containing versus decaffeinated coffee on serum clozapine concentrations in hospitalised patients. *Basic Clin Pharmacol Toxicol* (2004) 94, 13–18.
3. Carrillo JA, Herraiz AG, Ramos SI, Benitez J. Effects of caffeine withdrawal from the diet on the metabolism of clozapine in schizophrenic patients. *J Clin Psychopharmacol* (1998) 18, 311–16.
4. Vainer JL, Chouinard G. Interaction between caffeine and clozapine. *J Clin Psychopharmacol* (1994) 14, 284–5.
5. Odom-White A, de Leon J. Clozapine levels and caffeine. *J Clin Psychiatry* (1996) 57, 175–6.
6. Beale MD, Pritchett JT, Kellner CH. Supraventricular tachycardia in a patient receiving ECT, clozapine, and caffeine. *Convuls Ther* (1994) 10, 228–31.
7. Clozaril (Clozapine). Novartis Pharmaceuticals UK Ltd. UK Summary of product characteristics, March 2012.

Caffeine + Dexamethasone

The results of the dexamethasone suppression test can be falsified by the acute ingestion of caffeine, but chronic caffeine use does not appear to have an effect.

Evidence, mechanism, importance and management

In one study, 22 healthy subjects and 6 depressed patients were given a single 480-mg dose of caffeine or placebo at 2 pm following a single 1-mg dose of dexamethasone given at 11 pm the previous evening. Caffeine significantly increased the cortisol levels following the dexamethasone dose; cortisol levels taken at 4 pm were about 146 nanomol/L with caffeine, compared with about 64 nanomol/L with placebo.[1] Thus the equivalent of about 4 to 5 cups of coffee may effectively falsify the results of the dexamethasone suppression test. However, in a study in 121 patients with depression, there was no correlation between chronic low to high intake of caffeine (6 mg to 2.3 g daily) and cortisol levels at 8 am, 4 pm or 11 pm on the day after a 1-mg dose of dexamethasone given at 11 pm the previous evening. It was suggested that chronic caffeine intake produces tolerance to the effects of acute caffeine on the hypothalamic-pituitary adrenal (HPA) axis.[2]

Therefore, it appears that the results of the dexamethasone suppression test can be falsified by the acute ingestion of a high dose of caffeine but that chronic caffeine use does not appear to have an effect. As chronic intake of caffeine does not appear to affect this test, it does not seem necessary to advise patients to stop any regular intake of caffeine-containing herbs. However, bear the potential for an interaction with caffeine-containing herbs in mind should an unexpected response occur.

1. Uhde TW, Bierer LM, Post RM. Caffeine-induced escape from dexamethasone suppression. *Arch Gen Psychiatry* (1985) 42, 737–8.
2. Lee MA, Flegel P, Cameron OG, Greden JF. Chronic caffeine consumption and the dexamethasone suppression test in depression. *Psychiatry Res* (1988) 24, 61–5.

Caffeine + Dipyridamole

Caffeine may interfere with dipyridamole–thallium-201 myocardial scintigraphy tests.

Clinical evidence

Intravenous caffeine 4 mg/kg (roughly equivalent to 2 to 3 cups of coffee), given before dipyridamole–thallium-201 myocardial scintigraphy, caused a false-negative test result in a patient.[1] A further study in 8 healthy subjects confirmed that caffeine inhibits the haemodynamic response to an infusion of dipyridamole.[2]

Experimental evidence

Because of the quality of the clinical evidence (controlled pharmacokinetic studies), experimental data have not been sought.

Mechanism

It appears that caffeine might antagonise some of the haemodynamic effects of dipyridamole because it acts as a competitive antagonist of adenosine (an endogenous vasodilator involved in the action of dipyridamole).[1,2]

Importance and management

An interaction between caffeine and intravenous dipyridamole is established. Patients should abstain from caffeine from any source, including caffeine-containing herbal preparations, caffeine-containing beverages (tea, coffee, chocolate, cocoa, cola) and caffeine-containing analgesics,[1–3] for 24 hours[2,4] before dipyridamole testing. If during the test the haemodynamic response is low (e.g. no increase in heart rate) the presence of caffeine should be suspected.[2] Patients should be specifically prompted to discuss less obvious potential sources such as herbal medicines.

1. Smits P, Aengevaeren WRM, Corstens FHM, Thien T. Caffeine reduces dipyridamole-induced myocardial ischemia. *J Nucl Med* (1989) 30, 1723–6.
2. Smits P, Straatman C, Pijpers E, Thien T. Dose-dependent inhibition of the hemodynamic response to dipyridamole by caffeine. *Clin Pharmacol Ther* (1991) 50, 529–37.
3. Picano E. Safety of intravenous high-dose dipyridamole echocardiography. *Am J Cardiol* (1992) 70, 252–8.
4. Persantin Ampoules (Dipyridamole). Boehringer Ingelheim Ltd. UK Summary of product characteristics, July 2004.

Caffeine + Food; Caffeine-containing

The effects of dietary caffeine and caffeine from herbal medicines will be additive.

Evidence, mechanism, importance and management

The effects of caffeine from herbal medicines will be additive with that from caffeine-containing food (chocolate) and beverages (tea, coffee, cola). People who want to take a caffeine-containing herbal medicine should be aware of the possible increased risk of adverse effects, including headache, jitteriness, restlessness, and insomnia. They should be warned to reduce their caffeine intake if problems develop.

Caffeine + Herbal medicines; Bitter orange

The use of caffeine with bitter orange may lead to severe cardiac adverse effects. Bitter orange does not affect the metabolism of caffeine.

Clinical evidence

(a) Cardiovascular effects

Some evidence suggests that the haemodynamic effects of caffeine and bitter orange are synergistic. In a single-dose, crossover study in 10 healthy subjects, a combination product containing, amongst other ingredients bitter orange, maté, and cocoa (*Xenadrine* EFX), and a single-ingredient bitter orange product (*Advantra* Z, containing synephrine 15.6 mg), both increased heart rate (by 16.7 bpm and 11.4 bpm, respectively) when compared with placebo. *Xenadrine* EFX increased blood pressure (by 9.6/9.1 mmHg), whereas *Advantra* Z did not. *Advantra* Z contained eight times the dose of synephrine, a sympathomimetic alkaloid found in bitter orange, than *Xenadrine* (46.9 mg versus 5.5 mg), so it was concluded that caffeine and other stimulants in the *Xenadrine* must be acting synergistically with the synephrine.[1] Although this study did not find that bitter orange alone increased blood pressure, another single-dose study, in 13 healthy subjects, found that bitter orange (*Nature's Way Bitter Orange*, containing synephrine about 54 mg per capsule) increased systolic blood pressure by 7.3 mmHg and the heart rate by 4.2 bpm, when compared with placebo.[2]

Case reports suggest that this increase in blood pressure might be clinically important. For example, an ischaemic stroke occurred in a 38-year-old man with no relevant past medical history or risk factors for stroke or cardiovascular disease. The stroke occurred one week after he started taking one to two capsules per day of *Stacker 2 Ephedra Free* weight-loss supplement, which contains bitter orange, and cola nut extract, giving synephrine 6 mg and caffeine 200 mg per capsule.[3] Furthermore, from January 1998 to February 2004, Health Canada received 16 reports of serious cardiovascular adverse reactions (including tachycardia, cardiac arrest, ventricular fibrillation, transient collapse and blackout) that were suspected of being associated with bitter orange or supplements containing synephrine. In 15 of these cases, the product also contained caffeine: in 8 of those 15 cases the product also contained ephedra.[4] Note that the use of caffeine with ephedra has been associated with severe cardiac effects, see Ephedra + Caffeine, page 202. From March 2004 to October 2006, Health Canada noted an additional 21 reports, of which 15 were cardiovascular adverse effects.[5] One of these included a report of a myocardial infarction in a patient possibly precipitated by the use of a weight-loss supplement containing bitter orange 300 mg as well as guarananine and green tea (*Edita's Skinny Pill*).[6]

(b) Pharmacokinetics

In a study in 12 healthy subjects,[7] bitter orange 350 mg, standardised to synephrine 4%, was given twice daily for 28 days with a single 100-mg dose of caffeine before and at the end of the treatment with bitter orange. The metabolism of caffeine was not affected by the concurrent use of bitter orange, which suggests that bitter orange is unlikely to affect the metabolism of other drugs that are substrates of the cytochrome P450 isoenzymes CYP1A2.

Experimental evidence

Because of the extensive clinical evidence available, experimental data have not been sought.

Mechanism

Uncertain. Synephrine, a sympathetic alpha-adrenergic agonist, is one of the main constituents found in bitter orange, although the concentrations will vary between products. Simple additive hypertensive effects would seem to be part of the explanation. The

effects of caffeine may compound the effects of these sympathomimetic drugs on the cardiovascular and central nervous systems by blocking adenosine receptors (causing vasoconstriction) and also augmenting the release of catecholamines.

Importance and management

Fairly well established interactions. These studies and case reports illustrate the potential hazards of using caffeine-containing herbs with bitter orange, even in healthy individuals, therefore these preparations may pose a serious health risk to some users. The risk may be affected by individual susceptibility, the additive stimulant effects of caffeine, the variability in the contents of alkaloids in non-prescription dietary supplements, or pre-existing medical conditions,[8] including compromised cardiac function.[9] Ephedra was banned by the FDA in the US in 2004 and as a result of this, many manufacturers replaced it with bitter orange which contains a similar sympathomimetic alkaloid, synephrine. Evidence shows that these products are no safer than ephedra products when used in a similar way. It would be prudent to avoid using herbal products containing combinations of bitter orange and caffeine or caffeine-containing herbs, especially in patients with risk factors such as heart conditions, diabetes, thyroid disease, or hypertension.

1. Haller CA, Benowitz NL, Jacob P. Hemodynamic effects of ephedra-free weight-loss supplements in humans. *Am J Med* (2005) 118, 998–1003.
2. Bui LT, Nguyen DT, Ambrose PJ. Blood pressure and heart rate effects following a single dose of bitter orange. *Ann Pharmacother* (2006) 40, 53–7.
3. Bouchard NC, Howland MA, Greller HA, Hoffman RS, Nelson LS. Ischemic stroke associated with use of an ephedra-free dietary supplement containing synephrine. *Mayo Clin Proc* (2005) 80, 541–5.
4. Jordan S, Murty M, Pilon K. Products containing bitter orange or synephrine: suspected cardiovascular adverse reactions. *Can Adverse React News* (2004) 14, 3–4.
5. Jack S, Desjarlais-Renaud T, Pilon K. Bitter orange or synephrine: update on cardiovascular adverse reactions. *Can Adverse React News* (2007) 17, 2–3.
6. Nykamp DL, Fackih MN, Compton AL. Possible association of acute lateral-wall myocardial infarction and bitter orange supplement. *Ann Pharmacother* (2004) 38, 812–15.
7. Gurley BJ, Gardner SF, Hubbard MA, Williams DK, Gentry WB, Carrier J, Khan IA, Edwards DJ, Shah A. In vivo assessment of botanical supplementation on human cytochrome P450 phenotypes: *Citrus aurantium*, *Echinacea purpurea*, milk thistle, and saw palmetto. *Clin Pharmacol Ther* (2004) 76, 428–40.
8. Haller CA, Benowitz NL. Adverse cardiovascular and central nervous system events associated with dietary supplements containing ephedra alkaloids. *N Engl J Med* (2000) 343, 1833–8.
9. Haller CA, Jacob P, Benowitz NL. Enhanced stimulant and metabolic effects of combined ephedrine and caffeine. *Clin Pharmacol Ther* (2004) 75, 259–73.

Caffeine + Lithium

The heavy consumption of caffeine-containing drinks can cause a small reduction in serum lithium levels.

Clinical evidence

In a single-dose study in 8 healthy subjects, lithium carbonate 300 mg was given 14 hours before placebo or caffeine 400 mg (given orally as 100 mg every 30 minutes). Caffeine was associated with a 29% greater decrease in plasma lithium concentration (measured one hour after completion of caffeine administration), and a 32% increase in the urinary excretion of lithium.[1] Similarly, a study in 11 psychiatric patients taking lithium 600 mg to 1.2 g daily who were also regular coffee drinkers (4 to 8 cups daily containing 70 to 120 mg of caffeine per cup), serum lithium levels *rose* by an average of 24% when the coffee was *withdrawn*, although the levels of 3 patients did not change.[2] In addition, an early single-dose study found that the intake of xanthines such as caffeine caused an increase in lithium excretion.[3]

These findings are consistent with a report of 2 patients with lithium-induced tremors that were aggravated when they stopped drinking large amounts of coffee. One of the patients had a 50% rise in lithium levels, and required a reduction in the dose of lithium from 1.5 g daily to 1.2 g daily.[4]

In contrast, a single-dose study did not find any changes in the urinary clearance of lithium in 6 subjects given caffeine 200 mg four times daily compared with a caffeine-free control period.[5]

C

C

Experimental evidence

Because of the quality of the clinical evidence (controlled pharmacokinetic studies), experimental data have not been sought.

Mechanism

It is not clear exactly how caffeine affects the excretion of lithium by the renal tubules, but other xanthines have a similar effect. It has been suggested that caffeine acts as an antagonist at renal adenosine A_1 receptors, inhibiting the proximal tubular reabsorption of lithium, but maintaining the glomerular filtration rate.[1]

Importance and management

The weight of evidence suggests that, although there is no need for those taking lithium to avoid caffeine (from caffeine-containing herbs, coffee, tea, cola drinks etc.), they should not exceed a moderate intake. In cases where a reduction in caffeine intake is desirable, it should be withdrawn cautiously. This is particularly important in those whose serum lithium levels are already high, because of the risk of toxicity. When caffeine is withdrawn it might be necessary to reduce the dose of lithium. In addition, remember that there is a caffeine-withdrawal syndrome (headache and fatigue being the major symptoms) that might worsen some of the major psychiatric disorders (such as affective and schizophrenic disorders),[2] for which lithium is given. Although the evidence is for caffeine and coffee, all caffeine-containing herbal medicines would be expected to have similar effects, and similar caution should be applied to their use.

1. Shirley DG, Walter SJ, Noormohamed FH. Natriuretic effect of caffeine: assessment of segmental sodium reabsorption in humans. *Clin Sci* (2002) 103, 461–6.
2. Mester R, Toren P, Mizrachi I, Wolmer L, Karni N, Weizman A. Caffeine withdrawal increases lithium blood levels. *Biol Psychiatry* (1995) 37, 348–50.
3. Thomsen K, Schou M. Renal lithium excretion in man. *Am J Physiol* (1968) 215, 823–7.
4. Jefferson JW. Lithium tremor and caffeine intake: two cases of drinking less and shaking more. *J Clin Psychiatry* (1988) 49, 72–3.
5. Bikin D, Conrad KA, Mayersohn M. Lack of influence of caffeine and aspirin on lithium elimination. *Clin Res* (1982) 30, 249A.

Caffeine + Nicotine

Caffeine may increase some of the stimulant effects of nicotine, and under certain conditions, some of the cardiovascular effects of caffeine and nicotine may be additive. Caffeine appears to cause a small, if any, rise in nicotine levels.

Clinical evidence

In a placebo-controlled study in 10 healthy non-smokers, a single 250-mg intravenous dose of caffeine increased resting blood pressure and reduced heart rate, whereas nicotine 4 mg (given as chewing gum) increased both blood pressure and heart rate. When given together, the effects of caffeine with nicotine on blood pressure were additive, resulting in an increase in blood pressure of 10.8/12.4 mmHg. However, during physical and mental stress (standing up and mental arithmetic, respectively) the cardiovascular effects were less than additive.[1] In contrast, a study in 20 non-smokers found that nicotine 2 or 4 mg (given as a chewing gum) increased heart rate and subjective effects but these effects were not influenced by oral caffeine 75 or 150 mg.[2]

In a study in 21 smokers who regularly drank one to six cups of coffee daily, a 50-mg tablet of caffeine increased self-ratings of 'stimulated', 'alert' and 'jittery' at various doses of nicotine chewing gum (0.25 mg, 0.5 mg and 1 mg) when compared with the nicotine gum alone.[3] In a placebo-controlled study, 12 healthy subjects were given nicotine 1 mg or 2 mg with caffeine 50 mg or 100 mg, both as a chewing gum. Both nicotine and caffeine alone increased energy expenditure; however, adding caffeine 50 mg to nicotine 1 mg had almost double the effects of increasing the nicotine dose from 1 to 2 mg. Similar effects were seen in both smokers and non-smokers. No adverse effects were reported with either nicotine 1 mg alone or given with caffeine.[4] In another similar study by the same authors, caffeine enhanced the appetite-suppressant effects of nicotine.[5] In another study in 13 smokers who regularly drank at least one cup of coffee daily, pre-treatment with oral caffeine 2.5 or 5 mg/kg (added to 180 mL of decaffeinated coffee) did not alter the subjects ability to discriminate between nasal nicotine and placebo, and did not alter the amount of caffeine they self-administered during a period of smoking cessation. Caffeine pre-treatment caused a modest dose-related increase in nicotine levels (maximum 21%).[6] In a study in 12 smokers, two doses of caffeine 150 mg (given in a decaffeinated cola drink before and during smoking) had no effect on the plasma levels of nicotine achieved by smoking 5 cigarettes.[7]

Experimental evidence

Because of the quality of the clinical evidence (controlled pharmacokinetic studies), experimental data have not been sought.

Mechanism

Not understood.

Importance and management

The interaction between caffeine and nicotine appears to be established but the effects of concurrent use are less certain, although the effects of caffeine and nicotine on blood pressure may be additive under certain conditions. Caffeine may boost some of the stimulant effects of nicotine (energy consumption, appetite suppression, but also adverse effects such as jitteriness), but it only appears to cause a small, if any, rise in nicotine levels. Bear the potential for this increase in effects in mind should a patient receiving nicotine replacement therapy and also taking medicines formulated with caffeine (such as some analgesics) or consuming caffeine-containing drinks (e.g. tea, coffee, cola drinks) develop troublesome nicotine-related adverse effects.

1. Smits P, Temme L, Thien T. The cardiovascular interaction between caffeine and nicotine in humans. *Clin Pharmacol Ther* (1993) 54, 194–204.
2. Blank MD, Kleykamp BA, Jennings JM, Eissenberg T. Caffeine's influence on nicotine's effects in nonsmokers. *Am J Health Behav* (2007) 31, 473–83.
3. Duka T, Tasker R, Russell K, Stephens DN. Discriminative stimulus properties of nicotine at low doses: the effects of caffeine preload. *Behav Pharmacol* (1998) 9, 219–29.
4. Jessen AB, Toubro S, Astrup A. Effect of chewing gum containing nicotine and caffeine on energy expenditure and substrate utilization in men. *Am J Clin Nutr* (2003) 77, 1442–7.
5. Jessen A, Buemann B, Toubro S, Skovgaard IM, Astrup A. The appetite-suppressant effect of nicotine is enhanced by caffeine. *Diabetes Obes Metab* (2005) 7, 327–33.
6. Perkins KA, Fonte C, Stolinski A, Blakesley-Ball R, Wilson AS. The influence of caffeine on nicotine's discriminative stimulus, subjective, and reinforcing effects. *Exp Clin Psychopharmacol* (2005) 13, 275–81.
7. Gilbert DG, Dibb WD, Plath LC, Hiyane SG. Effects of nicotine and caffeine, separately and in combination, on EEG topography, mood, heart rate, cortisol, and vigilance. *Psychopharmacology (Berl)* (2000) 37, 583–95.

Caffeine + Paracetamol (Acetaminophen)

Caffeine appears to increase the rate of absorption of paracetamol, and has been reported to increase the bioavailability of paracetamol, although one study found a decrease and another found no change in paracetamol bioavailability.

Evidence, mechanism, importance and management

In a study in 10 healthy subjects, caffeine citrate 120 mg increased the AUC of a single 500-mg dose of paracetamol by 29%, increased its maximum plasma levels by 15% and decreased its total body clearance by 32%. The decrease in time to maximum level and increase in absorption rate were not statistically significant.[1] A randomised, crossover study in 24 healthy subjects compared the effects of a single 1 g dose of paracetamol alone and with caffeine 130 mg. The overall bioavailability was the same with or without caffeine, but paracetamol had a faster rate of absorption in the presence of caffeine, shown by an increase in the AUC of paracetamol over the first 20 minutes.[2] There was also an increase in analgesic effects (using a pain model) throughout the observation period from about one to 3.5 hours.[2] In another study, although caffeine increased the rate of absorption of paracetamol, it had no effect on the extent of absorption.[3] However, a further study states that caffeine *decreased* both the plasma levels and AUC of paracetamol, and increased paracetamol elimination in healthy men.[4]

Caffeine is commonly included in paracetamol preparations as an analgesic adjuvant, although its potential benefits and the exact mechanism for its action are still unclear. However, note that if paracetamol formulated with caffeine is given there is the potential for additive caffeine adverse effects (such as headache, jitteriness, restlessness, and insomnia) with dietary caffeine. Caffeine intake should be reduced if this occurs.

1. Iqbal N, Ahmad B, Janbaz KH, Gilani A-UH, Niazi SK. The effect of caffeine on the pharmacokinetics of acetaminophen in man. *Biopharm Drug Dispos* (1995) 16, 481–7.
2. Renner B, Clarke G, Grattan T, Beisel A, Mueller C, Werner U, Kobal G, Brune K. Caffeine accelerates absorption and enhances the analgesic effect of acetaminophen. *J Clin Pharmacol* (2007) 47, 715–26.
3. Tukker JJ, Sitsen JMA, Gusdorf CF. Bioavailability of paracetamol after oral administration to healthy volunteers. Influence of caffeine on rate and extent of absorption. *Pharm Weekbl (Sci)* (1986) 8, 239–43.
4. Raińska-Giezek T. Influence of caffeine on toxicity and pharmacokinetics of paracetamol [Article in Polish]. *Ann Acad Med Stetin* (1995) 41, 69–85.

Caffeine + Phenylpropanolamine

Phenylpropanolamine can raise blood pressure and in some cases this may be further increased by caffeine. Combined use has resulted in hypertensive crises in a few individuals. An isolated report describes the development of acute psychosis when caffeine was given with phenylpropanolamine. Phenylpropanolamine greatly raises caffeine levels.

Clinical evidence

In a placebo-controlled study, the mean blood pressure of 16 healthy subjects rose by 11/12 mmHg after they took caffeine 400 mg, by 12/13 mmHg after they took phenylpropanolamine 75 mg, and by 12/11 mmHg when both drugs were taken. Phenylpropanolamine 150 mg caused a greater rise of 36/18 mmHg. One of the subjects had a hypertensive crisis after taking phenylpropanolamine 150 mg and again 2 hours after taking caffeine 400 mg. This needed antihypertensive treatment.[1] The same group of workers describe a similar study in which the AUC of caffeine 400 mg increased by more than threefold, and the mean peak caffeine concentration increased almost fourfold (from 2.1 to 8 micrograms/mL) after phenylpropanolamine 75 mg was given.[2] Additive increases in blood pressure are described in another report.[3]

A review describes 41 severe adverse reactions to phenylpropanolamine. Of these cases, caffeine was also taken by 15 subjects, with outcomes such as stroke and seizure. However, it should be noted that these effects were similar to those seen in patients who had taken phenylpropanolamine alone.[4]

Experimental evidence

Because of the quality of the clinical evidence (controlled pharmacokinetic studies), experimental data have not been sought.

Mechanism

Additive pharmacological effects.

Importance and management

Evidence is limited and an adverse effect is not fully established, especially as hypertensive episodes, stroke and seizures have been reported with the use of phenylpropanolamine alone. One possible explanation for the lack of reports could be that these interactions may go unrecognised or be attributed to one drug only e.g. phenylpropanolamine, whereas caffeine has also been taken in beverages (often not reported). The risk may be affected by individual susceptibility, the additive stimulant effects of caffeine, the variability in the contents of caffeine and other sympathomimetic alkaloids in non-prescription dietary supplements, or pre-existing medical conditions, such as cardiovascular disease. Note that, phenylpropanolamine was available formulated with caffeine. Phenylpropanolamine is no longer available in the US and UK, and its use has been restricted in many other countries.

The authors of one report[1] advised that users of phenylpropanolamine should be warned about the over-use of phenylpropanolamine, and also about taking caffeine at the same time, because of the possible risk of intracranial haemorrhage secondary to severe hypertension.[1] It would therefore seem prudent to also avoid the use of caffeine-containing herbal medicines. If both drugs are given there is the potential for increased caffeine adverse effects (such as headache, jitteriness, restlessness, and insomnia). Caffeine intake should be reduced if this occurs.

1. Lake CR, Zaloga G, Bray J, Rosenberg D, Chernow B. Transient hypertension after two phenylpropanolamine diet aids and the effects of caffeine: a placebo-controlled follow-up study. *Am J Med* (1989) 86, 427–32.
2. Lake CR, Rosenberg DB, Gallant S, Zaloga G, Chernow B. Phenylpropanolamine increases plasma caffeine levels. *Clin Pharmacol Ther* (1990) 47, 675–85.
3. Brown NJ, Ryder D, Branch RA. A pharmacodynamic interaction between caffeine and phenylpropanolamine. *Clin Pharmacol Ther* (1991) 50, 363–71.
4. Lake CR, Gallant S, Masson E, Miller P. Adverse drug effects attributed to phenylpropanolamine: a review of 142 case reports. *Am J Med* (1990) 89, 195.

Caffeine + Theophylline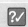

The consumption of caffeine-containing beverages can raise theophylline levels. Similarly, removal of caffeine-containing foods from the diet might reduce the half-life of theophylline.

Clinical evidence

Caffeine can decrease the clearance of theophylline by 18 to 29%, prolong its half-life by up to 44% and increase its average serum levels by up to 23%.[1–3] In addition, plasma caffeine levels were increased about twofold when theophylline was given, and this might have caused the headaches and nausea reported in 2 subjects who did not usually drink coffee.[2] In these studies, caffeine was given in the form of tablets[1,2] or as 2 to 7 cups of instant coffee.[3] Another study found that, when 4 healthy subjects removed methylxanthines from their diet, the half-life of theophylline was reduced from 9.8 hours to 7 hours.[4]

Experimental evidence

Because of the quality of the clinical evidence (controlled pharmacokinetic studies), experimental data have not been sought.

Mechanism

Unknown. It has been suggested that as theophylline and caffeine are both metabolised by CYP1A2 and a proportion of caffeine is converted to theophylline, saturation of theophylline metabolism or competition for metabolism by CYP1A2 may occur.[3] However, note that interactions by substrate competition are rarely clinically relevant.

Importance and management

An interaction between caffeine and theophylline is reasonably well studied and established. There would, however, seem to be no good reason for patients taking theophylline to avoid caffeine (in herbal preparations, beverages such as coffee, tea, cola drinks, or medications, etc.), but if otherwise unexplained adverse effects occur it might be worth checking if caffeine is responsible. Removal of caffeine from the diet might have a modest effect on theophylline levels, but the clinical relevance of this is unclear. There appears to be no direct evidence regarding aminophylline, but as it is metabolised to theophylline, it would be expected to interact similarly.

1. Loi CM, Jue SG, Bush ED, Crowley JJ, Vestal RE. Effect of caffeine dose on theophylline metabolism. *Clin Res* (1987) 35, 377A.
2. Jonkman JHG, Sollie FAE, Sauter R, Steinijans VW. The influence of caffeine on the steady-state pharmacokinetics of theophylline. *Clin Pharmacol Ther* (1991) 49, 248–55.
3. Sato J, Nakata H, Owada E, Kikuta T, Umetsu M, Ito K. Influence of usual intake of dietary caffeine on single-dose kinetics of theophylline in healthy human subjects. *Eur J Clin Pharmacol* (1993) 44, 295–8.
4. Monks TJ, Caldwell J, Smith RL. Influence of methylxanthine-containing foods on theophylline metabolism and kinetics. *Clin Pharmacol Ther* (1979) 26, 513–24.

C

Calamus

Acorus calamus L. (Acoraceae)

Synonym(s) and related species

Myrtle flag, Sweet flag, Sweet sedge.

Calamus aromaticus.

There are various types of calamus, mainly reflecting geographical origin: type I is an American diploid variety; type II is a European triploid; and types III and IV are subtropical tetraploids.

Constituents

The main active constituents of calamus are found in the volatile oil, but considerable qualitative and quantitative differences are found between different species and varieties. Tetraploid (subtropical, specifically Indian) species contain 96% β-asarone (isoasarone), whereas triploid (European) species contain 5% and diploid (North American) species do not contain any. In addition, α-asarone, acolamone, acoragermacrone, calamenol, calamene, calamone, eugenol, galangin, methyl eugenol and isoacolamone are present in varying amounts.

Use and indications

Calamus is traditionally used as a carminative and spasmolytic, in acute and chronic dyspepsia, gastritis and gastric ulcer, intestinal colic and anorexia, and for respiratory disorders. However, note that β-asarone is considered to be toxic (based on the results of *animal* studies) and it is recommended that oils containing this substance should be avoided.

Pharmacokinetics

In a preliminary study[1] using *rat* liver microsomes, extracts of calamus were found to be moderate inhibitors of CYP3A4 and CYP2D6 when compared to the recognised potent inhibitors ketoconazole and quinidine, respectively. However, *in vitro* studies cannot be directly extrapolated to the clinical situation, and there do not appear to be any clinical reports that support the findings. Further study is needed.

Interactions overview

No interactions with calamus found.

1. Pandit S, Mukherjee PK, Ponnusankar S, Venkatesh M, Srikanth N. Metabolism mediated interaction of α-asarone and *Acorus calamus* with CYP3A4 and CYP2D6. *Fitoterapia* (2011) 82, 369–74.

Calendula

Calendula officinalis L. (Asteraceae)

Synonym(s) and related species

Gold-bloom, Marigold, Marybud, Pot Marigold.

Caltha officinalis.

Pharmacopoeias

Calendula Flower (*BP 2012, PhEur 7.5*).

Constituents

Calendula flower extracts contain mainly **triterpenes**. **Oleanolic acid** and its saponins calendulosides C–H, sterols, carotenoids and a sesquiterpene glycoside (arvoside A) are also present. **Flavonoids** in the form of flavonol glycosides of quercetin (isoquercitrin and rutin) and isorhamnetin have also been identified.

Use and indications

Calendula is often used in externally-applied products for the treatment of cuts, bruises, burns and scalds, and topically for conjunctivitis. It has also been used to treat gastric and duodenal ulcers, haemorrhoids and varicose veins.

Pharmacokinetics

No relevant pharmacokinetic data found for calendula extracts, but the pharmacokinetics of **oleanolic acid** have been evaluated in preliminary studies. Incubation with *rat* liver microsomes suggests that **oleanolic acid** is likely to be extensively metabolised in the liver by hydroxylation, but the exact sites for this were not determined.[1] For information on the pharmacokinetics of individual flavonoids present in calendula, see under flavonoids, page 213.

Interactions overview

It has been reported that calendula has possible sedative effects, which theoretically could be additive if given with conventional drugs that cause sedation. However, the evidence for this is extremely limited. For information on the interactions of individual flavonoids present in calendula, see under flavonoids, page 213.

1. Jeong DW, Kim YH, Kim HH, Ji HY, Yoo SD, Choi WR, Lee SM, Han C-K, Lee HS. Dose-linear pharmacokinetics of oleanolic acid after intravenous and oral administration in rats. *Biopharm Drug Dispos* (2007) 28, 51–7.

Cannabis

Cannabis sativa L. (Cannabaceae)

Synonym(s) and related species

Bhang, Dagga, Ganja, Hashish, Indian hemp, Marihuana, Marijuana.

Cannabis indica Lam.

Constituents

Cannabis herb contains a wide range of cannabinoids, which are the major active compounds. The main psychoactive constituent is Δ^9-**tetrahydrocannabinol** (THC; dronabinol), and it is the cause of many of the pharmacological effects elicited by the consumption of cannabis. However other cannabinoids, which do not possess psychoactive properties, such as cannabidiol, cannabinol (a decomposition product of Δ^9-**tetrahydrocannabinol**), cannabigerol, and cannabichromene, are increasingly being investigated for their pharmacological and therapeutic properties. Cannabinoids are often found in the plant as their acid metabolites, e.g. 11-nor-9-carboxy-Δ^9-tetrahydrocannabinol, cannabidiol acid and others, especially if the plant has been grown in a cooler climate. These decarboxylate to the parent cannabinoid at high temperatures, such as during smoking. Most medicinal cannabis products have been heat-treated to ensure the cannabinoids are present only in the non-acid form.

Use and indications

Cannabis has no current established use in herbal medicine because of its legal position in most parts of the world. However, medicinal cannabis is increasingly being used to treat chronic conditions, as an adjunct, or where other treatments may be inadequate. For example, a buccal spray preparation of cannabis, containing mainly dronabinol (the medicinal name for Δ^9-tetrahydrocannabinol) with cannabidiol, is available as an adjunctive treatment for the symptomatic relief of neuropathic pain in multiple sclerosis in adults. It is also being investigated for use as an analgesic in other disease states such as diabetic neuropathy and rheumatoid arthritis, and to relieve spasticity in multiple sclerosis and spinal cord injury. Dronabinol and nabilone (a synthetic cannabinol) are used as antiemetics in patients receiving cancer chemotherapy, and dronabinol has been used as an appetite stimulant in AIDS. Cannabis is a widely used illicit drug because of its psychoactive properties, and has a long history of such use, including by those with chronic illnesses.

Varieties of *Cannabis sativa* that contain very little cannabinoids (often referred to as hemp) have been cultivated for their fibre and seeds, and these, and the oil derived from the seeds, may be found in some herbal products.

Pharmacokinetics

The most important pharmacokinetic effects of cannabis depend on whether the herb (or its extracts) are smoked or taken orally. When smoked, cannabinoid acids are decarboxylated by the high temperature, and reach the lung as active free cannabinoids. Psychotropic effects start from within seconds to a few minutes, reach a maximum after 20 to 30 minutes, and taper off within 3 to 4 hours. If the same preparation were to be taken orally however, cannabinoid acid absorption would be lower and much less predictable,[1] with psychotropic effects starting after a delay of 30 to 90 minutes, reaching their maximum after 2 to 4 hours and lasting for about 6 hours.

The metabolism of cannabis is complex, resulting in both active and inactive compounds. The cannabinoids are extensively metabolised by cytochrome P450, in particular, by the isoenzymes CYP2C9 and CYP3A4.[2] Smoking cannabis may induce CYP1A2, see theophylline, page 123, and also clozapine, page 120. Dronabinol has also been shown to inhibit CYP1A1, despite increasing its expression.[3] Cannabis also induces the expression of CYP2E1 and CYP2D6 in *mice*.[4]

Research suggests that some constituents of cannabis can affect others. Cannabidiol, an active but non-psychotropic cannabinoid, has been shown to partially inhibit the hydroxylation of dronabinol, probably by CYP2C.[5] There is limited evidence that some cannabinoids might inhibit P-glycoprotein[6] or reduce P-glycoprotein expression.[7]

Interactions overview

Most of the drug interaction data relate to smoking cannabis. Smoking cannabis has been shown to decrease levels of theophylline, chlorpromazine and probably clozapine. Use of transdermal nicotine with cannabis enhances tachycardia, and increases the stimulant effect of cannabis. Tachycardia has also been seen with combined use of tricyclic antidepressants and cannabis. Cannabis might increase the effects of opioids such as morphine. Cannabis opposes the stimulant effects of ecstasy, but long-term users of both drugs may potentially experience cumulative CNS impairment and additive immunomodulation. Δ^9-tetrahydrocannabinol may prolong the hyperthermic effects of ecstasy. The concurrent use of cannabis or synthetic cannabinoids and amfetamines may lead to adverse cardiac effects. Isolated cases of hypomania have been seen when cannabis was used with disulfiram and with fluoxetine, and a man taking cannabis and sildenafil had a myocardial infarction. Other case reports have attributed a fatal stroke in a young man who received cisplatin, and bleeding in a patient taking warfarin, to concurrent cannabis smoking. Indometacin might antagonise some of the effects of smoking cannabis. Smoking cannabis does not appear to affect the pharmacokinetics or antiviral efficacy of indinavir or nelfinavir, and oral cannabis does not appear to affect the pharmacokinetics of docetaxel or irinotecan.

Interactions monographs

1. Williamson EM, Evans FJ. Cannabinoids in clinical practice. *Drugs* (2000) 60, 1303–14.
2. Watanabe K, Yamaori S, Funahashi T, Kimura T, Yamamoto I. Cytochrome P450 enzymes involved in the metabolism of tetrahydrocannabinols and cannabinol by human hepatic microsomes. *Life Sci* (2007) 80, 1415–19.
3. Roth MD, Marques-Magallanes JA, Yuan M, Sun W, Tashkin DP, Hankinson O. Induction and regulation of the carcinogen-metabolizing enzyme CYP1A1 by marijuana smoke and Δ^9-tetrahydrocannabinol. *Am J Respir Cell Mol Biol* (2001) 24, 339–44.
4. Sheweita SA. Narcotic drugs change the expression of cytochrome P450 2E1 and 2C6 and other activities of carcinogen-metabolizing enzymes in the liver of male mice. *Toxicology* (2003) 191, 133–42.
5. Nadulski T, Pragst F, Weinberg G, Roser P, Schnelle M, Fronk E-M, Stadelmann AM. Randomized, double-blind, placebo-controlled study about the effects of cannabidiol (CBD) on the pharmacokinetics of Δ^9-tetrahydrocannabinol (THC) after oral application of THC verses standardized cannabis extract. *Ther Drug Monit* (2005) 27, 799–810.
6. Zhu H-J, Wang J-S, Markowitz JS, Donovan JL, Gibson BB, Gefroh HA, DeVane CL. Characterization of P-glycoprotein inhibition by major cannabinoids from marijuana. *J Pharmacol Exp Ther* (2006) 317, 850–857.
7. Holland ML, Panetta JA, Hoskins JM, Bebawy M, Roufogalis BD, Allen JD, Arnold JC. The effects of cannabinoids on P-glycoprotein transport and expression in multidrug resistant cells. *Biochem Pharmacol* (2006) 71, 1146–54.

Cannabis + Alcohol

The detrimental effects of drinking alcohol and smoking cannabis might be additive on some aspects of driving performance. However, there is some evidence that regular cannabis use *per se* does not potentiate the effects of alcohol. Smoking cannabis can alter the bioavailability of alcohol.

Evidence and mechanism

a) CNS effects

Simultaneous use of alcohol and oral Δ^9-tetrahydrocannabinol (THC, the major active ingredient of cannabis) reduced the performance of psychomotor tests, suggesting that those who use both drugs together should expect the deleterious effects to be additive.[1] Additive effects were found in other studies,[2] but in one,[2] additive effects occurred mainly in the first 40 minutes, but in later test periods (at 100 and 160 minutes) the depressant effects of oral Δ^9-tetrahydrocannabinol were not as marked as expected and for some tests, including standing steadiness, the effect of Δ^9-tetrahydrocannabinol alone was greater than that when it was given with alcohol, suggesting an antagonistic effect.[2]

In a placebo-controlled study, subjects smoked cannabis containing 100 or 200 micrograms/kg of Δ^9-tetrahydrocannabinol and drank alcohol (to achieve an initial blood level of 70 mg%, with further drinks taken to maintain levels at 40 mg%) 30 minutes before driving. They found that cannabis, even in low to moderate doses, negatively affected driving performance in real traffic situations. Further, the effect of combining moderate doses of both alcohol and cannabis resulted in dramatic performance impairment as great as that observed with blood-alcohol levels of 140 mg% alone.[3,4] Similar results (including a suggestion of a synergistic impairment of performance[5]) have been found in a number of other studies,[5–8] including different doses of cannabis and regular cannabis users.[6]

A study in 22 healthy subjects, who occasionally used cannabis cigarettes and drank moderate amounts of alcohol, found that the number of euphoric events in response to a cannabis cigarette was greater after alcohol ingestion, and the duration of euphoric events was longer. The speed of onset of the effects of cannabis was also faster when it was smoked after the ingestion of alcohol.[9]

One study in 14 regular cannabis users (long-term daily use) and 14 infrequent cannabis users found that regular use reduced the disruptive effects of alcohol on some psychomotor skills relevant to driving, whereas infrequent use did not have this effect. In this study, neither group had smoked any cannabis in the 12 hours before the alcohol test.[10] Another study found that moderate doses of alcohol and cannabis, consumed either alone or in combination, did not produce significant behavioural or subjective impairment the following day.[11]

A study in 12 healthy subjects who regularly used both cannabis and alcohol found that alcohol 0.5 g/kg significantly increased break latency without affecting body sway, whereas cannabis given as a cigarette containing tetrahydrocannabinol 3.33%, increased body sway but did not affect brake latency. There were no significant additive effects on brake latency, body sway, or mood when the two drugs were used together.[12] A population-based study of 2,777 drivers involved in fatal road crashes, who drank alcohol and/or used cannabis, found that although both cannabis and alcohol increased the risk of being responsible for a fatal crash, no statistically significant interaction was observed between the two drugs.[13]

b) Pharmacokinetic studies

Fifteen healthy subjects given alcohol 0.7 g/kg developed peak plasma alcohol levels of about 78 mg% at 50 minutes, but if they smoked a cannabis cigarette 30 minutes after the drink, their peak plasma alcohol levels were only 55 mg% and they occurred 55 minutes later. In addition, their subjective experience of the drugs decreased when used together.[14] However, another study found that smoking cannabis 10 minutes before alcohol

consumption did not affect blood-alcohol levels.[11] A further study found that blood-alcohol levels were not affected by Δ^9-tetrahydrocannabinol given orally one hour before alcohol.[1,15,2] A study in 22 healthy subjects, who occasionally used cannabis cigarettes and drank moderate amounts of alcohol, found that plasma Δ^9-tetrahydrocannabinol levels were higher when alcohol was consumed before smoking a cannabis cigarette.[9]

Importance and management

Several studies have found that cannabis and alcohol produce additive detrimental effects on driving performance, but other studies have not found any potentiation. This is probably due to the variety of simulated driving tests used and possibly the time lag between the administration of alcohol and cannabis; behavioural impairment after cannabis has been reported to peak within 30 minutes of smoking.[11] Nevertheless, both drugs have been shown to affect some aspects of driving performance and increase the risk of fatal car accidents. Of concern, one study found that drivers are willing to drive despite being aware of the effects of alcohol and/or cannabis and the only consideration that affected their risk taking was the urgency of the drive.[8] Concurrent use of cannabis and alcohol before driving should therefore be avoided.

1. Bird KD, Boleyn T, Chesher GB, Jackson DM, Starmer GA, Teo RKC. Intercannabinoid and cannabinoid-ethanol interactions and their effects on human performance. *Psychopharmacology (Berl)* (1980) 71, 181–8.
2. Chesher GB, Franks HM, Jackson DM, Starmer GA, Teo RKC. Ethanol and Δ^9-tetrahydrocannabinol interactive effects on human perceptual, cognitive and motor functions. II. *Med J Aust* (1977) 1, 478–81.
3. National Highway Traffic Safety Administration. Marijuana and alcohol combined severely impede driving performance. *Ann Emerg Med* (2000) 35, 398–9.
4. Jolly BT. Commentary: drugged driving–different spin on an old problem. *Ann Emerg Med* (2000) 35, 399–400.
5. Perez-Reyes M, Hicks RE, Burnberry J, Jeffcoat AR, Cook CE. Interaction between marihuana and ethanol: effects on psychomotor performance. *Alcohol Clin Exp Res* (1988) 12, 268–76.
6. Marks DF, MacAvoy MG. Divided attention performance in cannabis users and non-users following alcohol and cannabis separately and in combination. *Psychopharmacology (Berl)* (1989) 99, 397–401.
7. Hansteen RW, Miller RD, Lonero L, Reid LD, Jones B. Effects of cannabis and alcohol on automobile driving and psychomotor tracking. *Ann N Y Acad Sci* (1976) 282, 240–256.
8. Ronen A, Chassidim HS, Gershon P, Parmet Y, Rabinovich A, Bar-Hamburger R, Cassuto Y, Shinar D. The effect of alcohol, THC and their combination on perceived effects, willingness to drive and performance of driving and non-driving tasks. *Accid Anal Prev* (2010) 42, 1855–65.
9. Lukas SE, Orozco S. Ethanol increases plasma Δ^9-tetrahydrocannabinol (THC) levels and subjective effects after marihuana smoking in human volunteers. *Drug Alcohol Depend* (2001) 64, 143–9.
10. Wright KA, Terry P. Modulation of the effects of alcohol on driving-related psychomotor skills by chronic exposure to cannabis. *Psychopharmacology (Berl)* (2002) 160, 213–19.
11. Chait LD, Perry JL. Acute and residual effects of alcohol and marijuana, alone and in combination, on mood and performance. *Psychopharmacology (Berl)* (1994) 115, 340–349.
12. Liguori A, Gatto CP, Jarrett DB. Separate and combined effects of marijuana and alcohol on mood, equilibrium and simulated driving. *Psychopharmacology (Berl)* (2002) 163, 399–405.
13. Laumon B, Gadeqbeku B, Martin J-L, Biecheler M-B. Cannabis intoxication and fatal road crashes in France: population based case-control study. *BMJ* (2005) 331, 1371–6.
14. Lukas SE, Benedikt R, Mendelson JH, Kouri E, Sholar M, Amass L. Marihuana attenuates the rise in plasma ethanol levels in human subjects. *Neuropsychopharmacology* (1992) 7, 77–81.
15. Belgrave BE, Bird KD, Chesher GB, Jackson DM, Lubbe KE, Starmer GA, Teo RKC. The effect of (−) trans-Δ^9-tetrahydrocannabinol, alone and in combination with ethanol, on human performance. *Psychopharmacology (Berl)* (1979) 62, 53–60.

Cannabis + Amfetamines

Cannabis opposes the stimulant effects of ecstasy, but long-term users of both drugs may potentially experience cumulative CNS impairment and additive immunomodulation. The effects of ecstasy and Δ^9-tetrahydrocannabinol on heart rate may be additive and Δ^9-tetrahydrocannabinol may prolong the hyperthermic effects of ecstasy. A report describes severe arterial ischaemia in a patient who regularly abused amfetamines and cannabis. The concurrent use of amfetamines and synthetic cannabinoids may lead to adverse cardiac effects.

Clinical evidence

In a study, 16 healthy subjects who were regular users of **ecstasy** (MDMA, methylenedioxymethamfetamine) were given a single 100-mg oral dose of ecstasy or placebo and inhaled Δ^9-tetrahydrocannabinol (THC, the major active ingredient of cannabis) 4 mg to ensure tolerability. Subsequent doses of Δ^9-tetrahydrocannabinol 6 mg were given by inhalation 90 and 120 minutes after **ecstasy** 100 mg. Heart rate was increased by both substances (**ecstasy** 20.4 bpm; Δ^9-tetrahydrocannabinol 14.2 bpm), and this effect appeared to be roughly additive on concurrent use (29.9 bpm). **Ecstasy**-induced temperature increases (about 0.3°C over time) were not prevented by Δ^9-tetrahydrocannabinol but it delayed the onset and prolonged the duration of temperature elevation.[1]

In a study in 23 cannabis users, 37 cannabis and **ecstasy** users and a control group of 34 subjects who used neither drug, there was enhanced immunomodulation in those who used both **ecstasy** and cannabis, similar to that induced in stress conditions or mediated by other drugs of abuse. Cannabis alone produced less immunomodulation. A higher rate of mild infections was found in regular users of **ecstasy** and cannabis compared with occasional users, those who used cannabis only, and those who did not use either drug.[2]

A study in 18 cannabis users, 11 cannabis and **ecstasy** users, and 31 subjects who had used neither drug, found that users of cannabis and users of cannabis with **ecstasy** performed similarly in most CNS tests. However, these subjects performed less well than non-drug users on tests of memory, learning, word fluency, speed of processing and manual dexterity. Furthermore, the deficits were more closely related to cannabis usage than **ecstasy** usage.[3] Similar results were reported in another study.[4] A further self-rated study found that moderate cannabis use might help to improve or mask **ecstasy**-induced aggression and somatic symptoms (e.g. headache, chronic tiredness). However, heavy cannabis and **ecstasy** use appeared to be associated with problems such as paranoia or cognitive disorders, which might emerge after a period of abstinence from both drugs.[5] Another study found that self-reported psychological problems in **ecstasy** users were predominantly attributable to concurrent cannabis use. Abstinence from cannabis was found to be a predictor for remission of psychological problems in **ecstasy** users.[6]

A 22-year-old woman who smoked cigarettes and had regularly abused amfetamine derivatives such as **metamfetamine** and ecstasy together with cannabis, experienced severe arterial ischaemia leading to claudication and ulceration of the feet.[7]

Experimental evidence

An *animal* study found that pretreatment with cannabidiol, a major constituent of cannabis, did not affect the levels of ecstasy in the brain of *mice*.[8] Δ^9-tetrahydrocannabinol (THC, the major active ingredient of cannabis) prevented ecstasy-induced hyperthermia in studies in *mice*[9] and *rats*.[10] Various cannabinoids, including Δ^9-tetrahydrocannabinol, given in high doses, were also found to attenuate hyperactivity and some measures of the anxiety-inducing effects of ecstasy in *rats*.[10] In a further study, ecstasy attenuated Δ^9-tetrahydrocannabinol withdrawal symptoms in *mice*.[11]

Mechanism

Both cannabis and ecstasy may cause additive CNS impairment. Enhanced immunomodulation due to regular use of both ecstasy and cannabis may result in poorer general health and increased susceptibility to infection.[2] The additive effects of ecstasy appear to be due the effects of ecstasy on catecholamines and the direct cannabinoid (CB_1) agonism in cardiac tissue.[1]

In the case report describing ischaemia it was suggested that the amfetamine derivatives might have induced vasculitis of the arteries with cannabis possibly adding to the effect on the microcirculation.[7]

Importance and management

The majority of recreational ecstasy users (up to 98%[12]) also take cannabis and this combined drug usage appears to reflect the opposing effects of the two drugs: ecstasy is a powerful stimulant whereas cannabis is a relaxant. Therefore cannabis may modulate the acute reactions to ecstasy.[12] Ecstasy is hyperthermic and although cannabis is reported to be hypothermic,[12] one study suggests Δ^9-tetrahydrocannabinol may prolong the duration of ecstasy-associated temperature increases.[1] Ecstasy increases oxidative stress whereas cannabinoids are antioxidant, but one report suggests enhanced immunomodulation on concurrent use.[2] The chronic effects of each drug may be functionally damaging, so that using both drugs may be associated with a variety of psychological problems.[12,13] Furthermore, regular cannabis use seems to be necessary for the development and maintenance of symptoms of mental illness in ecstasy users.[13,6]

Note that synthetic cannabinoids are available as licensed medicinal products. The manufacturers of two such products, nabilone and dronabinol (synthetic Δ^9-tetrahydrocannabinol), suggest that the concurrent use of amfetamines may lead to additive hypertension, tachycardia, and possible cardiotoxicity.[14,15] The clinical relevance of these predictions does not appear to have been studied, and therefore, until more is known, it would be prudent to monitor the cardiac effects of concurrent use, particularly in those with pre-existing cardiovascular disease.

1. Dumont GJ, Kramers C, Sweep FC, Touw DJ, van Hasselt JG, de Kam M, van Gerven JM, Buitelaar JK, Verkes RJ. Cannabis coadministration potentiates the effects of "ecstasy" on heart rate and temperature in humans. *Clin Pharmacol Ther* (2009) 86, 160–166.
2. Pacifici R, Zuccaro P, Farré M, Poudevida S, Abanades S, Pichini S, Langohr K, Segura J, de la Torre R. Combined immunomodulating properties of 3,4-methylenedioxymethamphetamine (MDMA) and cannabis in humans. *Addiction* (2007) 102, 931–6.
3. Croft RJ, Mackay AJ, Mills ATD, Gruzelier JGH. The relative contributions of ecstasy and cannabis to cognitive impairment. *Psychopharmacology (Berl)* (2001) 153, 373–9.
4. Fisk JE, Montgomery C, Wareing M, Murphy PN. The effects of concurrent cannabis use among ecstasy users: neuroprotective or neurotoxic? *Hum Psychopharmacol* (2006) 21, 355–66.
5. Milani RM, Parrott AC, Schifano F, Turner JJD. Pattern of cannabis use in ecstasy polydrug users: moderate cannabis use may compensate for self-rated aggression and somatic symptoms. *Hum Psychopharmacol* (2005) 20, 249–61.
6. Daumann J, Hensen G, Thimm B, Rezk M, Till B, Gouzoulis-Mayfrank E. Self-reported psychopathological symptoms in recreational ecstasy (MDMA) users are mainly associated with regular cannabis use: further evidence from a combined cross-sectional/longitudinal investigation. *Psychopharmacology (Berl)* (2004) 173, 398–404.
7. Leithäuser B, Langheinrich AC, Rau WS, Tillmanns H, Matthias FR. A 22-year-old woman with lower limb arteriopathy, Buerger's disease, or methamphetamine- or cannabis-induced arteritis? *Heart Vessels* (2005) 20, 39–43.
8. Reid MJ, Bornheim LM. Cannabinoid-induced alterations in brain disposition of drugs of abuse. *Biochem Pharmacol* (2001) 61, 1357–67.
9. Touriño C, Zimmer A, Valverde O. THC prevents MDMA neurotoxicity in mice. *PLoS One* (2010) 5, e9143.
10. Morley KC, Li KM, Hunt GE, Mallet PE, McGregor IS. Cannabinoids prevent the acute hyperthermia and partially protect against the 5-HT depleting effects of MDMA ("Ecstasy") in rats. *Neuropharmacology* (2004) 46, 954–65.
11. Touriño C, Maldonado R, Valverde O. MDMA attenuates THC withdrawal syndrome in mice. *Psychopharmacology (Berl)* (2007) 193, 75–84.
12. Parrott AC, Milani RM, Gouzoulis-Mayfrank E, Daumann J. Cannabis and ecstasy/MDMA (3,4-methylenedioxymethamphetamine): an analysis of their neuropsychobiological interactions in recreational users. *J Neural Transm* (2007) 114, 959–68.
13. Sala M, Braida D. Endocannabinoids and 3,4-methylenedioxymethamphetamine (MDMA) interaction. *Pharmacol Biochem Behav* (2005) 81, 407–16.
14. Cesamet Nabilone. Valeant US Prescribing information, March 2009.
15. Marinol Dronabinol. Solvay Pharmaceuticals, Inc US Prescribing information, March 2008.

Cannabis + Chlorpromazine

Smokers of cannabis may possibly need larger doses of chlorpromazine than non-smokers.

Clinical evidence

A study in 31 patients found that the clearance of chlorpromazine was increased by 38% by tobacco smoking, by 50% by cannabis smoking, and by 107% when both tobacco and cannabis were smoked.[1]

Experimental evidence

No relevant data found.

Mechanism

Not established. The probable reason is that some of the components of tobacco smoke act as enzyme inducers, which increase the rate at which the liver metabolises chlorpromazine, thereby reducing its serum levels and clinical effects. Cannabis appears to have additional effects.

Importance and management

An established interaction but of uncertain clinical importance. Be alert for the need to increase the doses of chlorpromazine and possibly other phenothiazines in patients who smoke cannabis, and reduce the doses if smoking is stopped.

1. Chetty M, Miller R, Moodley SV. Smoking and body weight influence the clearance of chlorpromazine. *Eur J Clin Pharmacol* (1994) 46, 523–6.

Cannabis + Ciclosporin

Cannabidiol, an important constituent of cannabis, may increase ciclosporin levels. This interaction is based on experimental evidence only.

Clinical evidence

No interactions found.

Experimental evidence

An *in vitro* study found that the incubation of human and *mouse* liver microsomes with cannabidiol, an active but non-psychoactive constituent of cannabis, resulted in inhibition of ciclosporin metabolism. The production of ciclosporin metabolites was reduced by 73 to 83%. Similar results were found in studies in *mice*.[1]

Mechanism

Cannabidiol may inhibit the cytochrome P450 subfamily CYP3A, and so increase ciclosporin levels. However, cannabis does not affect the metabolism of other CYP3A4 substrates, see Cannabis + Irinotecan, page 121.

Importance and management

These preclinical data suggest that one constituent of cannabis might possibly raise ciclosporin levels. These data require confirmation in humans. Until such data are available, bear in mind the possibility that irregular use of cannabis might be a factor in unstable ciclosporin levels. It might be unwise for patients taking ciclosporin to use cannabis.

1. Jaeger W, Benet LZ, Bornheim LM. Inhibition of cyclosporine and tetrahydrocannabinol metabolism by cannabidiol in mouse and human microsomes. *Xenobiotica* (1996) 26, 275–84.

Cannabis + Cisplatin

A case report describes a fatal stroke when a young man receiving cisplatin smoked cannabis.

Evidence, mechanism, importance and management

A 27-year-old man who smoked cannabis and tobacco daily developed tinnitus and paraesthesias after receiving the first course of chemotherapy consisting of cisplatin, **etoposide** and **bleomycin** for testicular cancer. Following the second course of chemotherapy, the patient reported distal paresis of the right arm and, 2 days later, about 30 minutes after cannabis inhalation, he developed headache, paresis of his right leg and aphasia. A large thrombus was found in the carotid artery. The patient died the next day. He had no cardiovascular risk factors apart from the smoking (about 4 cigarettes per day).[1]

Cisplatin is known to carry a small risk of stroke, and cases have also been reported for cannabis smoking alone. In this case it was

suggested that the use of cannabis may have also contributed to the adverse outcome in this patient.[1] It might be prudent for patients receiving cisplatin to avoid smoking cannabis.

1. Russmann S, Winkler A, Lövblad KO, Stanga Z, Bassetti C. Lethal ischemic stroke after cisplatin-based chemotherapy for testicular carcinoma and cannabis inhalation. *Eur Neurol* (2002) 48, 178–80.

Cannabis + Clozapine

Patients who give up smoking cannabis might develop higher blood concentrations of clozapine and be at risk of adverse reactions, since plasma concentrations of clozapine are lower in smokers than in non-smokers.

Clinical evidence

A 37-year-old man who smoked both tobacco and cannabis daily, and took clozapine 700 mg daily, experienced elevated clozapine plasma concentrations and signs of clozapine toxicity, one month after he stopped smoking both tobacco and cannabis. One week after reducing the dose of clozapine to 500 mg daily, his psychotic symptoms disappeared and plasma concentrations returned to normal.[1]

Experimental evidence

No relevant data found.

Mechanism

Tobacco smoke contains aromatic hydrocarbons that are potent inducers of CYP1A2, by which clozapine is metabolised. Smoking therefore increases clozapine metabolism and lower concentrations result. The contribution of cannabis smoking to this case is unknown, but cannabis smoking alone is also known to induce CYP1A2, independent of tobacco. See Cannabis + Theophylline, page 123.

Importance and management

It is known that patients who smoke tobacco might experience lower serum clozapine concentrations, and, although there is no direct evidence, this might equally apply to cannabis smoking. Irregular smoking of cannabis might cause fluctuations in clozapine concentrations.

1. Zullino DF, Delessert D, Eap CB, Preisig M, Baumann P. Tobacco and cannabis smoking cessation can lead to intoxication with clozapine or olanzapine. *Int Clin Psychopharmacol* (2002) 17, 141–3.

Cannabis + Disulfiram

Two isolated case reports describe hypomanic-like reactions when patients taking disulfiram used cannabis, whereas no unusual interaction with the combination was seen in other subjects.

Evidence, mechanism, importance and management

A man with a 10-year history of drug abuse (alcohol, amfetamines, cocaine, cannabis) taking disulfiram 250 mg daily, experienced a hypomanic-like reaction (euphoria, hyperactivity, insomnia, irritability) on two occasions, associated with the concurrent use of cannabis. The patient said that he felt as though he had been taking amfetamine.[1] One other similar case has been reported.[2] The reason for this reaction is not understood. In a randomised study in alcohol-dependent subjects who had previously used cannabis, no unusual interaction effects were found in a group of 11 subjects receiving disulfiram and smoking cannabis twice weekly for

4 weeks.[3] Therefore the interaction described in the two case reports would not appear to be of general significance.

1. Lacoursiere RB, Swatek R. Adverse interaction between disulfiram and marijuana: a case report. *Am J Psychiatry* (1983) 140, 243–4.
2. Mackie J, Clark D. Cannabis toxic psychosis while on disulfiram. *Br J Psychiatry* (1994) 164, 421.
3. Rosenberg CM, Gerrein JR, Schnell C. Cannabis in the treatment of alcoholism. *J Stud Alcohol* (1978) 39, 1955–8.

Cannabis + Docetaxel

The pharmacokinetics of docetaxel are not altered by a herbal tea containing cannabis.

Clinical evidence

In a study investigating the effects of cannabis on docetaxel pharmacokinetics, 12 patients were given 200 mL of a herbal tea containing cannabis 1 g/L each day for 15 days. The tea was prepared from medicinal-grade cannabis (*Cannabis sativa* L. Flos, Bedrocan®) containing the cannabinoids Δ^9-tetrahydrocannabinol 18% and cannabidiol 0.8%. The clearance and the AUC of docetaxel given on day 12 of the cannabis tea were not significantly altered, when compared with docetaxel given before the cannabis tea. The dose of docetaxel used was 180 mg, reduced to 135 mg in 3 patients who experienced dose-related docetaxel toxicity.[1]

Experimental evidence

No relevant data found.

Mechanism

Docetaxel is metabolised by CYP3A4, and this does not appear to be affected by oral cannabis.

Importance and management

This study suggests that cannabis taken orally will not affect the pharmacokinetics of docetaxel. No dose adjustments are likely to be needed if docetaxel is given with cannabis tea.[1]

1. Engels FK, de Jong FA, Sparreboom A, Mathot RA, Loos WJ, Kitzen JJEM, de Bruijn P, Verweij J, Mathijssen RHJ. Medicinal cannabis does not influence the clinical pharmacokinetics of irinotecan and docetaxel. *Oncologist* (2007) 12, 291–300.

Cannabis + Fluoxetine

An isolated report describes mania when a patient taking fluoxetine smoked cannabis.

Evidence, mechanism, importance and management

A 21-year-old woman with a 9-year history of bulimia and depression was taking fluoxetine 20 mg daily. A month later, about 2 days after smoking two 'joints' of cannabis (marijuana), she experienced a persistent sense of well-being, increased energy, hypersexuality and pressured speech. These symptoms progressed into grandiose delusions, for which she was hospitalised. Her mania and excitement were controlled with lorazepam and perphenazine, and she largely recovered after about 8 days. The reasons for this reaction are not understood but the authors of the report point out that one of the active components of cannabis, dronabinol (Δ^9-tetrahydrocannabinol) is, like fluoxetine, a potent inhibitor of serotonin uptake. Thus a synergistic effect on central serotonergic neurones might have occurred.[1] This seems to be the first and only report of an apparent adverse interaction between cannabis and fluoxetine, but it emphasises the risks of concurrent use.

1. Stoll AL, Cole JO, Lukas SE. A case of mania as a result of fluoxetine-marijuana interaction. *J Clin Psychiatry* (1991) 52, 280–281.

Cannabis + Food

No interactions found.

Cannabis + Herbal medicines

No interactions found.

Cannabis + HIV-protease inhibitors

The short-term use of cannabis cigarettes or dronabinol (Δ^9-tetrahydrocannabinol) did not appear to adversely affect indinavir or nelfinavir levels or viral loads in HIV-positive patients.

Clinical evidence

In 9 HIV-positive patients on a stable regimen containing **indinavir** (mostly 800 mg every 8 hours), smoking a cannabis cigarette (3.95% tetrahydrocannabinol) three times daily before meals for 14 days resulted in a median 14% decrease in AUC and maximum level and a 34% decrease in minimum **indinavir** level. However, only the change in maximum level was statistically significant.[1] Similarly, dronabinol (Δ^9-tetrahydrocannabinol) 2.5 mg three times daily for 14 days had no significant effect on **indinavir** pharmacokinetics.[1]

In another 11 patients on a stable regimen containing **nelfinavir** 750 mg three times daily, there was a non-significant 10% decrease in AUC, 17% decrease in maximum level, and 12% decrease in minimum **nelfinavir** level after 14 days of cannabis cigarettes.[1] Similarly, dronabinol 2.5 mg three times daily for 14 days had no significant effect on **nelfinavir** pharmacokinetics.[1]

There was no adverse effect on viral load or CD4 count in the patients receiving cannabis cigarettes or dronabinol.[2]

Experimental evidence

No relevant data found.

Mechanism

No mechanism expected.

Importance and management

Short-term use of cannabis cigarettes or dronabinol does not appear to have any important effect on levels of indinavir or nelfinavir, nor on markers of HIV infection.

1. Kosel BW, Aweeka FT, Benowitz NL, Shade SB, Hilton JF, Lizak PS, Abrams DI. The effects of cannabinoids on the pharmacokinetics of indinavir and nelfinavir. *AIDS* (2002) 16, 543–50.
2. Abrams DI, Hilton JF, Leiser RJ, Shade SB, Elbeik TA, Aweeka FT, Benowitz NL, Bredt BM, Kosel B, Aberg JA, Deeks SG, Mitchell TF, Mulligan K, Bacchetti P, McCune JM, Schambelan M. Short-term effects of cannabinoids in patients with HIV-1 infection: a randomized, placebo-controlled clinical trial. *Ann Intern Med* (2003) 139, 258–66.

Cannabis + Irinotecan

In one study the pharmacokinetics of irinotecan were not altered by a herbal tea containing cannabis.

Clinical evidence

In a crossover study, 24 patients were given intravenous irinotecan 600 mg before and 12 days after starting a 15-day course of 200 mL daily of a herbal tea containing cannabis 1 g/L. This was prepared from medicinal-grade cannabis (*Cannabis sativa* L. Flos, Bedrocan®) containing Δ^9-tetrahydrocannabinol 18% and cannabidiol 0.8% (both cannabinoids). The clearance and the AUC of irinotecan and its metabolites, SN-38 (the active metabolite) and SN-38G (the inactive glucuronide metabolite of SN-38), were not notably altered by the presence of cannabis.[1]

Experimental evidence

No relevant data found.

Mechanism

Irinotecan is partly metabolised by CYP3A4 to inactive metabolites, but this isoenzyme does not appear to be affected by oral cannabis. The formation of the active metabolite, SN-38, via carboxylesterases; and SN-38G (the inactive glucuronide metabolite of SN-38) via UGT1A1 also seems to be unaffected by cannabis.

Importance and management

This study suggests that cannabis taken orally will not affect the pharmacokinetics of irinotecan. No dose adjustments are likely to be needed if irinotecan is given with cannabis tea.

1. Engels FK, de Jong FA, Sparreboom A, Mathot RAA, Loos WJ, Kitzen JJEM, de Bruijn P, Verweij J, Mathijssen RHJ. Medicinal cannabis does not influence the clinical pharmacokinetics of irinotecan and docetaxel. *Oncologist* (2007) 12, 291–300.

Cannabis + Nicotine

The effects of transdermal nicotine and cannabis smoking on increasing the heart rate are additive, and nicotine increased the stimulant effect of cannabis. Combined use might increase the addictive potential of both drugs.

Clinical evidence

In a study in 20 healthy subjects who smoked either a low-dose or high-dose cannabis cigarette 4 hours after the application of a placebo or a 21 mg nicotine patch, nicotine enhanced the maximum increase in heart rate seen with cannabis. The increase in heart rate for nicotine alone was between 10 and 15 bpm, for cannabis alone 32 and 42 bpm, for women and men, respectively, and for the combination, 45 and 58 bpm, respectively. In addition, the duration of tachycardia after smoking the low-dose cannabis was prolonged by 30 minutes by nicotine, but was not changed after the high-dose cannabis. Nicotine increased the subjective stimulant effects of cannabis, but the reported duration of effects of cannabis were shortened by nicotine. Plasma levels of nicotine and Δ^9-tetrahydrocannabinol (THC) did not differ on concurrent use. The cannabis cigarettes were standardised to 1.99% THC (low dose) and 3.51% THC (high dose).[1]

Experimental evidence

Studies in *mice* found that nicotine enhanced the effects of Δ^9-tetrahydrocannabinol in terms of hypolocomotion, hypothermia, antinociceptive responses. Somatic signs of withdrawal from Δ^9-tetrahydrocannabinol were more severe in *mice* that had received nicotine.[2]

Mechanism

Unknown. The additive effect on heart rate may be due to sympathetic activity of both drugs, and might also involve cannabinoid receptors.[1]

Importance and management

Cannabis is often smoked with tobacco. The findings of the clinical study show that transdermal nicotine has additive effects with cannabis on heart rate, and increased the stimulant effect of cannabis. The clinical significance of these findings is uncertain.

1. Penetar DM, Kouri EM, Gross MM, McCarthy EM, Rhee CK, Peters EN, Lukas SE. Transdermal nicotine alters some of marihuana's effects in male and female volunteers. *Drug Alcohol Depend* (2005) 79, 211–23.
2. Valjent E, Mitchell JM, Besson M-J, Caboche J, Maldonado R. Behavioural and biochemical evidence for interactions between Δ9-tetrahydrocannabinol and nicotine. *Br J Pharmacol* (2002) 135, 564–78.

Cannabis + NSAIDs

Indometacin appears to antagonise some of the effects of cannabis, and cannabis might antagonise the analgesic efficacy of NSAIDs.

Clinical evidence

Four healthy subjects were given placebo or **indometacin** 25 mg three times daily for one day, and then a single-dose 2 hours before smoking cannabis 400 micrograms/kg on the following day. **Indometacin** did not alter the pharmacokinetics of Δ^9-tetrahydrocannabinol. Subjective measures of heart rate acceleration and intoxication were modestly attenuated by **indometacin**. Subjects also reported that the effects of marihuana on time perception were antagonised by **indometacin**.[1]

Experimental evidence

In a study *rabbits* received placebo or 2% **indometacin** applied topically to both eyes one hour prior to an intravenous injection of Δ^9-tetrahydrocannabinol. The fall in intraocular pressure caused by Δ^9-tetrahydrocannabinol was inhibited by topical **indometacin**.

In an *animal* model of analgesia, chronic treatment with Δ^9-tetrahydrocannabinol markedly reduced the efficacy of **aspirin**, **celecoxib**, **indometacin**, **ketorolac** and **naproxen**, and reduced the potency of **diclofenac** and **paracetamol (acetaminophen)**.[2]

Mechanism

It is suggested that prostaglandins have some part to play in some of the effects of cannabis, and that these are antagonised by indometacin, which is a prostaglandin inhibitor.[1,3] Similarly, cannabis antagonises the effects of NSAIDs.[2]

Importance and management

The effects of indometacin on the subjective measures and intraocular pressure lowering effects of Δ^9-tetrahydrocannabinol are probably not of clinical significance. However, the relevance of the finding that chronic use of Δ^9-tetrahydrocannabinol might result in reduced efficacy and potency of NSAIDs requires further study.

1. Perez-Reyes M, Burstein SH, White WR, McDonald SA, Hicks RE. Antagonism of marihuana effects by indometacin in humans. *Life Sci* (1991) 8, 507–15.
2. Anikwue R, Huffman JW, Martin ZL, Welch SP. Decrease in efficacy and potency of nonsteroidal anti-inflammatory drugs by chronic delta(9)-tetrahydrocannabinol. administration. *J Pharmacol Exp Ther* (2002) 303, 340–346.
3. Green K, Kearse EC, McIntyre OL. Interaction between delta-9-tetrahydrocannabinol and indomethacin. *Ophthalmic Res* (2001) 33, 217–20.

Cannabis + Opioids

Low doses of cannabis enhanced the effect of morphine in three patients. *Animal* studies have shown that cannabinoids may enhance the potency of opioids.

Evidence, mechanism, importance and management

A report of 3 patients with chronic pain (due to multiple sclerosis, HIV-related peripheral neuropathy, and lumbar spinal damage) found that small doses of smoked cannabis potentiated the antinociceptive effects of **morphine**. The patients were able to decrease the dose of opioid by 60 to 100%.[1] Studies in *animals* have shown that Δ^9-tetrahydrocannabinol, the major psychoactive constituent of cannabis, enhances the potency of opioids such as **morphine**, **codeine**, **hydromorphone**, **methadone**, **oxymorphone** and **pethidine (meperidine)**.[2–4] It has been suggested that low doses of Δ^9-tetrahydrocannabinol given with low doses of **morphine** may increase opioid potency without increasing adverse effects.[5] Cannabis use in **methadone**-maintained patients did not appear to affect treatment progress, although some psychological difficulties were slightly more prevalent.[6] However, other workers have suggested that heavy cannabis use is associated with poorer progress when methadone is given in the treatment of opioid addiction.[7]

1. Lynch ME, Clark AJ. Cannabis reduces opioid dose in the treatment of chronic non-cancer pain. *J Pain Symptom Manage* (2003) 25, 496–8.
2. Smith FL, Cichewicz D, Martin ZL, Welch SP. The enhancement of morphine antinociception in mice by Δ9-tetrahydrocannabinol. *Pharmacol Biochem Behav* (1998) 60, 559–66.
3. Cichewicz DL, Martin ZL, Smith FL, Welch SP. Enhancement of μ opioid antinociception by oral Δ9-tetrahydrocannabinol: dose-response analysis and receptor identification. *J Pharmacol Exp Ther* (1999) 289, 859–67.
4. Cichewicz DL, McCarthy EA. Antinociceptive synergy between Δ9-tetrahydrocannabinol and opioids after oral administration. *J Pharmacol Exp Ther* (2003) 304, 1010–1015.
5. Cichewicz DL. Synergistic interactions between cannabinoid and opioid analgesics. *Life Sci* (2004) 74, 1317–24.
6. Epstein DH, Preston KL. Does cannabis use predict poor outcome for heroin-dependent patients on maintenance treatment? Past findings and more evidence against. *Addiction* (2003) 98, 269–79.
7. Nixon LN. Cannabis use and treatment outcome in methadone maintenance. *Addiction* (2003) 98, 1321–2.

Cannabis + Phencyclidine

The interaction between cannabis and phencyclidine is based on experimental evidence only.

Clinical evidence

No interactions found.

Experimental evidence

An *animal* study found that pretreatment with cannabidiol significantly increased the levels of phencyclidine in the brain and blood of *mice*. Behavioural tests indicated that the increase in brain levels led to an increase in intoxication caused by phencyclidine. When the study was repeated using Δ9-tetrahydrocannabinol in doses of 120 mg/kg, the brain levels of phencyclidine were increased twofold. Lower doses of Δ9-tetrahydrocannabinol did not result in such an effect.[1]

Mechanism

Unknown.

Importance and management

This preclinical study provides some evidence that cannabis might increase the abuse potential of phencyclidine.

1. Reid MJ, Bornheim LM. Cannabinoid-induced alterations in brain disposition of drugs of abuse. *Biochem Pharmacol* (2001) 61, 1357–67.

Cannabis + Phenytoin

There is one *in vitro* study suggesting that Δ9-tetrahydrocannabinol, a major constituent of cannabis, might induce phenytoin metabolism. Note that, in clinical use dronabinol has induced seizures.

Clinical evidence

No interactions found.

Experimental evidence

In an *in vitro* study in which human liver microsomes were incubated with phenytoin alone, or phenytoin and Δ9-tetrahydrocannabinol, a major constituent of cannabis, the rate of metabolism of phenytoin was slightly increased in a dose-dependent manner. The rate of metabolism of Δ9-tetrahydrocannabinol to its 11-hydroxy metabolite was not altered by phenytoin.[1]

Various cannabinoids have shown antiepileptic effects in *animal* studies. In one study, the antiepileptic effect of phenytoin was increased when combined with cannabidiol.[2]

Mechanism

The *in vitro* data suggests that Δ9-tetrahydrocannabinol induces the cytochrome P450 isoenzyme CYP2C9.[1]

Importance and management

This appears to be the only evidence that cannabis might affect phenytoin levels, and is only *in vitro* data. As such, it requires confirmation before any recommendations can be made. Note also that there are no reports in the literature of cannabis use affecting phenytoin levels. Note that oral dronabinol (Δ9-tetrahydrocannabinol) has caused seizures in clinical use, and the manufacturer recommends caution in those with a seizure disorder.[3]

1. Bland TM, Haining RL, Tracy TS, Callery PS. CYP2C-catalyzed delta(9)-tetrahydrocannabinol metabolism: kinetics, pharmacogenetics and interaction with phenytoin. *Biochem Pharmacol* (2005) 70, 1096–1103.
2. Consroe P, Wolkin A. Cannabidiol - antiepileptic drug comparisons and interactions in experimentally induced seizures in rats. *J Pharmacol Exp Ther* (1977) 201, 26–32.
3. Marinol (Dronabinol). Solvay Pharmaceuticals, Inc. US Prescribing information, March 2008.

Cannabis + Sildenafil

Myocardial infarction has been reported in a man who had smoked cannabis and taken sildenafil.

Clinical evidence

A 41-year old man with no history of cardiac disease experienced a myocardial infarction after smoking cannabis and recreationally taking a tablet of sildenafil (strength not specified). Later tests showed that he had no evidence of inducible ischaemia.[1]

Experimental evidence

No relevant data found.

Mechanism

Myocardial infarction is a rare adverse effect of sildenafil alone. It was suggested that the metabolism of sildenafil by CYP3A4 might be inhibited by constituents of cannabis such as cannabidiol, thereby increasing the risk of adverse events. However, in clinical studies, oral cannabis did not alter levels of other CYP3A4 substrates. These included Cannabis + Irinotecan, page 121, and Cannabis + Docetaxel, page 121.

Importance and management

An interaction between sildenafil and cannabis is not established. The vasodilatory effects of sildenafil necessitate caution in its use in patients with cardiovascular disease: myocardial infarction has rarely been associated with its use. The contribution of an interaction between sildenafil and cannabis to this case is unclear.

1. McLeod AL, McKenna CJ, Northridge DB. Myocardial infarction following the combined recreational use of Viagra® and cannabis. *Clin Cardiol* (2002) 25, 133–4.

Cannabis + Theophylline

Smoking cannabis appears to increase the clearance of theophylline.

Evidence, mechanism, importance and management

One study found that tobacco or cannabis smoking caused similar higher total clearances of theophylline (given as oral aminophylline) than occurred in non-smokers (about 74 mL/kg per hour compared with 52 mL/kg per hour), and that clearance was even higher (93 mL/kg per hour) in those who smoked both.[1] A later analysis by the same authors, of factors affecting theophylline clearance, found that smoking two or more joints of cannabis weekly was

C

associated with a higher total clearance of theophylline than non-use (82.9 mL/kg per hour versus 56.1 mL/kg per hour).[2] A study in which 16 of 49 healthy subjects admitted to smoking cannabis in the months before taking a single 4-mg/kg oral dose of theophylline found that cannabis use did not have a significant effect on the pharmacokinetics of theophylline. Their use was considered not to exceed normal social use of one joint per week.[3]

Both tobacco and cannabis smoke contain polycyclic hydrocarbons, which act as inducers of CYP1A2, the isoenzyme by which theophylline is metabolised, and therefore theophylline might be cleared more quickly in those who smoke these substances.

Evidence for an effect of smoking cannabis on theophylline levels is limited, but be alert for the need to increase the theophylline dose in regular cannabis users. Note also that irregular cannabis use might cause fluctuations in theophylline levels. An additional problem in interpreting this interaction is that the quantity of interacting constituent might vary between different sources of cannabis, and between different batches from the same source.

There appears to be no direct evidence regarding aminophylline, but as it is metabolised to theophylline, it seems likely that it will be similarly affected by cannabis.

1. Jusko WJ, Schentag JJ, Clark JH, Gardner M, Yurchak AM. Enhanced biotransformation of theophylline in marihuana and tobacco smokers. *Clin Pharmacol Ther* (1978) 24, 406–10.
2. Jusko WJ, Gardner MJ, Mangione A, Schentag JJ, Koup JR, Vance JW. Factors affecting theophylline clearances: age, tobacco, marijuana, cirrhosis, congestive heart failure, obesity, oral contraceptives, benzodiazepines, barbiturates, and ethanol. *J Pharm Sci* (1979) 68, 1358–66.
3. Gardner MJ, Tornatore KM, Jusko WJ, Kanarkowski R. Effects of tobacco smoking and oral contraceptive use on theophylline disposition. *Br J Clin Pharmacol* (1983) 16, 271–80.

Cannabis + Tricyclic antidepressants

Tachycardia has been described when patients taking tricyclic antidepressants smoked cannabis.

Evidence, mechanism, importance and management

A 21-year-old woman taking **nortriptyline** 30 mg daily experienced marked tachycardia (an increase from 90 to 160 bpm) after smoking a cannabis cigarette. It was controlled with propranolol.[1] A 26-year-old complained of restlessness, dizziness and tachycardia (120 bpm) after smoking cannabis while taking **imipramine** 50 mg daily.[2] Four adolescents aged 15 to 18 taking tricyclic antidepressants for attention-deficit hyperactivity disorder had transient cognitive changes, delirium and tachycardia after smoking cannabis.[3]

Increased heart rates are well-documented adverse effects of both the tricyclic antidepressants and cannabis, and what occurred was probably due to the additive beta-adrenergic and antimuscarinic effects of the tricyclics, with the beta-adrenergic effect of the cannabis. Direct information is limited but it has been suggested that concurrent use should be avoided.[1]

1. Hillard JR, Vieweg WVR. Marked sinus tachycardia resulting from the synergistic effects of marijuana and nortriptyline. *Am J Psychiatry* (1983) 140, 626–7.
2. Kizer KW. Possible interaction of TCA and marijuana. *Ann Emerg Med* (1980) 9, 444.
3. Wilens TE, Biederman J, Spencer TJ. Case study: adverse effects of smoking marijuana while receiving tricyclic antidepressants. *J Am Acad Child Adolesc Psychiatry* (1997) 36, 45–8.

Cannabis + Warfarin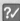

A case report describes an increased INR and bleeding in a patient who smoked cannabis while taking warfarin.

Clinical evidence

A 56-year-old man taking warfarin was admitted to hospital with black, tarry stools and was found to have an INR of 10.41. Although was also taking a number of potentially interacting drugs (including aspirin, carbamazepine and sertraline) he had been stable on these for 6 months, and had also been stable since starting clopidogrel about one month earlier. Further, he had recently had a small increase to his warfarin dose but his INR (measured subsequent to the dose increase and 5 days before he was hospitalised) had been 3.25. The raised INR was managed by temporarily stopping warfarin, aspirin and clopidogrel, giving vitamin K and fresh frozen plasma, and he was subsequently discharged. About 15 days after being discharged the patient was readmitted following an increased amount of bruising and a nosebleed: his INR was found to be 11.55. Again, he had recently had a dose increase of his warfarin because of an INR of 1.94, but the dose increase was small, from 3 mg daily to 3.25 mg daily. On both occasions it turned out that the patient had more than doubled the quantity of cannabis he was smoking.[1]

Experimental evidence

No relevant data found.

Mechanism

Unknown. *In vitro* data suggest that Δ^9-tetrahydrocannabinol, a major constituent of cannabis, induces the cytochrome P450 isoenzyme CYP2C9, see Cannabis + Phenytoin, page 123, but as the *S*-isomer of warfarin is metabolised by this route, this would be expected to increase the metabolism of warfarin and reduce its effects, which is in contrast to the case report.

Importance and management

Evidence for an interaction between cannabis and warfarin is limited and as such the general relevance of this case, which attributed a raised INR in a patient taking warfarin to cannabis smoking is unknown. Because of the many other factors influencing anticoagulant control, it is not possible to reliably ascribe a change in INR specifically to a drug interaction in a single case report without other supporting evidence. It may be better to advise patients to discuss the use of any herbal products they wish to try, and to increase monitoring if this is thought advisable. Cases of uneventful use should be reported, as they are as useful as possible cases of adverse effects.

1. Yamreudeewong W, Wong HK, Brausch LM, Pulley KR. Probable interaction between warfarin and marijuana smoking. *Ann Pharmacother* (2009) 43, 1347–53.

Capsicum

Capsicum species (Solanaceae)

Synonym(s) and related species

Caspic, Cayenne, Cayenne pepper, Chili pepper, Chilli pepper, Hot pepper, Paprika, Red pepper, Tabasco pepper.

Capsicum annuum L., *Capsicum baccatum* L., *Capsicum chinense* Jacq., *Capsicum frutescens* L., *Capsicum minimum* Roxb., *Capsicum pubescens* Ruiz & Pav.

Pharmacopoeias

Capsicum (*BP 2012, PhEur 7.5, USP35–NF30 S1*); Capsicum oleoresin (*USP35–NF30 S1*); Refined and quantified capsicum oleoresin (*BP 2012, PhEur 7.5*); Standardised capsicum tincture (*BP 2012, PhEur 7.5*).

Constituents

The pungent principles of capsicum are the capsaicinoids (to which it may be standardised), present in concentrations up to 1.5%, but more usually around 0.1%. The major components are capsaicin, 6,7-dihydrocapsaicin, nordihydrocapsaicin, homodihydrocapsaicin and homocapsaicin. Other constituents include the carotenoid pigments (capsanthin, capsorubin, carotene, lutein), vitamins including A and C, and a small amount of volatile oil.

Use and indications

Capsicum possesses stimulant, antispasmodic, carminative and counterirritant effects, which has led to its use in conditions such as colic and flatulent dyspepsia, and to increase peripheral circulation. Topical preparations are used for neuralgia including rheumatic pains and unbroken chilblains.

Capsicum is frequently eaten as part of the diet, and in particular, diets that contain spicy foods. It has been estimated that the average consumption of dietary spice from capsicum fruit is 2.5 g/person per day in India and 5 g/person per day in Thailand. As the capsaicin content in capsicum fruit is approximately 1%, the daily dietary intake of capsaicin may range from 0.5 to 1 mg/kg per day for a 50 kg person.[1]

Pharmacokinetics

In vitro study suggests that many of the cytochrome P450 enzymes are involved in the metabolism of capsaicinoids,

by dehydrogenation, oxygenation, hydroxylation, and *O*-demethylation. Principal isoenzymes thought to be involved are CYP2C9, CYP2E1 and to some extent CYP3A4.

Some metabolites of the capsaicinoids are thought to inhibit CYP2E1,[2] and a study with phenazone, page 127, a probe drug for hepatic enzyme activity, suggests that capsaicin may inhibit hepatic enzymes, although the lack of interaction seen with theophylline, page 128, a substrate for CYP1A2, suggests that this isoenzyme is not significantly affected. A further *in vitro* study has shown that the acute use of capsaicin inhibits P-glycoprotein whereas long-term exposure induces P-glycoprotein, see digoxin, page 126.

Interactions overview

Capsicum has the potential to decrease the absorption of aspirin, increase the absorption of ciprofloxacin and theophylline, and alter the absorption of cefalexin and digoxin. However, the clinical effects of these changes are unknown, not established or not clinically significant. Capsicum may also decrease the metabolism of pentobarbital and phenazone, but it does not alter the metabolism of theophylline or quinine, which suggests that it has selective effects on hepatic enzymes.

Interactions monographs

- Aspirin, page 126
- Cefalexin, page 126
- Ciprofloxacin, page 126
- Digoxin, page 126
- Food, page 127
- Herbal medicines, page 127
- Iron compounds, page 127
- Pentobarbital, page 127
- Phenazone (Antipyrine), page 127
- Quinine, page 127
- Theophylline, page 128

1. Axsain (Capsaicin). Cephalon Ltd. UK Summary of product characteristics, October 2007.
2. Reilly CA, Yost GS. Metabolism of capsaicinoids by P450 enzymes: a review of recent findings on reaction mechanisms, bio-activation, and detoxification processes. *Drug Metab Rev* (2006) 38, 685–706.

Capsicum + Aspirin

The interaction between capsicum and aspirin is based on experimental evidence only.

Clinical evidence

No interactions found.

Experimental evidence

A study in *rats* given oral aspirin 20 mg/kg found that the acute administration of a standardised extract of *Capsicum annuum* 100 mg/kg (equivalent to 10 mg/kg capsaicin) reduced the AUC and maximum serum levels of salicylic acid by 44% and 26%, respectively. The effect was dose-related, with a 300-mg/kg dose of *Capsicum annuum* reducing the AUC and maximum serum levels of salicylic acid by 59% and 51%, respectively. Similar, but greater, results were found when aspirin was given to *rats* that had been treated with *Capsicum annuum* extract for 4 weeks.[1]

Mechanism

It seems likely that capsaicin alters gastric motility, which reduces aspirin absorption and results in decreased salicylic acid levels.[1]

Importance and management

Evidence is limited, but capsaicin appears to decrease aspirin bioavailability. However, the clinical significance of this effect is unclear, especially as the capsaicin dose used in the study is 10-fold greater than the expected dietary intake in countries that typically eat a spicy diet, and many times higher than the expected exposure if capsaicin is given as a cream, or ingested as a medicinal product. More study is needed before any clinical recommendations can be made.

1. Cruz L, Castañeda-Hernández G, Navarrete A. Ingestion of chilli pepper (*Capsicum annuum*) reduces salicylate bioavailability after oral aspirin administration in the rat. *Can J Physiol Pharmacol* (1999) 77, 441–6.

Capsicum + Cefalexin

The interaction between capsicum and cefalexin is based on experimental evidence only.

Clinical evidence

No interactions found.

Experimental evidence

An *in vitro* study using *animal* tissue found that high concentrations of capsaicin instilled into *rat* intestines resulted in a lower rate of absorption of cefalexin.[1]

Mechanism

It was suggested that the capsaicin affected the transport channels in the intestine through which cefalexin is absorbed.[1]

Importance and management

Evidence appears to be limited to this study. Although the rate of cefalexin absorption was decreased the total amount of cefalexin absorbed was not studied, and therefore no conclusions can be drawn on the possible clinical relevance of the findings.

1. Komori Y, Aiba T, Sugiyama R, Nakai C, Kawasaki H, Kurosaki Y. Effects of capsaicin on intestinal cephalexin absorption in rats. *Biol Pharm Bull* (2007) 30, 547–51.

Capsicum + Ciprofloxacin

The interaction between capsicum and ciprofloxacin is based on experimental evidence only.

Clinical evidence

No interactions found.

Experimental evidence

A study in which *rats* were given oral ciprofloxacin 20 mg/kg with placebo, or capsaicin in concentrations of 0.01%, 0.1%, 0.5% or 1%, found that the maximum levels and AUC of ciprofloxacin increased with increasing concentrations of capsaicin up to 0.5%. The increase in AUC was 49%, 51%, 68% and 15% for capsaicin, 0.01%, 0.1%, 0.5% or 1%, respectively.[1]

Mechanism

It is possible that the irritant nature of the capsaicin increased blood flow to the gastrointestinal absorption site, or alternatively, the rate of gastric emptying was increased, so ciprofloxacin reached the duodenum more quickly, where the pH enhances its absorption.

Importance and management

Evidence appears to be limited to this study. The doses of the antibacterial and capsaicin were chosen to reflect those likely to be encountered clinically, and those encountered within dietary levels, respectively. Therefore if these findings are replicated in humans it seems possible that a clinically relevant rise in ciprofloxacin levels could occur; however, given the magnitude of the rise, the effect seems most likely to be beneficial rather than adverse, although more study is needed to establish this.

1. Sumano-López H, Gutiérrez-Olvera L, Aguilera-Jiménez R, Gutiérrez-Olvera C, Jiménez-Gómez F. Administration of ciprofloxacin and capsaicin in rats to achieve higher maximal serum concentrations. *Arzneimittelforschung* (2007) 57, 286–90.

Capsicum + Digoxin

The interaction between capsicum and digoxin is based on experimental evidence only.

Clinical evidence

No interactions found.

Experimental evidence

In an *in vitro* study, P-glycoprotein function was assessed by looking at the transport of digoxin, a known substrate of this transporter protein. In the presence of capsaicin the transport of digoxin across cells was enhanced, suggesting that capsaicin induces P-glycoprotein.[1]

Mechanism

Capsaicin may induce P-glycoprotein.

Importance and management

Evidence is limited and difficult to extrapolate to a clinical situation. The study found that the acute use of capsaicin inhibited P-glycoprotein, whereas long-term exposure induced P-glycoprotein. Clinically, P-glycoprotein induction has resulted in reduced digoxin absorption from the intestine, and increased biliary excretion; the end result being a reduction in digoxin levels. Whether capsaicin would initially raise then subsequently lower digoxin levels remains to be established, but it may be prudent to consider the possibility of this effect if large doses of capsaicin are given systemically.

1. Han Y, Tan TMC, Lim L-Y. Effects of capsaicin in P-gp function and expression in Caco-2 cells. *Biochem Pharmacol* (2006) 71, 1727–34.

Capsicum + Food

No interactions found. Capsicum is widely used as a spice in food.

Capsicum + Herbal medicines

No interactions found.

Capsicum + Iron compounds

Capsicum modestly reduces the absorption of dietary iron.

Clinical evidence

In a randomised, crossover study, 30 healthy women were given a standard Thai meal (fortified with about 4 mg of isotopically labelled ferrous sulfate), with soup, to which 4.2 g of ground *Capsicum annuum* had been added. *Capsicum annuum* reduced iron absorption by about 38%.[1]

Experimental evidence

No relevant data found.

Mechanism

Uncertain. It was thought that polyphenols in *Capsicum annuum* may inhibit iron absorption.

Importance and management

The study suggests that capsicum inhibits the absorption of dietary levels of iron. The levels of capsicum used were high, but they are not unusual in a typical Thai meal. However, the effects of capsicum on iron supplementation (e.g. ferrous sulfate in doses of 200 mg) does not appear to have been studied, so it is difficult to predict the effect of the use of capsicum as a herbal medicine on iron replacement therapy. However, consider this interaction if a patient taking capsicum supplements has a poor response to iron replacement therapy.

1. Tuntipopipat S, Judprasong K, Zeder C, Wasantwisut E, Winichagoon P, Charoenkiatkul S, Hurrell R, Walczyk T. Chili, but not turmeric, inhibits iron absorption in young women from an iron-fortified composite meal. *J Nutr* (2006) 136, 2970–2974.

Capsicum + Pentobarbital

The interaction between capsicum and pentobarbital is based on experimental evidence only.

Clinical evidence

No interactions found.

Experimental evidence

In a placebo-controlled study, *rats* were given a single 10-mg/kg subcutaneous dose of capsaicin followed 6 hours later by pentobar-

bital. The sleeping time of *rats* in response to the pentobarbital was more than doubled by capsaicin.[1]

Mechanism

It is thought that capsaicin may inhibit the cytochrome P450-mediated metabolism of pentobarbital.

Importance and management

Evidence is limited to this study in *rats*. If the findings are replicated in humans it seems likely that capsaicin could increase the response to pentobarbital. Therefore if patients taking pentobarbital are given systemic capsicum it may be prudent to warn them that prolonged drowsiness may occur.

1. Miller MS, Brendel K, Burks TF, Sipes IG. Interaction of capsaicinoids with drug-metabolizing systems: relationship to toxicity. *Biochem Pharmacol* (1983) 32, 547–51.

Capsicum + Phenazone (Antipyrine)

The interaction between capsicum and phenazone is based on experimental evidence only.

Clinical evidence

No interactions found.

Experimental evidence

In a placebo-controlled study, *rats* were given capsaicin 25 mg/kg daily for 7 days, followed by a single 10-mg intravenous dose of phenazone. It was found that capsaicin increased the half-life of phenazone by 28%, and increased the AUC of phenazone by 43%.[1]

Mechanism

Capsaicin inhibits the metabolism of phenazone by hepatic enzymes.[1]

Importance and management

Evidence is limited to this study in *rats*. Although rises in phenazone levels of this magnitude may be of clinical relevance, the dose of capsicum used in the study was very high, so it seems unlikely that these effects would be reproduced with clinical or dietary quantities of capsaicin.

1. Wanwimolruk S, Nyika S, Kepple M, Ferry DG, Clark CR. Effects of capsaicin on the pharmacokinetics of antipyrine, theophylline and quinine in rats. *J Pharm Pharmacol* (1993) 45, 618–21.

Capsicum + Quinine

The information regarding the use of capsicum with quinine is based on experimental evidence only.

Clinical evidence

No interactions found.

Experimental evidence

In a placebo-controlled study, *rats* were given capsaicin 25 mg/kg daily for 7 days, followed by a single 25-mg/kg intravenous dose of quinine. It was found that capsaicin had no effect on the pharmacokinetics of quinine.[1]

Mechanism

No mechanism expected.

Importance and management

The available evidence suggests that no pharmacokinetic interaction would be expected between capsaicin and quinine.

1. Wanwimolruk S, Nyika S, Kepple M, Ferry DG, Clark CR. Effects of capsaicin on the pharmacokinetics of antipyrine, theophylline and quinine in rats. *J Pharm Pharmacol* (1993) 45, 618–21.

Capsicum + Theophylline

Although capsicum may slightly increase the absorption of theophylline, it does not appear to be clinically relevant.

Clinical evidence

A study in 6 healthy subjects found that the absorption of theophylline 400 to 500 mg was increased after they ate a spicy meal, when compared with a European standard meal: the AUC_{0-6} and AUC_{0-12} were increased by 23% and 15%, respectively.[1]

Experimental evidence

In a study, *rabbits* were given a single intravenous 12-mg/kg dose of theophylline with either a single dose of ground capsicum suspension, or after 7 days of treatment with ground capsicum suspension. Capsicum did not affect the pharmacokinetics of theophylline, apart from a 40% increase in the elimination rate constant after the single dose of capsicum.[2]

A previous study by the same authors found that a ground capsicum fruit suspension, given at the time of the theophylline dose and 11 hours later, increased the AUC of a 20-mg/kg oral dose of theophylline, and increased peak theophylline levels by 33%.[3]

In contrast, a placebo-controlled study in *rats* given capsaicin 25 mg/kg daily for 7 days followed by a single 10-mg/kg intravenous dose of theophylline, given as aminophylline, found that capsaicin did not affect the pharmacokinetics of theophylline.[4]

Mechanism

Capsaicin has been shown in *animal* studies to increase mesenteric blood flow, which may result in increased absorption of theophylline.[3]

Importance and management

The evidence suggests that capsaicin has only modest effects on the pharmacokinetics of theophylline. The clinical study found an increase in the theophylline AUC of about 20%, which would not generally be expected to be clinically relevant. It would therefore appear that no specific additional precautions are necessary if patients taking theophylline also take capsicum.

1. Bouraoui A, Toumi A, Bouchacha S, Boukef K, Brazier JL. Influence de l'alimentation épicée et piquante sur l'absorption de la théophylline. *Therapie* (1986) 41, 467–71.
2. Bouraoui A, Brazier JL, Zouaghi H, Rousseau M. Theophylline pharmacokinetics and metabolism in rabbits following single and repeated administration of *Capsicum* fruit. *Eur J Drug Metab Pharmacokinet* (1995) 20, 173–8.
3. Bouraoui A, Toumi A, Ben Mustapha H, Brazier JL. Effects of capsicum fruit on theophylline absorption and bioavailability in rabbits. *Drug Nutr Interact* (1988) 5, 345–50.
4. Wanwimolruk S, Nyika S, Kepple M, Ferry DG, Clark CR. Effects of capsaicin on the pharmacokinetics of antipyrine, theophylline and quinine in rats. *J Pharm Pharmacol* (1993) 45, 618–21.

Carnitine derivatives

Synonym(s) and related species

Acetyl-L-carnitine: Acetylcarnitine, Levacecarnine.

Carnitine: Vitamin B_T.

L-carnitine: Levocarnitine. Note that the general term **carnitine** is sometimes used to describe both L-carnitine and acetyl-L-carnitine as well as other derivatives.

Types, sources and related compounds

Carnitine is an amino acid derivative, synthesised in the brain, liver and kidney from the essential amino acids lysine and methionine. It is normally synthesised in sufficient quantities to meet human requirements but is present in dietary sources such as meat and dairy products. It is an essential cofactor of fatty acid metabolism and exists as distinct L- and D-isomers, with L-carnitine being the form naturally occurring in the body. Acetylcarnitine is the most abundant acylated ester of carnitine in the body. Dietary supplements may contain L-carnitine or a mixture of both D- and L-isomers.

Pharmacopoeias

Levocarnitine (*BP 2012, PhEur 7.5, USP35–NF30 S1*); Levocarnitine Injection (*USP35–NF30 S1*), Levocarnitine Oral Solution (*USP35–NF30 S1*), Levocarnitine Tablets (*USP35–NF30 S1*).

Use and indications

Carnitine and its derivatives are used in the treatment of primary carnitine deficiency or deficiency caused by defects in intermediary metabolism or from haemodialysis. Among a wide variety of conditions, they are also occasionally used to treat cardiac disorders including angina, to improve exercise performance, to improve fatigue (including use in chronic fatigue syndrome) and to treat Alzheimer's disease, but there is little clinical evidence to support most of these uses.

It has been suggested that L-carnitine, rather than the DL-form, should be used therapeutically, as the two isomers differ in their actions, with D-carnitine possibly inhibiting the activity of L-carnitine.

Pharmacokinetics

L-carnitine, when given as an oral supplement, is absorbed slowly and incompletely from the small intestine. Bioavailability is low, about 10 to 18%, with peak plasma concentrations achieved about 3 to 4 hours after an oral dose. After intravenous doses, L-carnitine undergoes minimal metabolism and does not appear to bind to plasma proteins.

Interactions overview

Isolated case reports describe a substantial increase in the anticoagulant effect of acenocoumarol when given with L-carnitine. Drugs that reduce carnitine levels might reduce the efficacy of L-carnitine, and DL-carnitine might interact similarly. Acetyl-L-carnitine and propionyl-L-carnitine are predicted to undergo the same interactions as L-carnitine.

Interactions monographs

- Antidiabetics, page 130
- Carnitine, page 130
- Drugs that reduce carnitine levels, page 130
- Food, page 131
- Herbal medicines, page 131
- Warfarin and related drugs, page 131

C

C

L-carnitine (Levocarnitine) + Antidiabetics

Oral L-carnitine appears to have little effect on glucose control in patients taking antidiabetics.

Clinical evidence

Carnitine derivatives have been tested in patients with diabetes for a variety of indications, including diabetic neuropathy and to improve lipid profiles, as well as to try to improve insulin sensitivity. The possible effects on diabetic control are discussed here.

In one randomised, placebo-controlled study in 35 patients with type 2 diabetes taking **metformin** or **glibenclamide (glyburide)**, oral L-carnitine 1 g three times daily for 12 weeks decreased fasting blood glucose levels (by 13%), but had no effect on HbA_{1c} levels.[1] In another randomised, placebo-controlled study in 12 patients with type 2 diabetes not taking any antidiabetic medication, oral L-carnitine 1 g three times daily before meals for 4 weeks, had no effect on insulin sensitivity or lipid profile.[2] In contrast, a continuous 3-hour intravenous infusion of L-carnitine increased insulin sensitivity in 15 type 2 diabetic patients, in whom diabetes was controlled by rapid action insulin from one week before the study.[3] In two other randomised controlled studies in patients with poorly controlled diabetes taking oral antidiabetics or insulin, the addition of oral L-carnitine 2 g daily to either sibutramine or orlistat slightly improved diabetic control (a 0.4 to 0.9 further reduction in HbA_{1c} % at 9 to 12 months) compared with sibutramine or orlistat alone.[4,5] In those studies reporting adverse effects, there was no mention of hypoglycaemia.[2,5]

Experimental evidence

Because of the clinical evidence available, experimental data have not been sought.

Mechanism

L-carnitine is thought to stimulate glucose oxidation.[3] However, note that hypoketotic hypoglycaemia is one symptom of primary carnitine deficiency, for which L-carnitine is a treatment.

Importance and management

The available clinical evidence cited here indicates that in most patients with diabetes, oral L-carnitine has little effect on diabetic control, and hypoglycaemia does not appear to have been reported. Nevertheless, in some of its products, the UK manufacturer notes that giving L-carnitine to diabetic patients receiving either insulin or oral antidiabetics might result in hypoglycaemia. They advise regular monitoring of plasma glucose concentrations in these patients in order to adjust the hypoglycaemic treatment immediately, if required.[6] However, in the US, the manufacturer gives no such warning, and makes no comment about any precautions in diabetes.[7]

1. Rahbar AR, Shakerhosseini R , Saadat N, Taleban F, Pordal A, Gollestan B. Effect of L-carnitine on plasma glycemic and lipidemic profile in patients with type II diabetes mellitus. *Eur J Clin Nutr* (2005) 59, 592–6.
2. González-Ortiz M, Hernández-González SO, Hernández-Salazar E, Martínez-Abundis E. Effect of oral L-carnitine administration on insulin sensitivity and lipid profile in type 2 diabetes mellitus patients. *Ann Nutr Metab* (2008) 52, 335–8.
3. Mingrone G, Greco AV, Capristo E, Benedetti G, Giancaterini A, De Gaetano A, Gasbarrini G. L-carnitine improves glucose disposal in type 2 diabetic patients. *J Am Coll Nutr* (1999) 18, 77–82.
4. Derosa G , Maffioli P, Salvadeo SA, Ferrari I, Gravina A, Mereu R, D'Angelo A, Palumbo I, Randazzo S, Cicero AF. Sibutramine and L-carnitine compared to sibutramine alone on insulin resistance in diabetic patients. *Intern Med* (2010) 49, 1717–25.
5. Derosa G, Maffioli P, Ferrari I, D'Angelo A, Fogari E, Palumbo I, Randazzo S, Cicero AF. Orlistat and L-carnitine compared to orlistat alone on insulin resistance in obese diabetic patients. *Endocr J* (2010) 57, 777–86.
6. Carnitor oral single dose L-Carnitine. Sigma-tau Pharma Ltd UK UK Summary of product characteristics, September 2008.
7. Carnitor Levocarnitine. Sigma-tau Pharmaceuticals, Inc. US Prescribing information, May 2007.

L-carnitine (Levocarnitine) + Carnitine

The D-isomer of carnitine (present in racemic carnitine) might reduce the activity of L-carnitine.

Clinical evidence, mechanism, importance and management

Naturally occurring carnitine exists as the L-isomer (levocarnitine), which is biologically active. Carnitine supplements contain either L-carnitine or the racemic DL-carnitine. D-carnitine can reduce the activity of L-carnitine. Therefore, to ensure adequate biological activity, if carnitine supplementation is required, it might be prudent to use L-carnitine, and to avoid DL-carnitine.

L-carnitine (Levocarnitine) + Drugs that reduce carnitine levels

Pivalic acid-containing drugs such as pivampicillin and pivmecillinam, can reduce carnitine levels on long-term use. Reduced carnitine levels have also been seen with other drugs, such as valproate and certain cytotoxic antineoplastics.

Clinical evidence

Pivalic acid-containing drugs can reduce serum carnitine levels, especially on long-term or repeated use at doses that release considerable amounts of pivalic acid. For example, in 17 children taking **pivampicillin** with **pivmecillinam** for more than one year, the mean total serum and muscle carnitine levels fell by 90%, to a level similar to those in patients with primary carnitine deficiency. High-dose carnitine was required to reverse this deficiency, with replenishment taking a number of months.[1] In a short-term study in healthy subjects, high-dose **pivmecillinam** 1.2 g daily for 12 days reduced serum carnitine levels by 73% without affecting muscle levels; however, impaired ketogenesis occurred in 2 out of 6 of the subjects.[2]

Of other antibacterials given as the pivoxil, **cefditoren pivoxil** 400 mg twice daily for 14 days decreased the plasma carnitine levels by about 80% in healthy subjects,[3] and one case of severe carnitine deficiency has been reported in an 18-month-old who had received **cefditoren pivoxil** for about 6 months.[4] Reduced carnitine levels have also been seen with **cefetamet pivoxil** [5] and **cefteram pivoxil**.[6]

Very high doses of **adefovir dipivoxil** (120 mg daily) formerly studied for HIV infection were associated with reduced serum carnitine levels and carnitine supplementation was recommended.[7] However, doses of **adefovir dipivoxil** currently used for hepatitis B are 12 times lower than this (10 mg daily). The UK manufacturer of **adefovir dipivoxil** notes that on extended treatment, a decrease in serum carnitine levels occurred in 3 to 6% of patients.[8]

The antiepileptic drug **valproate** has caused carnitine deficiency.[9] Reduced carnitine levels have also been reported with cytotoxic antineoplastics such as **cisplatin**,[10,11] **doxorubicin**[10] and **ifosfamide**.[10,12]

Experimental evidence

The antiepileptic drug valproate has caused carnitine deficiency.[9] Reduced carnitine levels have also been reported with cytotoxic antineoplastics such as cisplatin,[10,11] doxorubicin[10] and ifosfamide.[10,12]

Mechanism

Drugs given as esters of pivalic acid are hydrolysed in the body to form the active drug and pivalic acid. Pivalic acid is excreted as its carnitine ester (pivaloylcarnitine), which depletes the body of carnitine. It is uncertain why valproate and some cytotoxics reduce carnitine levels.

Importance and management

It is well recognised that drugs such as pivampicillin can reduce carnitine levels, although this is rarely clinically important unless the drug is given long-term. L-carnitine has been given with drugs that are pivalic acid esters, to reduce this effect. In patients who are taking L-carnitine supplements, bear in mind the possibility that drugs that are pivalic acid esters, especially if used long term, might reduce the efficacy of the L-carnitine. If L-carnitine supplementation is clinically important, and long-term antibacterial treatment is required, it would seem prudent to consider using a drug that does not contain pivalic acid.

1. Holme E, Jodal U, Linstedt S, Nordin I. Effects of pivalic acid-containing prodrugs on carnitine homeostasis and on response to fasting in children. *Scand J Clin Lab Invest* (1992) 52, 361–72.
2. Abrahamsson K, Eriksson BO, Holme E, Jodal U, Lindstedt S, Nordin I. Impaired ketogenesis in carnitine depletion caused by short-term administration of pivalic acid prodrug. *Biochem Med Metab Biol* (1994) 52, 18–21.
3. Brass EP, Mayer MD, Mulford DJ, Stickler TK, Hoppel CL. Impact on carnitine homeostasis of short-term treatment with the pivalate prodrug cefditoren pivoxil. *Clin Pharmacol Ther* (2003) 73, 338–47.
4. Makino Y, Sugiura T, Ito T, Sugiyama N, Koyama N. Carnitine-associated encephalopathy caused by long-term treatment with an antibiotic containing pivalic acid. *Pediatrics* (2007) 120, E739–E741.
5. Nakashima M, Kosuge K, Ishii I, Ohtsubo M. Influence of multiple-dose administration of cefetamet pivoxil on blood and urinary concentrations of carnitine and effects of simultaneous administration of carnitine with cefetamet pivoxil. *Jpn J Antibiot* (1996) 49, 966–79.
6. Ito T, Sugiyama N, Kobayashi M, Kidouchi K, Itoh T, Uemura O, Sugiyama K, Togari H. Alteration of ammonia and carnitine levels in short-term treatment with pivalic acid-containing prodrug. *Tohoku J Exp Med* (1995) 175, 43–53.
7. Noble S, Goa KL. Adefovir dipivoxil. *Drugs* (1999) 58, 479–87.
8. Hepsera 10 mg Tablets Adefovir dipivoxil. Gilead Sciences Ltd UK Summary of product characteristics, January 2011.
9. Verrotti A, Greco R, Morgese G, Chiarelli F. Carnitine deficiency and hyperammonemia in children receiving valproic acid with and without other anticonvulsant drugs. *Int J Clin Lab Res* (1999) 29, 36–40.
10. Hockenberry MJ, Hooke MC, Gregurich M, McCarthy K. Carnitine plasma levels and fatigue in children/adolescents receiving cisplatin, ifosfamide, or doxorubicin. *J Pediatr Hematol Oncol* (2009) 31, 664–9.
11. Heuberger W, Berardi S, Jacky E, Pey P, Krähenbühl S. Increased urinary excretion of carnitine in patients treated with cisplatin. *Eur J Clin Pharmacol* (1998) 54, 503–8.
12. Marthaler NP, Visarius T, Küpfer A, Lauterburg BH. Increased urinary losses of carnitine during ifosfamide chemotherapy. *Cancer Chemother Pharmacol* (1999) 44, 170–172.

L-carnitine (Levocarnitine) + Food

No interactions found.

L-carnitine (Levocarnitine) + Herbal medicines

No interactions found. Note that supplements containing D-carnitine might antagonise the effect of L-carnitine and acetyl L-carnitine, see L-carnitine (Levocarnitine) + Carnitine, page 130

For mention of a case of stroke in a man taking a supplement containing L-carnitine, but for which the most likely explanation was the combination of ephedra and caffeine, see Creatine + Herbal medicines; Ephedra with Caffeine, page 180.

L-carnitine (Levocarnitine) + Warfarin and related drugs

Two isolated reports describe a substantial increase in the anticoagulant effects of acenocoumarol in patients taking L-carnitine, one of which was associated with melaena.

Clinical evidence

A woman who had taken **acenocoumarol** for 17 years because of aortic and mitral prosthetic valves, was admitted to hospital with melaena within 5 days of starting to take L-carnitine 1 g daily, which she was prescribed for congestive heart failure. Her INR had risen from 2.1 to 7. Endoscopy and colonoscopy revealed diffuse bleeding from superficial erosions in the gut. She was discharged 10 days later with the same dose of **acenocoumarol** and an INR of 2.1 without the L-carnitine.[1] A similar case has been described in a man stabilised on **acenocoumarol** (INR 1.99 to 2.94) who had a rise in his INR to 4.65 despite a dose correction. The increases in INR occurred when he was using L-carnitine 1 g daily for 10 weeks in the form of a drink (*Maximize*) promoted for bodybuilding and fitness training. When this product was discontinued, the INR returned to the therapeutic range.[2]

Experimental evidence

No relevant data found.

Mechanism

The reason for this apparent interaction is not known.

Importance and management

These seem to the only recorded cases of an interaction between a coumarin anticoagulant and L-carnitine, but it might be prudent to bear this interaction in mind if L-carnitine is taken with acenocoumarol, and possibly any coumarin anticoagulant, being alert for an increased response.

1. Martinez E, Domingo P, Roca-Cusachs A. Potentiation of acenocoumarol action by L-carnitine. *J Intern Med* (1993) 233, 94.
2. Bachmann HU, Hoffmann A. Interaction of food supplement L-carnitine with oral anticoagulant acenocoumarol. *Swiss Med Wkly* (2004) 134, 385.

Cascara

Frangula purshiana (DC.) A.Gray (Rhamnaceae)

Synonym(s) and related species

Cascara sagrada, Chittem bark, Rhamnus, Sacred bark.

Rhamnus purshiana DC.

Pharmacopoeias

Cascara (*BP 2012, PhEur 7.5*); Standardised Cascara Dry Extract (*BP 2012, PhEur 7.5*); Cascara Sagrada (*USP35–NF30 S1*).

Constituents

Anthraquinone glycosides are major components of cascara and include cascarosides A, B, C, D, E and F, aloins A and B, and chrysaloins A and B. Aloe-emodin, barbaloin, crysophanol, emodin, frangulin and physcion are also present in small amounts, as are resins and tannins.

Use and indications

Cascara bark is used as a laxative.

Pharmacokinetics

For information on the pharmacokinetics of an anthraquinone glycoside present in cascara, see under aloes, page 27.

Interactions overview

No interactions with cascara found; however, cascara (by virtue of its anthraquinone content) is expected to share some of the interactions of a number of other anthraquinone-containing laxatives, such as aloes, page 27 and senna, page 423. Of particular relevance are the interactions with corticosteroids, digitalis glycosides, and potassium-depleting diuretics.

Cassia

Cinnamomum cassia Blume

Synonym(s) and related species

Chinese cinnamon, False cinnamon, *Cassia lignea*, *Cinnamomum aromaticum Nees*, *Cinnamomum pseudomelastoma* auct. non Liao.

Cassia bark is the bark of *Cinnamomum cassia*, and is also known as Cortex Cinnamomi.

Pharmacopoeias

Cassia oil (*BP 2012, PhEur 7.5*)

Constituents

The bark of *Cinnamomum cassia* contains volatile oil mainly composed of *trans*-cinnamaldehyde, with cinnamylacetate, phenylpropylacetate, salicylaldehyde and methyleugenol. Diterpenes including cinncassiols, and tannins such as cinnamtannins are also present.

Use and indications

Cassia is mainly used for digestive disorders such as diarrhoea, and flatulent colic or dyspepsia. Cassia has also been used for the common cold, and the oil may have antiseptic activity. It has been used in Chinese medicine for circulatory disorders.

Pharmacokinetics

No relevant pharmacokinetic data found.

Interactions overview

It has been suggested that cassia may interfere with the control of diabetes by conventional antidiabetic drugs, but controlled studies do not appear to support this suggestion. Cassia is a constituent of various Chinese herbal medicines, see under bupleurum, page 98, for information.

Interactions monographs

- Antidiabetics, page 134
- Food, page 134
- Herbal medicines, page 134

Cassia + Antidiabetics

Although one study suggests that cassia may enhance the blood-glucose-lowering effects of conventional antidiabetics, a meta-analysis of controlled studies suggests otherwise.

Clinical evidence

In a placebo-controlled study, patients with type 2 diabetes were given cassia 1 g, 3 g or 6 g daily (total of 30 patients) for a total of 40 days in addition to their normal medications.[1] Blood-glucose levels were decreased by 2.9 mmol/L, 2 mmol/L and 3.8 mmol/L in the 1 g, 3 g and 6 g groups, respectively. Changes in blood-glucose levels were only significant at 20 days in the 6 g group (blood-glucose decreased by 2.8 mmol/L). No particular adverse effects were reported.[1]

Experimental evidence

No relevant data found.

Mechanism

Unknown.

Importance and management

Evidence is limited. The study cited above, which was not designed to investigate a potential drug interaction, seems to suggest that cassia has the potential to enhance the blood-glucose-lowering effects of conventional antidiabetic medication (unnamed). However, recent meta-analysis of randomised, controlled studies,[2] which included the study cited above, found that cassia does not appear to improve the control of type 1 or type 2 diabetes (glycosylated haemoglobin, fasting blood glucose and lipids assessed). However, note that this review included studies of both cassia (*Cinnamomum cassia*) and cinnamon (*Cinnamomum zeylancium*).

In general therefore, cassia would not be expected to markedly affect the control of diabetes with conventional antidiabetic drugs. If any effect does occur, it is likely to be picked up by standard blood-glucose monitoring, as high doses of cassia only had a significant effect on blood-glucose after 40 days of concurrent use.[1]

1. Khan A, Safdar M, Ali Khan MM, Khattak KN, Anderson RA. Cinnamon improves glucose and lipids of people with type 2 diabetes. *Diabetes Care* (2003) 26, 3215–18.
2. Baker WL, Gutierrez-Williams G, White CM, Kluger J, Coleman CI. Effect of cinnamon on glucose control and lipid parameters. *Diabetes Care* (2008) 31, 41–3.

Cassia + Carbamazepine

For mention that saiko-ka-ryukotsu-borei-to, of which cassia bark (cortex cinnamomi) is one of 10 constituents, did not affect the pharmacokinetics of carbamazepine in an *animal* study, see Bupleurum + Carbamazepine, page 99.

Cassia + Food

No interactions found. Cassia bark and oil are used as a flavouring in foods.

Cassia + Herbal medicines

No interactions found.

Cassia + Ofloxacin

For mention that sairei-to, of which cassia bark (cortex cinnamomi) is one of 12 constituents, did not affect the pharmacokinetics of ofloxacin, see Bupleurum + Ofloxacin, page 99.

Cat's claw

Uncaria tomentosa DC., *Uncaria guianensis* J.F.Gmel. (Rubiaceae)

Synonym(s) and related species

Life-giving vine of Peru, Samento, Savéntaro, Uña de gato.

Pharmacopoeias

Cat's Claw (*USP35–NF30 S1*); Powdered Cat's Claw (*USP35–NF30 S1*); Powdered Cat's Claw Extract (*USP35–NF30 S1*); Cat's Claw Tablets (*USP35–NF30 S1*); Cat's Claw Capsules (*USP35–NF30 S1*).

Constituents

The main constituents of both the closely related species of cat's claw include the tetracyclic oxindole alkaloids, isorhynchophylline and rhynchophylline; and the indole alkaloids, dihydrocorynantheine, hirsutine, and hirsuteine. Quinovic acid glycosides have also been isolated.

Note that there are two chemotypes of *Uncaria tomentosa,* one primarily containing the tetracyclic oxindole alkaloids, isorhynochophylline and rhynchopylline, and one primarily containing the pentacyclic oxindole alkaloids, (iso)pteropodine and (iso)mitraphylline.

Use and indications

Cat's claw roots, bark and leaves have been used for gastric ulcers, arthritis, gonorrhoea, dysentry, herpes zoster, herpes simplex, HIV, and as a contraceptive. In various preclinical studies, antiviral, anti-inflammatory, antirheumatic, immunostimulating, antimutagenic, antitumour, and hypotensive properties have been shown. There is some evidence that the tetracyclic oxindole alkaloids antagonise the immunomodulating effects of the pentacyclic oxindole alkaloids, and some preparations for arthritis are standardised to contain little or no tetracyclic oxindole alkaloids. Other preparations are essentially free of oxindole alkaloids.

Pharmacokinetics

In two *in vitro* studies,[1,2] alcoholic extracts of *Uncaria tomentosa* were found to be potent inhibitors of CYP3A4. Inhibitory effects on CYP2D6, CYP2C9, and CYP2C19 were minor (in order of decreasing potency).[2] It was suggested that *Uncaria tomentosa* might have the potential to interfere with the metabolism of substrates of CYP3A4,[1] but note that St John's wort was an *inhibitor* of CYP3A4 in this study, whereas clinically (multiple dose use), it is an *inducer* of CYP3A4. This serves as a reminder that *in vitro* studies cannot be directly extrapolated to the clinical situation, and that the findings need confirmation in a clinical setting.

Interactions overview

Cat's claw has some antiplatelet and antihypertensive effects, which may be additive with those of conventional drugs. Data from a clinical study suggests that cat's claw may safely be given with sulfasalazine and hydroxychloroquine. An isolated case reports an increase in the levels of atazanavir, ritonavir and saquinavir in a patient also taking cat's claw.

Interactions monographs

- Antihypertensives, page 136
- Antiplatelet drugs, page 136
- Antirheumatics, page 136
- Food, page 136
- Herbal medicines, page 136
- HIV-protease inhibitors, page 136

1. Budzinski JW, Foster BC, Vandenhoek S, Arnason JT. An *in vitro* evaluation of human cytochrome P450 3A4 inhibition be selected commercial herbal extracts and tinctures. *Phytomedicine* (2000) 7, 273–82.
2. Foster BC, Vandenhoek S, Hana J, Krantis A, Akhtar MH, Bryan M, Budzinski JW, Ramputh A, Arnason JT. *In vitro* inhibition of human cytochrome P450-mediated metabolism of marker substrates by natural products. *Phytomedicine* (2003) 10, 334–42.

C

Cat's claw + Antihypertensives

The interaction between cat's claw and antihypertensives is based on experimental evidence only.

Clinical evidence

No interactions found.

Experimental evidence

Isorhynchophylline 10 mg/kg, a tetracyclic oxindole alkaloid from cat's claw, given intravenously was found to lower systolic arterial blood pressure, diastolic arterial blood pressure and heart rate by about 9%, 21% and 14%, respectively, in normotensive *rats* and about 9%, 6% and 19%, respectively, in hypertensive *rats* in an experimental study.[1] The effect appears to be dose-dependent because isorhynchophylline 20 mg/kg, given via the duodenum, lowered the systolic pressure by about 25%, diastolic pressure by about 38%, and heart rate by about 25% in normotensive *rats*. A similar effect was seen in *dogs*.[1]

Mechanism

It is suggested that the hypotensive effect is mainly due to a vasodilating effect and transient reduction in the heart rate and force of cardiac contraction.[1] Additive blood pressure-lowering effects with conventional antihypertensives might therefore occur.

Importance and management

Evidence appears to be limited to experimental data and an interaction is not established. *Uncaria* species are commonly used in traditional medicine for hypertension, and the preclinical evidence shows that isorhynchophylline, a tetracyclic oxindole alkaloid from cat's claw, has antihypertensive activity. However, not all varieties of *Uncaria tomentosa* contain isorhynchophylline, and some preparations are specifically standardised not to contain this constituent, so not all cat's claw products will interact. Nevertheless, despite the lack of clinical evidence, there is the potential for an additive blood pressure-lowering effect if cat's claw containing isorhynchophylline is given with any antihypertensive. Concurrent use need not be avoided, but patients should be made aware of the possibility of increased antihypertensive effects.

1. Shi J-S, Liu G-X, Qin WU, Zhang W, Huang X-N. Hypotensive and hemodynamic effects of isorhynchophylline in conscious rats and anaesthetised dogs. *Chin J Pharmacol Toxicol* (1989) 3, 205–10.

Cat's claw + Antiplatelet drugs

The interaction between cat's claw and antiplatelet drugs is based on experimental evidence only.

Clinical evidence

No interactions found.

Experimental evidence

A study in *rabbits*[1] found that rhynchophylline, a tetracyclic oxindole alkaloid from cat's claw, caused a concentration-dependent inhibition of platelet aggregation by up to about 78%. Rhynchophylline also inhibited venous thrombosis by up to about 70% in *rats*. Similar results were seen in a second experimental study in *rats*.[2]

Mechanism

The authors suggest that the antiplatelet effect may be due to the suppression of the release of arachidonic acid (an inducer of platelet aggregation) from platelet membranes, and the reduction of other release products.[1,2] Theoretically, additive antiplatelet effects are possible with antiplatelet drugs, which might increase the risk of bleeding.

Importance and management

Evidence is limited to these experimental studies. Any interaction is complicated because not all varieties of *Uncaria tomentosa* contain rhynchophylline, and some preparations are specifically standardised not to contain this constituent, so not all cat's claw products will necessarily interact. What is known suggests that some cat's claw products may possibly have antiplatelet effects, which may be additive with conventional antiplatelet drugs. Concurrent use need not be avoided (indeed combinations of antiplatelet drugs are often prescribed together) but it may be prudent to be aware of the potential for increased bleeding if cat's claw is given with other antiplatelet drugs such as **aspirin** and **clopidogrel**. Warn patients to discuss any episode of prolonged bleeding with a healthcare professional.

1. Chen C-X, Jin R-M, Li Y-K, Zhong J, Yue L, Chen S-C, Zhou J-Y. Inhibitory effect of rhynchophylline on platelet aggregation and thrombosis. *Acta Pharmacol Sin* (1992) 13, 126–30.
2. Jin RM, Chen CX, Li YK, Xu PK. Effect of rhynchophylline on platelet aggregation and experimental thrombosis. *Acta Pharmacol Sin* (1991) 26, 246–9.

Cat's claw + Antirheumatics

No additional adverse effects appear to occur when cat's claw is taken with sulfasalazine or hydroxychloroquine.

Evidence, mechanism, importance and management

A cat's claw preparation (without tetracyclic oxindole alkaloids) was used for 52 weeks in a small clinical study in patients taking **sulfasalazine** or **hydroxychloroquine**. There were no safety concerns from the use of the combination when compared with placebo, and a modest clinical benefit.[1] Although this study does not exclude the possibility of a drug interaction, it provides some evidence that cat's claw can be combined with these established drugs without a problem.

1. Mur E, Hartig F, Eibl G, Schirmer M. Randomized double blind trial of an extract from the pentacyclic alkaloid-chemotype of Uncaria tomentosa for the treatment of rheumatoid arthritis. *J Rheumatol* (2002) 29, 678–81.

Cat's claw + Food

No interactions found.

Cat's claw + Herbal medicines

No interactions found.

Cat's claw + HIV-protease inhibitors

An isolated case report describes raised atazanavir, ritonavir and saquinavir levels following the use of cat's claw.

Clinical evidence

An HIV-positive woman awaiting liver transplantation, taking **atazanavir** 300 mg daily, **ritonavir** 100 mg daily and **saquinavir** 1 g daily, in combination with abacavir 600 mg daily and lamivudine 300 mg daily, was found to have an increased trough level of all three HIV-protease inhibitors. Atazanavir trough levels were 1.22 micrograms/mL (expected range of 0.15 to 0.18 micrograms/mL), ritonavir trough levels were

6.13 micrograms/mL (expected level of 2.1 micrograms/mL), and saquinavir trough levels were 3.4 micrograms/mL (expected range 0.1 to 0.25 micrograms/mL). On further questioning, the patient reported no change in her compliance with the medication but reported that she been taking a herbal supplement containing cat's claw for the previous 2 months. No evidence of HIV-protease inhibitor related toxicity was found and the patient reported no adverse effects. The supplement was stopped and by day 15 the levels of all three drugs had returned to within normal limits.[1]

Experimental evidence

No relevant data found.

Mechanism

Some *in vitro* studies suggest that cat's claw may inhibit the cytochrome P450 isoenzyme CYP3A4, the main isoenzyme responsible for the metabolism of atazanavir, ritonavir and saquinavir; however, the results of one of these studies are questionable. See under pharmacokinetics, page 135.

Importance and management

Evidence appears to be limited to one case report from which it is difficult to draw general conclusions. What it illustrates is that more research is needed into the use of cat's claw with HIV-protease inhibitors. Patients taking drugs for serious conditions such as HIV-infection should carefully consider the risks and benefits of adding herbal medicines to their existing regimen, where the outcome of concurrent use is unknown.

1. López Galera RM, Ribera Pascuet E, Esteban Mur JI, Montoro Ronsano JB, Juárez Giménez. Interaction between cat's claw and protease inhibitors atazanavir, ritonavir and saquinavir. *Eur J Clin Pharmacol* (2008) 64, 1235–6.

Celery

Apium graveolens L. (Apiaceae)

Synonym(s) and related species

Apium, Celery fruit, Celery seed, Smallage, Wild celery.

Not to be confused with celery stem, which is commonly eaten as a salad vegetable.

Constituents

The fruits of celery (usually referred to as 'seeds') contain a volatile oil mainly composed of limonene (about 60%), and selinene. Other important constituents are the **flavonoids** (notably apigenin and isoquercitrin), and **natural coumarins** (bergapten, isoimperatorin, osthenol, umbelliferone and 8-hydroxy-5-methoxypsoralen), some of which may cause photosensitivity; however, celery seed oil has been reported to be non-phototoxic in humans. Note that celery stem contains much lower levels of the phototoxic **natural coumarins**, even so, cases of phototoxicity have been reported.

Use and indications

Celery seed is traditionally used for joint inflammation (including rheumatism), gout, and urinary tract inflammation.

Pharmacokinetics

No relevant pharmacokinetic data found for celery seed, but see flavonoids, page 213, and natural coumarins, page 356, for information on these constituents present in the herb.

Interactions overview

No interactions with celery seed found. For information on the interactions of individual flavonoids present in celery seed, see flavonoids, page 213. Although celery seed contains natural coumarins, the quantity of these constituents is not established, and therefore the propensity of celery seed to interact with other drugs because of their presence is unclear. Consider natural coumarins, page 356, for further discussion of the interactions of coumarin-containing herbs.

Centaury

Centaurium erythraea Rafn. (Gentianaceae)

Synonym(s) and related species

Century, Common centaury, Feverwort.

Centaurium minus Auct. subsp. *minus*, *Centaurium minus* Moench, *Centaurium umbellatum* Gilib., *Erythraea centaurium* (L.) Pers.

Note that the synonym Feverwort has also been used for Boneset (*Eupatorium perfoliatum*), and it should also not be confused with Feverfew (*Tanacetum parthenium*).

Pharmacopoeias

Centaury (*BP 2012, PhEur 7.5*).

Constituents

The iridoids (bitters) are considered to be the main active constituents of centaury, and include **gentiopicroside** (about 2%), with centapicrin, gentioflavoside, sweroside and swertiamarin, and *m*-hydroxybenzoylesters of sweroside and catapicrin. Highly methylated xanthones, including eustomin and 8-demethyleustomin, have also been found. Alkaloids of the pyridine-type, including gentianine, gentianidine, gentioflavine, are also found in trace amounts. The triterpenoids α- and β-amyrin, erythrodiol, crataegolic acid, oleanolic acid and sitosterol are also present.

Use and indications

Centaury is used for disorders of the upper digestive tract, mainly dyspepsia. It is also used in the treatment of anorexia and it has reported anti-inflammatory activity. It should not be taken by patients with peptic ulceration.

Pharmacokinetics

No relevant pharmacokinetic data found.

Interactions overview

No interactions with centaury found.

Chamomile, German

Matricaria recutita L. (Asteraceae)

Synonym(s) and related species

Chamomile, Chamomilla, Hungarian chamomile, Matricaria flower, Scented mayweed, Single chamomile, Sweet false chamomile, Wild chamomile.

Chamomilla recutita (L.) Rauschert, *Chamomilla vulgaris* SF Gray, *Matricaria chamomilla* L.

Consider also Chamomile, Roman, page 142 (*Chamaemelum nobile*), which is a distinct species that is used similarly and is also known as chamomile.

Pharmacopoeias

Chamomile (*USP35–NF30 S1*); Matricaria Flower (*PhEur 7.5*); Matricaria Flowers (*BP 2012*); Matricaria Liquid Extract (*BP 2012, PhEur 7.5*); Matricaria Oil (*BP 2012, PhEur 7.5*).

Constituents

The flowerheads of German chamomile contain essential oil composed mainly of (−)-α-bisabolol. Sesquiterpenes and proazulenes (e.g. matricarin and matricin) are also present. Chamazulene (1 to 15%), another volatile oil found in chamomile, is formed from matricin during steam distillation of the oil. Other constituents present in chamomile include **flavonoids** (apigenin, luteolin, quercetin, rutin), and the natural coumarins umbelliferone and its methyl ether, heniarin.

Use and indications

German chamomile is used for dyspepsia, flatulence and travel sickness, especially when the gastrointestinal disturbance is associated with nervous disorders. It is also used for nasal catarrh and restlessness. German chamomile is widely used in babies and children as a mild sedative, and to treat colic and teething pain. It has been used topically for haemorrhoids, mastitis and leg ulcers.

Pharmacokinetics

In vitro studies have found that a commercial ethanolic extract of *Matricaria chamomilla* and a crude *Matricaria recutita* essential oil extract inhibited the cytochrome P450 isoenzyme CYP3A4.[1,2] However, the effects were weak when compared with the known potent CYP3A4 inhibitor ketoconazole.[2]

A crude *Matricaria recutita* essential oil extract has also been found to moderately inhibit CYP1A2 *in vitro*.[2] Similarly, a study using liver microsomes from *rats* pretreated with chamomile tea 2% for 4 weeks (*Vita Fit Nutrition*, made from the dried flower heads of *Matricaria chamomilla* and *Matricaria recutita*) found that CYP1A2 activity was reduced to 39%, when compared with the control group.[3]

A crude *Matricaria recutita* essential oil extract had no significant effect on the cytochrome P450 isoenzymes CYP2C9 and CYP2D6.[2]

For information on the pharmacokinetics of individual flavonoids present in German chamomile, see under flavonoids, page 213.

Interactions overview

An isolated case of bleeding in a patient taking warfarin and using chamomile products has been reported and chamomile tea (an infusion of *Matricaria recutita*) caused a minor reduction in iron absorption. No other relevant drug interactions have been found for German chamomile. For information on the interactions of individual flavonoids present in German chamomile, see under flavonoids, page 213.

Interactions monographs

- Food, page 141
- Herbal medicines, page 141
- Iron compounds, page 141
- Warfarin, page 141

1. Budzinski JW, Foster BC, Vandenhoek S, Arnason JT. An *in vitro* evaluation of human cytochrome P450 3A4 inhibition by selected commercial herbal extracts and tinctures. *Phytomedicine* (2000) 7, 273–82.
2. Ganzera M, Schneider P, Stuppner H. Inhibitory effects of the essential oil of chamomile (*Matricaria recutita* L.) and its major constituents on human cytochrome P450 enzymes. *Life Sci* (2006) 78, 856–61.
3. Maliakal PP, Wanwimolruk S. Effect of herbal teas on hepatic drug metabolizing enzymes in rats. *J Pharm Pharmacol* (2001) 53, 1323–9.

Chamomile, German + Food

No interactions found.

Chamomile, German + Herbal medicines

No interactions found.

Chamomile, German + Iron compounds

Chamomile tea (an infusion of *Matricaria recutita*) caused a modest reduction in iron absorption. An infusion of *Matricaria chamomilla* did not affect iron absorption.

Clinical evidence

In a study in 10 healthy subjects, a 275 mL serving of chamomile tea (an infusion of *Matricaria recutita*) reduced the absorption of iron in a 50 g bread roll by 47%. The tea was prepared by adding 300 mL of boiling water to 3 g of the herbal tea, then infusing for 10 minutes before straining and serving. In this study, the inhibitory effect of chamomile tea on iron absorption was less than that of black tea (Assam tea, *Camellia sinensis* L.), which is well known to inhibit iron absorption.[1] Consider also, Tea + Iron compounds, page 467.

In contrast, a study in 13 healthy subjects found that chamomile tea (an infusion of *Matricaria chamomilla*) sweetened with *panela* (an unrefined cane sugar sweetener containing fructose) did not affect the absorption of iron from an iron-fortified bread, when compared with the absorption of iron from the bread alone.[2]

Experimental evidence

No relevant data found.

Mechanism

The polyphenols in chamomile may bind to iron in the intestine and influence its absorption. The tannin content of the chamomile tea in the second study,[2] was reported to be 24.5 mg in 100 mL. This is much less than the tannin content of black tea, which is known to reduce iron absorption (see Tea + Iron compounds, page 467). This level of tannins did not appear to affect iron absorption in this particular study.

Importance and management

Evidence is limited to these two studies, which used different *Matricaria* species and found different effects on iron absorption. This is somewhat problematic, as either species are acceptable in some pharmacopoeial preparations labelled as chamomile. Therefore, despite the suggestion that some *Matricaria* species may not affect iron absorption it would seem prudent to consider any chamomile tea to be capable of reducing iron absorption. However, the clinical relevance of this effect is unclear, as the effect on absorption was smaller than that of black tea (Assam tea, *Camellia sinensis* L.), which is known to inhibit iron absorption to a clinically relevant extent (see Tea + Iron compounds, page 467). Until more is known it may be prudent to consider chamomile tea intake in patients requiring iron supplementation and in patients that are particularly unresponsive to iron replacement therapy.

1. Hurrell RF, Reddy M, Cook JD. Inhibition of non-haem iron absorption in man by polyphenolic-containing beverages. *Br J Nutr* (1999) 81, 289–95.
2. Olivares M, Pizarro F, Hertrampf E, Fuenmayor G, Estévez E. Iron absorption from wheat flour: effects of lemonade and chamomile infusion. *Nutrition* (2007) 23, 296–300.

Chamomile, German + Warfarin

A single case report describes a woman stabilised on warfarin who developed a marked increase in her INR with bleeding complications five days after she started using two chamomile products.

Clinical evidence

A 70-year-old woman stabilised on warfarin with an INR of 3.6 started drinking 4 to 5 cups of chamomile tea (an infusion of *Matricaria chamomilla*) daily for chest congestion, and using a chamomile-based skin lotion 4 to 5 times daily for foot oedema. About 5 days later she developed ecchymoses and was found to have an INR of 7.9, a retroperitoneal haematoma and other internal haemorrhages.[1]

Experimental evidence

No relevant data found.

Mechanism

German chamomile contains the natural coumarin compounds, umbelliferone and heniarin. However, these compounds do not possess the minimum structural requirements (a C-4 hydroxyl substituent and a C-3 non-polar carbon substituent) required for anticoagulant activity. German chamomile essential oil extracts do not appear to significantly affect the cytochrome P450 isoenzyme CYP2C9, the main isoenzyme involved in the metabolism of warfarin, but the effects of chamomile tea do not appear to have been studied.

Importance and management

This appears to be the first report of an interaction between warfarin and German chamomile. There seem to be no reports of German chamomile alone causing anticoagulation, and the natural coumarin constituents of German chamomile do not appear to possess anticoagulant activity, which might suggest that the risk of an additive effect is small. Furthermore, a pharmacokinetic basis for this interaction has not been established. Because of the many other factors influencing anticoagulant control, it is not possible to reliably ascribe a change in INR specifically to a drug interaction in a single case report without other supporting evidence. It may be better to advise patients to discuss the use of any herbal products they wish to try, and to increase monitoring if this is thought advisable. Cases of uneventful use should be reported, as they are as useful as possible cases of adverse effects.

1. Segal R, Pilote L. Warfarin interaction with *Matricaria chamomilla*. *CMAJ* (2006) 174, 1281–2.

C

Chamomile, Roman

Chamaemelum nobile All (Asteraceae)

Synonym(s) and related species

Chamomile, Double chamomile, English chamomile, Manzanilla.

Anthemis nobilis L.

Consider also Chamomile, German, page 140 (*Matricaria recutita*), which is a distinct species that is used similarly and is also known as chamomile.

Pharmacopoeias

Chamomile Flowers (*BP 2012*); Chamomile Flower, Roman (*PhEur 7.5*).

Constituents

The flowerheads contain an essential oil composed mainly of esters of angelic and tiglic acid, with 1,8-cineole, *trans*-pinocarveol, *trans*-pinocarvone, chamazulene, farnesol, nerolidol, various germacranolide-type sesquiterpene lactones, amyl and isobutyl alcohols, and anthemol. The **flavonoids** apigenin, luteolin, quercetin with their glyco-sides, and the natural coumarin scopoletin-7-glucoside, are also present. Chamazulene is formed from a natural precursor during steam distillation of the oil.

Use and indications

Roman chamomile is used as a carminative, anti-emetic, antispasmodic, and sedative for dyspepsia, nausea and vomiting, anorexia, and dysmenorrhoea. It is widely used as a topical preparation for the hair.

Pharmacokinetics

No relevant pharmacokinetic data found. For information on the pharmacokinetics of individual flavonoids found in Roman chamomile, see under flavonoids, page 213.

Interactions overview

No interactions with Roman chamomile found, but for information on the interactions of individual flavonoids found in Roman chamomile, see under flavonoids, page 213.

Chaparral

Larrea tridentata Coville (Zygophyllaceae)

Synonym(s) and related species

Creosote bush.

Larrea divaricata Cav. (formerly regarded as the same species as *Larrea tridentata*), *Larrea mexicana* Moric., *Larrea tridentata* var. *glutinosa* Jeps.

Constituents

Chaparral contains lignans, the major compound being **nordihydroguaiaretic acid** (**NDGA**). The herb also contains **flavonoids**, which include isorhamnetin, kaempferol and quercetin, and their derivatives. There is also a volatile oil present containing calamene, eudesmol, limonene, α- and β-pinene, and 2-rossalene. A cytotoxic naphthoquinone derivative, larreantin, has been isolated from the roots.

Use and indications

Chaparral has been used in the treatment of bowel cramps, arthritis, rheumatism and colds. It has also been used to treat other diseases such as cancer, venereal disease and tuberculosis. Its use as a herbal remedy is not recommended due to reports of hepatotoxicity and renal toxicity.

Pharmacokinetics

No relevant pharmacokinetic data found. For information on the pharmacokinetics of individual flavonoids present in chaparral, see under flavonoids, page 213.

Interactions overview

Chaparral contains digoxin-like constituents, which could, in theory, have additive effects with digoxin or digitoxin, or interfere with their assays, but the clinical relevance of this is unclear. For information on the interactions of individual flavonoids present in chaparral, see under flavonoids, page 213.

Interactions monographs

- Digitalis glycosides, page 144
- Food, page 144
- Herbal medicines, page 144

Chaparral + Digitalis glycosides

Many herbal medicines contain cardiac glycosides, which could in theory have additive effects with digoxin or digitoxin, or interfere with their assays. However, there appear to be few such interactions reported.

Evidence, mechanism, importance and management

In an *in vitro* study, 46 commercially packaged herb teas and 78 teas prepared from herbs were assayed for digoxin-like factors by their cross-reactivity with digoxin antibody, and these values were used to give approximate equivalent daily doses of digoxin. Chaparral was found to contain greater than 30 micrograms of digoxin equivalents per cup and it was suggested that this would provide a therapeutic daily dose of digoxin if 5 cups of chaparral tea a day were drunk.[1] However, note that some common teas sampled in this study (e.g. English Breakfast, Earl Grey) contained over 20 micrograms of digoxin equivalents per cup. Given that these teas are commonly consumed in the UK, and an interaction with digoxin has not been reported, the interpretation of the findings of this study is unclear. Theoretical interactions with herbal medicines are not always translated into practice. On the basis of this one study, no special precautions would be expected to be necessary in patients taking digoxin who drink chaparral tea. However, note that the use of chaparral as a herbal remedy is not recommended due to reports of hepatotoxicity and renal toxicity.

1. Longerich L, Johnson E, Gault MH. Digoxin-like factors in herbal teas. *Clin Invest Med* (1993) 16, 210–218.

Chaparral + Food

No interactions found.

Chaparral + Herbal medicines

No interactions found.

Chinese angelica

Angelica sinensis (Oliv.) Diels (Apiaceae)

Synonym(s) and related species

Dang Gui (Chinese), Danggui, Dong quai.

Angelica polymorpha var. *sinensis*.

Other species used in oriental medicine include *Angelica dahurica*.

Not to be confused with Angelica, which is *Angelica archangelica* L.

Pharmacopoeias

Angelica Sinensis Root (*PhEur 7.5*); Angelica Sinensis Root for use in THM (*BP 2012*); Processed Angelica Sinensis Root for use in THMP (*BP 2012*).

Constituents

The major constituents include **natural coumarins** (angelicin, archangelicin, bergapten, osthole, psoralen, and xanthotoxin), and volatile oils. Other constituents include caffeic and chlorogenic acids, and ferulic acid. *Angelica sinensis* also contains a series of phthalides (n-butylidenephthalide, ligustilide, n-butylphthalide).

Use and indications

One of the most common uses of Chinese angelica root is for the treatment of menopausal symptoms and menstrual disorders. It has also been used for rheumatism, ulcers, anaemia, constipation, psoriasis, the management of hypertension, and to relieve allergic conditions.

Pharmacokinetics

Evidence is limited to experimental studies, which suggest that the effects of *Angelica dahurica* and *Angelica sinen-* sis may not be equivalent.[1] Most of the evidence relates to *Angelica dahurica,* which may inhibit the cytochrome P450 isoenzymes CYP2C9 (see tolbutamide, page 147), CYP2C19 (see diazepam, page 146), and CYP3A4 (see nifedipine, page 146). If all these effects are found to be clinically relevant then Chinese angelica (where *Angelica dahurica* is used) has the potential to raise the levels of a wide range of conventional drugs.

Interactions overview

Angelica dahurica may raise the levels of diazepam and tolbutamide, thereby increasing their effects. More limited evidence suggests that nifedipine may be similarly affected. Case reports suggest that Chinese angelica may increase the bleeding time in response to warfarin, and may possess oestrogenic effects, which could be of benefit, but which may also, theoretically, oppose the effects of oestrogen antagonists, such as tamoxifen.

Interactions monographs

- Diazepam, page 146
- Food, page 146
- Herbal medicines, page 146
- Nifedipine, page 146
- Oestrogens or Oestrogen antagonists, page 146
- Tolbutamide, page 147
- Warfarin and related drugs, page 147

1. Guo L-Q, Taniguchi M, Chen Q-Y, Baba K, Yamazoe Y. Inhibitory potential of herbal medicines on human cytochrome P450-mediated oxidation: Properties of *Umbelliferous* or *Citrus* crude drugs and their relative prescriptions. *Jpn J Pharmacol* (2001) 85, 399–408.

Chinese angelica + Diazepam

The interaction between *Angelica dahurica* and diazepam is based on experimental evidence only.

Clinical evidence

No interactions found.

Experimental evidence

In a study in *rats*,[1] *Angelica dahurica* had little effect on the pharmacokinetics of intravenous diazepam 10 mg/kg. However, when diazepam 5 mg/kg was given orally, the AUC of diazepam was markedly increased from levels below detection to detectable levels, and the maximum plasma level, was increased fourfold. In a mobility study, *Angelica dahurica* potentiated the muscle relaxant effects of intravenous diazepam.[1]

Mechanism

In *rats*, diazepam is principally metabolised in the liver by cytochrome P450 isoenzymes including CYP2C19. It is thought that this isoenzyme is inhibited by *Angelica dahurica*. It was also suggested by the authors that there was a considerable effect of *Angelica dahurica* on the first-pass metabolism of diazepam.[1]

Importance and management

Although the data are from *animal* studies, because of the potential for increased levels and effects of diazepam, until more is known, it may be prudent to advise caution when giving *Angelica dahurica* with oral diazepam. Warn patients that they may experience increased sedation.

Note that it may not be appropriate to extrapolate from *Angelica dahurica* to other species such as *Angelica sinensis*, since, in one study, *Angelica sinensis* had much less effect on CYP3A4 than *Angelica dahurica*, see under nifedipine, below.

1. Ishihara K, Kushida H, Yuzurihara M, Wakui Y, Yanagisawa T, Kamei H, Ohmori S, Kitada M. Interaction of drugs and chinese herbs: Pharmacokinetic changes of tolbutamide and diazepam caused by extract of *Angelica dahurica*. *J Pharm Pharmacol* (2000) 52, 1023–9.

Chinese angelica + Food

No interactions found.

Chinese angelica + Herbal medicines

No interactions found.

Chinese angelica + Nifedipine

The interaction between Chinese angelica and nifedipine is based on experimental evidence only.

Clinical evidence

No interactions found.

Experimental evidence

In a study, *rats* were given an extract of *Angelica dahurica*, and then *rat* liver microsomes were prepared and incubated with nifedipine. *Angelica dahurica* was found to inhibit the activity of nifedipine oxidase 1 to 6 hours after administration, by about 30 to 40%.[1]

Mechanism

Nifedipine oxidation is mediated by the cytochrome P450 isoenzyme CYP3A4.[1] This activity of *Angelica dahurica* was shown to be related to furanocoumarin constituents. Other *in vitro* studies suggest that an alcoholic extract of *Angelica dahurica* more potently inhibited CYP3A4 than an aqueous decoction, whereas extracts of *Angelica sinensis* had no significant effect on CYP3A4.[2]

Importance and management

Evidence is limited to experimental studies, but what is known suggests that any CYP3A4 inhibitory effects of Chinese angelica depend on the species and the type of extract used. The results are difficult to reliably extrapolate to the use of Chinese angelica with nifedipine in humans, but it is possible that alcoholic extracts of *Angelica dahurica* may decrease nifedipine metabolism, and therefore increase its levels and effects. Be aware of this possibility if both substances are given.

1. Ishihara K, Kushida H, Yuzurihara M, Wakui Y, Yanagisawa T, Kamei H, Ohmori S, Kitada M. Interaction of drugs and chinese herbs: Pharmacokinetic changes of tolbutamide and diazepam caused by extract of *Angelica dahurica*. *J Pharm Pharmacol* (2000) 52, 1023–9.
2. Guo L-Q, Taniguchi M, Chen Q-Y, Baba K, Yamazoe Y. Inhibitory potential of herbal medicines on human cytochrome P450-mediated oxidation: Properties of *Umbelliferous* or *Citrus* crude drugs and their relative prescriptions. *Jpn J Pharmacol* (2001) 85, 399–408.

Chinese angelica + Oestrogens or Oestrogen antagonists

Chinese angelica may contain oestrogenic compounds. This may result in additive effects with oestrogens or it may oppose the effects of oestrogens. Similarly, Chinese angelica may have additive effects with oestrogen antagonists or oppose the effects of oestrogen antagonists (e.g. tamoxifen).

Clinical evidence

A letter in the Medical Journal of Australia[1] draws attention to the fact that some women with breast cancer receiving chemotherapy or hormone antagonists who develop menopausal symptoms have found relief from hot flushes by taking a Chinese herb 'dong quai' (or 'danggui' root), which has been identified as *Angelica sinensis*. A possible explanation is that this and some other herbs (agnus castus, hops flower, ginseng root, and black cohosh) have significant oestrogen-binding activity and physiological oestrogenic actions.[2]

The oestrogenic potential of Chinese angelica is however somewhat unclear. A phytoestrogenic preparation containing soy extract 75 mg, black cohosh 25 mg and *Angelica polymorpha* (a species related to Chinese angelica) 50 mg taken twice daily reduced the average frequency of menstrually-associated migraine attacks in a 15 week period by 54% in a randomised, placebo-controlled study in 42 women.[3] The preparation used in this study was standardised to content of isoflavones from soy, ligustilide from *Angelica polymorpha*, and triterpenes from black cohosh. In contrast, in another randomised, placebo-controlled study, *Angelica sinensis* root 4.5 g daily did not produce significant oestrogen-like responses in endometrial thickness or vaginal maturation and did not relieve menopausal symptoms in 71 postmenopausal women.[4] The *Angelica sinensis* preparation in this study was standardised to content of ferulic acid.

Experimental evidence

In various *in vitro* and *animal* studies, Chinese angelica extract has been shown to inhibit the binding of estradiol to the oestrogen receptor and increase uterine growth (oestrogenic effects). However, it also *decreased* uterine c-myc mRNA levels (which is induced by oestrogens).[2]

Mechanism

If Chinese angelica has oestrogenic actions, which are not established, then it might directly stimulate breast cancer growth and oppose the actions of competitive oestrogen receptor antagonists such as tamoxifen. See also Isoflavones + Tamoxifen, page 304.

Importance and management

One clinical study and the anecdotal cases mentioned in the letter suggests that Chinese angelica, either alone, or with other phytoestrogens, may possess estrogenic properties. In contrast, in a well-controlled study, Chinese angelica alone did not produce oestrogen-like responses. The concern is that if Chinese angelica does have oestrogenic effects, it might stimulate breast cancer growth and antagonise the effects of hormone antagonists used to treat cancer. Until more is known, it may be prudent to avoid using herbs with purported oestrogenic effects in women with oestrogen sensitive cancers. This is more strictly a disease-herb interaction. See also Isoflavones + Tamoxifen, page 304.

1. Boyle FM. Adverse interaction of herbal medicine with breast cancer treatment. *Med J Aust* (1997) 167, 286.
2. Eagon CL, Elm MS, Teepe AG, Eagon PK. Medicinal botanicals: estrogenicity in rat uterus and liver. *Proc Am Assoc Cancer Res* (1997) 38, 293.
3. Burke BE, Olson RD, Cusack BJ. Randomized, controlled trial of phytoestrogen in the prophylactic treatment of menstrual migraine. *Biomed Pharmacother* (2002) 56, 283–8.
4. Hirata JD, Swiersz LM, Zell B, Small R, Ettinger B. Does dong quai have estrogenic effects in postmenopausal women? A double-blind, placebo-controlled trial. *Fertil Steril* (1997) 68, 981–6.

Chinese angelica + Tolbutamide

The interaction between *Angelica dahurica* and tolbutamide is based on experimental evidence only.

Clinical evidence

No interactions found.

Experimental evidence

In a study, *rats* were given an extract of *Angelica dahurica,* and then *rat* liver microsomes were prepared and incubated with tolbutamide. *Angelica dahurica* was found to inhibit the activity of tolbutamide hydroxylase 1 to 6 hours after administration, by up to about 60%. In further experiments in *rats,* the AUC of intravenous tolbutamide 10 mg/kg was increased 2.5-fold by *Angelica dahurica* 1 g/kg.[1]

Mechanism

Angelica dahurica inhibits the activity of the cytochrome P450 CYP2C subfamily of isoenzymes, which are involved in the metabolism of tolbutamide.[1]

Importance and management

Although there is a lack of clinical evidence, because of the potential for increased levels of tolbutamide, it may be prudent to exercise some caution when using medicines containing *Angelica dahurica* in patients taking tolbutamide. Patients may wish to consider increasing the frequency of blood-glucose monitoring. It may not be appropriate to extrapolate from *Angelica dahurica* to other species such as *Angelica sinensis,* because in one study *Angelica sinensis* did not possess the same enzyme inhibitory properties as *Angelica dahurica,* see nifedipine, page 146.

1. Ishihara K, Kushida H, Yuzurihara M, Wakui Y, Yanagisawa T, Kamei H, Ohmori S, Kitada M. Interaction of drugs and chinese herbs: Pharmacokinetic changes of tolbutamide and diazepam caused by extract of *Angelica dahurica. J Pharm Pharmacol* (2000) 52, 1023–9.

Chinese angelica + Warfarin and related drugs

Two case reports describe a very marked increase in the anticoagulant effects of warfarin when Chinese angelica was given.

Clinical evidence

A 46-year-old African-American woman with atrial fibrillation taking warfarin had a greater than twofold increase in her prothrombin time and INR after taking Chinese angelica for 4 weeks. The prothrombin time and INR had returned to normal 4 weeks after stopping Chinese angelica.[1] In another case, a woman who had been taking warfarin for 10 years developed widespread bruising and an INR of 10, a month after starting to take Chinese angelica.[2]

A further report describes spontaneous subarachnoid haemorrhage in a 53-year-old woman not taking anticoagulants, which was attributed to a herbal supplement containing Chinese angelica root 100 mg and a number of other herbs. See Red clover + Anticoagulants, page 399.

Experimental evidence

In a study in *rabbits,* Chinese angelica aqueous extract 2 g/kg twice daily for 3 days significantly decreased the prothrombin time in response to a single 2-mg/kg dose of warfarin without altering the plasma warfarin concentrations. However, when the study was repeated with warfarin at steady state, prothrombin times tended to be increased after the addition of Chinese angelica, although as with the single-dose study, warfarin plasma levels were not significantly altered.[3] In an *in vitro* study, Chinese angelica extract alone slightly increased prothrombin time.[4]

Mechanism

The reasons for this interaction are not fully understood but Chinese angelica is known to contain natural coumarin derivatives, which may possibly have anticoagulant properties: these could be additive with those of warfarin. However, note that many coumarins do not have anticoagulant effects, see coumarins, page 356. The data suggest that alteration of warfarin levels is not involved, but other studies suggest that the herb may inhibit the cytochrome P450 isoenzyme CYP2C9, which is the main route of warfarin metabolism. See tolbutamide, above.

Importance and management

Clinical evidence for an interaction between Chinese angelica and warfarin appears to be limited to the case reports cited, and an interaction is not fully established. Nevertheless, it would seem prudent to warn patients taking warfarin, and possibly other coumarin anticoagulants, of the potential risks of also taking Chinese angelica. For safety, the use of Chinese angelica should be avoided unless the effects on anticoagulation can be monitored. More study is needed.

1. Page RL, Lawrence JD. Potentiation of warfarin by dong quai. *Pharmacotherapy* (1999) 19, 870–876.
2. Ellis GR, Stephens MR. Untitled report. *BMJ* (1999) 319, 650.
3. Lo ACT, Chan K, Yeung JHK, Woo KS. Dangui (*Angelica sinensis*) affects the pharmacodynamics but not the pharmacokinetics of warfarin in rabbits. *Eur J Drug Metab Pharmacokinet* (1995) 20, 55–60.
4. Jones SC, Miederhoff P, Karnes HT. The development of a human tissue model to determine the effect of plant-derived dietary supplements on prothrombin time. *J Herb Pharmacother* (2001) 1, 21–34.

Chirata

Swertia chirayita (Roxb.) H.Karst. (Gentianaceae)

Synonym(s) and related species

Brown chirata, Chirayta, Chiretta, White chirata.

Agathotes chirayita (Roxb.) D.Don ex G.Don,
Gentiana chirayita Roxb.,
Ophelia chirayita (Roxb.) Griseb, *Swertia chirata* C.B.Clarke.

Not to be confused with Andrographis, page 33 (*Andrographis paniculata*), which may be referred to as Green chiretta.

Constituents

Chirata contains iridoids such as amarogentin (chiratin), amaroswerin, sweroside and swertiamarin; the xanthone glycosides mangiferin, swerchirin, swertianin and others; and alkaloids such as gentianine and gentiocrucine.

Use and indications

Chirata is used as a bitter tonic and for dyspepsia, anorexia and diabetes. It is reported to have hypoglycaemic, anti-inflammatory and antiprotozoal properties.

Pharmacokinetics

No relevant pharmacokinetic data found.

Interactions overview

No interactions with chirata found.

Chitosan

Swertia chirayita (Roxb.) H.Karst. (Gentianaceae)

Types, sources and related compounds

Poliglusam.

Pharmacopoeias

Chitosan *(USP35–NF30 S1)*; Chitosan Hydrochloride (*BP 2012, PhEur 7.5*).

Constituents

Chitosan is a polysaccharide composed of polymers of glucosamine and *N*-acetylglucosamine. It is obtained from the partial deacetylation of chitin obtained from the shells of crustaceans such as shrimps and crabs. It is available in different molecular weights, viscosity grades and degrees of deacetylation.

Use and indications

Chitosan is used as a dietary supplement for obesity and hypercholesterolaemia. Pharmaceutically, chitosan and various derivatives are used, or being investigated, as excipients in drug formulations including oral or nasal dosage forms and gene carrier systems.

Pharmacokinetics

Chitosan is an absorption enhancer and increases the permeability of hydrophilic drugs across intestinal and mucosal epithelia, which has implications for drug delivery systems.[1] A thiolated chitosan derivative is also reported to inhibit the activity of P-glycoprotein, which has possible applications for improving the bioavailability of P-glycoprotein substrates,[2] but note that this derivative does not appear to be used as a dietary supplement.

Interactions overview

Chitosan appears to alter the rate of absorption of water-insoluble drugs such as indometacin and griseofulvin, but it is doubtful whether this is of general clinical significance. A case report describes two women taking valproate, who developed seizures and undetectable valproate levels after chitosan was started, and another case report suggests that chitosan may increase the effects of warfarin, and possible other related anticoagulants.

Interactions monographs

- Cefalexin, page 150
- Food, page 150
- Griseofulvin, page 150
- Herbal medicines, page 150
- Indometacin, page 150
- Paracetamol (Acetaminophen), page 150
- Valproate, page 151
- Warfarin and related drugs, page 151

1. Thanou M, Verhoef JC, Junginger HE. Oral drug absorption enhancement by chitosan and its derivatives. *Adv Drug Deliv Rev* (2001) 52, 117–26.
2. Werle M, Hoffer M. Glutathione and thiolated chitosan inhibit multidrug resistance P-glycoprotein activity in excised small intestine. *J Control Release* (2006) 111, 41–6.

C

Chitosan + Cefalexin

The information regarding the use of chitosan with cefalexin is based on experimental evidence only.

Clinical evidence

No interactions found.

Experimental evidence

There was no significant difference in the AUC and maximum levels of cefalexin 10 mg/kg given alone, and when *rats* were pretreated with oral chitosan 25 mg/kg.[1]

Mechanism

Chitosan does not appear to alter the gastrointestinal absorption of water-soluble drugs such as cefalexin.[1]

Importance and management

The evidence is limited to experimental data and the pharmacokinetics of cefalexin were unchanged. Therefore, no action is considered necessary.

1. Nadai M, Tajiri C, Yoshizumi H, Suzuki Y, Zhao YL, Kimura M, Tsunekawa Y, Hasegawa T. Effect of chitosan on gastrointestinal absorption of water-insoluble drugs following oral administration in rats. *Biol Pharm Bull* (2006) 29, 1941–6.

Chitosan + Food

No interactions found.

Chitosan + Griseofulvin

The information regarding the use of chitosan with griseofulvin is based on experimental evidence only.

Clinical evidence

No interactions found.

Experimental evidence

The AUC_{0-10} and maximum levels of griseofulvin 50 mg/kg were both reduced by about two-thirds when *rats* were pretreated with oral chitosan 25 mg/kg. The time to reach maximum levels was also prolonged.[1]

Mechanism

Little understood. The bioavailability of some formulations of griseofulvin are known to be enhanced when given with high-fat meals because the high levels of bile salts increase the solubilisation of this water-insoluble drug. The authors suggest that by binding to bile acids, chitosan inhibits this effect, which in turn affects the dissolution rate and the gastrointestinal absorption of griseofulvin.[1] This seems more likely than being due to a delay in gastric emptying, because chitosan did not alter the rate of absorption of paracetamol, below.

Importance and management

Evidence appears to be limited to the experimental study cited above, which suggests that the rate of absorption of griseofulvin is markedly reduced by chitosan. Furthermore, the extent of absorption might be reduced, although the sampling time was not long enough to conclude this. Making a clinical recommendation from these data alone is therefore difficult. It could be argued that chitosan is unlikely to affect conventional micronised formulations of griseofulvin, which are well absorbed when taken with food. Until more is known, an alternative cautious approach would be to advise patients to avoid chitosan while taking a course of griseofulvin, to minimise the risk of reduced griseofulvin efficacy.

1. Nadai M, Tajiri C, Yoshizumi H, Suzuki Y, Zhao YL, Kimura M, Tsunekawa Y, Hasegawa T. Effect of chitosan on gastrointestinal absorption of water-insoluble drugs following oral administration in rats. *Biol Pharm Bull* (2006) 29, 1941–6.

Chitosan + Herbal medicines

No interactions found.

Chitosan + Indometacin

The information regarding the use of chitosan with indometacin is based on experimental evidence only.

Clinical evidence

No interactions found.

Experimental evidence

There was no significant difference in the AUC and maximum levels of indometacin 10 mg/kg when *rats* were pretreated with oral chitosan 25 mg/kg although the rate of absorption (time to reach maximum levels) was prolonged.[1]

Mechanism

Little understood. The authors suggest that by binding to bile acids, chitosan inhibits the solubilisation and the gastrointestinal absorption of indometacin, which is not water soluble. They suggest the effect of chitosan is not due to a delay in gastric emptying,[1] because it did not alter the rate of absorption of paracetamol, below.

Importance and management

The evidence is limited to experimental data and the extent of indometacin absorption was unchanged. Therefore, no action is considered necessary.

1. Nadai M, Tajiri C, Yoshizumi H, Suzuki Y, Zhao YL, Kimura M, Tsunekawa Y, Hasegawa T. Effect of chitosan on gastrointestinal absorption of water-insoluble drugs following oral administration in rats. *Biol Pharm Bull* (2006) 29, 1941–6.

Chitosan + Paracetamol (Acetaminophen)

The information regarding the use of chitosan with paracetamol is based on experimental evidence only.

Clinical evidence

No interactions found.

Experimental evidence

There was no significant difference in the AUC and maximum levels of paracetamol 30 mg/kg when *rats* were pretreated with oral chitosan 25 mg/kg.[1]

Mechanism

Paracetamol absorption is dependent on the rate of gastric emptying, and it is often used to study this. The findings of this study suggest that chitosan does not alter the gastric emptying rate.[1]

Importance and management

The evidence is limited to experimental data and the pharmacokinetics of paracetamol were unchanged. Therefore, no action is considered necessary.

1. Nadai M, Tajiri C, Yoshizumi H, Suzuki Y, Zhao YL, Kimura M, Tsunekawa Y, Hasegawa T. Effect of chitosan on gastrointestinal absorption of water-insoluble drugs following oral administration in rats. *Biol Pharm Bull* (2006) 29, 1941–6.

Chitosan + Valproate

A case report describes two women taking valproate, who developed seizures and undetectable valproate levels after chitosan was started, which resolved when it was stopped.

Clinical evidence

A 35-year-old woman who had been seizure-free taking valproate 500 mg twice daily and phenobarbital for 3 years started to take chitosan 500 mg twice daily. Her seizures suddenly re-emerged, but then resolved after the chitosan was stopped. Three months later, the same reaction occurred 5 days after she again started to take chitosan. This time valproate levels were measured and were found to be undetectable. The seizures resolved on stopping the chitosan and within 4 days her valproate levels had returned to baseline (50 micrograms/mL).[1] The authors of this report also describe a second similar case, in which the re-emergence of seizures and undetectable valproate levels developed one week after chitosan 500 mg daily was started, and resolved when chitosan was stopped.[1]

Experimental evidence

No relevant data found.

Mechanism

Little understood. It has been suggested that by binding to bile acids, chitosan inhibits the solubilisation and gastrointestinal absorption of lipophilic drugs, such as valproate.

Importance and management

The general relevance of the isolated cases is unclear: they appear to be the only reports of an interaction. Whilst the evidence is not sufficiently strong to suggest that chitosan should be avoided by any patients taking valproate, some caution would be prudent and patients should be aware of the possibility of seizure recurrence after starting chitosan. Until more is known it may also be prudent to consider the possibility of an interaction if valproate levels are lowered in patients taking chitosan.

1. Striano P, Zara F, Minetti C, Striano S. Chitosan may decrease serum valproate and increase the risk of seizure reappearance. *BMJ* (2009) 339, b3751.

Chitosan + Warfarin and related drugs

An isolated report describes an increase in the INR of an elderly man taking warfarin when he also took chitosan.

Clinical evidence

A case report describes an 83-year-old man, with type 2 diabetes who was receiving warfarin (2.5 mg daily for one year, with an INR of between 2 and 3) for atrial fibrillation. At a routine blood test his INR was found to be about 3.7, and, although the dose of warfarin was halved, 3 days later his INR was more than 9. On discussion, it was established that he had recently started taking chitosan 1.2 g twice daily. He was advised to stop this supplement and was subsequently restabilised on warfarin. About one month later, the patient restarted the chitosan, which again resulted in a raised INR.[1]

Experimental evidence

No relevant data found.

Mechanism

Chitosan *sulfate* has been reported to have anticoagulant activity, but this has not been found with chitosan. The authors therefore suggest that chitosan impaired the absorption of fat soluble vitamins, including vitamin K. Warfarin is a vitamin-K antagonist and a reduction in vitamin K would be expected to enhance its effects.

Importance and management

Evidence is limited to this case, and the mechanism is largely speculative; however an interaction seems probable. The evidence is too slim to forbid patients taking warfarin from also taking chitosan, but it would seem prudent to discuss the possible outcome and advise an increase in the frequency of anticoagulant monitoring; measuring the INR after a few days of concurrent use seems reasonable. There appears to be no evidence regarding other anticoagulants, but if the mechanism is correct, all vitamin K antagonists (**coumarins** and **indanediones**) would be expected to be similarly affected.

1. Huang S-S, Sung S-H, Chiang C-E. Chitosan potentiation of warfarin effect. *Ann Pharmacother* (2007) 41, 1912–14.

C

Chondroitin

Swertia chirayita (Roxb.) H.Karst. (Gentianaceae)

Types, sources and related compounds

Chondroitin sulfate sodium.

Pharmacopoeias

Chondroitin Sulfate Sodium (*BP 2012, PhEur 7.5, USP35–NF30 S1*); Chondroitin Sulfate Sodium Tablets (*USP35–NF30 S1*).

Use and indications

Chondroitin is an acid mucopolysaccharide and is found naturally in cartilage and connective tissue. Supplemental chondroitin is used for the management of arthritis and is often given with glucosamine, page 260, for osteoarthritis.

Pharmacokinetics

Chondroitin is rapidly adsorbed from the gastrointestinal tract and the absolute bioavailability of an oral dose is about 15%. It is distributed into numerous tissues, with a particular affinity to articular cartilage and synovial fluid.[1]

Interactions overview

No interactions with chondroitin taken alone found, but chondroitin is often given with glucosamine. For information on these interactions, see under glucosamine, page 260.

1. Ronca F, Palmieri L, Panicucci P, Ronca G. Anti-inflammatory activity of chondroitin sulfate. *Osteoarthritis Cartilage* (1998) 6 (Suppl A), 14–21.

Clivers

Galium aparine L. (Rubiaceae)

Synonym(s) and related species

Cleavers, Galium, Goosegrass.

Constituents

Clivers contains the iridoids asperuloside, deacetylasperuloside and monotropein, polyphenolic acids, unspecified tannins based on gallic acid, and **flavonoids**. Anthraquinones have been found in the roots, but not the aerial parts.

Use and indications

Clivers is traditionally used for dysuria, cystitis, lymphadenitis, psoriasis and as a diuretic.

Pharmacokinetics

No relevant pharmacokinetic data found.

Interactions overview

No interactions with clivers found.

Clove

Syzygium aromaticum (L.) Merr. & L.M.Perry (Myrtaceae)

Synonym(s) and related species

Caryophyllus aromaticus L., *Eugenia aromatica* (L.) Baill., *Eugenia caryophyllata* Thunb., *Eugenia caryophyllus* (Spreng.) Bull. & Harr.

Pharmacopoeias

Clove (*BP 2012, PhEur 7.5*); Clove Oil (*BP 2012, PhEur 7.5*).

Constituents

Extracts of clove flower buds are often standardised to contain a minimum of 15% (w/v) essential oil (*BP 2012, PhEur 7.5*) composed mainly of the phenylpropanoid **eugenol** (85 to 90%), with methyleugenol, acetyleugenol, beta-caryophyllene, methyl salicylate, benzaldehyde, cadinenes, cubebenes and alpha-humulene also present. The buds also contain the tannins eugeniin, casuarictin, tellimagrandin I and others; chromones including bifiorin and isobifiorin; flavonoids; and sterols.

Clove oil is extracted from the unopened buds and is often standardised to contain 75 to 88% **eugenol** (*BP 2012, PhEur 7.5*).

Clove leaf oil may also be used and contains similar constituents.

Use and indications

Clove and clove oil are traditionally considered to have stimulant and carminative properties and have been used to treat digestive disorders. The oil has antiseptic and mild analgesic properties and is used in dental preparations for toothache. Note that clove oil should only be ingested in small quantities (less than 0.2 mL). Cloves are widely used in cooking as a flavouring.

Pharmacokinetics

No relevant pharmacokinetic data found.

Interactions overview

Experimental evidence suggests that clove oil and its constituents may have antiplatelet effects similar to aspirin, but these will not be relevant to topical use, and are unlikely to be clinically relevant at small oral doses. Clove oil may enhance the absorption of drugs applied to the skin, such as ibuprofen.

Interactions monographs

- Anticoagulant or Antiplatelet drugs, page 155
- Food, page 155
- Herbal medicines, page 155
- Miscellaneous, page 155

Clove + Anticoagulant or Antiplatelet drugs

The interaction between clove and anticoagulants or antiplatelet drugs is based on experimental evidence only.

Evidence, mechanism, importance and management

In *in vitro* studies, clove oil[1] and its main constituents eugenol[2,3] and acetyl eugenol[2] inhibited human platelet aggregation induced by arachidonic acid. Eugenol was a more potent inhibitor of arachidonic acid-induced platelet aggregation than aspirin,[2,3] and the effects were similar to indometacin.[2] In a study in *rabbits*, intraperitoneal administration of clove oil 100 mg/kg partially protected against arachidonic acid-induced pulmonary thrombosis, whereas aspirin 50 mg/kg completely protected against this.[1]

The constituents of clove oil appear to have antiplatelet effects and in theory, these effects have the potential to be additive with those of conventional antiplatelet drugs. However, any interaction between clove and anticoagulants or antiplatelet drugs would not be relevant to the topical use of clove or clove oil, and it is also unlikely to be important at small oral doses equivalent to the amounts used in foods.

1. Saeed SA, Gilani AH. Antithrombotic activity of clove oil. *JPMA* (1994) 44, 112–15.
2. Srivastava KC. Antiplatelet principles from a food spice clove (Syzygium aromaticum L). *Prostaglandins Leukot Essent Fatty Acids* (1993) 48, 363–72.
3. Raghavendra RH, Naidu KA. Spice active principles as the inhibitors of human platelet aggregation and thromboxane biosynthesis. *Prostaglandins Leukot Essent Fatty Acids* (2009) 81, 73–8.

Clove + Food

No interactions found. Cloves are commonly used as a flavouring in foods.

Clove + Herbal medicines

No interactions found.

Clove + Miscellaneous

The interaction between clove oil and topical ibuprofen or topical paracetamol (acetaminophen) is based on experimental evidence only.

Evidence, mechanism, importance and management

In a study in *rabbits*, clove oil 3% (w/v) increased the absorption of **ibuprofen** applied to the skin, which resulted in a 2.4-fold increase in the AUC of **ibuprofen**. This effect was much less than that seen *in vitro*.[1] In another *in vitro* study, clove oil 2% promoted the transdermal penetration of **paracetamol (acetaminophen)**.[2]

Essential oils such as clove are known to have skin permeation-enhancing effects, which could increase the absorption of topically applied drugs if used at the same time. Bear in mind that if clove oil and topical formulations of drugs are applied to the skin at the same time, there may be an increase in the absorption of the drug. The clinical effects of this may not necessarily be adverse.

1. Shen Q, Li W, Li W. The effect of clove oil on the transdermal delivery of ibuprofen in the rabbit by in vitro and in vivo methods. *Drug Dev Ind Pharm* (2007) 33, 1369–74.
2. Zheng X, Wang H, Cheng K, Liang Q. Evaluation of promoting effect of several transdermal enhancers with fuzzy matter-element model. *Zhongguo Zhong Yao Za Zhi* (2009) 34, 2599–2603.

Cocoa

Theobroma cacao L. (Sterculiaceae)

Synonym(s) and related species

Cacao, Chocolate, Chocolate tree, Theobroma.

Pharmacopoeias

Cocoa butter (*USP35–NF30 S1*); Chocolate (*USP35–NF30 S1*); Theobroma Oil (*BP 2012*).

Constituents

Cocoa seeds contain **xanthine derivatives**, principally **theobromine** (1% to 4%), with small amounts of **caffeine** (up to about 0.4%) and other alkaloids. They are also rich in **flavonoids** from the flavanol and procyanidin groups, mainly catechin and epicatechin and their polymers. The nibs (cotyledons) are a rich source of cocoa butter (theobroma oil), which contains oleic, stearic, palmitic and linoleic acids.

Use and indications

The seeds roasted and powdered are the source of cocoa, which is mainly used as a food (in chocolate). Medicinal uses include as a stimulant and as a diuretic; effects that can be attributed to the xanthine content. However, note that theobromine is a much weaker xanthine than caffeine. Cocoa butter is used as an emollient and pharmaceutical excipient.

More recently, there has been interest in the possible beneficial effects of cocoa consumption on cardiovascular health, because of its high content of flavonoids.

Pharmacokinetics

The pharmacokinetics of caffeine are discussed under caffeine, page 106. In one study, caffeine absorption from chocolate was slower with a lower maximum concentration than from capsules, whereas theobromine absorption was faster with higher maximum concentration than from capsules.[1] For information on the pharmacokinetics of individual flavonoids present in cocoa, see under flavonoids, page 213.

Interactions overview

Although the use of cocoa supplements has been cautioned by some in diabetic patients, there seems little evidence to support this. Dark chocolate may slightly decrease blood pressure in hypertensive patients, but caffeine from cocoa may have the opposite effect. Famotidine and foods have no effect, or only modest effects, on the absorption of flavanols from cocoa. Cocoa may reduce the absorption of iron.

Cocoa contains small amounts of caffeine compared with some other caffeine-containing herbs. Although it contains high levels of theobromine, this has weak xanthine effects when compared with caffeine. Nevertheless, when taken in sufficient quantities, cocoa could produce levels of caffeine sufficient to cause interactions, see caffeine, page 106.

For information on the interactions of individual flavonoids present in cocoa, see under flavonoids, page 213. Of particular note are studies showing that cocoa flavanols, might have antiplatelet effects, and that these might be additive with aspirin, see Flavonoids + Anticoagulant or Antiplatelet drugs, page 215.

Interactions monographs

- Antidiabetics, page 157
- Antihypertensives, page 157
- Famotidine, page 157
- Food, page 157
- Herbal medicines, page 157
- Iron compounds, page 158

1. Mumford GK, Benowitz NL, Evans SM, Kaminski BJ, Preston KL, Sannerud CA, Silverman K, Griffiths RR. Absorption rate of methylxanthines following capsules, cola and chocolate. *Eur J Clin Pharmacol* (1996) 51, 319–25.

Cocoa + Anticoagulant or Antiplatelet drugs

For studies showing that cocoa flavanols might have antiplatelet effects, and that these might be additive with aspirin, see Flavonoids + Anticoagulant or Antiplatelet drugs, page 215.

Cocoa + Antidiabetics

Although the use of cocoa supplements has been cautioned by some in diabetic patients, there seems little evidence to support this.

Evidence, mechanism, importance and management

The traditional advice in diabetes is to avoid or limit intake of chocolate. This is principally because of the high calorific value of chocolate, and its high sugar content (particularly milk chocolates). In one study, an isomalt-based chocolate (about 45% w/w) had a lower glycaemic effect than a sucrose-based chocolate (about 45% w/w), which confirms the concerns regarding the sucrose content.[1]

Conversely, in *animal* studies, cocoa extract containing high levels of procyanidins had beneficial effects on blood-glucose levels.[2,3] In addition, in one study in patients with untreated essential hypertension, an improvement in glucose and insulin responses was found during an oral glucose tolerance test, and a slightly lower fasting blood-glucose level was seen, after subjects ate 100 g of dark chocolate daily for 15 days (substituted for food of similar energy and macronutrient composition). This effect was not seen with 90 g of white chocolate daily.[4] Taken together, the evidence suggests that cocoa *per se*, and cocoa supplements, should not be a problem in diabetics and should not interfere with blood-glucose control.

1. Gee JM, Cooke D, Gorick S, Wortley GM, Greenwood RH, Zumbe A, Johnson IT. Effects of conventional sucrose-based, fructose-based and isomalt-based chocolates on postprandial metabolism in non-insulin-dependent diabetics. *Eur J Clin Nutr* (1991) 45, 561–6.
2. Ruzaidi A, Amin I, Nawalyah AG, Hamid M, Faizul HA. The effect of Malaysian cocoa extract on glucose levels and lipid profiles in diabetic rats. *J Ethnopharmacol* (2005) 98, 55–60.
3. Tomaru M, Takano H, Osakabe N, Yasuda A, Inoue K, Yanagisawa R, Ohwatari T, Uematsu H. Dietary supplementation with cacao liquor proanthocyanidins prevents elevation of blood glucose levels in diabetic obese mice. *Nutrition* (2007) 23, 351–5.
4. Grassi D, Necozione S, Lippi C, Croce G, Valeri L, Pasqualetti P, Desideri G, Blumberg JB, Ferri C. Cocoa reduces blood pressure and insulin resistance and improves endothelium-dependent vasodilation in hypertensives. *Hypertension* (2005) 46, 398–405.

Cocoa + Antihypertensives

Dark chocolate may slightly decrease blood pressure in hypertensive patients, but caffeine from cocoa may have the opposite effect.

Evidence, mechanism, importance and management

There has been some interest in the possible beneficial effects of cocoa consumption on cardiovascular health, because of its high content of flavonoids. In a meta-analysis of five short-term randomised controlled studies, daily consumption of high doses (46 to 100 g daily) of dark chocolate, or 105 g daily of milk chocolate, all containing high levels of flavonoids, caused a modest 4.7 and 2.8 mmHg reduction in systolic and diastolic blood pressure, respectively.[1] Another study with a lower dose (6.3 g daily) showed a smaller effect (2.9/1.9 mmHg reduction).[2]

These studies show that high doses of dark chocolate 100 g daily, modestly *decreases* blood pressure; an effect attributed to

its flavonoid content.[1–3] This suggests that blood pressure control is unlikely to be significantly affected by cocoa supplements in patients with hypertension. None of the patients in these studies were taking antihypertensive medication so some caution would still be needed. Theoretically, the caffeine content in cocoa could result in increases in blood pressure, and therefore large quantities of cocoa supplements could be inadvisable in patients with hypertension, see Caffeine + Antihypertensives, page 108.

1. Taubert D, Roesen R, Schömig E. Effect of cocoa and tea intake on blood pressure: a meta-analysis. *Arch Intern Med* (2007) 167, 626–34.
2. Taubert D, Roesen R, Lehmann C, Jung N, Schömig E. Effects of low habitual cocoa intake on blood pressure and bioactive nitric oxide: a randomized controlled trial. *JAMA* (2007) 298, 49–60.
3. Grassi D, Necozione S, Lippi C, Croce G, Valeri L, Pasqualetti P, Desideri G, Blumberg JB, Ferri C. Cocoa reduces blood pressure and insulin resistance and improves endothelium-dependent vasodilation in hypertensives. *Hypertension* (2005) 46, 398–405.

Cocoa + Famotidine

Famotidine has no effect on the absorption of flavanols from cocoa.

Evidence, mechanism, importance and management

In a study in 6 healthy subjects, a single 20-mg dose of famotidine given one hour before consumption of sugar-free, flavanol-rich cocoa had no effect on the AUC of flavanols.[1] It was concluded that alteration of gastric pH had no effect on flavanol absorption. No special precautions appear to be necessary.

1. Schramm DD, Karim M, Schrader HR, Holt RR, Kirkpatrick NJ, Polagruto JA, Ensunsa JL, Schmitz HH, Keen CL. Food effects on the absorption and pharmacokinetics of cocoa flavanols. *Life Sci* (2003) 73, 857–69.

Cocoa + Food

Food has no effect, or only modest effects, on the absorption of flavanols from cocoa.

Evidence, mechanism, importance and management

In a series of studies in 6 healthy subjects, high-carbohydrate foods (**bread** or **sugar**) increased the flavanol AUC by about 40% after consumption of 125 micrograms/kg of sugar-free, flavanol-rich cocoa. Lipid and protein-rich foods (**butter** or **steak**) and **whole milk** had little effect on flavanol absorption. **Grapefruit juice** had a minor effect (20% increase), which was attributed to its carbohydrate content.[1]

This study demonstrated that carbohydrates can increase oral flavanol absorption from cocoa. However, the extent is modest, and probably of little clinical relevance.

1. Schramm DD, Karim M, Schrader HR, Holt RR, Kirkpatrick NJ, Polagruto JA, Ensunsa JL, Schmitz HH, Keen CL. Food effects on the absorption and pharmacokinetics of cocoa flavanols. *Life Sci* (2003) 73, 857–69.

Cocoa + Herbal medicines

The caffeine content of cocoa suggests that it may interact with other herbal medicines in the same way as caffeine, see Caffeine + Herbal medicines; Bitter orange, page 111, and Ephedra + Caffeine, page 202.

Cocoa + Iron compounds

Cocoa may reduce the absorption of iron.

Clinical evidence

In a study in 10 healthy subjects[1] a 275 mL serving of cocoa beverage reduced the absorption of radiolabelled iron from a 50 g bread roll by about 70%. In this study, the inhibitory effect of cocoa beverage on iron absorption was only slightly less that of black tea (Assam tea, *Camellia sinensis*).Note that black tea is known to inhibit iron absorption, see Tea + Iron compounds, page 467.

Experimental evidence

No relevant data found.

Mechanism

The polyphenols in cocoa may bind to iron in the gastrointestinal tract and reduce its absorption.[1]

Importance and management

Evidence appears to be limited to this one study, but be aware that some beverages such as cocoa might reduce iron absorption similarly to conventional tea. See Tea + Iron compounds, page 467, for further discussion of the possible impact of this interaction.

1. Hurrell RF, Reddy M, Cook JD. Inhibition of non-haem iron absorption in man by polyphenolic-containing beverages. *Br J Nutr* (1999) 81, 289–95.

Coenzyme Q$_{10}$

Theobroma cacao L. (Sterculiaceae)

Types, sources and related compounds

Ubidecarenone, Ubiquinone.

Pharmacopoeias

Ubidecarenone (*BP 2012, PhEur 7.5, USP35–NF30 S1*); Ubidecarenone capsules (*USP35–NF30 S1*); Ubidecarenone tablets (*USP35–NF30 S1*).

Use and indications

Coenzyme Q$_{10}$ is a naturally-occurring enzyme co-factor that has a fundamental role in electron transport in mitochondria, and is also an antioxidant. It is often taken orally as a supplement to aid in the treatment of cardiovascular disorders such as congestive heart failure, angina, and hypertension. It has also been used to maintain the levels of endogenous coenzyme Q$_{10}$ during treatment with conventional drugs that reduce these, particularly the statins.

Coenzyme Q$_{10}$ has also been used alongside treatment for breast cancer, Huntington's disease and Parkinson's disease, and may help to prevent migraines.

Pharmacokinetics

The absorption of coenzyme Q$_{10}$ is relatively slow and is dependent on postprandial lipids in the gastrointestinal tract, see food, page 160.

Interactions overview

Coenzyme Q$_{10}$ did not interact with warfarin in a controlled study, but there are a few isolated reports describing either increased or decreased warfarin effects in patients taking coenzyme Q$_{10}$. Coenzyme Q$_{10}$ may decrease the effects of aldosterone and alter the levels of the major cytotoxic metabolite of doxorubicin. Pepper (*Piper nigrum*) may modestly increase the levels of coenzyme Q$_{10}$.

Interactions monographs

- Aldosterone, page 160
- Doxorubicin, page 160
- Food, page 160
- Herbal medicines; Pepper, page 160
- Warfarin and related drugs, page 160

C

Coenzyme Q_{10} + Aldosterone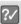

The interaction between coenzyme Q_{10} and aldosterone is based on experimental evidence only.

Evidence, mechanism, importance and management

In experimental studies in *rats* and *dogs,* single-dose coenzyme Q_{10} *increased* the sodium reabsorption stimulated by exogenous aldosterone, but in contrast, in *rats* and *dogs* pretreated for 3 weeks with multiple doses, increasing the dose of coenzyme Q_{10} *reduced* the sodium reabsorption caused by aldosterone. Potassium excretion remained unaffected throughout.[1]

This study suggests that long-term use of coenzyme Q_{10} might have some diuretic activity, and might oppose the effects of aldosterone. However, the clinical relevance of this is uncertain.

1. Igarashi T, Kobayashi M, Sugiyama K, Sagami F, Ohtake S. Effect of coenzyme Q10 on electrolyte metabolism and the interaction with aldosterone in rats and dogs. *Proc West Pharmacol Soc* (1975) 18, 399–402.

Coenzyme Q_{10} + Doxorubicin

The interaction between coenzyme Q_{10} and doxorubicin is based on experimental evidence only.

Evidence, mechanism, importance and management

In a study in *rats,* oral coenzyme Q_{10} 20 mg/kg for 6 days had no significant effect on the pharmacokinetics of intravenous doxorubicin 10 mg/kg or its major cytotoxic metabolite doxorubicinol. However, there was a twofold increase in the AUC of the doxorubicinolone metabolite.[1] The findings from this study suggest that coenzyme Q_{10} is unlikely to reduce the efficacy of doxorubicin via a pharmacokinetic mechanism. The reason for the significant rise in doxorubicinolone concentration and its impact is unknown. Note that the possible use of coenzyme Q_{10} to reduce doxorubicin-induced cardiotoxicity has been investigated.

1. Zhou Q, Chowbay B. Effect of coenzyme Q_{10} on the disposition of doxorubicin in rats. *Eur J Drug Metab Pharmacokinet* (2002) 27, 185–92.

Coenzyme Q_{10} + Food

The interaction between coenzyme Q_{10} and food is based on experimental evidence only.

Clinical evidence

No interactions found.

Experimental evidence

Food increased the maximum serum levels and AUC of oral coenzyme Q_{10} 25 mg/kg, given as an emulsion, by about fivefold and twofold respectively in *rats*. Coenzyme Q_{10} given as an emulsion showed greater increases than coenzyme Q_{10} given in suspension.[1]

Mechanism

Coenzyme Q_{10} has a large molecular weight and is relatively hydrophobic, which results in slow absorption in the gastrointestinal tract. Taking the supplement with food and/or as a lipid-based emulsion increases its water solubility and enhances its absorption.

Importance and management

Data regarding the effects of food on coenzyme Q_{10} absorption appears to be limited. The absorption of coenzyme Q_{10} is relatively slow and is dependent on postprandial lipids in the gastrointestinal

tract. Coenzyme Q_{10} supplements therefore often contain a lipid vehicle and it is recommended that they are taken with fatty meals.[2]

1. Ochiai A, Itagaki S, Kurokawa T, Kobayashi M, Hirano T, Iseki K. Improvement in intestinal coenzyme Q10 absorption by food intake. *Yakugaku Zasshi* (2007) 127, 1251–4.
2. Pepping J. Coenzyme Q_{10}. *Am J Health-Syst Pharm* (1999) 56, 519–21.

Coenzyme Q_{10} + Herbal medicines; Pepper

Pepper (*Piper nigrum*) may modestly increase the levels of coenzyme Q_{10}.

Clinical evidence

In a single-dose, placebo-controlled study in 12 healthy subjects, there was no change in pharmacokinetics of coenzyme Q_{10} (AUC and maximum level or time to maximum level) when **piperine** 5 mg (*Bioperine*) from pepper (*Piper nigrum*) was given with coenzyme Q_{10} 90 mg. Similarly, giving **piperine** 5 mg with coenzyme Q_{10} 90 mg daily for 14 days did not alter the AUC of coenzyme Q_{10}. However, when **piperine** 5 mg was given with coenzyme Q_{10} 120 mg daily for 21 days, the plasma levels of coenzyme Q_{10} were increased by 32% and the AUC was increased by 30%.[1]

Experimental evidence

No relevant data found.

Mechanism

It was suggested that piperine increased the absorption of coenzyme Q_{10} from the gastrointestinal tract, but the exact mechanism is unclear.

Importance and management

The modest increase in coenzyme Q_{10} levels seen in this study with piperine (an alkaloid derived from black pepper) is unlikely to be clinically important, since coenzyme Q_{10} is a ubiquitous compound, generally regarded as safe. Note that a combination product has been marketed.

1. Badmaev V, Majeed M, Prakash L. Piperine derived from black pepper increases the plasma levels of coenzyme Q10 following oral supplementation. *J Nutr Biochem* (2000) 11, 109–13.

Coenzyme Q_{10} + Warfarin and related drugs

Ubidecarenone did not alter the INR or required warfarin dose in a controlled study on warfarin. However, two reports describe reduced anticoagulant effects of warfarin in four patients taking ubidecarenone. A transient increase in INR has been reported in one patient taking ubidecarenone and warfarin. A 4-month prospective, longitudinal study describes an increased risk of self-reported bleeding events in patients taking coenzyme Q_{10} with warfarin.

Clinical evidence

In a randomised, crossover study in 21 patients stabilised on warfarin, coenzyme Q_{10} 100 mg daily (*Bio-Quinone*) for 4 weeks did not alter the INR or the required dose of warfarin, when compared with placebo.[1] Similarly, 2 patients taking coenzyme Q_{10} to treat alopecia caused by warfarin treatment did not have any notable changes in INR, except that one had a transient INR *increase* when coenzyme Q_{10} was started.[2]

In a 4-month prospective, longitudinal study of 78 patients taking warfarin and a herbal product or dietary supplement, there was a statistically significant *increased* risk of self-reported bleeding events in 14 patients taking warfarin and coenzyme Q_{10} (57 bleeding events, none major, in a total of 181 weeks of combined use for an odds ratio of 3.7).[3] There were 4 elevated INRs (specific values not given) for 55 weeks of combined use, but this was not a statistically significant increase in risk. Note that the coenzyme Q_{10} products used were not mentioned. The authors acknowledge that their finding might be due to chance and not a true interaction.

In contrast, another report describes 3 patients taking warfarin who had a reduction in their INR while taking coenzyme Q_{10}. In two of these, INR reductions from about 2.5 to 1.4 occurred when they took coenzyme Q_{10} 30 mg daily for 2 weeks. The INRs rapidly returned to normal when the coenzyme Q_{10} was stopped.[4] In two other cases, patients appeared to have a reduced response to warfarin while taking coenzyme Q_{10}, but responded normally when it was stopped.[5,6]

Experimental evidence

In a study in *rats,* coenzyme Q_{10} reduced the anticoagulant effect of warfarin and increased the clearance of both enantiomers of warfarin.[7]

Mechanism

Not known. Coenzyme Q_{10} may have some vitamin K-like activity, which would explain the decrease in INR. Explanations for the increase in bleeding or INRs are unknown.

Importance and management

The well-controlled study suggests that coenzyme Q_{10} does not interact with warfarin, and that no warfarin dose adjustment would be expected to be necessary in patients who take this substance. However, the contrasting findings of a *decrease* in warfarin effect in the case reports, and an *increase* in bleeding events reported in the epidemiological study, introduce a note of caution. Moreover, the authors of the controlled study recommend close monitoring of the INR if a patient decides to use coenzyme Q_{10}, because the underlying health problem resulting in them choosing to take this substance may alter their response to warfarin.[1] Until more is known it would seem prudent to increase the frequency of INR monitoring in patients taking warfarin if coenzyme Q_{10} is started.

1. Engelsen J, Nielsen JD, Winther K. Effect of coenzyme Q_{10} and ginkgo biloba on warfarin dosage in stable, long-term warfarin treated outpatients. A randomised, double blind, placebo-crossover trial. *Thromb Haemost* (2002) 87, 1075–6.
2. Nagao T, Ibayashi S, Fujii K, Sugimori H, Sadoshima S, Fujishima M. Treatment of warfarin-induced hair loss with ubidecarenone. *Lancet* (1995) 346, 1104–5.
3. Shalansky S, Lynd L, Richardson K, Ingaszewski A, Kerr C. Risk of warfarin-related bleeding events and supratherapeutic international normalized ratios associated with complementary and alternative medicine: a longitudinal analysis. *Pharmacotherapy* (2007) 27, 1237–47.
4. Spigset O. Reduced effect of warfarin caused by ubidecarenone. *Lancet* (1994) 344, 1372–3.
5. Landbo C, Almdal TP. Interaction mellem warfarin og coenzym Q10. *Ugeskr Laeger* (1998) 160, 3226–7.
6. Porterfield LM. Why did the response to warfarin change? *RN* (2000) 63, 107.
7. Zhou S, Chan E. Effect of ubidecarenone on warfarin anticoagulation and pharmacokinetics of warfarin enantiomers in rats. *Drug Metabol Drug Interact* (2001) 18, 99–122.

Coffee

Coffea L. species. (Rubiaceae)

Synonym(s) and related species

Arabian coffee is from *Coffea arabica*. Robusta coffee is from *Coffea canephora* (Pierre ex Froehner) also known as *Coffea robusta* (Linden ex De Wild.).

Other species include *Coffea liberica*.

Constituents

The kernel of the dried coffee bean contains xanthine derivatives, the main one being **caffeine** (1 to 2%), with some theobromine and theophylline. It also contains polyphenolic acids such as chlorogenic acids, and various diterpenes (e.g. kahweol, cafestrol).

Use and indications

Coffee has been used as a stimulant and diuretic. However, when roasted, coffee beans are most commonly used as a beverage.

Pharmacokinetics

The pharmacokinetics of caffeine are discussed under caffeine, page 106. Evidence suggests that chlorogenic acid is hydrolysed in the gastrointestinal tract to free caffeic acid, which is then conjugated to form the glucuronate or sulphate.[1]

Interactions overview

Coffee contains significant amounts of caffeine, therefore the interactions of caffeine, page 106, are relevant to coffee, unless the product is specified as decaffeinated. By virtue of its caffeine content, coffee may also cause serious adverse effects if used with other drugs or herbs with similar effects, such as ephedra, page 202. Evidence is conflicting, but in general the long-term use of coffee does not appear to be detrimental to the control of diabetes; however, coffee may have a small adverse effect on blood pressure control. Coffee may reduce the absorption of iron and the absorption of nicotine from chewing gum, but does not appear to affect the absorption of aspirin or tetracycline. A case report describes mania in a patient who drank coffee and took phenylpropanolamine. For the possible increase in clozapine effects with caffeine, sometimes from coffee, see Caffeine + Clozapine, page 109.

Interactions monographs

- Antidiabetics, page 163
- Antihypertensives, page 163
- Aspirin, page 163
- Food, page 163
- Herbal medicines, page 164
- Iron compounds, page 164
- Nicotine, page 164
- Phenylpropanolamine, page 164
- Tetracycline, page 164

1. Nardini M, Cirillo E, Natella F, Scaccini C. Absorption of phenolic acids in humans after coffee consumption. *J Agric Food Chem* (2002) 50, 5735–41.

Coffee + Antidiabetics

Evidence is conflicting, but in general the long-term use of coffee does not appear to be detrimental to the control of diabetes.

Evidence, mechanism, importance and management

There is a lot of epidemiological evidence that coffee consumption is associated with a reduced risk of type 2 diabetes (this has been the subject of a review[1]). In addition, a large prospective cohort study in Finland found that coffee drinking was associated with reduced total and cardiovascular disease mortality.[2]

In contrast, some short-term randomised studies have found that coffee consumption had detrimental effects on insulin sensitivity in healthy subjects (high consumption of filtered coffee over 4 weeks)[3] and increased postprandial hyperglycaemia in patients with type 2 diabetes taking unnamed oral antidiabetic drugs (caffeine added to decaffeinated coffee, single dose).[4]

The evidence is not conclusive, which makes it difficult to advise patients taking antidiabetics on use of coffee beverages or supplements. However the Finnish study does provides some reassurance that use of coffee may not be detrimental in the long-term, and may even be beneficial.

1. van Dam RM. Coffee and type 2 diabetes: from beans to beta-cells. *Nutr Metab Cardiovasc Dis* (2006) 16, 69–77.
2. Bidel S, Hu G, Qiao Q, Jousilahti P, Antikainen R, Tuomilehto J. Coffee consumption and risk of total and cardiovascular mortality among patients with type 2 diabetes. *Diabetologia* (2006) 49, 2618–26.
3. van Dam RM, Pasman WJ, Verhoef P. Effects of coffee consumption on fasting blood glucose and insulin concentrations: randomized controlled trials in healthy volunteers. *Diabetes Care* (2004) 27, 2990–2992.
4. Lane JD, Hwang AL, Feinglos MN, Surwit RS. Exaggeration of postprandial hyperglycemia in patients with type 2 diabetes by administration of caffeine in coffee. *Endocr Pract* (2007) 13, 239–43.

Coffee + Antihypertensives

Coffee may have a small adverse effect on blood pressure control.

Clinical evidence

Limited data is available on the effect of coffee on blood pressure in patients taking antihypertensives. In one study, two 150-mL cups of coffee (made from 24 g of coffee) increased the mean blood pressure of 12 healthy subjects taking **propranolol** 240 mg, **metoprolol** 300 mg or a placebo. Mean blood pressure rises were 7%/22% with **propranolol**, 7%/19% with **metoprolol** and 4%/16% with placebo. The beta blockers and placebo were given in divided doses over 15 hours before the test.[1] However, there are lots of short-term studies on the effect of coffee on blood pressure in healthy subjects or patients with untreated mild hypertension. In one meta-analysis of 18 randomised studies of coffee consumption, coffee drinking was associated with a very small 1.22/0.49 mmHg increase in blood pressure.[2]

One study found that blood pressure was higher in untreated hypertensives who drank coffee (5 cups daily, each containing approximately 60 mg caffeine) than in untreated hypertensives who did not drink coffee. However, coffee drinking reduced the potentially detrimental post-meal postural drop in systolic blood pressure in patients taking unnamed antihypertensives.[3]

The only long-term studies are of epidemiological type. In one large prospective cohort study in Finland, low to moderate daily consumption of coffee (2 to 7 cups daily) was associated with a small (about 24 to 29%) increased risk of requiring antihypertensive drug treatment.[4] In the Nurses Health prospective cohort, coffee consumption was not associated with an increased risk of developing hypertension.[5]

In contrast to some of the data on coffee, chlorogenic acids from coffee have been reported to reduce blood pressure. In one randomised study in patients with mild hypertension not receiving antihypertensives, **green coffee bean extract** 480 mg (containing 140 mg of chlorogenic acids) daily for 12 weeks was associated with a 10/7 mmHg reduction in blood pressure.[6] A dose related decrease in blood pressure with green coffee extract was seen in another study.[7] Note that green coffee is not roasted, and may therefore contain different constituents and have different effects than the usual roasted coffee, although the importance of this remains to be demonstrated.

Experimental evidence

Because of the extensive clinical evidence available, experimental data have not been sought.

Mechanism

Acute intake of caffeine raises blood pressure, but partial tolerance to this effect might possibly develop with regular consumption, see also Caffeine + Antihypertensives, page 108. Polyphenolic compounds in coffee might improve endothelial function, and might therefore lower blood pressure.

Importance and management

The evidence presented here is conflicting; however, most of the studies suggest that coffee might have a small adverse effect on blood pressure. It is possible that this does not extend to green (unroasted) coffee, and therefore supplements containing green coffee extract might not be expected to have a negative effect on blood pressure. Further study is needed.

For discussion of the adverse effect of caffeine on blood pressure, see Caffeine + Antihypertensives, page 108.

1. Smits P, Hoffmann H, Thien T, Houben H, van't Laar A. Hemodynamic and humoral effects of coffee after β1-selective and nonselective β-blockade. *Clin Pharmacol Ther* (1983) 34, 153–8.
2. Noordzij M, Uiterwaal CS, Arends LR, Kok FJ, Grobbee DE, Geleijnse JM. Blood pressure response to chronic intake of coffee and caffeine: a meta-analysis of randomized controlled trials. *J Hypertens* (2005) 23, 921–8.
3. Rakic V, Beilin LJ, Burke V. Effect of coffee and tea drinking on postprandial hypotension in older men and women. *Clin Exp Pharmacol Physiol* (1996) 23, 559–63.
4. Hu G, Jousilahti P, Nissinen A, Bidel S, Antikainen R, Tuomilehto J. Coffee consumption and the incidence of antihypertensive drug treatment in Finnish men and women. *Am J Clin Nutr* (2007) 86, 457–64.
5. Winkelmayer WC, Stampfer MJ, Willett WC, Curhan GC. Habitual caffeine intake and the risk of hypertension in women. *JAMA* (2005) 294, 233–5.
6. Watanabe T, Arai Y, Mitsui Y, Kusaura T, Okawa W, Kajihara Y, Saito I. The blood pressure-lowering effect and safety of chlorogenic acid from green coffee bean extract in essential hypertension. *Clin Exp Hypertens* (2006) 28, 439–49.
7. Kozuma K, Tsuchiya S, Kohori J, Hase T, Tokimitsu I. Antihypertensive effect of green coffee bean extract on mildly hypertensive subjects. *Hypertens Res* (2005) 28, 711–18.

Coffee + Aspirin

Coffee does not appear to affect aspirin absorption.

Evidence, mechanism, importance and management

A study in 5 healthy subjects found that 200 mL of coffee had no effect on the rate and extent of absorption of a single 500-mg dose of aspirin, whereas 200 mL of milk reduced the bioavailability and maximum concentration of salicylates from the same dose of aspirin by a modest 30%.[1]

No significant reduction in the bioavailability of aspirin would be expected with black coffee; however the addition of milk, depending on the quantity, may possibly reduce the absorption of aspirin.

Note that caffeine may enhance the analgesic effects of aspirin, see Caffeine + Aspirin or Diclofenac, page 108.

1. Odou P, Barthélémy C, Robert H. Influence of seven beverages on salicylate disposition in humans. *J Clin Pharm Ther* (2001) 26, 187–93.

Coffee + Food

No specific interactions found, however, the effects of caffeine from coffee or a coffee-containing herbal medicine will be additive with those of other caffeine-containing foods or beverages.

Coffee + Herbal medicines

The caffeine content of coffee suggests that it may interact with other herbal medicines in the same way as caffeine, see Caffeine + Herbal medicines; Bitter orange, page 111, and Ephedra + Caffeine, page 202.

Coffee + Iron compounds

C

Coffee may possibly contribute towards the development of iron-deficiency anaemia in pregnant women, and reduce the levels of iron in breast milk. As a result their babies may also be iron deficient.

Clinical evidence

In a series of studies in healthy subjects, drinking 200 mL of coffee with various test meals containing radiolabelled iron resulted in a 39% to 83% reduction in the absorption of iron. No decrease was observed if the coffee was drunk one hour before the meal, but when the coffee was given one hour after the meal the reduction was the same as taking it simultaneously with the meal. With one meal, the effect of coffee was about half that of tea.[1] In another study, a 275 mL serving of instant coffee reduced the absorption of radiolabelled iron from a 50 g bread roll, and this was not affected by milk.[2]

A controlled study among pregnant women in Costa Rica found that coffee consumption was associated with reductions in the haemoglobin levels and haematocrits of the mothers during pregnancy, and of their babies shortly after birth, despite the fact that the women were taking **ferric sulfate** 200 mg and 500 micrograms of folate daily. The babies also had a slightly lower birth weight (3189 g versus 3310 g). Almost a quarter of the mothers were considered to have iron-deficiency anaemia (haemoglobin levels of less than 11 g/dL), compared with none among the control group of non-coffee drinkers. Levels of iron in breast milk were reduced by about one-third. The coffee drinkers drank more than 450 mL of coffee daily, equivalent to more than 10 g of ground coffee.[3]

In a randomised study in Guatemalan infants, discontinuing coffee intake in those given an iron supplement led to a greater increase in serum ferritin than continuing coffee consumption (median 891 mL weekly). However, discontinuing coffee had no effect on changes in haemoglobin.[4]

Experimental evidence

Because of the extensive clinical evidence available, experimental data have not been sought.

Mechanism

It is suggested that polyphenolics in coffee might interfere with the absorption of iron.[4]

Importance and management

The general importance of these findings is uncertain, but be aware that coffee consumption may contribute to iron-deficiency anaemia. Note that coffee is not generally considered to be a suitable drink for babies and children, because of its effects on iron absorption. More study is needed. Consider also Tea + Iron compounds, page 467.

1. Morck TA, Lynch SR, Cook JD. Inhibition of food iron absorption by coffee. *Am J Clin Nutr* (1983) 37, 416–20.
2. Hurrell RF, Reddy M, Cook JD. Inhibition of non-haem iron absorption in man by polyphenolic-containing beverages. *Br J Nutr* (1999) 81, 289–95.
3. Muñoz LM, Lönnerdal B, Keen CL, Dewey KG. Coffee consumption as a factor in iron deficiency anemia among pregnant women and their infants in Costa Rica. *Am J Clin Nutr* (1988) 48, 645–51.
4. Dewey KG, Romero-Abal ME, Quan de, Serrano J, Bulux J, Peerson JM, Eagle P, Solomons NW. Effects of discontinuing coffee intake on iron status of iron-deficient Guatemalan toddlers: a randomized intervention study. *Am J Clin Nutr* (1997) 66, 168–76.

Coffee + Nicotine

Coffee drinking may reduce the absorption of nicotine from chewing gum.

Evidence, mechanism, importance and management

In a study in 8 otherwise healthy smokers, intermittent mouth rinsing with coffee substantially reduced salivary pH and nicotine absorption from nicotine polacrilex gum.[1] Buccal nicotine absorption is best in an alkaline environment, which is provided by the buffering agents in the nicotine gum. Consumption of coffee reduces the pH and therefore nicotine absorption.[1] The reduction in the absorption of buccal nicotine would apply only to beverages that affect buccal pH. Drinking coffee beverages during or immediately before nicotine gum use might therefore decrease the efficacy of this form of nicotine replacement therapy. See also Caffeine + Nicotine, page 112.

1. Henningfield JE, Radzius A, Cooper TM, Clayton RR. Drinking coffee and carbonated beverages blocks absorption of nicotine from nicotine polacrilex gum. *JAMA* (1990) 264, 1560–1564.

Coffee + Phenylpropanolamine

A case report describes mania in a patient who drank coffee and took phenylpropanolamine.

Evidence, mechanism, importance and management

A case report describes mania with psychotic delusions in a healthy woman (who normally drank 7 to 8 cups of coffee daily) within 3 days of her starting to take a phenylpropanolamine-containing decongestant. She recovered within one week of stopping both the coffee and the phenylpropanolamine.[1] This appears to be the only case report of an adverse interaction specifically between coffee and phenylpropanolamine. However, case reports have described other severe reactions with caffeine, see Caffeine + Phenylpropanolamine, page 113.

1. Lake CR. Manic psychosis after coffee and phenylpropanolamine. *Biol Psychiatry* (1991) 30, 401–4.

Coffee + Tetracycline

Coffee does not appear to affect the absorption of tetracycline.

Evidence, mechanism, importance and management

A study in 9 healthy subjects found that 200 mL of coffee (milk content, if any, unstated) did not significantly affect the bioavailability of a single 250-mg dose of tetracycline.[1]

Milk is well known to decrease the absorption of tetracyclines, and a study in 12 healthy subjects found that 16 mL of evaporated milk added to 200 mL of coffee still significantly reduced tetracycline absorption (by roughly half).[2] From the first study, it appears that coffee alone does not affect tetracycline absorption.

1. Jung H, Rivera O, Reguero MT, Rodrrguez JM, Moreno-Esparza R. Influence of liquids (coffee and orange juice) on the bioavailability of tetracycline. *Biopharm Drug Dispos* (1990) 11, 729–34.
2. Jung H, Peregrina AA, Rodriguez JM, Moreno-Esparza R. The influence of coffee with milk and tea with milk on the bioavailability of tetracycline. *Biopharm Drug Dispos* (1997) 18, 459–63.

Cola

Cola acuminata (P.Beauv.) Schott & Endl. or *Cola nitida* (Vent.) Schott & Endl. (Sterculiaceae)

Synonym(s) and related species

Guru nut, Kola.

Garcinia kola Heckel, *Sterculia acuminata* Beauv.

Pharmacopoeias

Cola (*BP 2012, PhEur 7.5*).

Constituents

Cola seed contains xanthine derivatives, mainly **caffeine** (1.5 to 3%) to which it may be standardised, with traces of theobromine and theophylline. Other constituents include **flavonoids** from the flavanol group (such as catechin and epicatechin), amines, an anthocyanin pigment (kola red) and betaine.

Use and indications

The main use of cola seed is as a stimulant for depression, tiredness and poor appetite, and as a diuretic. Both uses can be attributed to the caffeine content. Cola is also used as flavouring agent in the manufacture of soft drinks.

Pharmacokinetics

For the pharmacokinetics of caffeine, see caffeine, page 106. For information on the pharmacokinetics of individual flavonoids present in cola, see under flavonoids, page 213.

Interactions overview

Cola contains significant amounts of caffeine, therefore the interactions of caffeine, page 106, should be applied to cola, unless the product is specified as decaffeinated. By virtue of its caffeine content cola may also cause serious adverse effects if used with other drugs or herbs with similar effects, such as ephedra, page 202. Cola may reduce the bioavailability of halofantrine and increase the risk of developing hypertension. For information on the interactions of individual flavonoids present in cola, see under flavonoids, page 213.

Carbonated cola beverages are acidic, and they can therefore interact with drugs by altering gastric acidity. The best example of this is that they can increase the absorption of the azole antifungal drugs ketoconazole and itraconazole. However, this mechanism is not going to be applicable to herbal medicines containing cola extracts, and these interactions are not therefore covered here.

Interactions monographs

- Antihypertensives, page 166
- Food, page 166
- Halofantrine, page 166
- Herbal medicines, page 166

Cola + Antihypertensives

Cola appears to modestly increase the risk of developing hypertension.

Evidence, mechanism, importance and management

There is a possibility that the effect of cola on blood pressure might differ from that of pure caffeine. There appear to be very few published studies of the effect of cola on blood pressure; however, in the Nurses Health prospective cohort studies, both sugared cola and diet cola beverages were associated with an increased risk of developing hypertension with increased intake.[1] Whether patients taking antihypertensives should limit their intake of cola is unclear. However, the modest hypertensive effects of the caffeine content of cola may be of importance. See Caffeine + Antihypertensives, page 108, for further discussion of the adverse effect of caffeine on blood pressure.

1. Winkelmayer WC, Stampfer MJ, Willett WC, Curhan GC. Habitual caffeine intake and the risk of hypertension in women. *JAMA* (2005) 294, 233–5.

Cola + Food

No interactions found. Cola is used as a flavouring in carbonated drinks.

Note that the effects of caffeine from cola-containing herbal medicine or supplement will be additive with those of other caffeine-containing foods or beverages.

Cola + Halofantrine

Cola appears to moderately reduce the bioavailability of halofantrine.

Clinical evidence

In a study in 15 healthy subjects, a single 500-mg dose of halofantrine was given alone or with cola 12.5 g. Cola significantly reduced the maximum concentration and AUC of halofantrine by 45% and 31%, respectively. The overall clearance of halofantrine was reduced by 50%. Similar reductions were seen in the major metabolite of halofantrine, N-desbutylhalofantrine. No adverse effects were reported.[1]

Experimental evidence

No relevant data found.

Mechanism

The authors suggest that caffeine, or other constituents of cola such as catechins or tannins, may have formed a complex with halofantrine to reduce its absorption.

Importance and management

Evidence appears to be limited to this one study, which found a modest reduction in the bioavailability of halofantrine. However, the bioavailability of halofantrine can vary widely between patients. Nevertheless, as there is the potential that this interaction could lead to malaria treatment failure, it may be prudent to advise patients to avoid taking cola during treatment with halofantrine.

1. Kolade YT, Babalola CP, Olaniyi AA, Scriba GKE. Effect of kolanut on the pharmacokinetics of the antimalarial drug halofantrine. *Eur J Clin Pharmacol* (2008) 64, 77–81.

Cola + Herbal medicines

The caffeine content of cola suggests that it may interact with other herbal medicines in the same way as caffeine, see Caffeine + Herbal medicines; Bitter orange, page 111, and Ephedra + Caffeine, page 202.

Coltsfoot

Tussilago farfara L. (Asteraceae)

Synonym(s) and related species

Coughwort, Farfara, Foal's foot.

Constituents

The leaves and flowers of coltsfoot contain mucilage composed of polysaccharides, which include arabinose, fructose, galactose, glucose and xylose, and the carbohydrate inulin. **Flavonoids** (such as rutin, isoquercetin and hyperoside), polyphenolic acids, triterpenes and sterols are present, and sesquiterpenes including bisabolene derivatives and tussilagone may also be found. All parts of the plant may contain the pyrrolizidine alkaloids isotussilagine, senecionine, senkirkine and tussilagine in variable amounts. These are toxic but chemically very labile, and may be absent from some extracts.

Use and indications

Coltsfoot is traditionally used in cough and cold preparations as a demulcent and expectorant, and it is used in the treatment of asthma. Extracts have anti-inflammatory and antispasmodic activity and tussilagone alone has been found to be a cardiovascular and respiratory stimulant. The concentration of the most toxic pyrrolizidine alkaloid, senkirkine, is thought to be too low to cause toxicity if used infrequently, and tussilagine is unsaturated and therefore less toxic. However, care should be taken with prolonged use.

Pharmacokinetics

No relevant pharmacokinetic data found.

Interactions overview

No interactions with coltsfoot found.

C

Coptis

Coptis chinensis Franch. (Ranunculaceae)

Synonym(s) and related species

Gold thread, Mouth root, Vegetable gold.

Coptis deltoidea CY Cheng et Hasio, *Coptis groenlandica* (Oeder) Fernald, *Coptis teetoides* CY Cheng, *Coptis trifolia* (Salis).

Constituents

The thread-like rhizomes contain isoquinoline alkaloids, mainly **berberine** and coptisine.

Use and indications

Coptis species are used widely in Chinese medicine for infections, especially of the digestive tract, and for similar reasons as bloodroot, page 84 and berberis, page 66.

Pharmacokinetics

No relevant pharmacokinetic data found. For information on the pharmacokinetics of the alkaloid constituent, berberine, see under berberine, page 63.

Interactions overview

No interactions with coptis found. However, for the interactions of the alkaloid constituent, berberine, see under berberine, page 63.

Corn silk

Zea mays L. (Poaceae)

Synonym(s) and related species

Corn, Indian corn, Maize, Stigma maydis, Zea.

Pharmacopoeias

Corn Oil (*USP35–NF30 S1*); Maize Starch (*BP 2012, PhEur 7.5*); Refined Maize Oil (*BP 2012, PhEur 7.5*).

Constituents

The stigmas and styles contain phytosterols, including β-sitosterol and stigmasterol; the carotenoid cryptoxanthin; glycerides of linoleic, oleic, palmitic and stearic acids; **flavonoids** including maysin; **isoflavones** including genistein, and unspecified saponins and tannins.

Use and indications

Corn silk is derived from the stigmas and styles of unripe corn and is used traditionally as a diuretic and to reduce kidney and gall stones. It has also been used for a variety of urinary-tract disorders including cystitis, urethritis, nocturnal enuresis, prostatitis, and acute or chronic inflammation.

Pharmacokinetics

No relevant pharmacokinetic data found. For information on the pharmacokinetics of individual isoflavones present in corn silk, see under isoflavones, page 300.

Interactions overview

An isolated case of lithium toxicity has been reported in a patient who took a herbal diuretic containing corn silk among other ingredients, see under Parsley + Lithium, page 364. For information on the interactions of individual isoflavones present in corn silk, see under isoflavones, page 300.

Interactions monographs

- Food, page 170
- Herbal medicines, page 170

C

Corn silk + Food

No interactions found.

Corn silk + Herbal medicines

No interactions found.

Corn silk + Lithium

For mention of a case of lithium toxicity in a woman who had been taking a non-prescription herbal diuretic containing corn silk, *Equisetum hyemale,* juniper, buchu, parsley and bearberry, all of which are believed to have diuretic actions, see under Parsley + Lithium, page 364.

Cotton

Gossypium herbaceum L. (Malvaceae)

Synonym(s) and related species

Gossypium hirsutum L.

Pharmacopoeias

Cottonseed Oil, Hydrogenated (*BP 2012, Ph Eur 7.5*).

Constituents

The root bark and seed of cotton contain a fixed oil containing sesquiterpenes, the most important of these being **gossypol**. The root bark also contains 6-methoxygossypol and 6,6'-dimethoxygossypol, among others, and the seed also contains gossyfulvin and gossypurpurin.

Use and indications

Cotton root bark, cotton seed, and the oil extracted from cotton seed, have been used to induce abortion and have been tried as a male contraceptive. The root bark has also been used to treat menstrual disorders but the toxicity and teratogenicity of gossypol, the major constituent, make it unsuitable and cannot be recommended. Gossypol has been investigated for use in various diseases including the treatment of neoplastic diseases.

Pharmacokinetics

In vitro studies using liver microsomes from rats given gossypol for 5 days to 4 weeks found that cytochrome P450 activity was reduced by about 25% to 50%.[1-3] In one study, the effect of gossypol was inhibited by the con-current use of phenobarbital (a known, clinically relevant CYP3A4 inducer) and the authors suggest this could be due to increased metabolism of gossypol or prevention of its binding to microsomal membranes.[3] The clinical relevance of these findings is not clear. See under Cotton + Ethinylestradiol, page 172 and Cotton + Tolbutamide, page 172 for details of specific drug interaction studies using cytochrome P450 substrates.

Interactions overview

No clinical interactions found. However, *in vitro* and *animal* studies suggest that gossypol might reduce the metabolism of ethinylestradiol and increase its exposure, as well as inhibiting both alcohol dehydrogenase and aldehyde dehydrogenase, leading to the accumulation of alcohol.

Interactions monographs

- Alcohol, page 172
- Ethinylestradiol, page 172
- Food, page 172
- Herbal medicines, page 172
- Tolbutamide, page 172

1. Xiao-Nian M, Back DJ. Inhibition of hepatic microsomal enzymes by gossypol in the rat. *Contraception* (1984) 30, 89–97.
2. Johansen RL, Misra HP. Effects of gossypol on the hepatic drug metabolizing system in rats. *Contraception* (1990) 42, 683–90.
3. Gawai KR, Cox C, Jackson J, Dalvi RR. Changes in the activity of metabolic and non-metabolic liver enzymes in rats following co-administration of gossypol with phenobarbital. *Pharmacol Toxicol* (1995) 76, 289–91.

Cotton + Alcohol

The interaction between cotton and alcohol is based on experimental evidence only.

Evidence, mechanism, importance and management

Two *animal* studies, found that a single dose of gossypol, the major constituent of cotton root bark and cotton seed oil, inhibited alcohol dehydrogenase and aldehyde dehydrogenase, which the authors suggested could lead to accumulation of alcohol and necessitates the contraindication of gossypol with alcoholic beverages.[1,2]

The results of *animal* studies are difficult to reliably extrapolate to humans but given the increase in alcohol levels it may be prudent to heed this advice and avoid the concurrent use of products containing gossypol with alcoholic beverages.

1. Messiha FS. Effect of gossypol on kinetics of mouse liver alcohol and aldehyde dehydrogenase. *Gen Pharmacol* (1991) 22, 573–6.
2. Messiha FS. Behavioural and metabolic interaction between gossypol and ethanol. *Toxicol Lett* (1991) 57, 175–81.

Cotton + Ethinylestradiol

The interaction between cotton and ethinylestradiol is based on experimental evidence only.

Evidence, mechanism, importance and management

An *in vitro* study using *rat* liver microsomes, found that gossypol, the major constituent of cotton root bark and cotton seed oil, reduced the metabolism of ethinylestradiol to its main metabolite 2-hydroxyethinylestradiol by 82%.[1] Ethinylestradiol is metabolised by CYP3A4 and gossypol has been shown to reduce cytochrome P450 activity *in vitro*; so it is possible that gossypol is acting as a CYP3A4 inhibitor.

The results of *in vitro* studies are difficult to reliably extrapolate to humans and the use of gossypol is not recommended due to its abortifacient and teratogenic properties (see under *Use and indications*, page 171). Nevertheless, the concurrent use of gossypol and ethinylestradiol could potentially lead to increased ethinylestradiol

exposure and the possibility of an increased risk of adverse effects, such as nausea and breast tenderness. Bearing in mind the additional toxicity of gossypol, concurrent use of cotton products containing gossypol and ethinylestradiol should be avoided.

1. M Xiao-Nian, Back DJ. Inhibition of hepatic microsomal enzymes by gossypol in the rat. *Contraception* (1984) 30, 89–97.

Cotton + Food

No interactions found.

Cotton + Herbal medicines

No interactions found.

Cotton + Tolbutamide

The interaction between cotton and tolbutamide is based on experimental evidence only.

Evidence, mechanism, importance and management

An *in vivo* study in *rats* given gossypol, the major constituent of cotton root bark and cotton seed oil, as a single dose or daily for 2 weeks, found that the metabolism of tolbutamide was not altered when compared with controls.[1] Tolbutamide is metabolised by CYP2C9 and although gossypol has been shown to reduce cytochrome P450 activity *in vitro,* it seems unlikely that gossypol affects the isoenzyme CYP2C9. Although gossypol does not appear to affect the pharmacokinetics of tolbutamide, the use of gossypol is not recommended due to its toxicity and teratogenic properties (see under *Use and indications*, page 171).

1. M Xiao-Nian, Back DJ. Inhibition of hepatic microsomal enzymes by gossypol in the rat. *Contraception* (1984) 30, 89–97.

Cowslip

Primula veris L. (Primulaceae)

Synonym(s) and related species

Paigle, Peagle, Primula.

Primula officinalis Hill.

Oxlip (*Primula elatior* Hill) is a related species that can be substituted for *Primula veris* in some pharmacopoeial Primula root preparations. Primrose (*Primula vulgaris* Huds.) is also a related species and has been used in the same way as cowslip. Note that Primrose should not be confused with Evening primrose oil, page 206 (*Oenothera biennis*).

Pharmacopoeias

Primula Root (*BP 2012, PhEur 7.5*).

Constituents

The flowers and roots of cowslip contain the **flavonoids** apigenin, gossypetin, isorhamnetin, kaempferol, luteolin, quercetin, and a number of methoxylated flavones. Carbohydrates based on arabinose, galactose, galacturonic acid, glucose, rhamnose and xylose, and other polyphenolic compounds such as proanthocyanidin B2, epicatechin, epigallocatechin are also present.

A range of saponin glycosides based on the primulagenins are found in the root, such as primulaveroside (primulaverin) and primveroside, and although primula acid has been found in the sepals, saponins are otherwise absent from the flower. Primin and other quinones have also been isolated from cowslip.

Use and indications

Cowslip extracts are used in cough and cold preparations, and as a mild sedative. The saponins have been reported to have anti-inflammatory properties and to act as an expectorant. The flavonoids have been reported to have anti-inflammatory and antispasmodic properties. Primin is the cause of primula contact dermatitis, an allergic reaction caused by cowslip and other species.

Pharmacokinetics

No relevant pharmacokinetic data found. For information on the pharmacokinetics of individual flavonoids present in cowslip, see under flavonoids, page 213.

Interactions overview

No interactions with cowslip found. For information on the interactions of individual flavonoids present in cowslip see under flavonoids, page 213.

Cramp bark

Viburnum opulus L. (Caprifoliaceae)

Synonym(s) and related species

Guelder rose, Snowball tree.

Constituents

The chemistry of cramp bark is not well known. The bark reportedly contains hydroquinones including arbutin and methylarbutin; **natural coumarins** such as scopoletin and aesculetin (esculetin); triterpenes including oleanolic and ursolic acid derivatives; iridoid glycosides; and **flavonoids** based on kaempferol such as astragalin and paeonoside, and catechins.

Use and indications

Traditionally cramp bark has been used as a uterine tonic for menstrual cramps, preventing miscarriages and internal haemorrhages. The safety in pregnancy has not been established and there is little evidence to support its efficacy.

Pharmacokinetics

No relevant pharmacokinetic data found. For information on the pharmacokinetics of individual flavonoids and natural coumarins present in cramp bark, see under flavonoids, page 213 and natural coumarins, page 356, respectively.

Interactions overview

No interactions with cramp bark found. For information on the interactions of individual flavonoids present in cramp bark, see under flavonoids, page 213. Although cramp bark contains natural coumarins, the quantity of these constituents is not established, and therefore the propensity of cramp bark to interact with other drugs because of their presence is unclear. Consider natural coumarins, page 356, for further discussion of the interactions of natural coumarin-containing herbs.

Cranberry

Vaccinium macrocarpon Aiton (Ericaceae)

Synonym(s) and related species

Large cranberry (*Vaccinium macrocarpon*) is the cultivated species. European cranberry or Mossberry (*Vaccinium oxycoccus*) has also been used.

Pharmacopoeias

Cranberry Liquid Preparation (*USP35–NF30 S1*).

Constituents

The berries contain anthocyanins and proanthocyanidins (mainly oligomers of epicatechin), and organic acids including malic, citric, quinic and benzoic acids.

Note that, although salicylic acid does not appear as a constituent of the juice in many cranberry monographs, some studies have shown low levels of salicylates in commercial cranberry juice (e.g. 7 mg/L), which resulted in detectable plasma and urine levels of salicylic acid in women who drank 250 mL of cranberry juice three times daily.[1]

Use and indications

The main use of cranberries and cranberry juice is for the prevention and treatment of urinary tract infections, although they have also been used for blood and digestive disorders. Cranberries are commonly used in food and beverages.

Pharmacokinetics

There is high absorption and excretion of cranberry anthocyanins in human urine, as shown by a study where 11 healthy subjects drank 200 mL of cranberry juice containing 651 micrograms of total anthocyanins. The urinary levels of anthocyanins reached a maximum between 3 and 6 hours, and the recovery of total anthocyanins in the urine over 24 hours was estimated to be 5% of the amount consumed.[2]

Some *in vitro* and *animal* studies have suggested that cranberry may affect the cytochrome P450 isoenzymes CYP2C9 (see flurbiprofen, page 176,) and CYP3A4 (see nifedipine, page 176). However, clinical studies with tizanidine, page 177, (a substrate of CYP1A2), flurbiprofen, page 176, (a substrate of CYP2C9), and midazolam, page 176, (a substrate of CYP3A4) have found no evidence of a significant interaction in humans.

Interactions overview

Clinical studies suggest that cranberry juice and/or extracts do not affect the pharmacokinetics of ciclosporin, flurbiprofen, midazolam, tizanidine and warfarin. Despite this, there have been some case reports of raised INRs and significant bleeding with cranberry and warfarin. Cranberry juice is unlikely to affect the pharmacokinetics of nifedipine to a clinically relevant extent.

Interactions monographs

- Ciclosporin, page 176
- Flurbiprofen, page 176
- Food, page 176
- Herbal medicines, page 176
- Midazolam, page 176
- Nifedipine, page 176
- Tizanidine, page 177
- Warfarin and related drugs, page 177

1. Duthie GG, Kyle JA, Jenkinson AM. Increased salicylate concentrations in urine of human volunteers after consumption of cranberry juice. *J Agric Food Chem* (2005) 53, 2897–2900.
2. Ohnishi R, Ito H, Kasajima N, Kaneda M, Kariyama R, Kumon H, Hatano T, Yoshida T. Urinary excretion of anthocyanins in humans after cranberry juice ingestion. *Biosci Biotechnol Biochem* (2006) 70, 1681–7.

C

Cranberry + Ciclosporin

Occasional consumption of cranberry juice does not appear to affect the bioavailability of ciclosporin. Regular daily consumption has not been studied.

Evidence, mechanism, importance and management

In a well-controlled, single-dose study, 12 healthy fasted subjects were given a 200-mg dose of oral ciclosporin simultaneously with 240 mL of cranberry juice or water. Cranberry juice was found to have no clinically significant effect on the pharmacokinetics of ciclosporin.[1] In this study, the cranberry juice used was reconstituted from frozen concentrate (*Ocean Spray*).

This study suggests that cranberry juice does not affect the absorption of ciclosporin, and that drinking the occasional glass of cranberry juice with ciclosporin should not affect ciclosporin levels. However, note that a study of regular daily cranberry juice consumption is required to also rule out an interaction affecting ciclosporin elimination, which may have a bearing on the safety of regular (e.g. daily) intake of cranberry juice with ciclosporin.

1. Grenier J, Fradette C, Morelli G, Merritt GJ, Vranderick M, Ducharme MP. Pomelo juice, but not cranberry juice, affects the pharmacokinetics of cyclosporine in humans. *Clin Pharmacol Ther* (2006) 79, 255–62.

Cranberry + Flurbiprofen

Limited evidence suggests that cranberry juice does not appear to affect the pharmacokinetics of flurbiprofen.

Clinical evidence

In a study in 14 healthy subjects, 230 mL of cranberry juice taken the night before, and 30 minutes before a single 100-mg dose of flurbiprofen, had no significant effect on the pharmacokinetics of flurbiprofen. Fluconazole, used as a positive control, increased the flurbiprofen AUC by about 80%.[1] In this study, the cranberry juice used was *Ocean Spray* cranberry juice cocktail from concentrate containing 27% cranberry juice.

Experimental evidence

In an *in vitro* study, cranberry juice inhibited flurbiprofen hydroxylation by about 44%, which was less than that of the positive control sulfaphenazole (79%).[1]

Mechanism

Flurbiprofen is metabolised by the cytochrome P450 isoenzyme CYP2C9, and the clinical study appears to suggest that cranberry has no clinically relevant effect on this particular isoenzyme, despite the fact that it had some weak inhibitory effects *in vitro*.[1]

Importance and management

Both the study in humans and the supporting experimental metabolic data suggest that no pharmacokinetic interaction occurs between flurbiprofen and cranberry juice. Therefore no dosage adjustment appears to be necessary if patients taking flurbiprofen wish to drink cranberry juice.

Flurbiprofen is used as a probe drug for CYP2C9 activity, and therefore these results also suggest that a pharmacokinetic interaction as a result of this mechanism between cranberry juice and other CYP2C9 substrates is unlikely.

1. Greenblatt DJ, von Moltke LL, Perloff ES, Luo Y, Harmatz JS, Zinny MA. Interaction of flurbiprofen with cranberry juice, grape juice, tea, and fluconazole: in vitro and clinical studies. *Clin Pharmacol Ther* (2006) 79, 125–33.

Cranberry + Food

No interactions found. Note that cranberry juice is widely used in food and beverages.

Cranberry + Herbal medicines

No interactions found.

Cranberry + Midazolam

Limited evidence suggests that cranberry juice does not appear to affect the pharmacokinetics of midazolam.

Clinical evidence

In a randomised, crossover study in 10 healthy subjects, 200 mL of cranberry juice three times daily for 10 days had no significant effect on the pharmacokinetics of a single 500-microgram oral dose of midazolam taken on day 5. In this study, the cranberry juice used was a concentrate (*Kontiomehu sokeroitu karpalomehu*) diluted 1 to 4 with tap water before use.[1]

Experimental evidence

No relevant data found.

Mechanism

This study suggests that cranberry juice has no clinically relevant effect on CYP3A4 activity.

Importance and management

Although the evidence is limited to this particular study, there appears to be no need for special precautions when taking cranberry juice with midazolam.

Midazolam is used as a probe drug for CYP3A4 activity, and therefore these results also suggest that a pharmacokinetic interaction between cranberry juice and other CYP3A4 substrates is unlikely.

1. Lilja JJ, Backman JT, Neuvonen PJ. Effects of daily ingestion of cranberry juice on the pharmacokinetics of warfarin, tizanidine, and midazolam - probes of CYP2C9, CYP1A2, and CYP3A4. *Clin Pharmacol Ther* (2007) 81, 833–9.

Cranberry + Nifedipine

The interaction between cranberry juice and nifedipine is based on experimental evidence only.

Clinical evidence

No interactions found.

Experimental evidence

In a study in human liver microsomes and *rat* intestinal microsomes, cranberry juice slightly decreased the cytochrome P450 isoenzyme CYP3A4-mediated metabolism of nifedipine by around 12% to 18%. Similarly, intraduodenal administration of cranberry juice to *rats* appeared to reduce the apparent clearance and increase the AUC of nifedipine 30 mg/kg by 44% and 60%, respectively, when compared with a control group. However, other pharmacokinetic parameters such as the mean residence time, volume of distribution, and elimination rate constant were not significantly affected.[1]

Mechanism

The experimental evidence suggests that cranberry juice may slightly inhibit the cytochrome P450 isoenzyme CYP3A4 *in vitro* and in *rats*.[1] However, note that in a clinical study, cranberry had no effect on a single dose of midazolam, page 176, a well established probe CYP3A4 substrate.

Importance and management

Evidence appears to be limited to two experimental studies. Taken on its own, this evidence suggests the possibility of a modest interaction, and therefore some caution might be warranted in patients taking nifedipine who drink cranberry juice. However, a clinical study with midazolam, page 176, a sensitive, specific substrate for CYP3A4, found no evidence of an interaction, and this suggests that cranberry juice would be unlikely to affect the pharmacokinetics of nifedipine to a clinically relevant extent.

1. Uesawa Y, Mohri K. Effects of cranberry juice on nifedipine pharmacokinetics in rats. *J Pharm Pharmacol* (2006) 58, 1067–72.

Cranberry + Tizanidine

Limited evidence suggests that cranberry juice does not appear to affect the pharmacokinetics of tizanidine.

Clinical evidence

In a randomised, crossover study in 10 healthy subjects 200 mL of cranberry juice three times daily for 10 days had no significant effect on the pharmacokinetics of a single 1-mg oral dose of tizanidine taken on day 5. In this study, the cranberry juice used was a concentrate (*Kontiomehu sokeroitu karpalomehu*) diluted 1 to 4 with tap water before use.[1]

Experimental evidence

No relevant data found.

Mechanism

This study suggests that cranberry juice has no clinically relevant effect on CYP1A2 activity.

Importance and management

Although the evidence is limited to this particular study, there appears to be no need for any special precautions when taking cranberry juice with tizanidine.

Tizanidine is used as a probe drug for CYP1A2 activity, and therefore these results also suggest that a pharmacokinetic interaction between cranberry juice and other CYP1A2 substrates is unlikely.

1. Lilja JJ, Backman JT, Neuvonen PJ. Effects of daily ingestion of cranberry juice on the pharmacokinetics of warfarin, tizanidine, and midazolam - probes of CYP2C9, CYP1A2, and CYP3A4. *Clin Pharmacol Ther* (2007) 81, 833–9.

Cranberry + Warfarin and related drugs

A number of case reports suggest that cranberry juice can increase the INR of patients taking warfarin, and one patient has died as a result of this interaction. Other patients have developed unstable INRs, or, in one isolated case, a *reduced* INR. However, in four controlled studies, cranberry juice did not alter the anticoagulant effect of warfarin, or had only very minor effects on the INR. Neither cranberry juice nor the extract altered warfarin pharmacokinetics.

Clinical evidence

(a) Case reports

In September 2003, the MHRA/CSM in the UK noted that they had received 5 reports suggesting an interaction between warfarin and cranberry juice since 1999 (3 cases of INR increases, one case of unstable INR and one case of a decrease in INR).[1] By October 2004, the MHRA/CSM reported that they had now received 12 reports of a suspected interaction, including 5 additional cases of bleeding episodes and two additional cases of unstable INRs in patients drinking cranberry juice while taking warfarin.[2] The most serious case involved a man taking **warfarin** whose INR markedly increased (INR greater than 50) 6 weeks after starting to drink cranberry juice. He died from gastrointestinal and pericardial haemorrhages.[1,3] Further details of this case included that he had recently been treated with cefalexin (not known to interact) for a chest infection, and had been eating virtually nothing for at least 2 weeks,[3] a fact that would have contributed to the increase in anticoagulation.

In a further published case report, a patient stabilised on warfarin was found to have INRs of 10 to 12 in the surgical procedure, although he had no previous record of an INR greater than 4. Vitamin K was given, and heparin was substituted for warfarin. When warfarin was restarted postoperatively, the INR quickly rose to 8 and then to 11 with haematuria, and postoperative bleeding. The patient was drinking almost 2 litres of cranberry juice daily, because of recurrent urinary tract infections, and was advised to stop drinking this. Three days later the INR had stabilised at 3 with no further intervention.[4] Another case of fluctuating INR (between 1 and 10) in a patient taking warfarin has been attributed to cranberry juice.[5]

In the US, a case of major bleeding and a high INR has been reported in a man taking warfarin, which occurred shortly after cranberry juice 710 mL daily was started.[6] Another case, describes an increase in the INR of a patient receiving warfarin, from below 3 to 6.45, without bleeding, after the patient drank about 2 litres of cranberry/apple juice over the last week. Of note, the patient was subsequently re-stabilised on a lower dose of warfarin and may have taken an extra dose of warfarin in the week before the raised INR was measured.[7]

(b) Controlled studies

In one controlled crossover study, 7 male patients with atrial fibrillation who were taking stable doses of **warfarin** drank 250 mL of cranberry juice or placebo [daily] for a week without any significant change in their INR from baseline values.[8] The same finding was reported in another very similar study in patients taking **warfarin**.[9] However, note that the daily volume of cranberry juice in these studies was lower than the daily volume in the couple of case reports where cranberry juice intake is known. Nevertheless, in another controlled study in 10 healthy subjects, a higher volume of cranberry juice (200 mL three times daily) for 10 days did not alter the effect of a single 10-mg dose of **warfarin** (given on day 5) on the maximum thromboplastin time or AUC of the thromboplastin time.[10] In addition, cranberry juice had no effect on warfarin pharmacokinetics, except that there was a slight non-significant 7% *decrease* in the AUC of *S*-warfarin.

In yet another study in 12 healthy subjects, cranberry juice concentrate 2 capsules three times daily for 21 days (equivalent to 57 g of fruit daily)had no effect on the maximum INR after a single 25-mg dose of **warfarin** given on day 15 (2.8 versus 2.6). However, the AUC of the INR was slightly increased by 28%, which was statistically significant, but the clinical relevance of this measure is uncertain. The cranberry concentrate had no effect on platelet aggregation, and had no effect on the pharmacokinetics of either *R*- or *S*-warfarin.[11]

Experimental evidence

Because of the quality of the clinical evidence (controlled pharmacokinetic studies), experimental data have not been sought.

Mechanism

Not known. It was originally suggested that one or more of the constituents of cranberry juice might inhibit the metabolism of warfarin by the cytochrome P450 isoenzyme CYP2C9, thereby reducing its clearance from the body and increasing its effects.[1] However, four studies have shown that cranberry juice or cranberry extracts do not alter the pharmacokinetics of warfarin, and cranberry juice had no effect on flurbiprofen pharmacokinetics, a drug used as a surrogate index of CYP2C9 activity.[12] See also flurbiprofen, page 176. An interaction might therefore be via a pharmacodynamic mechanism. For example, the salicylate constituent of commercial cranberry juice might cause hypoprothrombinaemia.[13]

Importance and management

An interaction is not established. Controlled studies have not found a pharmacokinetic interaction, and only one of four studies found any evidence for an increase in warfarin effect. Moreover, the clinical relevance of the finding of this study of a 0.2 increase in INR and 28% increase in AUC of the INR is likely to be slight at most, and does not fit with the sometimes marked increase in INR seen in some case reports. This might be explained if the interaction is dose dependent (in one of the cases where cranberry intake was mentioned a quantity of 2 litres daily was being consumed), or if it is product dependent (i.e. due to a constituent present in the cranberry juice that is not standardised for and varies widely). However, it could also be that there is no specific interaction, and that the case reports just represent idiosyncratic reactions in which other unknown factors (e.g. altered diet) were more important.

In 2004, on the basis of the then available case reports and lack of controlled studies, the CSM/MHRA in the UK advised that patients taking warfarin should avoid drinking cranberry juice unless the health benefits are considered to outweigh any risks. They recommended increased INR monitoring for any patient taking warfarin and who has a regular intake of cranberry juice.[2] They also advised similar precautions with other cranberry products (such as capsules or concentrates).[2] These might still be prudent precautions, although the controlled studies now available do provide some reassurance that, in otherwise healthy individuals, moderate doses of cranberry juice are unlikely to have an important impact on anticoagulation control.

1. Committee on Safety of Medicines/Medicines and Healthcare products Regulatory Agency Possible interaction between warfarin and cranberry juice. *Current Problems* (2003) 29, 8.
2. Committee on Safety of Medicines/Medicines and Healthcare products Regulatory Agency Interaction between warfarin and cranberry juice: new advice. *Current Problems* (2004) 30, 10.
3. Suvarna R, Pirmohamed M, Henderson L. Possible interaction between warfarin and cranberry juice. *BMJ* (2003) 327, 1454.
4. Grant P. Warfarin and cranberry juice: an interaction? *J Heart Valve Dis* (2004) 13, 25–6.
5. Walsh KM. Getting to yes. *J Am Geriatr Soc* (2005) 53, 1072.
6. Rindone JP, Murphy TW. Warfarin-cranberry juice interaction resulting in profound hypoprothrombinemia and bleeding. *Am J Ther* (2006) 13, 283–4.
7. Paeng CH, Sprague M, Jackevicius CA. Interaction between warfarin and cranberry juice. *Clin Ther* (2007) 29, 1730–1735.
8. Li Z, Seeram NP, Carpenter CL, Thames G, Minutti C, Bowerman S. Cranberry does not affect prothrombin time in male subjects on warfarin. *J Am Diet Assoc* (2006) 106, 2057–61.
9. Ansell J, McDonough M, Jarmatz JS, Greenblatt DJ. A randomized, double-blind trial of the interaction between cranberry juice and warfarin. *J Thromb Thrombolysis* (2008) 25, 112.
10. Lilja JJ, Backman JT, Neuvonen PJ. Effects of daily ingestion of cranberry juice on the pharmacokinetics of warfarin, tizanidine, and midazolam – probes of CYP2C9, CYP1A2, and CYP3A4. *Clin Pharmacol Ther* (2007) 81, 833–9.
11. Mohammed Abdul MI, Jiang X, Williams KM, Day RO, Roufogalis BD, Liauw WS, Xu H, McLachlan AJ. Pharmacodynamic interaction of warfarin with cranberry but not with garlic in healthy subjects. *Br J Pharmacol* (2008) 154, 1691–1700.
12. Greenblatt DJ, von Moltke LL, Perloff ES, Luo Y, Harmatz JS, Zinny MA. Interaction of flurbiprofen with cranberry juice, grape juice, tea, and fluconazole: in vitro and clinical studies. *Clin Pharmacol Ther* (2006) 79, 125–33.
13. Isele H. Tödliche Blutung unter Warfarin plus Preiselbeersaft. Liegt's an der Salizylsäure? *MMW Fortschr Med* (2004) 146, 13.

Creatine

N-(Aminoiminomethyl)-*N*-methylglycine

Types, sources and related compounds

Creatine monohydrate. Creatine phosphate is also used.

Use and indications

Creatine supplements are taken most often to improve exercise performance and increase muscle mass. They are also used for the treatment of cardiac disorders and have possible uses for motor neurone disease, muscular dystrophies, Huntington disease, and Parkinson's disease.

Creatine is found in foods, most abundantly in meat and fish, and is also synthesised endogenously.

Excessive intake of creatine, by the use of supplements, has, very rarely, been reported to cause acute renal impairment.[1]

Pharmacokinetics

Creatine is distributed throughout the body, with the majority being found in skeletal muscle. Creatine is degraded to creatinine, and both creatine and creatinine are excreted via the kidneys. Absorption of creatine is likely to be an active process, and may follow nonlinear kinetics with the ingestion of high doses because of saturation of skeletal muscle stores, although this has not been confirmed experimentally. The maximum plasma level of creatine is reached less than 2 hours after the ingestion of doses of under 10 g, but after more than 3 hours for doses over 10 g, and may vary with the ingestion of carbohydrate, see food, page 180. Clearance of creatine would appear to be dependent on both skeletal muscle and renal function.[2]

Interactions overview

There are no established interactions with creatine, but there is some evidence that caffeine might counteract its beneficial effects, and a high carbohydrate intake might increase its retention. There is an isolated report of stroke in a patient taking a creatine supplement with caffeine plus ephedra, although the role of creatine in this case is uncertain. There is a possibility that creatine supplements might complicate interpretation of serum creatinine measurement.

Interactions monographs

- Caffeine, page 180
- Food, page 180
- Herbal medicines; Ephedra with Caffeine, page 180
- Laboratory tests; Serum creatinine, page 180

1. Yoshizumi WM, Tsourounis C. Effects of creatine supplementation on renal function. *J Herb Pharmacother* (2004) 4, 1–7.
2. Persky AM, Brazeau GA, Hochhaus G. Pharmacokinetics of the dietary supplement creatine. *Clin Pharmacokinet* (2003) 42, 557–74.

C

Creatine + Caffeine

Limited evidence suggests that the performance-enhancing effects of creatine may be reduced by caffeine.

Clinical evidence

Nine healthy subjects given a creatine supplement 500 mg/kg daily for 6 days and caffeine capsules 5 mg/kg daily for 3 days beginning on the fourth day, experienced a lack of performance-enhancing effects of creatine during knee extension exercises, when compared with creatine given alone. One subject experienced some gastrointestinal discomfort during concurrent use.[1]

These findings were replicated in a later study in 9 healthy subjects. Caffeine 5 mg/kg reduced phosphocreatine resynthesis during rest from a period of exercise when given with creatine 25 g daily for 2 or 5 days.[2]

Experimental evidence

No relevant data found.

Mechanism

Caffeine appears to inhibit the resynthesis of endogenous phosphocreatine during recovery from a period of strenuous exercise, which in turn, delays the formation of the energy source, ATP.

Importance and management

These studies are preliminary and there seem to be no further reports of an interaction. However, those taking creatine supplements to enhance exercise performance should perhaps reduce caffeine intake from beverages and other sources. Note that caffeine is also present in a number of herbal medicines, consider also caffeine-containing herbs, page 106.

1. Vandenberghe K, Gillis N, van Leemputte M, van Hecke P, Vanstapel F, Hespel P. Caffeine counteracts the ergogenic action of muscle creatine loading. *J Appl Physiol* (1996) 80, 452–7.
2. Vandenberghe K, van Hecke P, van Leemputte M, Vanstapel F, Hespel P. Inhibition of muscle phosphocreatine resynthesis by caffeine after creatine loading. *Med Sci Sports Exerc* (1997) 29, 249.

Creatine + Food

Limited evidence suggests that a high carbohydrate intake may increase creatine retention.

Clinical evidence

In a study, 22 healthy male subjects were given 5 g creatine alone, or with 500 mL *Lucozade* (which provided a source of glucose and simple sugars) every 4 to 5 hours, giving a total dose of creatine of 20 g daily for 2 days. Subjects who received creatine alone continued their normal diet, whereas those receiving creatine with *Lucozade* received a high-carbohydrate diet. The peak plasma concentration and AUC of creatine was higher in those who had not received the glucose load (as *Lucozade*), but this group also demonstrated the highest urinary creatine excretion.[1] In a similar study, the effect of about 50 g of protein plus 50 g of carbohydrate on the retention of creatine from supplements was similar to that of high carbohydrate (100 g carbohydrate).[2]

Experimental evidence

No relevant data found.

Mechanism

The authors suggested that their findings indicate that the ingestion of carbohydrate with creatine led to an increase in insulin secretion, resulting in an increased uptake of creatine by skeletal muscle,[1] and that protein/carbohydrate might have a similar effect.[2]

Importance and management

These studies suggest that patients who are taking creatine to improve their muscle creatine stores might experience better results if the creatine is taken at the same time as high amounts of carbohydrates or protein/carbohydrates. However, this requires further study.

1. Green AL, Simpson EJ, Littlewood JJ, Macdonald IA, Greenhaff PL. Carbohydrate ingestion augments creatine retention during creatine feeding in humans. *Acta Physiol Scand* (1996) 158, 195–202.
2. Steenge GR, Simpson EJ, Greenhaff PL. Protein- and carbohydrate-induced augmentation of whole body creatine retention in humans. *J Appl Physiol* (2000) 89, 1165–71.

Creatine + Herbal medicines; Ephedra with Caffeine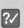

There is an isolated report of stroke in a patient taking a creatine supplement with ephedra plus caffeine, although the role of creatine in this case is uncertain.

Evidence, mechanism, importance and management

A 33-year-old fit man with no vascular risk factors had a stroke 6 weeks after starting to take two supplements to aid body building. The first contained ephedra alkaloids (from ma huang), caffeine, L-carnitine (levocarnitine), and chromium, and the second contained creatine, taurine, inosine and coenzyme Q_{10}. His daily consumption was estimated to be 40 to 60 mg of ephedra alkaloids, 400 to 600 mg of caffeine and 6 g of creatine.[1] Note that serious adverse events such as stroke have been reported with caffeine and dietary supplements containing ephedra alkaloids, and ephedra is banned in some countries. See Ephedra + Caffeine, page 202. Therefore, this case could be attributed to this supplement alone, and the role of creatine is unclear.

Note that caffeine might counteract some beneficial effects of creatine. Consider caffeine, above.

1. Vahedi K, Domigo V, Amarenco P, Bousser M-G. Ischaemic stroke in a sportsman who consumed MaHuang extract and creatine monohydrate for body building. *J Neurol Neurosurg Psychiatry* (2000) 68, 112–13.

Creatine + Laboratory tests

There is a possibility that creatine supplements might complicate the interpretation of serum creatinine measurement.

Evidence, mechanism, importance and management

Creatinine is produced in muscles from the breakdown of creatine, and is excreted by the kidneys. Blood levels of creatinine are therefore used as one measure to estimate renal function.

It is possible that dietary supplementation with creatine could lead to increased serum levels of creatinine, and this might be particularly so in patients with impaired renal function and with long-term use.[1] Note that, it has been suggested that the long-term, high-dose use of creatine supplements might actually contribute to worsening renal function,[1] although further study is needed to establish this.

It would be sensible for individuals taking creatine supplements to tell their health provider this fact, if they need to have renal function tests.

1. Yoshizumi WM, Tsourounis C. Effects of creatine supplementation on renal function. *J Herb Pharmacother* (2004) 4, 1–7.

C

Damiana

Turnera diffusa Willd. ex Schult. (Turneraceae)

Synonym(s) and related species

Turnera aphrodisiaca Ward, *Turnera diffusa* var *aphrodisiaca* (Ward) Urb, *Turnera microphylla*.

Constituents

Damiana leaves contain **flavonoids** including trimethoxy-flavone derivatives. The hydroquinone arbutin, a cyanogenetic glycoside tetraphylline B, and the phytosterol β-sitosterol have also been reported. The volatile oil contains, among other components, α- and β-pinene, thymol, α-copaene, δ-cadinene and calamene.

Use and indications

Damiana is used most often as an aphrodisiac, but, although there are some *animal* studies, there is no clinical evidence to support this use. It is also reported to be mildly sedative and antidepressant.

Pharmacokinetics

No relevant pharmacokinetic data found.

Interactions overview

No interactions with damiana found.

Dandelion

Taraxacum officinale F.H.Wigg. (Asteraceae)

Synonym(s) and related species

Lion's tooth, Taraxacum.

Leontodon taraxacum L., *Taraxacum dens-leonis* Desf., *Taraxacum palustre* (Lyons) Lam & DC. *Taraxacum mongolicum* Hand.–Mazz. is used in Chinese medicine.

Pharmacopoeias

Dandelion Herb with Root (*BP 2012, PhEur 7.5*); Dandelion Root (*BP 2012, PhEur 7.5*).

Constituents

The root and leaf of dandelion contain sesquiterpene lactones including taraxinic acid, dihydrotaraxinic acid, taraxacoside, taraxacolide and others; caffeic, chlorogenic and cichoric acids; the natural coumarins cichoriin and aesculin; and **flavonoids** based on luteolin. The phytosterols sitosterol, stigmas terol, taraxasterol and homotaraxasterol; the triterpenes β-amyrin, taraxol and taraxerol; carotenoids, and vitamin A are also found.

Use and indications

Dandelion has been widely used as a diuretic, and also for its purported laxative, anti-inflammatory, choleretic (to increase bile secretion) and blood-glucose-lowering activity. Some of these activities have been demonstrated in some, but not all, *animal* studies, and no human studies appear to have been published.[1] Dandelion has been used as a foodstuff (the leaf in salads, and the ground root as a coffee substitute). A prebiotic effect has been suggested for the root.

Pharmacokinetics

In a study in *rats* pre-treated for 4 weeks with a dandelion tea solution 2%, the solution inhibited the cytochrome P450 isoenzymes CYP1A2 and CYP2E by 85% and 52%, respectively, when compared with a control group, but did not change CYP2D and CYP3A activity. An increase in UDP-glucuronyl transferase activity of 244% was also reported in the *rats* given dandelion tea.[2] The findings of *animal* studies cannot be directly extrapolated to humans, but positive findings such as these suggest that clinical studies are required. For information on the pharmacokinetics of individual flavonoids present in dandelion, see under flavonoids, page 213.

Interactions overview

No interactions specific to dandelion, although there is limited evidence from *animals* that *Taraxacum mongolicum* (the species used in Chinese medicine) might alter the absorption of ciprofloxacin. For information on the interactions of individual flavonoids present in dandelion, see under flavonoids, page 213.

Interactions monographs

- Ciprofloxacin, page 183
- Food, page 183
- Herbal medicines, page 183

1. Schütz K, Carle R, Schieber A. *Taraxacum* – A review on its phytochemical and pharmacological profile. *J Ethnopharmacol* (2006) 107, 313–23.
2. Maliakal PP, Wanwimolruk S. Effect of herbal teas on hepatic drug metabolizing enzymes in rats. *J Pharm Pharmacol* (2001) 53, 1323–9.

Dandelion + Ciprofloxacin

The interaction between *Taraxacum mongolicum* and ciprofloxacin is based on experimental evidence only.

Clinical evidence

No interactions found.

Experimental evidence

In a study in *rats*, an aqueous extract of *Taraxacum mongolicum* (2 g crude drug/kg) significantly reduced the maximum concentration of a single 20-mg/kg oral dose of ciprofloxacin by 73% when compared with administration of oral ciprofloxacin alone. The overall tissue distribution and half-life were also increased, although the AUC was not different. The *Taraxacum mongolicum* extract used was analysed and found to have a high concentration of magnesium, calcium and iron.[1]

Mechanism

Cations such as magnesium, calcium, and iron are known to chelate with ciprofloxacin and modestly reduce its overall absorption. However, in this study, the overall absorption of ciprofloxacin was unchanged. The reason for the reduced maximum level and prolonged elimination half-life is uncertain.

Importance and management

The general significance of this *animal* study is unclear, especially as the overall absorption of ciprofloxacin did not appear to be affected. Further study is required to discover if, and under what circumstances, dandelion might interact with ciprofloxacin in clinical use. Also, study is needed to see whether the effects of the dandelion species used in this study (*Taraxacum mongolicum*) apply to *Taraxacum officinalis*.

1. Zhu M, Wong PY, Li RC. Effects of *Taraxacum mongolicum* on the bioavailability and disposition of ciprofloxacin in rats. *J Pharm Sci* (1999) 88, 632–4.

Dandelion + Food

No interactions found.

Dandelion + Herbal medicines

No interactions found.

Danshen

Salvia miltiorrhiza Bunge (Lamiaceae)

Synonym(s) and related species

Chinese salvia, Dan-Shen, Red root sage, Tan-Shen.

Constituents

Danshen products may be standardised according to the content of tanshinones (diterpene quinones), tanshinone IIA and tanshinone IIB; the polyphenolic acid, salvianolic acid B; and the related compound danshensu (3,4-dihydroxyphenyllactic acid). Other constituents include fatty-acid (oleoyl) derivatives, lithospermic acid B, and salvinal (a benzofuran) and nitrogen-containing compounds such as salvianen.

Use and indications

The dried root of danshen is traditionally used in Chinese medicine for cardiovascular and cerebrovascular diseases, specifically angina pectoris, hyperlipidaemia, and acute ischaemic stroke, but also palpitations, hypertension, thrombosis and menstrual problems. It is also used as an antiinflammatory and for the treatment of cancer and liver disease.

Pharmacokinetics

Limited *in vitro* and *animal* studies suggest that danshen extracts affect the activities of various cytochrome P450 isoenzymes. However, these effects do not appear to be clinically relevant. In a study in *mice,* a commercial pharmaceutical extract of danshen induced the activity of the cytochrome P450 isoenzyme CYP1A2 (assessed by 7-methoxyresorufin *O*-demethylation) by about 60%. An *aqueous* extract had no effect, whereas an *ethyl acetate* extract, which is not used in pharmaceutical preparations, had a very marked four- to eightfold increase in CYP1A2 activity. A purified extract of tanshinone IIA had a similar effect in this study,[1] and in one of two *mice* models in another study.[2] Conversely, in another study using *mice* and human liver microsomes, tanshinone IIA (extracted in *ethyl acetate*) inhibited CYP1A2.[3] Any potent effects of danshen extracts on CYP1A2 therefore appear to be limited to ethyl extracts of danshen, which are not used clinically. The more modest effects found with the commercial pharmaceutical extract may not be clinically relevant, as clinical studies with theophylline, page 187, a substrate of CYP1A2 did not find a clinically relevant interaction.

The extracts of danshen that are used pharmaceutically do not appear to have clinically relevant effects on CYP2C9 (see tolbutamide, page 187), and only weak effects on CYP3A4 (see calcium-channel blockers, page 185 and midazolam, page 186).

Some extracts of danshen may inhibit P-glycoprotein, see under digoxin, page 185.

Interactions overview

Some case reports and *animal* data indicate that danshen can, rarely, increase the effects of warfarin, resulting in bleeding. The antiplatelet activity of danshen may be partly responsible, and therefore additive antiplatelet effects might occur if danshen is taken with conventional antiplatelet drugs, which may also increase the risk of bleeding. Danshen can falsify the results of serum immunoassay methods for digoxin, and experimental evidence suggests that danshen could raise digoxin levels. Additive blood-pressure-lowering effects could, in theory, occur if danshen is taken with nifedipine, but no clinically relevant pharmacokinetic interaction appears to occur. Clinical evidence suggests that danshen has only weak effects on midazolam metabolism and does not affect the pharmacokinetics of theophylline Experimental evidence suggests that danshen does not affect the pharmacokinetics of alcohol or tolbutamide.

Interactions monographs

- Alcohol, page 185
- Calcium-channel blockers, page 185
- Digoxin, page 185
- Food, page 185
- Herbal medicines, page 185
- Laboratory tests, page 186
- Midazolam, page 186
- Salicylates, page 186
- Theophylline, page 187
- Tolbutamide, page 187
- Warfarin and related drugs, page 187

1. Kuo Y-H, Lin Y-L, Don M-J, Chen R-M, Ueng Y-F. Induction of cytochrome P450-dependent monooxygenase by extracts of the medicinal herb *Salvia miltiorrhiza*. *J Pharm Pharmacol* (2006) 58, 521–7.
2. Ueng Y-F, Kuo Y-H, Wang S-Y, Lin Y-L, Chen C-F. Induction of CYP1A by a diterpene quinone tanshinone IIA isolated from a medicinal herb *Salvia miltiorrhiza* in C57BL/6J but not in DBA/2J mice. *Life Sci* (2004) 74, 885–96.
3. Ueng Y-F, Kuo Y-H, Peng H-C, Chen T-L, Jan W-C, Guengerich FP, Lin Y-L. Diterpene quinine tanshinone IIA selectively inhibits mouse and human cytochrome P4501A2. *Xenobiotica* (2003) 33, 603–13.

Danshen + Alcohol

The interaction between danshen and alcohol is based on experimental evidence only.

Clinical evidence

No interactions found.

Experimental evidence

An oral danshen extract 200 mg/kg inhibited the oral absorption of alcohol in *rats*. Blood-alcohol levels were reduced by up to 60% in comparison to control *rats*. Danshen had no effect on blood-alcohol levels when ethanol was injected intraperitoneally. The danshen used in this study was standardised to contain 13% tanshinone IIA.[1]

Mechanism

Unknown.

Importance and management

Evidence for an interaction between alcohol and danshen appears to be limited to one study in *rats*. Even if these results are replicated in humans, any effect is probably not clinically relevant, and danshen is certainly not proven for use as an aid to reducing alcohol absorption or lowering blood-alcohol levels.

1. Colombo G, Agabio R, Lobina C, Reali R, Morazzoni P, Bombardelli E, Gessa GL. *Salvia miltiorrhiza* extract inhibits alcohol absorption, preference, and discrimination in sP rats. *Alcohol* (1999) 18, 65–70.

Danshen + Calcium-channel blockers

The interaction between danshen and calcium-channel blockers is based on experimental evidence only.

Clinical evidence

No interactions found.

Experimental evidence

In a study in *mice,* a commercial pharmaceutical extract and an aqueous extract of danshen had no effect on nifedipine oxidation. In contrast an ethyl acetate extract of danshen (which is not used as a pharmaceutical preparation) caused a threefold increase in nifedipine oxidation.[1] Another study found that purified tanshinone IIA, present in ethyl acetate extracts, caused a *decrease* in nifedipine oxidation in *mice,*[2] whereas a third study reported no change in nifedipine oxidation by tanshinone IIA in human liver microsomes.[3]

Studies in the *rat* femoral artery have shown that danshen extracts cause vasorelaxant effects.[4]

Mechanism

Contradictory findings have been reported on the effect of ethyl acetate danshen extracts on nifedipine oxidation, which is mediated by the cytochrome P450 isoenzyme CYP3A4. This could be increased, decreased or unchanged.

Importance and management

Evidence for an interaction between nifedipine and danshen appears to be limited to experimental studies, which suggest the type of danshen extract used is important in determining whether or not an interaction may occur. In general a clinically important interaction with pharmaceutical extracts seems unlikely. Ethyl acetate extracts may decrease nifedipine metabolism, but as these are not used pharmaceutically, this is of little clinical relevance. A pharmacodynamic interaction may occur, because both nifedipine and danshen have calcium-channel blocking effects. Until more is known, some caution might be warranted if patients take nifedipine (and possibly any

calcium-channel blocker) with danshen, as additive blood pressure-lowering effects could, in theory, occur.

1. Kuo Y-H, Lin Y-L, Don M-J, Chen R-M, Ueng Y-F. Induction of cytochrome P450-dependent monooxygenase by extracts of the medicinal herb *Salvia miltiorrhiza*. *J Pharm Pharmacol* (2006) 58, 521–7.
2. Ueng Y-F, Kuo Y-H, Wang S-Y, Lin Y-L, Chen C-F. Induction of CYP1A by a diterpene quinone tanshinone IIA isolated from a medicinal herb *Salvia miltiorrhiza* in C57BL/6J but not in DBA/2J mice. *Life Sci* (2004) 74, 885–96.
3. Ueng Y-F, Kuo Y-H, Peng H-C, Chen T-L, Jan W-C, Guengerich FP, Lin Y-L. Diterpene quinine tanshinone IIA selectively inhibits mouse and human cytochrome P4501A2. *Xenobiotica* (2003) 33, 603–13.
4. Lam FFY, Yeung JHK, Cheung JHY, Or PMY. Pharmacological evidence for calcium channel inhibition by danshen (*Salvia miltiorrhiza*) on rat isolated femoral artery. *J Cardiovasc Pharmacol* (2006) 47, 139–45.

Danshen + Digoxin

The interaction between danshen and digoxin is based on experimental evidence only.

Clinical evidence

No interactions found.

Experimental evidence

Two *in vitro* studies[1,2] have assessed the effects of tanshinone IIA and tanshinone IIB (major constituents of danshen) on the uptake of digoxin by P-glycoprotein. Both extracts exhibited concentration-dependent inhibitor effects on P-glycoprotein. Tanshinone IIA had the greatest effects of the two extracts, inhibiting the P-glycoprotein-mediated transport of digoxin in a similar manner to verapamil, a known clinically relevant P-glycoprotein inhibitor. The effects of tanshinone IIB were modest in comparison.

Mechanism

Tanshinone IIA appears to be a clinically relevant inhibitor of P-glycoprotein, of which digoxin is a substrate.

Importance and management

The available data appears to be from experimental studies in which specific constituents of danshen were used. This makes it difficult to extrapolate the data to the use of the herb in a clinical setting. What is known suggests that danshen may inhibit the transport of digoxin by P-glycoprotein, which could lead to raised digoxin levels. Therefore if danshen is taken by a patient receiving digoxin it may be prudent to be alert for symptoms of raised digoxin levels, such as bradycardia, and consider monitoring levels, should this occur. However, note that danshen may interfere with some of the tests used to assess digoxin levels, see also Laboratory tests, page 186.

1. Yu X-Y, Lin S-G, Zhou Z-W, Chen X, Liang J, Liu P-Q, Duan W, Chowbay B, Wen J-Y, Li C-G, Zhou S-F. Role of P-glycoprotein in the intestinal absorption of tanshinone IIA, a major active ingredient in the root of *Salvia miltiorrhiza* Bunge. *Curr Drug Metab* (2007) 8, 325–40.
2. Yu X-Y, Zhou Z-W, Lin S-G, Chen X, Yu X-Q, Liang J, Duan W, Wen J-Y, Li X-T, Zhou S-F. Role of ATP-binding cassette drug transporters in the intestinal absorption of tanshinone IIB, one of the major active diterpenoids from the root of *Salvia miltiorrhiza*. *Xenobiotica* (2007) 37, 375–415.

Danshen + Food

No interactions found.

Danshen + Herbal medicines

No interactions found.

Danshen + Laboratory tests

Danshen can falsify the results of serum immunoassay methods for digoxin.

Evidence, mechanism, importance and management

Danshen can falsify some laboratory measurements of digoxin because it contains digoxin-like immunoreactive components. A study found that a fluorescent polarization immunoassay method (Abbott Laboratories) for digoxin gave falsely high readings in the presence of danshen, whereas a microparticle enzyme immunoassay (Abbott Laboratories) gave falsely low readings. These, or similar findings have been reported elsewhere.[1] These false readings could be eliminated by monitoring the free (i.e. unbound) digoxin concentrations[2] or by choosing assay systems that are unaffected by the presence of danshen (said to be the Roche and Beckman systems[3] or an enzyme linked chemiluminescent immunosorbent digoxin assay by Bayer HealthCare[1,4]). Similarly, when assaying serum from patients taking digoxin, to which a variety of danshen extracts were added, the use of a fluorescent polarization immunoassay gave variable results, whereas the results were more consistent with a chemiluminescent assay, the EMIT 2000 digoxin assay and the Randox digoxin assay.[5] It would therefore seem prudent, wherever possible, to use a chemiluminescent assay for digoxin in patients also taking danshen.

1. Dasgupta A, Actor JK, Olsen M, Wells A, Datta P. In vivo digoxin-like immunoreactivity in mice and interference of Chinese medicine Danshen in serum digoxin measurement: elimination of interference by using a chemiluminescent assay. *Clin Chim Acta* (2002) 317, 231–4.
2. Wahed A, Dasgupta A. Positive and negative in vitro interference of Chinese medicine dan shen in serum digoxin measurement. Elimination by monitoring free digoxin concentration. *Am J Clin Pathol* (2001) 116, 403–8.
3. Chow L, Johnson M, Wells A, Dasgupta A. Effect of the traditional Chinese medicines Chan Su, Lu-Shen-Wan, Dan Shen, and Asian ginseng on serum digoxin measurement by Tina-quant (Roche) and Synchron LX System (Beckman) digoxin immunoassays. *J Clin Lab Anal* (2003) 17, 22–7.
4. Dasgupta A, Kang E, Olsen M, Actor JK, Datta P. New enzyme-linked chemiluminescent digoxin assay is free from interference of Chinese medicine DanShen. *Ther Drug Monit* (2006) 28, 775–8.
5. Datta P, Dasgupta A. Effect of Chinese medicines Chan Su and Danshen on EMIT 2000 and Randox digoxin immunoassays: wide variation in digoxin-like immunoreactivity and magnitude of interference in digoxin measurement by different brands of the same product. *Ther Drug Monit* (2002) 24, 637–44.

Danshen + Midazolam

Danshen slightly decreases the exposure to midazolam.

Clinical evidence

In a pharmacokinetic study, 12 healthy subjects were given a single 15-mg oral dose of midazolam before and after taking four danshen tablets three times daily for 14 days. Danshen decreased the AUC and maximum levels of midazolam by 28% and 36%, respectively.[1]

In this study, the tablets were analysed, and each tablet was found to contain cryptotanshinone 260 micrograms, tanshinone I 500 micrograms, tanshinone IIA 370 micrograms, protocatechuic aldehyde 670 micrograms, danshenu 1.7 mg and salvianolic acid B 13.5 mg.[1]

Experimental evidence

In vitro study suggests that a constituent of danshen, protocatechuic aldehyde is a weak *inhibitor* of midazolam metabolism by the cytochrome P450 isoenzyme CYP3A4.[2]

Mechanism

Midazolam is known to be metabolised by the cytochrome P450 isoenzyme CYP3A4. It was suggested that danshen induced CYP3A4 in the intestine, resulting in lower midazolam exposure.[1]

Importance and management

Evidence for an interaction between danshen and midazolam is limited, but an interaction would appear to be established. However, the reduction in midazolam exposure was small and is expected to be of only of modest clinical relevance. No immediate action is necessary on concurrent use, but if a patient receiving danshen shows a reduced response to midazolam, it may be prudent to consider an interaction as a possible cause.

Midazolam is used as a probe drug for CYP3A4 activity, and therefore these results also suggest that a pharmacokinetic interaction between danshen and other CYP3A4 substrates is possible. See Drugs and herbs affecting or metabolised by the cytochrome P450 isoenzyme CYP3A4, page 7, for a list of known CYP3A4 substrates.

1. Qiu F, Wang G, Zhang R, Sun J, Jiang J, Ma Y. Effect of danshen extract on the activity of CYP3A4 in healthy volunteers. *Br J Clin Pharmacol* (2010) 69, 656–62.
2. Qiu F, Zhang R, Sun J, A J, Hao H, Peng Y, Ai H, Wang G. Inhibitory effects of seven components of danshen extract on catalytic activity of cytochrome P450 enzyme in human liver microsomes. *Drug Metab Dispos* (2008) 36, 1308–14.

Danshen + Salicylates

The interaction between danshen and salicylates is based on experimental evidence only.

Clinical evidence

No interactions found.

Experimental evidence

(a) Protein binding

In vitro experiments show that danshen can increase free salicylate concentration by displacing salicylate from binding to albumin proteins. In contrast, unexpectedly, salicylate significantly decreased free danshen concentrations at full anti-inflammatory concentrations of salicylate (150 micrograms/mL and above). However, no significant change in free danshen concentrations was observed when salicylate concentrations were less than this (up to 100 micrograms/mL).[1]

(b) Pharmacodynamic

An active component of danshen (765-3) has been shown to inhibit human platelet aggregation via its effects on platelet calcium.[2]

Mechanism

In vitro many conventional drugs are capable of being displaced by others, but in the body the effects seem almost always to be buffered so effectively that the outcome is not normally clinically important. It would therefore seem that the importance of this interaction mechanism has been grossly over-emphasised. It is difficult to find an example of a clinically important interaction (with conventional drugs) due to this mechanism alone.

Additive antiplatelet effects might occur, which might increase the risk of bleeding.

Importance and management

In vitro evidence suggests that danshen displaces salicylate from protein binding sites at high doses, but the clinical relevance of this seems minimal. There may be a more clinically significant interaction with low-dose aspirin, as both it and danshen have antiplatelet activity. Concurrent use may therefore result in additive antiplatelet effects. Bear this possibility in mind if unexpected signs of bleeding, such as bruising, occur.

1. Gupta D, Jalali M, Wells A, Dasgupta A. Drug-herb interactions: unexpected suppression of free danshen concentrations by salicylate. *J Clin Lab Anal* (2002) 16, 290–294.
2. Wu H, Li J, Peng L, Teng B, Zhai Z. Effect of 764-3 on aggregation and calcium movements in aequorin-loaded human platelets. *Chin Med Sci J* (1996) 11, 49–52.

D

Danshen + Theophylline

Danshen does not appear to affect the pharmacokinetics of theophylline.

Clinical evidence

In a crossover study, 12 healthy subjects were given a single 100-mg dose of theophylline alone, and after taking four tablets, each containing an extract of 1-g of danshen, three times daily, for 14 days. Danshen slightly decreased the time to maximum theophylline levels, but this was not expected to be clinically relevant, and no other pharmacokinetic parameters were altered.[1]

Experimental evidence

No relevant data found.

Mechanism

Alcoholic extracts of danshen may have effects on cytochrome P450 CYP1A2, the isoenzyme by which theophylline is metabolised. See pharmacokinetics, page 184.

Importance and management

The available evidence is limited, but seems to suggest that the dose of theophylline will not need to be altered in patients also taking danshen extract tablets.

1. Qiu F, Wang G, Zhao Y, Sun H, Mao G, A J, Sun J. Effect of danshen extract on pharmacokinetics of theophylline in healthy volunteers. *Br J Clin Pharmacol* (2008) 65, 270–274.

Danshen + Tolbutamide

The information regarding the use of danshen with tolbutamide is based on experimental evidence only.

Clinical evidence

No interactions found.

Experimental evidence

In a study in *mice,* a commercial pharmaceutical extract of danshen had no effect on tolbutamide hydroxylation. Similarly, an aqueous extract had no effect, whereas the ethyl acetate extract (which is not used as a pharmaceutical preparation, and contained the greatest amount of tanshinone IIA) caused a twofold increase in tolbutamide hydroxylation.[1]

However, *in vitro,* tanshinone IIA did not affect the oxidation of tolbutamide in mouse or human liver microsomes.[2]

Mechanism

Tolbutamide is a substrate of the cytochrome P450 isoenzyme CYP2C9, and is also used as a probe substrate to assess the effects of other substances on this isoenzyme. The evidence suggests that the usual extracts of danshen do not affect tolbutamide metabolism, and therefore would not be expected to have clinically relevant effects on other substrates of CYP2C9.

Importance and management

Evidence appears to be limited to two experimental studies. However, they provide reasonably strong evidence to suggest that danshen will not affect the metabolism of tolbutamide. Therefore no dosage adjustments are expected to be needed if danshen is given to patients also taking tolbutamide. This study also suggests that danshen is unlikely to affect the metabolism of other drugs that are substrates of this isoenzyme.

1. Kuo Y-H, Lin Y-L, Don M-J, Chen R-M, Ueng Y-F. Induction of cytochrome P450-dependent monooxygenase by extracts of the medicinal herb *Salvia miltiorrhiza*. *J Pharm Pharmacol* (2006) 58, 521–7.

2. Ueng Y-F, Kuo Y-H, Peng H-C, Chen T-L, Jan W-C, Guengerich FP, Lin Y-L. Diterpene quinone tanshinone IIA selectively inhibits mouse and human cytochrome P4501A2. *Xenobiotica* (2003) 33, 603–13.

Danshen + Warfarin and related drugs

Three case reports and some *animal* data indicate that danshen can increase the effects of warfarin, resulting in bleeding.

Clinical evidence

A woman taking warfarin, furosemide and digoxin, who began to take danshen on alternate days, was hospitalised a month later with anaemia and bleeding (prothrombin time greater than 60 seconds, INR greater than 5.62). The anaemia was attributed to occult gastrointestinal bleeding and the over-anticoagulation to an interaction with the danshen. She was later restabilised on warfarin in the absence of the danshen with an INR of 2.5, and within 4 months her haemoglobin levels were normal.[1]

A man taking warfarin, digoxin, captopril and furosemide with an INR of about 3, developed chest pain and breathlessness about 2 weeks after starting to take danshen. He was found to have a massive pleural effusion, and an INR of more than 8.4. He was later discharged on his usual dose of warfarin with an INR stable at 3, in the absence of the danshen.[2]

Over-anticoagulation was investigated in Chinese patients admitted to a medica unit during a 9-month period in 1994/1995. An interaction with warfarin was reported in a patient using a medicated oil product that contained methyl salicylate 15%, and an "analgesic balm" that contained danshen, methyl salicylate 50% and diclofenac.[3]

Experimental evidence

In a study in *rats,* danshen aqueous extract 5 g/kg twice daily given intraperitoneally for 3 days prolonged the prothrombin time and increased the steady-state levels of both isomers of warfarin.[4] Similar findings were reported in another earlier study by the same group.[5] In contrast, in a study in *mice,* a commercial pharmaceutical extract of danshen had no effect on warfarin 7-hydroxylation (mediated by the cytochrome P450 isoenzyme CYP2C9). Similarly, an aqueous extract had no effect, but an ethyl acetate extract (which is not used as a pharmaceutical preparation, and contained the greatest amount of tanshinone IIA) *increased* warfarin 7-hydroxylation threefold, which would be expected to lead to a decrease in its anticoagulant effects.[6]

A study in *animals* found that high doses of Kangen-Karyu (a mixture of peony root, cnidium rhizome, safflower, cyperus rhizome, saussurea root and the root of danshen) 2 g/kg twice daily inhibited the metabolism and elimination of single doses of warfarin, and prolonged bleeding time. There was no interaction at a lower dose of 500 mg/kg, which suggests that a clinical interaction is unlikely at the recommended dose of 90 mg/kg of Kangen-Karyu daily.[7]

Mechanism

Danshen has antiplatelet actions, which may be additive with the anticoagulant effect of warfarin. The mechanism for the increase in warfarin levels is unknown, because the studies suggest that the usual extracts of danshen do not inhibit the cytochrome P450 isoenzyme CYP2C9, the main route of warfarin metabolism. Consider also tolbutamide, above, and for more information on the antiplatelet effects of danshen, see salicylates, page 186.

Importance and management

Evidence appears to be limited to three case studies, which alone would be insufficient to establish an interaction. The pharmacokinetic effects of the usual extracts of danshen seem to suggest that an interaction resulting in raised warfarin levels is unlikely in most patients. However, because danshen may have antiplatelet effects, an interaction between warfarin and danshen, resulting in increased

D

bleeding, is possible. Clinically the use of an antiplatelet drug with an anticoagulant should generally be avoided in the absence of a specific indication. It may therefore be prudent to advise against concurrent use. However, if concurrent use is felt desirable it would seem sensible to warn patients to be alert for any signs of bruising or bleeding, and report these immediately, should they occur.

1. Yu CM, Chan JCN, Sanderson JE. Chinese herbs and warfarin potentiation by 'Danshen'. *J Intern Med* (1997) 241, 337–9.
2. Izzat MB, Yim APC, El-Zufari MH. A taste of Chinese medicine. *Ann Thorac Surg* (1998) 66, 941–2.
3. Chan TYK. Drug interactions as a cause of overanticoagulation and bleedings in Chinese patients receiving warfarin. *Int J Clin Pharmacol Ther* (1998) 36, 403–5.
4. Chan K, Lo ACT, Yeung JHK, Woo KS. The effects of Danshen (*Salvia miltiorrhiza*) on warfarin pharmacodynamics and pharmacokinetics of warfarin enantiomers in rats. *J Pharm Pharmacol* (1995) 47, 402–6.
5. Lo ACT, Chan K, Yeung JHK, Woo KS. The effects of Danshen (*Salvia miltiorrhiza*) on pharmacokinetics and dynamics of warfarin in rats. *Eur J Drug Metab Pharmacokinet* (1992) 17, 257–62.
6. Kuo Y-H, Lin Y-L, Don M-J, Chen R-M, Ueng Y-F. Induction of cytochrome P450-dependent monooxygenase by extracts of the medicinal herb *Salvia miltiorrhiza*. *J Pharm Pharmacol* (2006) 58, 521–7.
7. Makino T, Wakushima H, Okamoto T, Okukubo Y, Deguchi Y, Kano Y. Pharmacokinetic interactions between warfarin and *kangen-karyu*, a Chinese traditional herbal medicine, and their synergistic action. *J Ethnopharmacol* (2002) 82, 35–40.

D

Devil's claw

Harpagophytum procumbens DC. (Pedaliaceae)

Synonym(s) and related species

Grapple plant, Harpagophytum, Wood spider.

Harpagophytum burchellii Decne.

Pharmacopoeias

Devil's Claw (*BP 2012*); Devil's Claw Dry Extract (*BP 2012, PhEur 7.5*), Devil's Claw Root (*PhEur 7.5*).

Constituents

Devil's claw is usually standardised to the content of the iridoid glycoside, **harpagoside**. Other iridoid glycosides include harpagide and procumbide, and other constituents include diterpenes, the phenolic glycosides 6-acetylacteoside and 2,6-diacetylacteoside, **flavonoids** (including kaempferol), triterpenes, and harpagoquinone.

Use and indications

The dried secondary root tuber is used as a stomachic and bitter tonic, and for inflammatory disorders including arthritis, gout, myalgia, fibrositis, lumbago and rheumatic disease.

Pharmacokinetics

In vitro, a Devil's claw extract moderately inhibited the activity of the cytochrome P450 isoenzymes, CYP2C8, CYP2C9, CYP2C19, and CYP3A4.[1] Devil's claw had the greatest effect on CYP2C9, but this was still, at best, a modest effect. For information on the pharmacokinetics of individual flavonoids present in Devil's claw, see under flavonoids, page 213.

Interactions overview

Limited evidence is available. Devil's claw does not appear to affect blood pressure, and its theoretical interaction with drugs with antiplatelet effects seems unlikely to be of practical relevance; however, it may increase the anticoagulant effects of drugs such as warfarin.

For information on the interactions of individual flavonoids present in Devil's claw, see under flavonoids, page 213.

Interactions monographs

- Antihypertensives, page 190
- Antiplatelet drugs and NSAIDs, page 190
- Food, page 190
- Herbal medicines, page 190
- Warfarin and related drugs, page 190

1. Unger M, Frank A. Simultaneous determination of the inhibitory potency of herbal extracts on the activity of six major cytochrome P450 enzymes using liquid chromatography/mass spectrometry and automated online extraction. *Rapid Commun Mass Spectrom* (2004) 18, 2273–81.

D

D

Devil's claw + Antihypertensives

Devil's claw does not appear to affect blood pressure and is therefore unlikely to interact with antihypertensives to a clinically relevant extent, although further study is needed to confirm this.

Clinical evidence

In a randomised placebo-controlled 4-week study,[1] a Devil's claw extract was studied for the possible treatment of low back pain in 109 patients. One patient had an episode of tachycardia while on holiday, and stopped taking the herbal medicine. When he returned from holiday, Devil's claw was restarted and was well tolerated. It was suggested that this adverse event was due to the change in climate rather than the medication. Furthermore, in the study, there was no significant change in systolic and diastolic blood pressure or heart rate between the beginning and the end of the study, and between Devil's claw and placebo recipients. The Devil's claw extract used in this study was given at a dose of 800 mg three times daily, equivalent to a daily dose of 50 mg of harpagoside.[1]

Experimental evidence

Crude methanolic extracts of Devil's claw, and isolated harpagoside, showed a significant and dose-dependent, protective action toward ventricular arrhythmias in *rat* hearts.[2,3] In other *animal* studies, high doses of Devil's claw has caused a reduction in blood pressure.[3,4]

Mechanism

No mechanism established.

Importance and management

Clinical evidence is limited to one study that was not specifically designed to assess interactions. However, the available data suggests that Devil's claw, used in standard doses, is unlikely to affect treatment with conventional antihypertensives, although this ideally needs confirmation in hypertensive patients. The reduction in blood pressure found in *animal* studies seems unlikely to be clinically relevant, due to the high doses used. Too little is known to be able to make any clinical recommendations regarding the potential antiarrhythmic effect of Devil's claw.

1. Chrubasik S, Zimpfer CH, Schütt U, Ziegler R. Effectiveness of *Harpagophytum procumbens* in treatment of acute low back pain. *Phytomedicine* (1996) 3, 1–10.
2. Costa-De-Pasquale R, Busa G, Circosta C, Iauk L, Ragusa S, Ficarra P, Occhiuto F. A drug used in traditional medicine: *Harpagophytum procumbens* DC. III. Effects on hyperkinetic ventricular arrhythmias by reperfusion. *J Ethnopharmacol* (1985) 13, 193–9.
3. Circosta C, Occhiuto F, Ragusa S, Trovato A, Tumino G, Briguglio F, de-Pasquale A. A drug used in traditional medicine: *Harpagophytum procumbens* DC. II. Cardiovascular activity. *J Ethnopharmacol* (1984) 11, 259–74.
4. Occhiuto F, De-Pasquale A. Electrophysiological and haemodynamic effects of some active principles of *Harpagophytum procumbens* DC. in the dog. *Pharmacol Res* (1990) 22 (Suppl 2), 1–2.

Devil's claw + Antiplatelet drugs and NSAIDs

The interaction between Devil's claw and antiplatelet drugs and NSAIDs is based on a prediction only.

Evidence, mechanism, importance and management

One licensed preparation for Devil's claw suggests that there is a theoretical increased risk of bleeding if Devil's claw is given with drugs that inhibit platelet aggregation, such as antiplatelet drugs and NSAIDs.[1] The exact basis for this recommendation is unclear and another subsequently licensed preparation does not carry this warning.[2] A case report suggests that Devil's claw may interact with warfarin, page 190, but this seems most likely to be due to a metabolic effect rather than intrinsic antiplatelet properties. Devil's claw appears to be contraindicated in peptic ulceration, and this could be taken to suggest that any antiplatelet effects it may have could increase the risks of bleeding from an ulcer. However, some sources suggest that this contraindication is because of the bitter properties of Devil's claw (implying that it may stimulate gastric secretions), and there are no documented cases of bleeding or ulceration with the use of Devil's claw. This warning with antiplatelet drugs and NSAIDs therefore appears to represent tremendous caution and it seems unlikely that the theoretical prediction will be of clinical importance.

1. Flexiherb Film-coated Tablets (Devil's claw root dry aqueous extract). MH Pharma (UK) Ltd. UK Summary of product characteristics, March 2007.
2. Atrosan Film-coated Tablets (Devil's claw root dry extract). Bioforce (UK) Ltd. UK Summary of product characteristics, January 2008.

Devil's claw + Food

No interactions found.

Devil's claw + Herbal medicines

No interactions found.

Devil's claw + Warfarin and related drugs

Devil's claw may increase the effects of warfarin, and possibly other coumarins.

Clinical evidence

A case report from a 5-year toxicological study[1] describes the development of purpura in a patient following the concurrent use of Devil's claw and warfarin.

Experimental evidence

In an *in vitro* study, a Devil's claw extract modestly inhibited the activity of the cytochrome P450 isoenzyme CYP2C9.[2]

Mechanism

Limited *in vitro* evidence suggests that Devil's claw may inhibit the cytochrome P450 isoenzyme CYP2C9.[2] Although the metabolism of warfarin is complex, CYP2C9 plays a significant role. Therefore it is possible that Devil's claw could inhibit the metabolism of warfarin, raising its levels and increasing its effect.

Importance and management

Evidence is limited to a case study, which reports minor adverse effects, and experimental data. An interaction seems possible, but it has not been conclusively demonstrated. Although only warfarin has been studied, all coumarins are metabolised by CYP2C9 to some extent, and therefore they also have the potential to be affected. The evidence is too sparse to make any firm recommendations, but it may be prudent to consider a possible interaction if a patient taking a coumarin develops otherwise unexplained bruising.

1. Shaw D, Leon C, Kolev S, Murray V. Traditional remedies and food supplements. A 5-year toxicological study (1991-1995). *Drug Safety* (1997) 17, 342–56.
2. Unger M, Frank A. Simultaneous determination of the inhibitory potency of herbal extracts on the activity of six major cytochrome P450 enzymes using liquid chromatography/mass spectrometry and automated online extraction. *Rapid Commun Mass Spectrom* (2004) 18, 2273–81.

Echinacea

Echinacea species (Asteraceae)

Synonym(s) and related species

Black sampson, Brauneria, Coneflower, Purple coneflower, Rudbeckia.

Echinacea angustifolia (DC) Heller, *Echinacea pallida* (Nutt.) Britt., *Echinacea purpurea* (L.) Moensch. Other names that have been used include *Brauneria pallida* (Nutt.) Britton, *Echinacea intermedia* Lindl., *Rudbeckia hispida* Hoffm, *Rudbeckia pallida* Nutt. *Rudbeckia purpurea* L. and *Rudbeckia serotina* (Nutt) Sweet.

Pharmacopoeias

Echinacea angustifolia: Powder and Powdered extract (*USP35–NF30 S1*); Root (*BP 2012*).

Echinacea pallida: Powder and Powdered extract (*USP35–NF30 S1*); Root (*BP 2012*).

Echinacea purpurea: Aerial Parts (*USP35–NF30 S1*); Herb (*BP 2012*); Powder and Powdered extract (*USP35–NF30 S1*); Root (*BP 2012, USP35–NF30 S1*).

Constituents

The constituents of the various species are slightly different and this leads to confusion as to the potential for drug interactions.

(a) Echinacea angustifolia

The **root** contains alkamides, mainly 2-monoene isobutylamides; and similar caffeic acid esters and glycosides to *Echinacea purpurea*, including the major component, echinacoside, and cynarin. Alkylketones, and the saturated pyrrolizidine alkaloids tussilagine and isotussilagine, are also present (these are not the unsaturated hepatotoxic type).

(b) Echinacea pallida

The **root** contains similar caffeic acid esters and glycosides to *Echinacea purpurea*, including the major component, echinacoside. Polyenes and polyacetylenes, including a range of ketoalkenes and ketopolyacetylenes, have been reported and polysaccharides and glycoproteins are also present.

(c) Echinacea purpurea

The **root** contains alkamides, mainly 2,4-dienoic isobutylamides of straight-chain fatty acids; caffeic acid derivatives including the major component, cichoric acid, with echinacoside, verbascoside, caffeoylechinacoside, chlorogenic acid, isochlorogenic acid and caftaric acid. The saturated pyrrolizidine alkaloids tussilagine and isotussilagine are present.

The **herb** contains similar alkamides, and cichoric acid is the major caffeic acid derivative present. Polysaccharides PS1 (a methylglucuronoarabinoxylan), PS2 (an acidic rhamnoarabinogalactan), a xyloglucan, and glycoproteins have been reported.

The **pressed juice** (from the aerial parts) contains heterogeneous polysaccharides, inulin-type compounds, arabinogalactan polysaccharides and glycoproteins.

Use and indications

Echinacea is mainly used for its immunostimulant (immunomodulatory) effects, particularly in the treatment and prevention of the common cold, influenza and other upper respiratory tract infections. It has a long history of medicinal use for infections, both bacterial and viral, especially in skin conditions such as acne and boils, and also in mild septicaemia.

Pharmacokinetics

Most work has been carried out using *Echinacea purpurea*, although other *Echinacea* species have been studied on selected isoenzymes. *In vitro* studies using non-drug probe substrates[1,2] suggest that *Echinacea purpurea* extracts (*Echinacare* and *Echinagard*) do not have any significant effects on the cytochrome P450 isoenzyme CYP2D6: a finding supported by *in vitro* and clinical studies using drugs as probe substrates, see dextromethorphan, page 193. Similarly, *in vitro* studies[1–3] suggest that *Echinacea purpurea* extracts (*Echinacare, Echinagard* and *Echinaforce*) either do not inhibit, or only weakly inhibit, CYP1A2, CYP2C9, and CYP2C19. These *in vitro* findings for CYP2C9 and CYP1A2 would be expected to be replicated in most patients, as suggested by clinical studies with the probe substrates tolbutamide, page 195, and caffeine, page 193, respectively.

The effects of echinacea on CYP3A4 are less clear. Some extracts of *Echinacea angustifolia, Echinacea pallida*, and *Echinacea purpura* (*Echinagard* and *Echinaforce*) weakly[2,3] or moderately[4] inhibited CYP3A4, whereas one extract of *Echinacea purpura* (*Echinacare*) caused both weak inhibition and induction of CYP3A4.[1] However, in one study[2] the inhibitory properties varied greatly (150-fold). This seemed to be related to the alkamide content of the extract, although *Echinacea pallida* contains only low concentrations of alkamides, so other constituents may also have a role in CYP3A4 inhibition. Indeed, one study found that the caffeic acid derivatives echinacoside and cichoric acid caused moderate and very weak CYP3A4 inhibition, respectively.[4] The findings of a clinical study using midazolam (a probe substrate for CYP3A4) were also somewhat complex (see midazolam, page 195), but appears to suggest only a clinically modest effect of echinacea on CYP3A4.

E

Interactions overview

Theoretically, echinacea may antagonise the effects of immunosuppressants. The use of echinacea has been studied with a number of drugs that are used as probe substrates for cytochrome P450 activity or P-glycoprotein. With the possible exceptions of midazolam and caffeine, and very possibly darunavir in some patients, no clinically relevant interactions have been identified. Echinacea seems to present a low risk for interactions occurring as a result of these mechanisms.

Interactions monographs

- Caffeine, page 193
- Dextromethorphan, page 193
- Digoxin, page 193
- Etravirine, page 194

- Fexofenadine, page 194
- Food, page 194
- Herbal medicines, page 194
- HIV-protease inhibitors, page 194
- Immunosuppressants, page 195
- Midazolam, page 195
- Tolbutamide, page 195
- Warfarin and related drugs, page 195

1. Yale SH, Glurich I. Analysis of the inhibitory potential of *Ginkgo biloba, Echinacea purpurea,* and *Serenoa repens* on the metabolic activity of cytochrome P450 3A4, 2D6, and 2C9. *J Altern Complement Med* (2005) 11, 433–9.
2. Modarai M, Gertsch J, Suter A, Heinrich M, Kortenkamp A. Cytochrome P450 inhibitory action of Echinacea preparations differs widely and co-varies with alkylamide content. *J Pharm Pharmacol* (2007) 59, 567–73.
3. Hellum BH, Hu Z, Nilsen OG. The induction of CYP1A2, CYP2D6 and CYP3A4 by six trade herbal products in cultured primary human hepatocytes. *Basic Clin Pharmacol Toxicol* (2007) 100, 23–30.
4. Budzinski JW, Foster BC, Vandehoek S, Arnason JT. An *in vitro* evaluation of human cytochrome P450 3A4 inhibition by selected commercial herbal extracts and tinctures. *Phytomedicine* (2000) 7, 273–82.

E

Echinacea + Caffeine

Echinacea appears to have a variable effect on the pharmacokinetics of caffeine. In most patients, echinacea is unlikely to raise caffeine levels.

Clinical evidence

In a pharmacokinetic study, 12 healthy subjects were given an 8-day course of *Echinacea purpurea* root 400 mg four times daily, with a single 200-mg oral dose of caffeine on day 6. The maximum serum concentration and AUC of caffeine were increased by about 30%. There was a large variation between subjects, with some having a 50% *increase* in caffeine clearance, and some a 90% *decrease*. However, the paraxanthine-to-caffeine ratio (a measure of CYP1A2 activity) was reduced by just 10%.[1] In another study in 12 healthy subjects given *Echinacea purpurea* 800 mg twice daily for 28 days, the paraxanthine-to-caffeine ratio was not significantly affected when a single 100-mg dose of caffeine was given at the end of the treatment with *Echinacea purpurea*.[2]

Experimental evidence

No relevant data found.

Mechanism

Echinacea is an inhibitor of the cytochrome P450 isoenzyme CYP1A2, which is involved in caffeine metabolism. Echinacea was therefore expected to raise caffeine levels. Although the studies found that caffeine levels were modestly raised by caffeine this did not appear to be due to an effect of echinacea on CYP1A2 (effects found were mild).

Importance and management

Evidence appears to be limited to the two studies cited, which suggest that in most patients echinacea is unlikely to raise caffeine levels by inhibiting CYP1A2. However, some patients did experience a decrease in caffeine clearance, which suggests that, rarely, caffeine levels may be raised. Some patients may therefore experience some increase in the adverse effects of caffeine, such as headache, tremor, and restlessness, particularly if they have a high caffeine intake. Should this occur, advise the patient to either stop taking echinacea and/or reduce their caffeine intake.

Caffeine is used as a probe drug for CYP1A2 activity, and therefore these results also suggest that a pharmacokinetic interaction between echinacea and other CYP1A2 substrates is unlikely.

1. Gorski JC, Huang S-M, Pinto A, Hamman MA, Hilligoss JK, Zaheer NA, Desai M, Miller M, Hall SD. The effect of echinacea (*Echinacea purpurea* root) on cytochrome P450 activity *in vivo*. *Clin Pharmacol Ther* (2004) 75, 89–100.
2. Gurley BJ, Gardner SF, Hubbard MA, Williams DK, Gentry WB, Carrier J, Khan IA, Edwards DJ, Shah A. In vivo assessment of botanical supplementation on human cytochrome P450 phenotypes: *Citrus aurantium, Echinacea purpurea,* milk thistle, and saw palmetto. *Clin Pharmacol Ther* (2004) 76, 428–40.

Echinacea + Dextromethorphan

Echinacea does not appear to have a clinically relevant effect on the pharmacokinetics of dextromethorphan.

Clinical evidence

In a study, 12 healthy subjects were given *Echinacea purpurea* root 400 mg four times daily for 8 days with a single 30-mg dose of dextromethorphan on day 6. In the 11 subjects who were of the cytochrome P450 isoenzyme CYP2D6 extensive metaboliser phenotype there were no changes in the pharmacokinetics of dextromethorphan. In contrast, the one subject who was a poor metaboliser had a 42% increase in the AUC of dextromethorphan and a 31% increase in its half-life.[1] In another study, in 12 healthy subjects given *Echinacea purpurea* 800 mg twice daily for 28 days,

there was no change in the **debrisoquine** urinary ratio after a single 5-mg dose of **debrisoquine**.[2]

Experimental evidence

In vitro studies found that an ethanol-based extract of *Echinacea purpura* (*Echinagard*) produced a slight, non-significant inhibition of dextromethorphan metabolism, a marker for CYP2D6 activity.[3,4] Similar effects have been found with other probe substrates of CYP2D6.[5]

Mechanism

In vitro studies suggest that echinacea has weak inhibitory effects on the cytochrome P450 isoenzyme CYP2D6, however, the *in vivo* study using debrisoquine (another probe substrate of CYP2D6) suggests that this is not of clinical relevance.

Importance and management

The available evidence seems to reliably suggest that in most patients echinacea does not affect the pharmacokinetics of dextromethorphan. Those that are lacking, or are deficient in CYP2D6 may experience a modest increase in dextromethorphan levels. However, dextromethorphan is generally considered to have a wide therapeutic range and the dose is not individually titrated. Therefore, the interaction is probably unlikely to be clinically relevant.

Dextromethorphan is used as a probe drug for CYP2D6 activity, and therefore these results (along with those for debrisoquine) also suggest that a clinically relevant pharmacokinetic interaction between echinacea and other CYP2D6 substrates is unlikely.

1. Gorski JC, Huang S-M, Pinto A, Hamman MA, Hilligoss JK, Zaheer NA, Desai M, Miller M, Hall SD. The effect of echinacea (*Echinacea purpurea* root) on cytochrome P450 activity *in vivo*. *Clin Pharmacol Ther* (2004) 75, 89–100.
2. Gurley BJ, Gardner SF, Hubbard MA, Williams DK, Gentry WB, Carrier J, Khan IA, Edwards DJ, Shah A. In vivo assessment of botanical supplementation on human cytochrome P450 phenotypes: *Citrus aurantium, Echinacea purpurea,* milk thistle, and saw palmetto. *Clin Pharmacol Ther* (2004) 76, 428–40.
3. Hellum BH, Nilsen OG. The *in vitro* inhibitory potential of trade herbal products on human CYP2D6-mediated metabolism and the influence of ethanol. *Basic Clin Pharmacol Toxicol* (2007) 101, 350–358.
4. Hellum BH, Hu Z, Nilsen OG. The induction of CYP1A2, CYP2D6 and CYP3A4 by six trade herbal products in cultured primary human hepatocytes. *Basic Clin Pharmacol Toxicol* (2007) 100, 23–30.
5. Gurley BJ, Swain A, Hubbard MA, Williams DK, Barone G, Hartsfield F, Tong Y, Carrier DJ, Cheboyina S, Battu SK. Clinical assessment of CYP2D6-mediated herb-drug interactions in humans: effects of milk thistle, black cohosh, goldenseal, kava kava, St John's wort, and *Echinacea*. *Mol Nutr Food Res* (2008) 52, 755–63.

Echinacea + Digoxin

Echinacea does not appear to affect the pharmacokinetics of digoxin.

Clinical evidence

In a study, 18 healthy subjects were given an extract containing *Echinacea purpurea* 195 mg and *Echinacea angustifolia* 72 mg three times daily for 14 days with a single 250-microgram dose of digoxin before and after the course of echinacea. The pharmacokinetics of digoxin were not affected by echinacea.[1]

Experimental evidence

An *in vitro* study found that *Echinacea purpurea* extract did not effect the pharmacokinetics of digoxin, a substrate for P-glycoprotein.[2]

Mechanism

No mechanism expected.

Importance and management

Echinacea does not appear to interact with digoxin, and no digoxin dose adjustments would seem necessary on concurrent use.

E

Digoxin is used as a probe substrate for P-glycoprotein, and therefore these results also suggest that a clinically relevant pharmacokinetic interaction between echinacea and other P-glycoprotein substrates is unlikely.

1. Gurley BJ, Swain A, Williams DK, Barone G, Battu SK. Gauging the clinical significance of P-glycoprotein mediated herb-drug interactions: Comparative effects of St Johns wort, Echinacea, clarithromycin, and rifampin on digoxin pharmacokinetics. *Mol Nutr Food Res* (2008) 52, 755–63.
2. Hellum BH, Nilsen OG. *In vitro* inhibition of CYP3A4 metabolism and P-glycoprotein-mediated transport by trade herbal products. *Basic Clin Pharmacol Toxicol* (2008) 102, 466–75.

Echinacea + Etravirine

Echinacea does not affect the pharmacokinetics of etravirine.

Clinical evidence

In a study in 14 HIV-positive patients who had been taking etravirine 400 mg daily for at least 4 weeks, the concurrent use of echinacea 500 mg three time daily had no effect on the pharmacokinetics of etravirine. In this study, echinacea was given as *Echinacea purpurea* root extract (*Arkocápsulas Echinácea*, Arkopharma).[1]

Experimental evidence

No relevant data found.

Mechanism

Etravirine is a substrate and an inducer of the cytochrome P450 isoenzyme CYP3A4. It had been suggested that echinacea might induce CYP3A4 and therefore induce etravirine metabolism.

Importance and management

Evidence for an interaction between echinacea and etravirine comes from one study, which shows that echinacea does not appear to affect etravirine pharmacokinetics. No etravirine dose adjustments would therefore be expected to be necessary if echinacea is also taken.

1. Moltó J, Valle M, Miranda C, Sedeño S, Negredo E, Clotet B. Herb-drug interaction between *Echinacea purpurea* and etravirine in HIV-infected patients *Antimicrobial Agents Chemother* (2012) 56, 5328–31.

Echinacea + Fexofenadine

Echinacea does not affect the pharmacokinetics of single-dose fexofenadine.

Clinical evidence

In a study, 12 healthy subjects were given a single 120-mg dose of oral fexofenadine before and after taking echinacea (*Echinamide®* USA) 500 mg three times daily for 4 weeks. Echinacea had no effect on the pharmacokinetics of fexofenadine.[1]

Experimental evidence

No relevant data found.

Mechanism

Fexofenadine, a P-glycoprotein substrate, was given in this study to assess the effects of echinacea on P-glycoprotein.

Importance and management

Evidence for an interaction between fexofenadine and echinacea is limited to one single-dose study, but what is known suggests that no dose adjustments of fexofenadine are likely to be necessary if patients also take echinacea.

1. Penzak SR, Robertson SM, Hunt JD, Chairez C, Malati CY, Alfaro RM, Stevenson JM, Kovacs JA. Echinacea purpurea significantly indices cytochrome P450 3A (CYP3A) but does not alter lopinavir-ritonavir exposure in healthy subjects. *Pharmacotherapy* (2010) 30, 797–805.

Echinacea + Food

No interactions found.

Echinacea + Herbal medicines

No interactions found.

Echinacea + HIV-protease inhibitors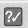

Echinacea does not affect the pharmacokinetics of lopinavir boosted with ritonavir.

Clinical evidence

In a study in 13 healthy subjects given lopinavir boosted with ritonavir 400/100 mg twice daily, the addition of echinacea for 2 weeks did not affect the pharmacokinetics of lopinavir or ritonavir. In this study echinacea was given as Echimamide® USA, containing Echinacea purpura, 500 mg three times daily.[1]

In another study in 15 HIV-positive subjects taking darunavir boosted with ritonavir 600/100 mg twice daily for at least 4 weeks, the addition of echinacea for 2 weeks did not affect the pharmacokinetics of darunavir or ritonavir. However, individual patients were noted to have decreases in darunavir trough concentrations of up to 40%. In this study echinacea was given as *Arkocápsulas Echinácea*, Spain, containing Echinacea purpura root, 500 mg three times daily.[2]

Experimental evidence

No relevant data found.

Mechanism

In the study with lopinavir, echinacea was found to be a weak CYP3A4 inducer; however, these effects were not apparent against the known, potent CYP3A4 inducing effects of ritonavir. The reason for the reduced darunavir concentrations in some patients is unclear.

Importance and management

Evidence for an interaction between echinacea and the HIV-protease inhibitors is based on two studies, one involving darunavir boosted with ritonavir, the other involving lopinavir boosted with ritonavir. In general, echainacea does not appear to affect the pharmacokinetics of these antiretrovirals, although the finding of reduced darunavir concentrations in some patients warrants further study. Patients taking drugs for serious conditions such as HIV-infection should carefully consider the risks and benefits of adding herbal medicines to their existing regimen, where the outcome of concurrent use is unknown.

1. Penzak SR, Roberstson SM, Hunt JD, Chairez C, Malati CY, Alfaro RM, Stevenson JM, Kovacs JA. *Echinacea purpurea* significantly indices cytochrome P450 3A (CYP3A) but does not alter lopinavir-ritonavir exposure in healthy subjects. *Pharmacotherapy* (2010) 30, 797–805.
2. Molto J, Valle M, Mirands C, Cedeno S, Negredo E, Barbanoj MJ, Clotet B. Herb-drug interaction between *Echinacea purpurea* and darunavir-ritonavir in HIV-infected patients. *Antimicrob Agents Chemother* (2011) 55, 326–30.

Echinacea + Immunosuppressants

The interaction between echinacea and immunosuppressants is based on a prediction only.

Evidence, mechanism, importance and management

Echinacea has immunostimulating effects. Theoretically therefore, echinacea may antagonise the effects of immunosuppressant drugs. The manufacturers of three echinacea products licensed by the MHRA in the UK advise against concurrent use with immunosuppressants and specifically name **ciclosporin** and **methotrexate**.[1-3] There do not appear to be any clinical reports of an interaction, but until more is known, it may be prudent to follow this advice.

1. Echinaflu Soft Capsules (Dried pressed juice from *Echinacea purpurea*). Swiss Caps GmbH. UK Summary of product characteristics, June 2008.
2. EchinEeze Tablets (Dry extract of *Echinacea purpurea* root). Natures Aid Health Products. UK Summary of product characteristics, July 2008.
3. Duchy Herbals Echina-Relief Tincture (Alcoholic dry extract of *Echinacea purpurea* root). Nelson and Co. Ltd. UK Summary of product characteristics, October 2008.

Echinacea + Midazolam

Echinacea does not appear to alter the AUC and clearance of oral midazolam, although the bioavailability may be increased. Clearance of intravenous midazolam may be modestly increased in patients taking echinacea.

Clinical evidence

In a pharmacokinetic study, 12 healthy subjects were given *Echinacea purpurea* root (*Nature's Bounty,* USA) 400 mg four times daily for 28 days, with a single 50-microgram/kg *intravenous* dose of midazolam on day 6, and, 24 hours later, a single 5-mg *oral* dose of midazolam. The clearance of intravenous midazolam was increased by 42%, and its AUC was reduced by 23%. In contrast, the clearance and AUC of oral midazolam were not significantly altered; however, the oral bioavailability of midazolam was increased by 50% but the oral bioavailability was still relatively low.[1] In another study, 12 healthy subjects were given a single 8-mg dose of oral midazolam before and after taking echinacea (Echinamide® Natural Factors, USA) 500 mg three times daily for 4 weeks. Echinacea decreased the AUC of midazolam by 27% and increased its oral clearance by 37%.[2] In a further study in 12 healthy subjects given *Echinacea purpurea* 800 mg twice daily for 28 days with a single 8-mg *oral* dose of midazolam, there was no difference in the ratio of midazolam to its 1-hydroxy metabolite.[3]

Experimental evidence

No relevant data found.

Mechanism

Midazolam is predominantly metabolised by the cytochrome P450 isoenzyme CYP3A4. It was suggested the echinacea may have exerted opposing effects on the cytochrome P450 isoenzyme CYP3A in the liver and the intestine, which resulted in this differences in its effects on oral and intravenous midazolam.[1]

Importance and management

Direct evidence about an interaction between midazolam and echinacea comes from three studies which suggest that echinacea is unlikely to interact to a clinically relevant extent with oral midazolam, as those studies that reported a change in the exposure to oral midazolam found only slight effects. The interaction of echinacea with intravenous midazolam is, at best, modest. As the dose of intravenous midazolam is usually tapered to the individual's response, the potential for a reduced effect should be accommodated. The

authors of one of the studies,[1] suggest that the effect of echinacea on CYP3A4 substrates may depend on whether they have high oral bioavailability and the degree of hepatic extraction, and is not easily predicted. More study is needed to establish if echinacea has any clinically relevant effects on a range of CYP3A4 substrates. See the table Drugs and herbs affecting or metabolised by the cytochrome P450 isoenzyme CYP3A4, page 7, for a list of known CYP3A4 substrates.

1. Gorski JC, Huang S-M, Pinto A, Hamman MA, Hilligoss JK, Zaheer NA, Desai M, Miller M, Hall SD. The effect of echinacea (*Echinacea purpurea* root) on cytochrome P450 activity in vivo. *Clin Pharmacol Ther* (2004) 75, 89–100.
2. Penzak SR, Roberstson SM, Hunt JD, Chairez C, Malati CY, Alfaro RM, Stevenson JM, Kovacs JA. Echinacea purpura significantly indices cytochrome P450 3A (CYP3A) but does not alter lopinavir-ritonavir exposure in healthy subjects. *Pharmacotherapy* (2010) 30, 797–805.
3. Gurley BJ, Gardner SF, Hubbard MA, Williams DK, Gentry WB, Carrier J, Khan IA, Edwards DJ, Shah A. In vivo assessment of botanical supplementation on human cytochrome P450 phenotypes: *Citrus aurantium, Echinacea purpurea,* milk thistle, and saw palmetto. *Clin Pharmacol Ther* (2004) 76, 428–40.

Echinacea + Tolbutamide

Echinacea does not appear to have a clinically relevant effect on the pharmacokinetics of tolbutamide.

Clinical evidence

In a pharmacokinetic study, 12 healthy subjects were given *Echinacea purpurea* root 400 mg four times daily for 8 days with a single 500-mg dose of tolbutamide on day 6. The AUC of tolbutamide was increased by 14%, and the time to maximum levels was increased from 4 to 6 hours.[1] The oral clearance was decreased by a mean of 11%, although 2 subjects had a 25% or greater reduction.

Experimental evidence

No relevant data found.

Mechanism

No mechanism expected.

Importance and management

This one study suggests that echinacea does not significantly affect the pharmacokinetics of tolbutamide, and therefore no tolbutamide dosage adjustments appear necessary if echinacea is also taken.

Tolbutamide is used as a probe substrate for CYP2C9, and therefore these results also suggest that a clinically relevant pharmacokinetic interaction between echinacea and other CYP2C9 substrates is unlikely.

1. Gorski JC, Huang S-M, Pinto A, Hamman MA, Hilligoss JK, Zaheer NA, Desai M, Miller M, Hall SD. The effect of echinacea (*Echinacea purpurea* root) on cytochrome P450 activity in vivo. *Clin Pharmacol Ther* (2004) 75, 89–100.

Echinacea + Warfarin and related drugs

Echinacea does not appear to affect the pharmacokinetics or pharmacodynamics of warfarin.

Clinical evidence

In a randomised study, 12 healthy subjects were given a single 25-mg dose of warfarin before and after taking echinacea for 14 days. Echinacea decreased the AUC of S-warfarin by 9% but did not affect the pharmacokinetics of *R*-warfarin, and in the 11 subjects assessed, there was no change in the INR in response to warfarin in the presence of echinacea. In this study echinacea was given as *MediHerb Premium Echinacea* tablets (containing a mixture of

E. angustifolia roots 600 mg and E. purpura roots 675 mg, standardised to contain 5.75 mg of total alkamides) four times daily for a total of 21 days.[1]

Experimental evidence

Echinacea purpurea extracts either do not inhibit, or only weakly inhibit, CYP2C9, the main isoenzyme involved in the metabolism of the more active isomer of warfarin, *S*-warfarin. See *Pharmacokinetics,* under Echinacea, page 191.

Mechanism

None. Echinacea does not appear to affect the metabolism of warfarin.

Importance and management

Evidence for an interaction between echinacea and warfarin appears to be limited to this one well-designed study, which suggests that echinacea does not interact with warfarin. Although other coumarins do not appear to have been studied, they are metabolised similarly to warfarin, and therefore would also seem unlikely to interact with echinacea. This study therefore suggests that no dose adjustments are likely to be necessary if a patient taking a coumarin also takes echinacea.

1. Abdul MIM, Jiang X, Williams KM, Day RO, Roufogalis BD, Liauw WS, Xu H, Matthias A, Lehmann RP, McLachlan AJ. Pharmacokinetic and pharmacodynamic interactions of echinacea and policosanol with warfarin in healthy subjects. *Br J Clin Pharmacol* (2010) 69, 508–15.

E

Eclipta

Eclipta alba Hassk. (Asteraceae)

Synonym(s) and related species

Trailing eclipta.

Eclipta prostrata (L.).

Constituents

Eclipta contains terthienyl derivatives, including α-formylterthienyl and a number of esterified 5-hydroxyterthienyl derivatives. The leaves and stem contain the **flavonoids** apigenin and luteolin, and the **isoflavones** orobol; wedelolactone and desmethylwedelolactone, as well as their glucosides, are present throughout the herb. Oleanane-type triterpenoids known as the ecliptasaponins, eclalbatin and the eclalbasaponins (based on echinocystic acid), and several steroidal alkaloids based on verazine and ecliptalbine, are also found in eclipta.

Use and indications

Eclipta is traditionally used for blood related diseases, including liver diseases such as hepatitis and jaundice. Pharmacological studies support these uses to some extent, but clinical data is lacking. It has also been used for alopecia, as an antiseptic and as an analgesic; its analgesic effects have been attributed to the alkaloid content.

Pharmacokinetics

No relevant pharmacokinetic data found. For information on the pharmacokinetics of individual flavonoids and isoflavones present in eclipta, see under flavonoids, page 213 and isoflavones, page 300, respectively.

Interactions overview

No interactions with eclipta found. For information on the interactions of individual flavonoids and isoflavones present in eclipta, see under flavonoids, page 213 and isoflavones, page 300, respectively.

E

Elder

Sambucus nigra L. (Caprifoliaceae)

Synonym(s) and related species

Black elder, European elder, Sambucus.

Not to be confused with American elder, which is *Sambucus canadensis* L.

Pharmacopoeias

Elder Flower (*BP 2012, PhEur 7.5*).

Constituents

The flowers and berries of elder are most often medicinally. The flowers contain triterpenes based on oleanolic and ursolic acids; the **flavonoids** rutin, quercetin, hyperoside, kaempferol, nicotoflorin and others; and linolenic and linoleic acids. The berries contain anthocyanins cyanidin-3-sambubioside and cyanidin-3-glucoside; the **flavonoids** quercetin and rutin; cyanogenic glycosides including sambunigrin; and vitamins. The unripe berries of elder contain toxic constituents, but these are lost on drying and/or heating, and are not present in the medicinal product. Elder extracts may be standardised to contain 0.8% **flavonoids** based on isoquercitroside (*BP 2012, PhEur 7.5*).

Use and indications

Elder extracts are used mainly to treat colds and flu. Several *in vitro* studies have shown that elder berry constituents have antidiabetic, antiviral and immune-modulating effects, enhance cytokine production and activate phagocytes, but clinical data are lacking.

Pharmacokinetics

No relevant pharmacokinetic data found. For information on the pharmacokinetics of individual flavonoids found in elder, see under flavonoids, page 213.

Interactions overview

There is some very weak experimental evidence to suggest that elder extracts may have additive effects with antidiabetic drugs and phenobarbital, and may antagonise the effects of morphine. For information on the interactions of individual flavonoids found in elder, see under flavonoids, page 213.

Interactions monographs

- Antidiabetics, page 199
- Food, page 199
- Herbal medicines, page 199
- Morphine, page 199
- Phenobarbital, page 199

E

Elder + Antidiabetics

The interaction between elder and antidiabetics is based on experimental evidence only.

Clinical evidence
No interactions found.

Experimental evidence
In an *in vitro* study, it was found that an aqueous elder flower extract enhanced glucose uptake by 70%, but had no additional effect on glucose uptake when insulin was also given. The extract also stimulated insulin secretion and glycogen synthesis.[1]

Mechanism
Elder is thought to enhance insulin secretion in a similar manner to the sulfonylureas. This study supports this suggestion as it found that diazoxide inhibited the effects of elder.

Importance and management
The *in vitro* study provides limited evidence of a possible blood-glucose-lowering effect of an aqueous elder flower extract. Because of the nature of the evidence, applying these results in a clinical setting is extremely difficult, and the effect of elder flower extracts given with conventional antidiabetic medication is unknown. However, if patients taking antidiabetic drugs want to take elder it may be prudent to discuss the potential for additive effects, and advise an increase in blood-glucose monitoring, should an interaction be suspected.

1. Gray AM, Abdel-Wahab YHA, Flatt PR. The traditional plant treatment, *Sambucus nigra* (elder), exhibits insulin-like and insulin-releasing actions in vitro. *J Nutr* (2000) 130, 15–20.

Elder + Food

No interactions found.

Elder + Herbal medicines

No interactions found.

Elder + Morphine

The interaction between elder and morphine is based on experimental evidence only.

Clinical evidence
No interactions found.

Experimental evidence
In a study in *rats* aqueous extracts of elder flower and elder berry were found to modestly decrease the analgesic effects of morphine 90 minutes after dosing. The elder extracts had no effect on the analgesic response to morphine at a subsequent time point (150 minutes), and had tended to increase the effects of morphine 10 minutes after dosing. The berry and flower extracts had no analgesic effect when given alone.[1]

Mechanism
Unknown.

Importance and management
Evidence for an interaction between extracts of elder flower and elder berry and morphine appears to be limited to this study in *rats,* which found only a modest decrease in analgesic effects at just one time point. It is unknown if this effect would occur in humans, but even if it does; it seems unlikely to be of much clinical relevance.

1. Jakovljević V, Popović M, Mimica-Dukić N, Sabo J. Interaction of *Sambucus nigra* flower and berry decoctions with the actions of centrally acting drugs in rats. *Pharm Biol* (2001) 39, 142–5.

E

Elder + Phenobarbital

The interaction between elder and phenobarbital is based on experimental evidence only.

Clinical evidence
No interactions found.

Experimental evidence
In a study in *rats* aqueous extracts of elder flower and elder berry were found to approximately halve the time to the onset of sleep and increase the sleeping time in response to phenobarbital (from about 190 minutes to 200 minutes).[1]

Mechanism
Unknown.

Importance and management
Evidence for an interaction between extracts of elder flower and elder berry and phenobarbital appears to be limited to this study in *rats,* which found only a very modest increase in sleeping time. It is unknown if this effect would occur in humans, but even if it does; it seems unlikely to be clinically relevant.

1. Jakovljević V, Popović M, Mimica-Dukić N, Sabo J. Interaction of *Sambucus nigra* flower and berry decoctions with the actions of centrally acting drugs in rats. *Pharm Biol* (2001) 39, 142–5.

Elecampane

Inula helenium L. (Asteraceae)

Synonym(s) and related species

Alant, Helenio, Horseheal, Inula, Scabwort, Yellow star-wort.

Aster helenium (L.) Scop., *Aster officinalis* All., *Helenium grandiflorum* Gilib.

Constituents

The root contains sesquiterpene lactones, mainly helenalin (alantolactone or elecampane camphor), isohelenalin, dihydroalantolactone, alantic acid, azulene, and a large amount of inulin. Phytosterols including β- and γ-sitosterols, stigmasterol and friedelin are also present.

Use and indications

Elecampane is used as an expectorant, antitussive and antiseptic, especially for catarrh and dry irritating cough in children.

Pharmacokinetics

No relevant pharmacokinetic data found.

Interactions overview

No interactions with elecampane found.

E

Ephedra

Ephedra sinica Stapf, *Ephedra gerardiana* Wall., *Ephedra equisetina* Bunge
(Ephedraceae)

Synonym(s) and related species

Ma huang.

Pharmacopoeias

Ephedra Herb (*BP 2012, PhEur 7.5*).

Constituents

The main active components of ephedra are the amines (sometimes referred to as alkaloids, or more properly pseudoalkaloids) **ephedrine**, **pseudoephedrine**, norephedrine, norpseudoephedrine, N-methylephedrine, ephedroxane, maokonine, a series of ephedradines and others. Other constituents include the diterpenes ephedrannin A and mahuannin, catechins, and a trace of volatile oil containing terpinen-4-ol, α-terpineol, linalool and other monoterpenes.

Use and indications

Ephedra is used traditionally for asthma, bronchitis, hayfever and colds, but recently the herb has become liable to abuse as a stimulant and slimming aid. For this reason the herb has been banned by the FDA in the US. Its main active constituents are ephedrine and pseudoephedrine; however, ephedra herb is claimed to have many more effects than those ascribed to ephedrine and its derivatives. It is these compounds that also give rise to the toxic effects of ephedra.

Pharmacokinetics

No relevant pharmacokinetic data found.

Interactions overview

Ephedra herb contains ephedrine and pseudoephedrine, and therefore has the potential to interact in the same manner as conventional medicines containing these substances. The most notable of these interactions is the potential for hypertensive crises with MAOI; it would therefore seem unwise to take ephedra during, or for 2 weeks after, the use of an MAOI. There do not seem to be any reports of drug interactions for ephedra itself, with the exception of caffeine.

Interactions monographs

- Caffeine, page 202
- Food, page 202
- Herbal medicines, page 202

E

Ephedra + Caffeine

Ephedrine can raise blood pressure and in some cases this may be further increased by caffeine. Combined use has resulted in hypertensive crises in a few individuals. Isolated reports describe the development of acute psychosis when caffeine was given with ephedra.

Clinical evidence

A review of reports from the FDA in the US revealed that several patients have experienced severe adverse effects (subarachnoid haemorrhage, cardiac arrest, hypertension, tachycardia and neurosis) after taking dietary supplements containing ephedrine or ephedra alkaloids with caffeine.[1] However, it is not possible to definitively say that these effects were the result of an interaction because none of the patients took either drug separately. Similarly, a meta-analysis assessing the safety of ephedra or ephedrine and caffeine found a two- to threefold increase in the risk of adverse events (including psychiatric symptoms and palpitations) with ephedra or ephedrine, but concluded that it was not possible to assess the contribution of caffeine to these events.[2]

Two episodes of acute psychosis occurred in a 32-year-old man after he took *Vigueur fit* tablets (containing ephedra alkaloids and caffeine), *Red Bull* (containing caffeine) and alcohol. He had no previous record of aberrant behaviour despite regularly taking 6 to 9 tablets of *Vigueur fit* daily (about twice the recommended dose). However, on this occasion, over a 10-hour period, he consumed 3 or 4 bottles of *Red Bull* (containing about 95 mg of caffeine per 250-mL bottle) and enough alcohol to reach a blood-alcohol level of about 335 mg%. No more episodes occurred after he stopped taking the *Vigueur fit* tablets. Ephedra alkaloids (ephedrine and pseudoephedrine) may cause psychosis and it appears that their effects may be exaggerated by an interaction with caffeine and alcohol.[3] In another case report, an ischaemic stroke that occurred in a 33-year-old man was thought to be due to taking a supplement called *Thermadrene,* (now reformulated, but which at the time contained ephedrine, guarana, caffeine, cayenne pepper and willow bark). The use of bupropion may have been a contributory factor.[4] A similar case of stroke is reported in a man who took a **creatine** supplement with ephedra plus caffeine. In this case, the interaction was attributed to **creatine**. See Creatine + Herbal medicines; Ephedra with Caffeine, page 180.

Experimental evidence

In a study, *rats* were given an oral solution of ephedra (containing up to 50 mg/kg ephedrine) with, and without, caffeine. Ephedra with caffeine increased the clinical signs of toxicity (salivation, hyperactivity, ataxia, lethargy, failure to respond to stimuli) in the treated *rats,* when compared with ephedra alone. Histological analysis for cardiotoxicity showed some evidence of haemorrhage, necrosis, and tissue degeneration within 2 to 4 hours of treatment. No statistical difference in the occurrence of cardiotoxic lesions was found when *animals* treated with *ephedrine* were compared with those treated with ephedra, indicating that the cardiotoxic effects of ephedra are due to ephedrine.[5]

Another study also reported that cardiac toxicity was observed in 7- and 14-week-old male *rats* administered ephedrine (25 mg/kg) in combination with caffeine (30 mg/kg) for one or two days. The ephedrine and caffeine dosage was approximately 12-fold and 1.4-fold, respectively, above average human exposure. Five of the seven treated 14-week-old *rats* died or were sacrificed 4 to 5 hours after the first dose, and massive interstitial haemorrhage was reported.[6]

Mechanism

Ephedrine and caffeine may cause catecholamine release and an increase in intracellular calcium release which leads to vasoconstriction. Myocardial ischaemia may occur as a result of this vasoconstriction (in the coronary artery), and this may result in myocardial necrosis and cell death.[5,6]

Importance and management

The interaction between ephedra alkaloids and caffeine is fairly well established. However, it has to be said that there seem to be few reports of adverse interactions specifically with ephedra alkaloids. One possible explanation for this could be that these interactions may go unrecognised or be attributed to one drug only, whereas caffeine may also have been taken either as part of the preparation or in beverages or foods (often not reported). Nevertheless, a number of serious adverse events have been reported and these preparations may pose a serious health risk to some users. The risk may be affected by individual susceptibility, the additive stimulant effects of caffeine, the variability in the contents of alkaloids, or pre-existing medical conditions.[1]

Note that the FDA has banned combinations of caffeine and herbal products containing ephedra. It would seem prudent to avoid concurrent use.

1. Haller CA, Benowitz NL. Adverse cardiovascular and central nervous system events associated with dietary supplements containing ephedra alkaloids. *N Engl J Med* (2000) 343, 1833–8.
2. Shekelle PG, Hardy ML, Morton SC, Maglione M, Mojica WA, Suttorp MJ, Rhodes SL, Jungvig L, Gagné J. Efficacy and safety of ephedra and ephedrine for weight loss and athletic performance: a meta-analysis. *JAMA* (2003) 280, 1537–45.
3. Tormey WP, Bruzzi A. Acute psychosis due to the interaction of legal compounds - ephedra alkaloids in 'Vigueur Fit' tablets, caffeine in 'Red Bull' and alcohol. *Med Sci Law* (2001) 41, 331–6.
4. Kaberi-Otarod J, Conetta R, Kundo KK, Farkash A. Ischemic stroke in a user of Thermadrene: a case study in alternative medicine. *Clin Pharmacol Ther* (2002) 72, 343–6.
5. Dunnick JK, Kissling G, Gerken DK, Vallant MA, Nyska A. Cardiotoxicity of Ma Huang/caffeine or ephedrine/caffeine in a rodent model system. *Toxicol Pathol* (2007) 35, 657–64.
6. Nyska A, Murphy E, Foley JF, Collins BJ, Petranka J, Howden R, Hanlon P, Dunnick JK. Acute hemorrhagic myocardial necrosis and sudden death of rats exposed to a combination of ephedrine and caffeine. *Toxicol Sci* (2005) 83, 388–96.

Ephedra + Food

No interactions found.

Ephedra + Herbal medicines

No interactions found.

Epimedium

Epimedium brevicornu Maxim. (Berberidaceae)

Synonym(s) and related species

Barrenwort, Horny goat weed, Yin Yang Huo.

There is some taxonomic confusion within the species, and most of the commercially available material has not been properly characterised. In Chinese medicine, a mixture of species (referred to as Herba Epimedii) is often used and includes the following species (some of which may be synonyms): *Epimedium koreanum* Nakai, *Epimedium pubescens* Maxim., *Epimedium sagittatum* (Sieb. Et Zucc) Maxim, and *Epimedium wushanense* T.S.Ying.

Constituents

The major constituents of all species of epimedium are prenylated **flavonoids** and **isoflavones**: the most important being **icariin**, epimedin A, B, and C, and 6-prenylchrysin. Apigenin, luteolin, kaempferol and quercetin are also present. A multitude of other constituents, of which the pharmaceutical relevance is unclear, have been identified.

Use and indications

Epimedium is used traditionally as an antirheumatic, tonic and to enhance bone health and treat osteoporosis. The isoflavones and prenylated flavones have oestrogenic activity.

The herb is also used to enhance sexual function. Legend has it that this use was discovered after a goat herd in China found that his animals became much more sexually active after eating the herb, hence the name horny goat weed. It has therefore been widely advertised as a 'herbal Viagra'.

Pharmacokinetics

In vitro, freeze-dried aqueous extracts of Herba Epimedii have been found to have some inhibitory effect on the cytochrome P450 isoenzyme CYP1A2, an effect thought to be related to the quercetin content of the herb.[1] Extracts of Herba Epimedii may also inhibit (in decreasing order of potency) CYP2C19, CYP2E1, CYP2C9, CYP3A4, and CYP2D6,[1] but the clinical relevance of this has not been established. See flavonoids, page 213, for information on the pharmacokinetics of individual flavonoids present in epimedium.

Interactions overview

Little is known. Epimedium may have additive effects with other medicines used for erectile dysfunction. For information on the interactions of the individual flavonoids present in epimedium, see flavonoids, page 213.

Interactions monographs

- Food, page 204
- Herbal medicines, page 204
- Phosphodiesterase type-5 inhibitors, page 204

1. Liu KH, Kim ML, Jeon BH, Shon JH, Cha IJ, Cho KH, Lee SS, Shin JG. Inhibition of human cytochrome P450 isoforms and NADPH-CYP reductase *in vitro* by 15 herbal medicines, including *Epimedii herba*. *J Clin Pharm Ther* (2006) 31, 83–91.

E

Epimedium + Food

No interactions found.

Epimedium + Herbal medicines

No interactions found.

Epimedium + Phosphodiesterase type-5 inhibitors

The interaction between epimedium and phosphodiesterase type-5 inhibitors is based on experimental evidence only.

Clinical evidence

No interactions found.

Experimental evidence

An *in vitro* study using *rabbit* corpus cavernosum tissue found that an aqueous extract of *Epimedium brevicornum* relaxed the smooth muscle of the corpus cavernosum. The extract also enhanced the relaxation caused by **sildenafil**, **tadalafil** and **vardenafil**.[1]

Mechanism

Epimedium appears to have a similar mode of action to the phosphodiesterase type-5 inhibitors. *In vitro,* an extract of *Epimedium brevicornum* and one of its constituents, icariin, have been found to inhibit phosphodiesterase type-5, although both had weaker effects than sildenafil.[2]

Importance and management

Evidence is limited to experimental studies, but what is known suggests that epimedium may potentiate the effects of the phosphodiesterase type-5 inhibitors, sildenafil, tadalafil and vardenafil. The results of *in vitro* studies are difficult to reliably extrapolate to humans. Nevertheless, the concurrent use of epimedium and a phosphodiesterase type-5 inhibitor could potentially lead to additive effects, which may be beneficial, but which could in theory also lead to adverse effects, such as priapism. It would therefore seem prudent to discuss concurrent use with patients, and warn them of the potential risks. Note that it is generally recommended that other agents for erectile dysfunction should be avoided in those taking sildenafil, tadalafil or vardenafil.

1. Chiu J-H, Chen K-K, Chien T-M, Chiou W-F, Chen C-C, Wang J-Y, Lui W-Y, Wu C-W. *Epimedium brevicornum* Maxim extract relaxes rabbit corpus cavernosum through multitargets on nitric oxide/cyclic guanosine monophosphate signaling pathway. *Int J Impot Res* (2006) 18, 335–42.
2. Dell'Agli M, Galli GV, Dal Cero E, Belluti F, Matera R, Zironi E, Pagliuca G, Bosisio E. Potent inhibition of human phosphodiesterase-5 by icariin derivatives. *J Nat Prod* (2008) 71, 1513–17.

European goldenrod

Solidago virgaurea L. (Asteraceae)

Synonym(s) and related species

Goldenrod.

The related species *Solidago canadensis* (Canadian goldenrod, Common goldenrod) and *Solidago gigantea* (Early goldenrod, Giant goldenrod, Smooth goldenrod, Tall goldenrod) are used similarly.

Varieties and subspecies of all the above are also used.

Note that European goldenrod may be referred to as Aaron's rod. However, this term has also been applied to a number of *Solidago* species as well as other unrelated species.

Pharmacopoeias

Solidago virgaurea: European Goldenrod (*BP 2012, PhEur 7.5*).

Solidago gigantea or *Solidago canadensis*: Goldenrod (*BP 2012, PhEur 7.5*).

Constituents

The active constituents of the goldenrod species are **saponins**, but the type may depend on the source. Virgaurea saponins, based on polygalic acid, have been isolated from European varieties and solidago saponins from Asian varieties. A series of clerodane diterpenes, the nature of which again depends on the origin, has also been found. Phenolic glycosides such as the virgaureosides; **flavonoids** based on quercetin, kaempferol, isorhamnetin and hyperoside; caffeic acid derivatives; and a small amount of volatile oil are also present.

Use and indications

European goldenrod is most commonly used for its anti-inflammatory, antimicrobial and diuretic properties. It is used in inflammatory disorders of the urinary tract, for the treatment of renal and bladder stones, and to treat inflammatory or degenerative rheumatic diseases (in combination with other herbs).

Pharmacokinetics

No relevant pharmacokinetic data found. For information on the pharmacokinetics of individual flavonoids present in European goldenrod, see under flavonoids, page 213.

Interactions overview

No interactions with European goldenrod found. For information on the interactions of individual flavonoids present in European goldenrod, see under flavonoids, page 213.

E

Evening primrose oil

Oenothera biennis L. (Onagraceae)

Synonym(s) and related species

Common evening primrose, King's cureall, Sun drop, Tree primrose.

Oenothera lamarkiana, *Onagra biennis* (L.) Scop.

Pharmacopoeias

Evening primrose oil (*BP 2012, PhEur 7.5*).

Constituents

The oil from evening primrose seeds contains the essential fatty acids of the omega-6 series, **linoleic acid** (about 65 to 85%) and **gamolenic acid** (gamma-linolenic acid, about 7 to 14%). Other fatty acids include oleic acid, alpha-linolenic acid, palmitic acid, and stearic acid.

Use and indications

Evening primrose oil is used as a food supplement to provide essential fatty acids. It is also used for atopic eczema and mastalgia; however, in the UK licenses for two prescription products containing gamolenic acid derived from evening primrose oil were withdrawn in 2002, due to lack of evidence in support of efficacy.

Other conditions for which it is used include rheumatoid arthritis, premenstrual syndrome, menopausal symptoms, chronic fatigue syndrome, and attention deficit hyperactivity disorder. Evening primrose oil has also been used topically as a cream, for the relief of dry or inflamed skin. Traditionally it has been used for asthma, whooping cough, gastrointestinal disorders, and as a sedative painkiller.

In manufacturing, evening primrose oil is used in soaps and cosmetics. The root of evening primrose has been used as a vegetable.

Pharmacokinetics

In *in vitro* experiments,[1] *cis*-linoleic acid, was found to be a modest inhibitor of the cytochrome P450 isoenzyme CYP2C9 (but this is not expected to result in clinically relevant effects on drug metabolism, see warfarin and related drugs, page 208), and a modest to minor inhibitor of, in order of potency, CYP1A2, CYP2C19, CYP3A4, and CYP2D6.

Interactions overview

Evening primrose oil has been predicted to interact with antiplatelet and anticoagulant drugs, but data supporting this prediction is limited. Although seizures have occurred in a few schizophrenics taking phenothiazines and evening primrose oil, no adverse effects were seen in others, and there appears to be no firm evidence that evening primrose oil should be avoided by epileptic patients. A case report describes raised lopinavir levels and persistent diarrhoea when evening primrose oil and a product containing aloes, rhubarb and liquorice were started.

Interactions monographs

- Antiplatelet drugs, page 207
- Food, page 207
- Herbal medicines, page 207
- Lopinavir, page 207
- NSAIDs, page 207
- Phenothiazines, page 208
- Warfarin and related drugs, page 208

1. Zou L, Harkey MR, Henderson GL. Effects of herbal components on cDNA-expressed cytochrome P450 enzyme catalytic activity. *Life Sci* (2002) 71, 1579–89.

Evening primrose oil + Antiplatelet drugs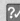

Evening primrose oil can inhibit platelet aggregation and increase bleeding time. It has therefore been suggested that it may have additive effects with other antiplatelet drugs, but evidence of this is generally lacking.

Clinical evidence

In 12 patients with hyperlipidaemia given evening primrose oil 3 g daily for 4 months, platelet aggregation decreased and bleeding time increased by 40%. The evening primrose oil was given in the form of six 500-mg soft-gel capsules and the daily dose contained **linoleic acid** 2.2 g and **gamolenic acid** 240 mg.[1]

Experimental evidence

Similar findings to the clinical study above have been reported in *animals* given evening primrose oil or **gamolenic acid**.[1,2]

Mechanism

Prostaglandin E_1 (which has antiplatelet properties) and thromboxane (which promotes platelet aggregation) are formed from gamolenic acid. Supplementing the diet with gamolenic acid has been shown to augment the production of prostaglandin E_1, and because prostaglandin E_1 is also preferentially formed (the conversion of gamolenic acid to thromboxane is slower), evening primrose oil could inhibit platelet aggregation. This effect could be additive with the effects of other antiplatelet drugs.

Importance and management

Information is limited to one clinical study, in which patients were not taking conventional antiplatelet drugs, and experimental data. Based on the potential antiplatelet effects of evening primrose oil, some authors[3] suggest that patients taking antiplatelet drugs should use evening primrose oil cautiously or not at all. This seems overly cautious because evening primrose oil is a widely used herbal product, and was formerly used as a prescription product in the UK, and clinical reports of an interaction have yet to come to light. Furthermore, the concurrent use of two conventional antiplatelet drugs is not uncommon.

1. Guivernau M, Meza N, Barja P, Roman O. Clinical and experimental study on the long-term effect of dietary gamma-linolenic acid on plasma lipids, platelet aggregation, thromboxane formation, and prostacyclin production. *Prostaglandins Leukot Essent Fatty Acids* (1994) 51, 311–16.
2. De La, Cruz JP, Martrn-Romero M, Carmona JA, Villalobos MA, Sánchez de la Cuesta F. Effect of evening primrose oil on platelet aggregation in rabbits fed an atherogenic diet. *Thromb Res* (1997) 87, 141–9.
3. Halat KM, Dennehy CE. Botanicals and Dietary Supplements in Diabetic Peripheral Neuropathy. *J Am Board Fam Pract* (2003) 16, 47–57.

Evening primrose oil + Food

No interactions found.

Evening primrose oil + Herbal medicines

No interactions found.

Evening primrose oil + Lopinavir

A case report describes raised lopinavir levels and persistent diarrhoea, which developed in an HIV-positive man after evening primrose oil and a product containing aloes, rhubarb and liquorice were started.

Clinical evidence

A case report[1] describes a 47-year-old HIV-positive man taking lopinavir boosted with ritonavir 533/133 mg twice daily, tenofovir 245 mg daily and lamivudine 150 mg twice daily who developed persistent diarrhoea (episodes occurring more than 5 times a day) and a raised lopinavir level of 15.2 mg/L (56% increase) after also taking *Efamol* (evening primrose oil), *Rheum frangula* [containing aloes, rhubarb, liquorice and peppermint] and *Colayur* (a bowel cleansing preparation). Lopinavir levels returned to baseline (within the normal range of 5 to 10 mg/L) six weeks after stopping all herbal preparations. The patient was re-challenged with *Efamol* for one week and his lopinavir level increased from 6.69 mg/L to 8.11 mg/L, with no adverse effects reported.

Experimental evidence

No relevant data found.

Mechanism

Unknown. The authors suggested that as evening primrose oil has been shown *in vitro* to inhibit the cytochrome P450 isoenzymes CYP3A4 and CYP2D6, which are involved in lopinavir metabolism, the raised levels may be a result of this inhibitory effect. However, evening primrose oil is only a minor inhibitor of these isoenzymes (see under *Pharmacokinetics*, page 206 for further information). Lopinavir commonly causes diarrhoea (and this may be associated with high levels), an effect that may be additive with the laxative properties of aloes, page 27, rhubarb, page 406 and liquorice, page 329, and the bowel cleansing product *Colayur*.

Importance and management

This is an isolated case report and as such no general recommendations can be made. However, evening primrose oil is unlikely to have clinically important effects as a result of cytochrome P450 isoenzyme inhibition and therefore an effect on lopinavir is unlikely. Nevertheless, patients taking drugs for serious conditions such as HIV-infection should carefully consider the risks and benefits of adding herbal medicines to their existing regimen, where the outcome of concurrent use is uncertain.

1. van den Bout-van den Beukel CJP, Bosch MEW, Burger DM, Koopmans PP, van der Ven AJAM. Toxic lopinavir concentrations in an HIV-1 infected patient taking herbal medications. *AIDS* (2008) 22, 1243–4.

Evening primrose oil + NSAIDs

The interaction between evening primrose oil and NSAIDs is based on a prediction only.

Evidence, mechanism, importance and management

Gamolenic acid, a major constituent of evening primrose oil, is a precursor of prostaglandin E_1, which inhibits the synthesis of tumour necrosis factor-alpha (which has an important effect in the inflammatory processes of rheumatoid arthritis). Supplementing the diet with **gamolenic acid** has been shown to augment the production of prostaglandin E_1, which has a rate-limiting step mediated by cyclooxygenase-2. Theoretically, the production of prostaglandin E_1, and therefore the anti-inflammatory effects of **gamolenic acid**, could be opposed by the concurrent use of NSAIDs because both selective and non-selective NSAIDs inhibit cyclooxygenase-2.[1] However, evening primrose oil is often used alongside conventional treatments for arthritis and two clinical studies found that high doses of **gamolenic acid** reduced pain and swelling of the joints of arthritic patients when given with usual

E

doses of NSAIDs. This theoretical interaction therefore appears to be of little clinical importance.[2,3]

1. Kast RE. Borage oil reduction of rheumatoid arthritis activity may be mediated by increased cAMP that suppresses tumor necrosis factor-alpha. *Int Immunopharmacol* (2001) 1, 2197–9.
2. Leventhal LJ, Boyce EG, Zurier RB. Treatment of rheumatoid arthritis with gammalinolenic acid. *Ann Intern Med* (1993) 119, 867–73.
3. Zurier RB, Rossetti RG, Jacobson EW, DeMarco DM, Liu NY, Temming JE, White BM, Laposata M. Gamma-linolenic acid treatment of rheumatoid arthritis. A randomized, placebo-controlled trial. *Arthritis Rheum* (1996) 39, 1808–17.

Evening primrose oil + Phenothiazines

Although seizures have occurred in a few schizophrenics taking phenothiazines and evening primrose oil, no adverse effects were seen in others, and there appears to be no firm evidence that evening primrose oil should be avoided by epileptic patients.

Clinical evidence

Twenty-three patients were enrolled in a placebo-controlled study of evening primrose oil in schizophrenia. During the treatment phase, patients were given 8 capsules of *Efamol* in addition to their normal medication. Seizures developed in 3 patients, one during treatment with placebo. The other two patients were taking evening primrose oil, one was receiving **fluphenazine decanoate** 50 mg once every 2 weeks and the other **fluphenazine decanoate** 25 mg once every 2 weeks with **thioridazine**, which was later changed to **chlorpromazine**.[1] In another study, 3 long-stay hospitalised schizophrenics were taking evening primrose oil. Their schizophrenia became much worse and all 3 patients showed EEG evidence of temporal lobe epilepsy.[2]

In contrast, no seizures or epileptiform events were reported in a crossover study in 48 patients (most of them schizophrenics) taking **phenothiazines** when they were given evening primrose oil for 4 months.[3] Concurrent use was also apparently uneventful in another study in schizophrenic patients.[4]

Experimental evidence

No relevant data found.

Mechanism

Not understood. One suggestion is that evening primrose oil possibly increases the well-recognised epileptogenic effects of the phenothiazines, rather than having an epileptogenic action of its own.[1] Another idea is that it might unmask temporal lobe epilepsy.[1,2]

Importance and management

The interaction between phenothiazines and evening primrose oil is not well established, nor is its incidence known, but clearly some caution is appropriate during concurrent use, because seizures may develop in a few individuals. There seems to be no way of identifying the patients at particular risk. The extent to which the underlying disease condition might affect what happens is also unclear.

No interaction between antiepileptics and evening primrose oil has been established and the reports cited above[1,2] appear to be the sole basis for the suggestion that evening primrose oil should be avoided by epileptics. No seizures appear to have been reported in patients taking evening primrose oil in the absence of phenoth-

iazines. One review,[5] analysing these two reports, goes as far as suggesting that formularies should now remove seizures or epilepsy as an adverse effect of evening primrose oil because the evidence for the seizures clearly point to the phenothiazines taken. Moreover, the manufacturers of *Epogam*, an evening primrose oil preparation, claim that it is known to have improved the control of epilepsy in patients previously uncontrolled with conventional antiepileptic drugs, and other patients are said to have had no problems during concurrent treatment.[6]

1. Holman CP, Bell AFJ. A trial of evening primrose oil in the treatment of chronic schizophrenia. *J Orthomol Psychiatry* (1983) 12, 302–4.
2. Vaddadi KS. The use of gamma-linolenic acid and linoleic acid to differentiate between temporal lobe epilepsy and schizophrenia. *Prostaglandins Med* (1981) 6, 375–9.
3. Vaddadi KS, Courtney P, Gilleard CJ, Manku MS, Horrobin DF. A double-blind trial of essential fatty acid supplementation in patients with tardive dyskinesia. *Psychiatry Res* (1989) 27, 313–23.
4. Vaddadi KS, Horrobin DF. Weight loss produced by evening primrose oil administration in normal and schizophrenic individuals. *IRCS Med Sci* (1979) 7, 52.
5. Puri BK. The safety of evening primrose oil in epilepsy. *Prostaglandins Leukot Essent Fatty Acids* (2007) 77, 101–3.
6. Scotia Pharmaceuticals Ltd. Personal communication. January 1991.

Evening primrose oil + Warfarin and related drugs

The information regarding the use of evening primrose oil with warfarin is based on experimental evidence only.

Clinical evidence

No interactions found.

Experimental evidence

In vitro, **cis**-linoleic acid was found to be a moderate inhibitor of the cytochrome P450 isoenzyme CYP2C9, which is the main isoenzyme involved in the metabolism of warfarin. However, it was 26-fold less potent than sulfaphenazole,[1] a drug known to have clinically relevant inhibitory effects on CYP2C9 *in vivo*.

Mechanism

Prostaglandin E_1 (which has antiplatelet properties) and thromboxane (which promotes platelet aggregation) are formed from gamolenic acid. Supplementing the diet with gamolenic acid has been shown to augment the production of prostaglandin E_1, and because prostaglandin E_1 is also preferentially formed (the conversion of gamolenic acid to thromboxane is slower), evening primrose oil could inhibit platelet aggregation. This effect could slightly increase the risk of bleeding with anticoagulants.

Importance and management

Evening primrose oil seems unlikely to alter the pharmacokinetics of warfarin. Other **coumarins** are metabolised by a similar route to warfarin, and are therefore also unlikely to be affected. However, based on the potential antiplatelet effects of evening primrose oil, some authors[2] suggest that patients taking anticoagulants should use evening primrose oil cautiously or not at all. This seems overly cautious because evening primrose oil is a widely used herbal product, and was formerly used as a prescription product in the UK, and clinical reports of an interaction have yet to come to light.

1. Zou L, Harkey MR, Henderson GL. Effects of herbal components on cDNA-expressed cytochrome P450 enzyme catalytic activity. *Life Sci* (2002) 71, 1579–89.
2. Halat KM, Dennehy CE. Botanicals and Dietary Supplements in Diabetic Peripheral Neuropathy. *J Am Board Fam Pract* (2003) 16, 47–57.

Fenugreek

Trigonella foenum-graecum L. (Fabaceae)

Synonym(s) and related species

Bird's foot, Bockshornsame, Foenugreek, Greek hay.

Not to be confused with Bird's foot trefoil, which is *Lotus corniculatus*.

Pharmacopoeias

Fenugreek (*PhEur 7.5*).

Constituents

Fenugreek seeds are about 25% protein (particularly lysine and tryptophan), and about 50% mucilaginous fibre. The seeds also contain **flavonoids** (luteolin, quercetin and vitexin). Saponins, natural coumarins and vitamins (nicotinic acid) are also present.

Use and indications

The seeds of fenugreek have been used as an appetite stimulant and for digestive disorders (including constipation, dyspepsia and gastritis). It has also been used in respiratory disorders and is said to be an expectorant. Topically, fenugreek has been used for wounds and leg ulcers, and as an emollient. It has been reported to have hypocholesterolaemic and hypoglycaemic activity.

Pharmacokinetics

No relevant pharmacokinetic data found. For information on the pharmacokinetics of individual flavonoids present in fenugreek, see under flavonoids, page 213.

Interactions overview

Fenugreek saponins may modestly enhance the antidiabetic effects of the sulfonylureas. For a case report describing a raised INR in a patient taking a herbal medicine containing boldo and fenugreek, see Boldo + Warfarin and related drugs, page 88. For information on the interactions of individual flavonoids present in fenugreek, see under flavonoids, page 213.

Interactions monographs

- Antidiabetics, page 210
- Food, page 210
- Herbal medicines, page 210

F

Fenugreek + Antidiabetics

In one study, fenugreek saponins had modest additional antidiabetic effects when they were added to established treatment with sulfonylureas.

Clinical evidence

Fenugreek seed appears to have been widely studied for its blood-glucose-lowering properties; however, studies on its effects in combination with conventional treatments for diabetes appear limited. In one randomised study,[1] 46 patients taking **sulfonylureas** (not named), with fasting blood-glucose levels of 7 to 13 mmol/L, were given **fenugreek saponins** 2.1 g three times daily after meals for 12 weeks. When compared with 23 similar patients given placebo it was found that **fenugreek saponins** decreased fasting blood-glucose levels by 23% (8.38 mmol/L versus 6.79 mmol/L). Diabetic control was also improved: glycosylated haemoglobin levels were about 20% lower in the treatment group (8.2% versus 6.56%). The **fenugreek saponin** preparation was an extract of total saponins of fenugreek given as capsules containing 0.35 mg per capsule, equivalent to 5.6 g of crude fenugreek.

Experimental evidence

The blood-glucose-lowering activity of fenugreek and its extracts has been well studied in *animal* models, however, there appears to be no data directly relating to interactions.

Mechanism

It is suggested that fenugreek decreases blood-glucose levels by affecting an insulin signalling pathway.

Importance and management

Evidence on the use of fenugreek with conventional antidiabetic medicines appears to be limited to this one study, which suggests that fenugreek may have some modest additional blood-glucose-lowering effects to those of the sulfonylureas. As these modest effects were apparent over a period of 12 weeks it seems unlikely that a dramatic hypoglycaemic effect will occur.

1. Lu F, Shen L, Qin Y, Gao L, Li H, Dai Y. Clinical observation on *Trigonella Foenumgraecum* L. total saponins in combination with sulfonylureas in the treatment of type 2 diabetes mellitus. *Chin J Integr Med* (2008) 14, 56–60.

Fenugreek + Food

No interactions found. Fenugreek is often used as a flavouring in foodstuffs.

Fenugreek + Herbal medicines

No interactions found.

Fenugreek + Warfarin and related drugs

For a case report describing a raised INR in a patient taking a herbal medicine containing boldo and fenugreek, see Boldo + Warfarin and related drugs, page 88.

Feverfew

Tanacetum parthenium Sch.Bip. (Asteraceae)

Synonym(s) and related species

Altamisa, Featherfew, Featherfoil, Midsummer daisy.

Chrysanthemum parthenium (L.) Bernh., *Leucanthemum parthenium* (L.) Gren & Godron, *Pyrethrum parthenium* (L.) Sm.

Not to be confused with Boneset (*Eupatorium perfoliatum*) or Centaury (*Centaurium erythraea*), which are both sometimes known as Feverwort.

Pharmacopoeias

Feverfew (*BP 2012, PhEur 7.5, USP35–NF30 S1*); Powdered feverfew (*USP35–NF30 S1*).

Constituents

The leaf and aerial parts contain sesquiterpene lactones, especially **parthenolide**, its esters and other derivatives, santamarin, reynosin, artemorin, partholide, chrysanthemonin and others. The volatile oil is composed mainly of α-pinene, bornyl acetate, bornyl angelate, costic acid, camphor and spirotekal ethers.

Use and indications

Feverfew is mainly used for the prophylactic treatment of migraine and tension headache, but it has antiplatelet and anti-inflammatory activity, and has been used for coughs, colds and rheumatic conditions. It can cause allergic and cytotoxic reactions due to the presence of sesquiterpene lactones with an α-methylene butyrolactone ring, as in parthenolide.

Pharmacokinetics

In a study investigating the *in vitro* inhibitory potency of an extract of feverfew using a commercially available mixture of cytochrome P450 isoenzymes, and established substrates of these isoenzymes, the feverfew extract modestly inhibited the activity of CYP1A2, CYP2C8, CYP2C9, CYP2C19 and CYP3A4.[1] The findings of *in vitro* studies cannot be directly extrapolated to humans, but positive findings such as these suggest that further study is required.

In an *in vitro* study, the transport of parthenolide, a constituent of feverfew, was not affected by the presence of MK-571, an inhibitor of P-glycoprotein.[2]

Interactions overview

Feverfew inhibits platelet aggregation *in vitro,* and theoretically, might increase the risk of bleeding in patients taking other drugs that increase bleeding such as aspirin or anticoagulants.

Interactions monographs

- Anticoagulants, page 212
- Antiplatelet drugs, page 212
- Food, page 212
- Herbal medicines, page 212

1. Unger M, Frank A. Simultaneous determination of the inhibitory potency if herbal extracts on the activity of six major cytochrome P450 enzymes using liquid chromatography/mass spectrometry and automated online extraction. *Rapid Commun Mass Spectrom* (2004) 18, 2273–81.
2. Khan SI, Abourashed EA, Khan IA, Walker LA. Transport of parthenolide across human intestinal cells (Caco-2). *Planta Med* (2003) 69, 1009–12.

F

Feverfew + Anticoagulants

The interaction between feverfew and anticoagulants is based on a prediction only.

Evidence, mechanism, importance and management

The manufacturer[1] advises that feverfew as a herbal medicine may theoretically interact with warfarin and increase the risk of bleeding on the basis of its *in vitro* antiplatelet effects (see Feverfew + Antiplatelet drugs, below). However, they note that the clinical relevance of this *in vivo* is unknown.[2] Some reviews also note this potential for an interaction and suggest that concurrent use should be avoided.[3] Clinically the use of an antiplatelet drug with an anticoagulant should generally be avoided in the absence of a specific indication. It may therefore be prudent to advise against concurrent use. However, if concurrent use is felt desirable, the risks and benefits of treatment should be considered. It would seem sensible to warn patients to be alert for any signs of bruising or bleeding, and report these immediately, should they occur.

1. Migraherb (Feverfew herb). MH Pharma (UK) Ltd. UK Summary of product characteristics, April 2007.
2. Schwabe Pharma (UK) Ltd. Personal communication. January 2009.
3. Heck AM, DeWitt BA, Lukes AL. Potential interactions between alternative therapies and warfarin. *Am J Health-Syst Pharm* (2000) 57, 1221–7.

Feverfew + Antiplatelet drugs

Feverfew inhibits platelet aggregation *in vitro*, and theoretically, might have additive effects with conventional antiplatelet drugs.

Clinical evidence

A letter briefly describes a study in which platelet aggregation was assessed in samples taken from 10 patients who had taken feverfew for at least 3.5 years. The platelets aggregated normally in response to thrombin and ADP; however, the response to serotonin and U46619 (a thromboxane mimetic) was attenuated, and only occurred at higher doses.[1]

Experimental evidence

In a number of early *in vitro* studies, mostly by the same research group, feverfew was found to inhibit platelet aggregation.[2–8] In these studies, feverfew extracts inhibited ADP, thrombin and collagen-induced platelet aggregation,[5–7] and inhibited the uptake[3] and release of arachidonic acid.[3,5,6] Parthenolide, a constituent of feverfew, has also been shown to inhibit platelet aggregation *in vitro*.[8]

Mechanism

Unclear. It was suggested that the mechanism of platelet inhibition is neutralisation of sulphahydryl groups within the platelets, although the exact sulphahydryl groups involved still need to be defined.[2]

Importance and management

There appears to be only one clinical study, which does not wholly substantiate the *in vitro* findings that feverfew inhibits platelet aggregation in response to certain chemical stimuli. However, the study does support the finding of somewhat reduced platelet responsiveness. It could be argued that any interaction should have come to light by now, since feverfew has been in fairly widespread use for the management of migraines, and, in this setting, it is likely to have been taken with aspirin and NSAIDs. On the other hand, the small increased risk of bleeding with low-dose aspirin has required very large retrospective comparisons to establish. Concurrent use need not be avoided (indeed combinations of antiplatelet drugs are often prescribed together) but it may be prudent to be aware of the potential for increased bleeding if feverfew is given with other antiplatelet drugs such as aspirin and clopidogrel. Patients should discuss any episode of prolonged bleeding with a healthcare professional.

1. Biggs MJ, Johnson ES, Persaud NP, Ratcliffe DM. Platelet aggregation in patients using feverfew for migraine. *Lancet* (1982) 2, 776.
2. Heptinstall S, Groenewegen WA, Spangenberg P, Lösche W. Inhibition of platelet behaviour by feverfew: a mechanism of action involving sulphydryl groups. *Folia Haematol Int Mag Klin Morphol Blutforsch* (1988) 115 (Suppl), 447–9.
3. Loesche W, Groenewegen WA, Krause S, Spangenberg P, Heptinstall S. Effects of an extract of feverfew (Tanacetum parthenium) on arachidonic acid metabolism in human blood platelets. *Biomed Biochim Acta* (1988) 47 (Suppl), S241–S243.
4. Loesche W, Mazurov AV, Voyno-Yasenetskaya TA, Groenewegen WA, Heptinstall S, Repin VS. Feverfew - an antithrombotic drug? *Folia Haematol Int Mag Klin Morphol Blutforsch* (1988) 115 (Suppl), 181–4.
5. Makheja AN, Bailey JM. A platelet phospholipase inhibitor from the medicinal herb feverfew (Tanacetum parthenium). *Prostaglandins Leukot Med* (1982) 8, 653–60.
6. Heptinstall S, White A, Williamson L, Mitchell JR. Extracts of feverfew inhibit granule secretion in blood platelets and polymorphonuclear leucocytes. *Lancet* (1985) 1, 1071–4.
7. Lösche W, Mazurov AV, Heptinstall S, Groenewegen WA, Repin VS, Till U. An extract of feverfew inhibits interactions of human platelets with collagen substrates. *Thromb Res* (1987) 48, 511–18.
8. Groenewegen WA, Heptinstall S. A comparison of the effects of an extract of feverfew and parthenolide, a component of feverfew, on human platelet activity in-vitro. *J Pharm Pharmacol* (1990) 42, 553–7.

Feverfew + Food

No interactions found.

Feverfew + Herbal medicines

No interactions found.

Flavonoids

Bioflavonoids

The flavonoids are a large complex group of related compounds, which are widely available in the form of dietary supplements, as well as in the herbs or foods they are originally derived from. They are the subject of intensive investigations and new information is constantly being published.

You may have come to this monograph via a herb that contains flavonoids. Note that the information in this general monograph relates to the individual flavonoids, and the reader is referred back to the herb (and *vice versa*) where appropriate. It is very difficult to confidently predict whether a herb that contains one of the flavonoids mentioned will interact in the same way. The levels of the flavonoid in the particular herb can vary a great deal between specimens, related species, extracts and brands, and it is important to take this into account when viewing the interactions described below.

Types, sources and related compounds

Flavonoids are a very large family of polyphenolic compounds synthesised by plants that are common and widely distributed. With the exception of the flavanols (e.g. catechins) and their polymers, the proanthocyanidins, they usually occur naturally bound to one or more sugar molecules (flavonoid glycosides) rather than as the free aglycones. The sub-groups of flavonoids, their main representatives, and their principal sources are as follows:

- *Flavones:* e.g. apigenin, luteolin; found in celery, page 138, and parsley, page 363. The rind of citrus fruits is rich in the polymethoxylated flavones, tangeretin (from tangerine), nobiletin, and sinensetin.
- *Flavonols:* e.g. **quercetin**, **kaempferol**, myricetin, isorhamnetin; widely distributed in berries, teas, broccoli, apples and onions. **Rutin** (sophorin), also known as quercetin-3-rutinoside is a common glycoside of quercetin; other glycosides include quercitrin, baicalin, and hyperin. **Morin** is a flavonol found in *Morus* species.
- *Flavanones:* e.g. hesperetin (from oranges), naringenin (from grapefruit), eriodictyol (from lemons); and their glycosides, hesperidin, **naringin**, and eriocitrin. They are most concentrated in the membranes separating the fruit segments and the white spongy part of the peel. Flavanone glycosides are often present in supplements as **citrus bioflavonoids**.
- *Flavanols (Flavan-3-ols):* monomers, e.g. **catechins** and gallic acid esters of catechins, **epicatechins** and gallic acid esters of epicatechins; found in teas, page 463, (particularly green and white), cocoa, page 156, grapes, berries, and apples. *Dimers* e.g. **theaflavins** and gallic acid esters of theaflavins, and thearubigins also found in teas, page 463, (particularly

black and oolong). **Proanthocyanidins** are polymers of flavanols, also known as condensed tannins, the most frequent being **procyanidins** (polymers of catechin and epicatechin). Found widely in cocoa, page 156, some berries and nuts, hops, page 293 and grapeseed, page 274.
- *Anthocyanins:* e.g. cyanidin, delphinidin, malvidin, pelargonidin, peonidin, and petunidin; found widely in chocolate, apples, red, blue and purple berries, red and purple grapes, and red wine.
- *Isoflavones (Isoflavonoids):* are a distinct group of flavonoids with phytoestrogenic effects and are considered elsewhere, see isoflavones, page 300.

Use and indications

Some prospective cohort studies show that a high dietary intake of flavonoid-rich foods is associated with a reduced risk of coronary heart disease,[1,2] but not all show this effect.[3] Other cohort and case-control studies show a reduced risk of some cancers.[4] However, there do not appear to be any studies to show whether isolated flavonoid supplements confer similar benefits to flavonoid-rich foods.

Many beneficial properties have been identified for flavonoids; one of the most popularly cited being their antioxidant activity. Other actions that are proposed to contribute to their biological effects include chelating metal ions, stimulating phase II detoxifying enzyme activity, inhibiting proliferation and inducing apoptosis, reducing inflammation, decreasing vascular cell adhesion molecule expression, increasing endothelial nitric oxide synthase (eNOS) activity, and inhibiting platelet aggregation.

Pharmacokinetics

The bioavailability of flavonoids is relatively low due to limited absorption and rapid elimination, and they are generally rapidly and extensively metabolised.[5,6] Flavonoid esters, glycosides or polymers require hydrolysis to the free aglycone before absorption, and this occurs by intestinal enzymes (e.g. beta-glucosidases) and colonic bacteria. During absorption, the aglycone is then conjugated by sulfation, glucuronidation or methylation. These conjugates are excreted back into the intestine by efflux pumps. Those absorbed are eventually excreted in the urine and bile, and may undergo enterohepatic recycling.[5,6] It appears that metabolism of flavonoids by cytochrome P450 isoenzymes is probably minor compared to conjugation reactions for flavonoids.[5]

The potential for flavonoids to alter drug metabolism by cytochrome P450 isoenzymes, in particular, and also intestinal and hepatic drug transporters, such as P-glycoprotein, has been extensively investigated *in vitro*.[5,7] There are also

F

some *animal* studies, but few human clinical pharmacokinetic studies, and those that are available have generally used very high doses of the flavonoids.

There is at present no reason to avoid flavonoids in the diet, or in the form of herbal medicines (most of which contain significant amounts of flavonoids naturally), and many positive reasons for including them. However, *very high* doses (such as the use of specific flavonoid supplements) could potentially alter the metabolism of other drugs that are substrates for CYP3A4 and/or P-glycoprotein, or OATP1B1, and increase or decrease the bioavailability of some drugs; for instance the statins, page 221; ciclosporin, page 217; benzodiazepines, page 216, such as midazolam; and digoxin, page 218.

Interactions overview

The interactions covered in this monograph relate to individual flavonoids. It may be possible to directly extrapolate some of these interactions to some flavonoid supplements, especially those regarding quercetin; however, caution must be taken when applying these interactions to herbs or foods known to contain the flavonoid in question. This is because the amount of the flavonoid found in the herb or food must be considered (this can be highly variable, and might not be known) and the other constituents present in the herb or food might affect the bioavailability or activity of the flavonoid (information that is usually unknown). Therefore, although data on isolated flavonoids is useful, it is no substitute for direct studies of the herb, food or dietary supplement in question.

Interactions monographs

- Aciclovir, page 215, (with quercetin)
- Antibacterials, page 215, (with baicalein or chrysin)
- Anticoagulant or Antiplatelet drugs, page 215, (with apigenin, flavanols, procyanidins or quercetin)
- Benzodiazepines, page 216, (with baicalin, hesperidin, kaempferol, naringenin, quercetin or tangeretin)
- Caffeine, page 216, (with naringin or naringenin)
- Calcium-channel blockers, page 216, (with morin, naringin or quercetin)
- Ciclosporin, page 217, (with baicalein, baicalin, morin or quercetin)
- Digoxin, page 218, (with quercetin or kaempferol)
- Enalapril, page 218, (with kaempferol or naringenin)
- Etoposide, page 218, (with morin or quercetin)
- Fexofenadine, page 219, (with hesperidin, naringin or quercetin)
- Food; Milk, page 219, (with catechins, kaempferol or quercetin)
- Herbal medicines, page 219
- Irinotecan or Topotecan, page 219, (with chrysin)
- Paclitaxel, page 220, (with morin, naringin or quercetin)
- Quinine or Quinidine, page 220, (with baicalin, kaempferol, naringenin, naringin or quercetin)
- Rosiglitazone, page 220, (with quercetin)
- Saquinavir, page 221, (with quercetin)
- Statins, page 221, (with apigenin, baicalin, kaempferol or naringenin or quercetin)
- Tamoxifen, page 221, (with catechins, quercetin or tangeretin)

1. Huxley RR, Neil HAW. The relation between dietary flavonol intake and coronary heart disease mortality: a meta-analysis of prospective cohort studies. *Eur J Clin Nutr* (2003) 57, 904–8.
2. Mink PJ, Scrafford CG, Barraj LM, Harnack L, Hong CP, Nettleton JA, Jacobs DR. Flavonoid intake and cardiovascular disease mortality: a prospective study in postmenopausal women. *Am J Clin Nutr* (2007) 85, 895–909.
3. Lin J, Rexrode KM, Hu F, Albert CM, Chae CU, Rimm EB, Stampfer MJ, Manson JE. Dietary Intakes of Flavonols and Flavones and Coronary Heart Disease in US Women. *Am J Epidemiol* (2007) 165, 1305–13.
4. Neuhouser ML. Dietary flavonoids and cancer risk: evidence from human population studies. *Nutr Cancer* (2004) 50, 1–7.
5. Cermak R, Wolffram S. The potential of flavonoids to influence drug metabolism and pharmacokinetics by local gastrointestinal mechanisms. *Curr Drug Metab* (2006) 7, 729–44.
6. Manach C, Scalbert A, Morand C, Remesy C, Jimenez L. Polyphenols: food sources and bioavailability. *Am J Clin Nutr* (2004) 79, 727–47.
7. Morris ME, Zhang S. Flavonoid-drug interactions: effects of flavonoids on ABC transporters. *Life Sci* (2006) 78, 2116–30.

F

Flavonoids + Aciclovir

The interaction between quercetin and aciclovir is based on experimental evidence only.

Evidence, mechanism, importance and management

Findings from an *in vitro* study suggest that **quercetin** might modestly increase the absorption of oral aciclovir by inhibiting intestinal P-glycoprotein. The effect of high-dose **quercetin** (80 mg/L) was equivalent to that of verapamil 10 mg/L,[1] which is an established, clinically relevant, inhibitor of P-glycoprotein. However, because aciclovir has a wide therapeutic index, even if this change is seen in practice, it is unlikely to be clinically important.

1. Yang ZG, Meng H, Zhang X, Li XD, Lv WL, Zhang Q. Effect of quercetin on the acyclovir intestinal absorption. *Beijing Da Xue Xue Bao* (2004) 36, 309–12.

Flavonoids + Antibacterials

The interaction between flavonoids and antibacterials is based on experimental evidence only.

Evidence, mechanism, importance and management

(a) Aminoglycosides

In a study, *rats* were given either the aglycone **baicalein** or the parent flavone **baicalin** orally. The bioavailability of **baicalein** from the parent flavone was reduced from 28% to about 8% in *rats* given **neomycin** and **streptomycin**, when compared with *rats* not given these antibacterials, but the antibacterials did not affect the bioavailability of administered **baicalein**.[1]

These antibacterials decimate colonic bacteria, which are involved in the hydrolysis of **baicalin** to **baicalein**. This study used the combination of **neomycin** and **streptomycin** because previous research had shown that this combination was most effective in reducing intestinal microflora, and that a single aminoglycoside did not have this effect.[1]

These findings are likely to have little clinical relevance, because individuals are rarely given combinations of aminoglycosides with such potent effects on colonic microflora. It would be of use to know the effect of standard broad-spectrum antibacterials in general clinical use. However, even these are only given for short courses, so any reduction in the effect of the flavonoid would be short-lived.

(b) Nitrofurantoin

In a study in *rats,* oral administration of high-dose **chrysin** 200 mg/kg increased the AUC of nitrofurantoin by about 76% and decreased its clearance by 42%, whereas low-dose **chrysin** 50 mg/kg had no effect on the pharmacokinetics of nitrofurantoin.[2]

Available evidence[2] suggests that **chrysin** increases the AUC of nitrofurantoin by inhibition of the transporter protein BCRP.

The doses used in this study were much greater than those likely to be encountered clinically, and therefore these data suggest that even high doses of **chrysin** used as dietary supplements (e.g. 3 g daily) are unlikely to have a clinically important effect on nitrofurantoin pharmacokinetics.

1. Xing J, Chen X, Sun Y, Luan Y, Zhong D. Interaction of baicalin and baicalein with antibiotics in the gastrointestinal tract. *J Pharm Pharmacol* (2005) 57, 743–50.
2. Wang X, Morris ME. Effects of the flavonoid chrysin on nitrofurantoin pharmacokinetics in rats: potential involvement of ABCG2. *Drug Metab Dispos* (2007) 35, 268–74.

Flavonoids + Anticoagulant or Antiplatelet drugs

The interaction between flavonoids and anticoagulant or antiplatelet drugs is based on a prediction only.

Clinical evidence

There are few clinical studies investigating whether the *in vitro* antiplatelet effect of flavonoids occurs in humans, and whether this effect could be clinically relevant, and findings are not consistent. Some studies are cited in the following section as examples to illustrate the differences.

Antiplatelet effects

In one randomised controlled study, a cocoa supplement (234 mg of **cocoa flavanols** and **procyanidins** daily) given for 28 days decreased collagen- and ATP-induced platelet aggregation when compared with placebo.[1] Similarly, onion soup high in **quercetin** (one 'dose' of about 69 mg) inhibited collagen-stimulated platelet aggregation.[2] However, in another study, neither dietary supplementation with onions 220 g daily (providing **quercetin** 114 mg daily) nor parsley 4.9 g daily (providing **apigenin** 84 mg daily) for 7 days affected platelet aggregation or other haemostatic variables.[3] Similarly, a supplement containing **quercetin** 1 g daily and other flavonoids did not affect platelet aggregation in a placebo-controlled study in healthy subjects.[4]

In a single-dose study in healthy subjects, a **flavanol**-rich **cocoa** beverage (897 mg total flavonoids in 300 mL) had a similar, but less marked, effect than aspirin 81 mg on epinephrine-stimulated platelet activation and function. The effect of the cocoa beverage and aspirin appeared to be additive.[5]

Experimental evidence

Numerous *in vitro* studies show that many flavonoids, and **flavanols** and **procyanidin** oligomers in particular, inhibit platelet aggregation,[6] and this has been suggested as a mechanism to explain why some epidemiological studies show that a diet high in flavonoids is associated with a reduced risk of cardiovascular disease.

Mechanism

Flavonoids might have antiplatelet effects, which, if confirmed, could be additive with other antiplatelet drugs. In addition, they might increase the risk of bleeding when used with anticoagulants.

Importance and management

There is a large amount of information regarding an interaction between flavonoids and antiplatelet drugs, but an interaction is not established. There is a well-established small increased risk of bleeding when aspirin at antiplatelet doses is combined with the anticoagulant drug warfarin. Theoretically, very high intakes of flavonoids (e.g. from supplements) might have similar clinically important antiplatelet effects, and could therefore increase the risk of bleeding when taken with any anticoagulant drug, and have additive effects with antiplatelet drugs. However, available evidence is conflicting, with some studies showing that a number of flavonoids have antiplatelet effects and others finding no antiplatelet effects. Until more is known, some caution might be appropriate with high-doses of flavonoid supplements. In practice this would mean being aware of an increased risk of bleeding, and patients being alert for symptoms of bleeding, such as petechiae and bruising. Modest doses of flavonoids are unlikely to cause any problems.

1. Murphy KJ, Chronopoulos AK, Singh I, Francis MA, Moriarty H, Pike MJ, Turner AH, Mann NJ, Sinclair AJ. Dietary flavanols and procyanidin oligomers from cocoa (*Theobroma cacao*) inhibit platelet function. *Am J Clin Nutr* (2003) 77, 1466–73.
2. Hubbard GP, Wolffram S, de Vos R, Bovy A, Gibbins JM, Lovegrove JA. Ingestion of onion soup high in quercetin inhibits platelet aggregation and essential components of the collagen-stimulated platelet activation pathway in man: a pilot study. *Br J Nutr* (2006) 96, 482–8.

F

3. Janssen K, Mensink RP, Cox FJJ, Harryvan JL, Hovenier R, Hollman PCH, Katan MB. Effects of the flavonoids quercetin and apigenin on hemostasis in healthy volunteers: results from an in vitro and a dietary supplement study. *Am J Clin Nutr* (1998) 67, 255–62.
4. Conquer JA, Maiani G, Azzini E, Raguzzini A, Holub BJ. Supplementation with quercetin markedly increases plasma quercetin concentration without effect on selected risk factors for heart disease in healthy subjects. *J Nutr* (1998) 128, 593–7.
5. Pearson DA, Paglieroni TG, Rein D, Wun T, Schramm DD, Wang JF, Holt RR, Gosselin R, Schmitz HH, Keen CL. The effects of flavanol-rich cocoa and aspirin on ex vivo platelet function. *Thromb Res* (2002) 106, 191–7.
6. Nardini M, Natella F, Scaccini C. Role of dietary polyphenols in platelet aggregation. A review of the supplementation studies. *Platelets* (2007) 18, 224–43.

Flavonoids + Benzodiazepines

In a study, tangerine juice, containing tangeretin, did not affect the pharmacokinetics of midazolam. However, grapefruit juice, which contains different flavonoids, does increase levels of some benzodiazepines.

Clinical evidence

In a crossover study in 8 healthy subjects, **tangerine juice** (which contains the flavone **tangeretin**) 100 mL, given 15 minutes before and with a single 15-mg dose of oral **midazolam**, had no effect on the AUC and elimination of midazolam. The only change was a slight delay in midazolam absorption.[1]

Note that grapefruit juice (a rich source of flavonoids) has a well-established inhibitory effect on the metabolism of some benzodiazepines, resulting in increased exposure (1.5- to 3.5-fold increase in AUC).

Experimental evidence

(a) Anxiolytic effect

In various *animal* models, the anxiolytic effects were additive for **diazepam** and **baicalin**,[2] and synergistic for **diazepam** and **hesperidin**.[3]

(b) Pharmacokinetics

In vitro, **tangeretin** (a flavone from tangerine) stimulated the hydroxylation of **midazolam** in human liver microsomes.[1] Conversely, in another study, **quercetin** was found to be an inhibitor of the metabolism of **midazolam**, with **kaempferol** and **naringenin** also having some effect.[4]

Mechanism

Theoretically, flavonoids might inhibit the metabolism of some benzodiazepines by the cytochrome P450 isoenzyme CYP3A4 (note that not all benzodiazepines are metabolised by this route). Some flavonoids have anxiolytic properties in *animal* models.

Importance and management

Contrary to what was predicted from *in vitro* studies using tangeretin, a single dose of tangerine juice did not appear to alter the pharmacokinetics of midazolam. In contrast, grapefruit juice, which contains different flavonoids, does increase levels of some calcium-channel blockers, but studies with the flavonoid **naringin**, have found no interaction, suggesting that naringin is not the primary active constituent of grapefruit juice (see calcium-channel blockers, below). Therefore individual flavonoids might *not* be anticipated to increase benzodiazepine levels. Furthermore, although evidence is preliminary, it is possible that high doses of some individual flavonoids such as hesperidin and baicalin might have additive anxiolytic effects with benzodiazepines, suggesting a possible pharmacodynamic interaction.

This suggests that, until more is known, some caution might be appropriate if citrus bioflavonoids are used with benzodiazepines, bearing in mind the possibility of increased benzodiazepine effects.

1. Backman JT, Mäenpää J, Belle DJ, Wrighton SA, Kivistö KT, Neuvonen PJ. Lack of correlation between in vitro and in vivo studies on the effects of tangeretin and tangerine juice on midazolam hydroxylation. *Clin Pharmacol Ther* (2000) 67, 382–90.
2. Xu Z, Wang F, Tsang SY, Ho KH, Zheng H, Yuen CT, Chow CY, Xue H. Anxiolytic-like effect of baicalin and its additivity with other anxiolytics. *Planta Med* (2006) 72, 189–92.
3. Fernández SP, Wasowski C, Paladini AC, Marder M. Synergistic interaction between hesperidin, a natural flavonoid, and diazepam. *Eur J Pharmacol* (2005) 512, 189–98.
4. Ha HR, Chen J, Leuenberger PM, Freiburghaus AU, Follath F. In vitro inhibition of midazolam and quinidine metabolism by flavonoids. *Eur J Clin Pharmacol* (1995) 48, 367–71.

Flavonoids + Caffeine

Naringin does not appear to affect the pharmacokinetics of caffeine.

Clinical evidence

In a crossover study in 10 healthy subjects, changes in caffeine pharmacokinetics and physiological responses (resting energy expenditure, oxygen consumption, and respiratory exchange ratio), were measured after an acute dose of caffeine 200 mg with or without **naringin** 100 or 200 mg. **Naringin** did not alter either the pharmacokinetics of caffeine or the physiological responses to caffeine.[1] Note that grapefruit juice (which is a rich source of flavonoids) either does not interact with caffeine,[2] or causes only clinically irrelevant increases in caffeine levels.[3]

Experimental evidence

In contrast to the clinical findings, *in vitro* evidence suggests that grapefruit juice and **naringenin** inhibit CYP1A2 activity in human liver microsomes.[3] Nevertheless, it is not unusual for *in vitro* effects to be less marked or not apparent when studied in humans.

Mechanism

Although *in vitro* studies[3] have suggested that grapefruit juice and one of its constituents, naringenin, may inhibit the metabolism of caffeine by the cytochrome P450 isoenzyme CYP1A2, this does not appear to occur in humans.

Importance and management

Although some of the data is conflicting, the balance of evidence suggests that flavonoids such as naringin would not be expected to alter the effects of caffeine or other substrates of CYP1A2 by a pharmacokinetic mechanism.

1. Ballard TL, Halaweish FT, Stevermer CL, Agrawal P, Vukovich MD. Naringin does not alter caffeine pharmacokinetics, energy expenditure, or cardiovascular haemodynamics in humans following caffeine consumption. *Clin Exp Pharmacol Physiol* (2006) 33, 310–314.
2. Maish WA, Hampton EM, Whitsett TL, Shepard JD, Lovallo WR. Influence of grapefruit juice on caffeine pharmacokinetics and pharmacodynamics. *Pharmacotherapy* (1996) 16, 1046–52.
3. Fuhr U, Klittich K, Staib AH. Inhibitory effect of grapefruit juice and its bitter principal, naringenin, on CYP1A2 dependent metabolism of caffeine in man. *Br J Clin Pharmacol* (1993) 35, 431–6.

Flavonoids + Calcium-channel blockers

Supplements of specific citrus bioflavonoids do not appear to affect the pharmacokinetics of calcium-channel blockers to a clinically relevant extent.

Clinical evidence

(a) Felodipine

In a crossover study in 9 healthy subjects, 200 mL of an aqueous solution of **naringin** 450 micrograms/mL had no effect on the mean AUC of a single 5-mg dose of felodipine. This contrasted with the effect of 200 mL of **grapefruit juice** (determined to have the same **naringin** level), which doubled the AUC of felodipine.[1] In another study, in 12 healthy subjects, the liquid fraction (after centrifugation and filtration) of **grapefruit juice**, which contained **naringin** 148 mg, had *less* effect on the AUC of felodipine than the particulate fraction (the sediment after centrifugation, which contained 7 mg of **naringin**; 20-fold less). The AUC of felodipine increased by about 50% with the liquid fraction and by about 100% with the particulate fraction.[2]

(b) Nifedipine

In a crossover study in 8 healthy subjects, high-dose **quercetin** 200 mg given the night before, 100 mg given on waking, and 100 mg given with nifedipine 10 mg, had no effect on the AUC of nifedipine. This contrasted with the effect of 200 mL of double-strength **grapefruit juice** (a rich source of flavonoids), which increased the AUC of nifedipine by about 50%.[3]

(c) Nisoldipine

In a crossover study in 12 healthy subjects, the AUC of a single 20-mg dose of nisoldipine was not altered by **naringin** 185 mg (given simultaneously), but was increased by 75% by 250 mL of **grapefruit juice** (a rich source of flavonoids).[4]

Experimental evidence

One research group has extensively investigated the effects of various flavonoids on the pharmacokinetics of various oral calcium-channel blockers in *rats* and *rabbits*.[5–10] In these studies, the flavonoids tested (**morin, naringin, quercetin**) caused dose-dependent increases in the AUC of **diltiazem** (30 to 120%),[5,6] **nimodipine** (47 to 77%),[7] and **verapamil** (27 to 72%).[8–10] No effect was seen on the elimination half-life. An interaction occurred when the flavonoid was given 30 minutes before the calcium-channel blocker, but not when it was given simultaneously.[7,10]

Mechanism

The increased bioavailability of calcium-channel blockers in *animals* pretreated with morin, naringin or quercetin may result from inhibition of P-glycoprotein and the cytochrome P450 isoenzyme CYP3A4. However, no individual flavonoids have had any effect on the bioavailability of calcium-channel blockers in humans. It is probable that furanocoumarins are more important for the grapefruit interaction in humans,[11] see also Natural coumarins + Felodipine, page 359.

Importance and management

Experimental evidence for an interaction is extensive, but less is known about any interaction between flavonoids and calcium-channel blockers in humans. In contrast to the effect of grapefruit juice, no individual flavonoid has had any effect on the pharmacokinetics of a calcium-channel blocker in clinical studies (naringin with felodipine, quercetin with nifedipine, naringin with nisoldipine). Although, high doses of these flavonoids have increased levels of several calcium-channel blockers in *animals*, the clinical data seems to suggest that this is not applicable to humans. Supplements of specific citrus bioflavonoids are therefore unlikely to interact with calcium-channel blockers; however, an interaction might occur with extracts of grapefruit if these contain constituents other than just the flavonoids (e.g. furanocoumarins such as bergamottin). Consider also Grapefruit + Calcium-channel blockers, page 272.

1. Bailey DG, Arnold JMO, Munoz C, Spence JD. Grapefruit juice-felodipine interaction: mechanism, predictability, and effect of naringin. *Clin Pharmacol Ther* (1993) 53, 637–42.
2. Bailey DG, Kreeft JH, Munoz C, Freeman DJ, Bend JR. Grapefruit juice-felodipine interaction: effect of naringin and 6',7'-dihydroxybergamottin in humans. *Clin Pharmacol Ther* (1998) 64, 248–56.
3. Rashid J, McKinstry C, Renwick AG, Dirnhuber M, Waller DG, George CF. Quercetin, an *in vitro* inhibitor of CYP3A, does not contribute to the interaction between nifedipine and grapefruit juice. *Br J Clin Pharmacol* (1993) 36, 460–463.
4. Bailey DG, Arnold JMO, Strong HA, Munoz C, Spence JD. Effect of grapefruit juice and naringin on nisoldipine pharmacokinetics. *Clin Pharmacol Ther* (1993) 54, 589–94.
5. Choi J-S, Han H-K. Pharmacokinetic interaction between diltiazem and morin, a flavonoid, in rats. *Pharmacol Res* (2005) 52, 386–91.
6. Choi J-S, Han H-K. Enhanced oral exposure of diltiazem by the concomitant use of naringin in rats. *Int J Pharm* (2005) 305, 122–8.
7. Choi JS, Burm JP. Enhanced nimodipine bioavailability after oral administration of nimodipine with morin, a flavonoid, in rabbits. *Arch Pharm Res* (2006) 29, 333–8.
8. Yeum C-H, Choi J-S. Effect of naringin pretreatment on bioavailability of verapamil in rabbits. *Arch Pharm Res* (2006) 29, 102–7.
9. Kim HJ, Choi JS. Effects of naringin on the pharmacokinetics of verapamil and one of its metabolites, norverapamil, in rabbits. *Biopharm Drug Dispos* (2005) 26, 295–300.
10. Choi J-S, Han H-K. The effect of quercetin on the pharmacokinetics of verapamil and its major metabolite, norverapamil, in rabbits. *J Pharm Pharmacol* (2004) 56, 1537–42.
11. Bailey DG, Dresser GK, Kreeft JH, Munoz C, Freeman DJ, Bend JR. Grapefruit-felodipine interaction: effect of unprocessed fruit and probable active ingredients. *Clin Pharmacol Ther* (2000) 68, 468–77.

Flavonoids + Ciclosporin

A study found that quercetin increased the bioavailability of ciclosporin.

Clinical evidence

In a study in 8 healthy subjects, a single 300-mg dose of ciclosporin was given four times: alone, with oral **quercetin** 5 mg/kg, 30 minutes after oral **quercetin** 5 mg/kg, or after a 3-day course of **quercetin** 5 mg/kg twice daily. It was found that the AUC of ciclosporin was *increased* by 16% when given with a single dose of **quercetin**, by 36% when given after single-dose **quercetin**, and by 46% when given after multiple-dose **quercetin**.[1]

Experimental evidence

(a) Nephrotoxicity

There are some data suggesting that flavonoids might reduce the renal toxicity of ciclosporin. For example, in one study in *rats*, **quercetin** given with ciclosporin for 21 days attenuated the renal impairment and morphological changes (such as interstitial fibrosis), when compared with ciclosporin alone.[2]

(b) Pharmacokinetics

In contrast to the clinical evidence above, in an *animal* study, giving single doses of oral ciclosporin with **quercetin** 50 mg/kg resulted in a 43% and 42% *decrease* in the AUC of ciclosporin in *rats* and *pigs,* respectively (note, this did not reach statistical significance in *pigs*).[3] In a further study in *rats,* onion (which is a rich source of **quercetin**) caused a 68% reduction in the levels of ciclosporin given orally, but had no effect on the AUC of ciclosporin given intravenously.[4]

Similarly, in another study, **morin** decreased levels of ciclosporin in blood by a modest 33%, and also decreased levels in other tissues (by 17% to 45%). However, despite this reduction, the ciclosporin-suppressed Th1 immune response was not reduced by **morin**.[5]

In yet another study, the individual flavonoids **baicalin** and **baicalein** markedly *increased* ciclosporin levels in *rats,* whereas the root of baical skullcap, which contains these flavonoids, *decreased* the AUC of ciclosporin by up to 82%.[6] In *rats,* ciclosporin halved the AUC of **baicalin** in blood, and increased its levels in bile by about 60%.[7]

Mechanism

Flavonoids might affect ciclosporin levels by their effects on P-glycoprotein or the cytochrome P450 isoenzyme CYP3A4. In *animal* studies both increased and decreased levels have been seen.[3–6]

Importance and management

Evidence for an interaction between flavonoids and ciclosporin is largely limited to experimental data. In the one clinical study, high-dose quercetin modestly increased ciclosporin levels. The interaction is not sufficiently severe to suggest that concurrent use should be avoided; however, it may make ciclosporin levels less stable as the quercetin content of different herbs and preparations is likely to vary. Concurrent use may therefore be undesirable. If concurrent use of ciclosporin and a quercetin-containing product is undertaken it should be monitored well.

In *animal* studies, both increases and decreases in ciclosporin levels have been seen with individual flavonoids. Until more is

F

known, it may be prudent to be cautious with any flavonoid supplement and ciclosporin, especially those containing high doses. Although the reduced nephrotoxicity is interesting, this has to be viewed in the context of possible adverse pharmacokinetic interactions.

1. Choi JS, Choi BC, Choi KE. Effect of quercetin on the pharmacokinetics of oral cyclosporine. *Am J Health-Syst Pharm* (2004) 61, 2406–9.
2. Satyanarayana PSV, Singh D, Chopra K. Quercetin, a bioflavonoid, protects against oxidative stress-related renal dysfunction by cyclosporine in rats. *Methods Find Exp Clin Pharmacol* (2001) 23, 175–81.
3. Hsiu S-L, Hou Y-C, Wang Y-H, Tsao C-W, Su S-F, Chao P-DL. Quercetin significantly decreased cyclosporin oral bioavailability in pigs and rats. *Life Sci* (2002) 72, 227–35.
4. Yang C-H, Chao PDL, Hou YC, Tsai SY, Wen KC, Hsiu SL. Marked decrease of cyclosporin bioavailability caused by coadministration of ginkgo and onion in rats. *Food Chem Toxicol* (2006) 44, 1572–8.
5. Fang S-H, Hou Y-C, Chao P-DL. Pharmacokinetic and pharmacodynamic interactions of morin and cyclosporin. *Toxicol Appl Pharmacol* (2005) 205, 65–70.
6. Lai M-Y, Hsiu S-L, Hou Y-C, Tsai S-Y, Chao P-DL. Significant decrease of cyclosporine bioavailability in rats caused by a decoction of the roots of *Scutellaria baicalensis*. *Planta Med* (2004) 70, 132–7.
7. Tsai P-L, Tsai T-H. Pharmacokinetics of baicalin in rats and its interactions with cyclosporin A, quinidine and SKF-525A: a microdialysis study. *Planta Med* (2004) 70, 1069–74.

Flavonoids + Digoxin

The interaction between flavonoids and digoxin is based on experimental evidence only.

Clinical evidence

No interactions found.

Experimental evidence

In a study in *pigs*, three *animals* were given digoxin 20 micrograms/kg with **quercetin** 50 mg/kg and three *animals* were given digoxin alone. Unexpectedly, two of the *pigs* receiving the combination died suddenly within 30 minutes. At 20 minutes, the serum digoxin levels of the *animals* receiving the combination were 2.6-fold higher than those in the *animals* given digoxin alone (6.73 nanograms/mL versus 2.54 nanograms/mL).[1] In a further crossover study in 4 *pigs*, **quercetin** at a slightly lower dose of 40 mg/kg increased the maximum level of digoxin fivefold and the AUC 2.7-fold.[1] The authors state that they specifically chose *pigs* for this study, as a preliminary study suggested that the pharmacokinetics of digoxin in *pigs* were similar to that in humans.

Mechanism

Quercetin is suspected to increase the oral absorption of digoxin by inhibiting intestinal P-glycoprotein. A study investigating the effects of **kaempferol** derivatives isolated from *Zingiber zerumbet*, a species related to ginger, found that some of these derivatives inhibited P-glycoprotein, with a potency similar to verapamil, a known clinically relevant P-glycoprotein inhibitor.[2] **Kaempferol** may therefore also raise digoxin levels.

Importance and management

Although there is just one *animal* study of quercetin, its findings of markedly increased levels of digoxin and toxicity suggest that caution would be appropriate with supplements containing quercetin in patients taking digoxin until further data become available. Monitor for digoxin adverse effects, such as bradycardia, and consider measuring digoxin levels if this occurs.

Note that there is currently no evidence of any clinically important interactions between digoxin and food, even for foods known to be rich sources of quercetin such as onions (about 7 to 34 mg/100 g),[3] which suggests that any interaction might require very high doses. The only possible evidence identified was one early pharmacokinetic paper, which reported a modest 43% increase in the peak level of digoxin after administration of acetyldigoxin with carob seed flour,[4] which is also a rich source of quercetin (about 39 mg/100 g).[3]

1. Wang Y-H, Chao P-DL, Hsiu S-L, Wen K-C, Hou Y-C. Lethal quercetin-digoxin interaction in pigs. *Life Sci* (2004) 74, 1191–7.
2. Chung SY, Jang DS, Han A-R, Jang JO, Kwon Y, Seo E-K, Lee HJ. Modulation of P-glycoprotein-mediated resistance by kaempferol derivatives isolated from *Zingiber zerumbet*. *Phytother Res* (2007) 21, 565–9.
3. USDA Database for the flavonoid content of selected foods, Release 2.1. http://www.nal.usda.gov/fnic/foodcomp/Data/Flav/Flav02-1.pdf (accessed 20/11/2008).
4. Kasper H, Zilly W, Fassl H, Fehle F. The effect of dietary fiber on postprandial serum digoxin concentration in man. *Am J Clin Nutr* (1979) 32, 2436–8.

Flavonoids + Enalapril

The interaction between flavonoids and enalapril is based on experimental evidence only.

Clinical evidence

No interactions found.

Experimental evidence

In *rats*, oral **kaempferol** 2 mg/kg and 10 mg/kg given with enalapril increased the AUC of enalaprilat (the active metabolite of enalapril) by 60% and 109%, respectively, but only the effect with 10 mg/kg was statistically significant. **Naringenin** 2 mg/kg and 10 mg/kg caused only a minor 18 to 38% increase in AUC of enalaprilat, which was not statistically significant.[1]

Mechanism

In vitro, both kaempferol and naringenin were shown to be potent esterase inhibitors. Esterases hydrolyse enalapril in the gut: esterase inhibition by these flavonoids may be expected to increase the stability of enalapril, increasing its absorption.[1]

Importance and management

Evidence appears to be limited to this experimental study. The effect of kaempferol would not be expected to be clinically important because enalapril has a wide therapeutic range. Naringenin does not appear to interact. No dosage adjustments would therefore be expected to be needed if either of these flavonoids is given with enalapril.

1. Li P, Callery PS, Gan L-S, Balani SK. Esterase inhibition by grapefruit juice flavonoids leading to a new drug interaction. *Drug Metab Dispos* (2007) 35, 1203–8.

Flavonoids + Etoposide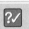

The interaction between flavonoids and etoposide is based on experimental evidence only.

Clinical evidence

No interactions found.

Experimental evidence

In an *in vitro* study using *rat* gut sacs, pre-treatment with **quercetin** or a natural diet (assumed to contain flavonoids) for 30 minutes increased etoposide absorption when compared with a flavonoid-free diet. However, there was no difference in etoposide absorption when *rats* were pretreated for one week with a natural diet (assumed to contain flavonoids) compared with a flavonoid-free diet.[1]

In another *animal* study, oral **morin** given 30 minutes before etoposide increased the AUC of oral etoposide by about 46% but had no effect on the AUC of intravenous etoposide.[2]

Mechanism

It is suggested that flavonoids might inhibit P-glycoprotein or the cytochrome P450 isoenzyme CYP3A4 in the gut, and thereby increase the absorption of etoposide, which is a substrate of CYP3A4 and/or P-glycoprotein.

F

Importance and management

A finding of a 50% increase in the AUC of etoposide might be clinically relevant in humans. However, these are *animal* data, and therefore some caution is required in extrapolating their findings. Also, the data suggest that the effect of continued use over one week might have little effect. Further study is needed before any specific recommendations can be made.

1. Lo Y-L, Huang J-D. Comparison of effects of natural or artificial rodent diet on etoposide absorption in rats. *In Vivo* (1999) 13, 51–5.
2. Li X, Yun J-K, Choi J-S. Effects of morin on the pharmacokinetics of etoposide in rats. *Biopharm Drug Dispos* (2007) 28, 151–6.

Flavonoids + Fexofenadine

Naringin and hesperidin may slightly reduce fexofenadine exposure whereas quercetin might slightly increase fexofenadine exposure.

Clinical evidence

In a crossover study in 12 healthy subjects, fexofenadine 120 mg was given with either 300 mL of grapefruit juice, an aqueous solution of **naringin** at roughly the same concentration found in the juice (1 210 micromol), or water. The AUC of fexofenadine with grapefruit juice and **naringin** solution was reduced by 45% and 25%, respectively, when compared with water.[1] In another study in 12 healthy subjects, fexofenadine was given with grapefruit juice, or water, at the same time, or 2 hours before, an aqueous suspension of the particulate fraction of grapefruit juice. The particulate fraction (i.e. the solid matter after centrifugation of the juice) is known to be rich in furanocoumarins, which are clinical inhibitors of intestinal CYP3A4, but relatively low in **naringin** (34 micromol). The AUC of fexofenadine was reduced by 43% by grapefruit juice, but was not affected by the particulate fraction (when compared with water).[1]

In a placebo-controlled study, 12 healthy subjects were given a single 60-mg dose of fexofenadine after taking **quercetin** 500 mg three times daily for 7 days. **Quercetin** increased the AUC and maximum plasma concentration of fexofenadine by 55% and 68%, respectively.[2]

Experimental evidence

An *in vitro* study found that the flavonoids in grapefruit (**naringin**) and orange (**hesperidin**) were potent inhibitors of intestinal OATP transport.[1]

Mechanism

The authors suggested that naringin directly inhibited enteric OATP1A2 to decrease oral fexofenadine bioavailability, and that inactivation of enteric CYP3A4 was probably not involved.[1] Quercetin was considered to have inhibited the intestinal transport of fexofenadine by P-glycoprotein, although some contribution from other transporter proteins was not excluded.[2]

Importance and management

The slight 25% reduction in AUC of fexofenadine with a high concentration of naringin is unlikely to be clinically important. No interaction would therefore be expected with naringin supplements. However, note that grapefruit juice and other fruit juices might cause clinically relevant reductions in fexofenadine levels in some individuals. See the table Summary of established drug interactions of grapefruit juice, page 271. Therefore an interaction with other extracts from these juices cannot be ruled out.

The studies of the effects of quercetin on fexofenadine disposition were conducted primarily to assess the potential for quercetin to inhibit P-glycoprotein. Nevertheless, the clinical data shows that it causes a slight increase in fexofenadine exposure, which is unlikely to be clinically relevant.

1. Bailey DG, Dresser GK, Leake BF, Kim RB. Naringin is a major and selective clinical inhibitor of organic anion-transporting polypeptide 1A2 (OATP1A2) in grapefruit juice. *Clin Pharmacol Ther* (2007) 81, 495–502.
2. Kim K-A, Park P-W, Park J-Y. Short-term effect of quercetin on the pharmacokinetics of fexofenadine, a substrate of p-glycoprotein, in healthy volunteers *Eur J Clin Pharmacol* (2009) 65, 609–14.

Flavonoids + Food; Milk

The addition of milk to tea did not alter the absorption of quercetin or kaempferol, or catechins, see Tea + Food, page 467.

Flavonoids + Herbal medicines

No interactions found. Flavonoids are a very large family of polyphenolic compounds synthesised by plants that are common and widely distributed.

Flavonoids + Irinotecan or Topotecan

Limited evidence suggests that high doses of chrysin are unlikely to cause an adverse interaction with irinotecan and possibly topotecan.

Clinical evidence

In a pilot study in patients with colorectal cancer receiving intravenous irinotecan 350 mg/m2 every 3 weeks, **chrysin** 250 mg twice daily for one week before, and one week after, irinotecan appeared to be associated with a low incidence of irinotecan-induced diarrhoea. There was no difference in the pharmacokinetics of irinotecan and its metabolites when compared with historical data for irinotecan. Survival data did not differ from historical data suggesting that **chrysin** did not reduce the efficacy of irinotecan.[1] However, note that this study was small and did not include a control group: therefore its findings require confirmation in a larger randomised study.

Experimental evidence

In vitro, **chrysin** has been found to be a potent inhibitor of the human transporter protein, BCRP. However, in a study in *rats* and *mice,* oral **chrysin** did not alter the pharmacokinetics of the BCRP substrate, topotecan. It was suggested that this may have been due to differences in *rat* and *mouse* BCRP compared with human BCRP.[2]

Mechanism

The flavonoid chrysin possibly acts as an inducer of the metabolism of irinotecan by glucuronidases. It may also be an inhibitor of human BCRP.

Importance and management

The available data suggest that high doses of chrysin are unlikely to cause an adverse interaction if given with irinotecan, and might possibly be beneficial, but more study is needed to establish this. It is too early to say whether chrysin might affect topotecan pharmacokinetics, but the study does highlight a problem with extrapolating *animal* data to humans when studying this potential interaction.

1. Tobin PJ, Beale P, Noney L, Liddell S, Rivory LP, Clarke S. A pilot study on the safety of combining chrysin, a non-absorbable inducer of UGT1A1, and irinotecan (CPT-11) to treat metastatic colorectal cancer. *Cancer Chemother Pharmacol* (2006) 57, 309–16.
2. Zhang S, Wang X, Sagawa K, Morris ME. Flavonoids chrysin and benzoflavone, potent breast cancer resistance protein inhibitors, have no significant effect on topotecan pharmacokinetics in rats or mdr1a/1b (-/-) mice. *Drug Metab Dispos* (2005) 33, 341–8.

F

Flavonoids + Paclitaxel

The interaction between morin, naringin or quercetin and paclitaxel is based on experimental evidence only.

Clinical evidence

No interactions found.

Experimental evidence

(a) Morin

The pharmacokinetics of paclitaxel were determined in *rats* after oral or intravenous administration of paclitaxel with or without morin (3.3 and 10 mg/kg).[1] Compared with paclitaxel alone, morin, given 30 minutes before oral paclitaxel, increased the maximum levels and AUC of paclitaxel by 70 to 90% and 30 to 70%, respectively, without any change in the time to reach maximum levels, or elimination half-life. In contrast, the pharmacokinetics of intravenous paclitaxel (3.3 mg/kg) were not altered significantly by morin.

(b) Naringin

A study to investigate the effects of oral naringin on the pharmacokinetics of intravenous paclitaxel in *rats* found that oral naringin (3.3 and 10 mg/kg), when given to rats 30 minutes before intravenous administration of paclitaxel (3 mg/kg), produced a significantly higher AUC for paclitaxel (about 41% and 49% for naringin doses of 3.3 and 10 mg/kg, respectively). Clearance was also delayed (29% and 33% decrease, respectively) when compared with the controls.[2] In a similar study using oral paclitaxel, oral naringin increased the AUC of paclitaxel by up to threefold, and increased the elimination half-life. The oral bioavailability of paclitaxel increased from 2.2% up to 6.8%.[3]

(c) Quercetin

In an *animal* study using oral paclitaxel, oral quercetin increased the AUC of paclitaxel by up to 3.3-fold, and increased the elimination half-life. The oral bioavailability of paclitaxel increased from 2% up to 6.6%.[4]

Mechanism

Paclitaxel is a substrate of P-glycoprotein and the hepatic cytochrome P450 subfamily CYP3A and isoenzyme CYP2C8. The flavonoids might inhibit the metabolism of paclitaxel by CYP3A and the transport of paclitaxel via intestinal P-glycoprotein, thereby increasing the AUC of paclitaxel. Note that there is evidence that quercetin does not inhibit CYP2C8, because it did not alter the metabolism of rosiglitazone, page 220, a specific substrate for CYP2C8.

Importance and management

The finding of increased *oral* absorption of paclitaxel with morin, naringin and quercetin is of little clinical relevance because paclitaxel is not used orally (it is poorly absorbed, even in the presence of the flavonoids).

Morin had no effect on the pharmacokinetics of *intravenous* paclitaxel, but the 50% increase in the AUC of intravenous paclitaxel caused by naringin would be clinically relevant in humans. However, these are *animal* data, and therefore some caution is required in extrapolating their findings. Further study is needed before any specific recommendations can be made.

1. Choi B-C, Choi J-S, Han H-K. Altered pharmacokinetics of paclitaxel by the concomitant use of morin in rats *Int J Pharm* (2006) 323, 81–5.
2. Lim S-C, Choi J-S. Effects of naringin on the pharmacokinetics of intravenous paclitaxel in rats. *Biopharm Drug Dispos* (2006) 27, 443–7.
3. Choi J-S, Shin S-C. Enhanced paclitaxel bioavailability after oral coadministration of paclitaxel prodrug with naringin to rats. *Int J Pharm* (2005) 292, 149–56.
4. Choi J-S, Jo B-W, Kim Y-C. Enhanced paclitaxel bioavailability after oral administration of paclitaxel or prodrug to rats pretreated with quercetin. *Eur J Pharm Biopharm* (2004) 57, 313–18.

Flavonoids + Quinine or Quinidine

The interaction between flavonoids and quinine or quinidine is based on experimental evidence only.

Clinical evidence

No interactions found.

Experimental evidence

In *rats,* **naringin** 25 mg/kg daily for 7 days increased the oral bioavailability of a single 25-mg/kg oral dose of quinine from 17% to 42%, but did not affect the pharmacokinetics of intravenous quinine.[1] In an *in vitro* study, **quercetin** and **naringenin** were modest inhibitors of quinine metabolism.[2]

In another *in vitro* study, **quercetin** was an inhibitor of quinidine metabolism, with **kaempferol** and **naringenin** also having an effect,[3] and in *rats,* quinidine approximately halved the AUC of **baicalin** in blood, and increased its levels in bile by 47%.[4]

Mechanism

Flavonoids are predicted to interact with quinine and quinidine via effects on cytochrome P450 isoenzymes or P-glycoprotein.

Importance and management

On the basis of *animal* and *in vitro* data, it is possible that high doses of quercetin, kaempferol and naringenin or naringin might increase quinine or quinidine levels, but any interaction is not firmly established. Furthermore, the rise in the quinine levels was modest, and unlikely to be clinically relevant if a similar effect were shown in practice. Note that grapefruit juice (a rich source of flavonoids), does not have a clinically relevant effect on the pharmacokinetics of quinine or quinidine. The clinical relevance of the effects of quinidine on biacalin disposition are unclear.

1. Zhang H, Wong CW, Coville PF, Wanwimolruk S. Effect of the grapefruit flavonoid naringin on pharmacokinetics of quinine in rats. *Drug Metabol Drug Interact* (2000) 17, 351–63.
2. Ho P-C, Saville DJ, Wanwimolruk S. Inhibition of human CYP3A4 activity by grapefruit flavonoids, furanocoumarins and related compounds. *J Pharm Pharm Sci* (2001) 4, 217–27.
3. Ha HR, Chen J, Leuenberger PM, Freiburghaus AU, Follath F. In vitro inhibition of midazolam and quinidine metabolism by flavonoids. *Eur J Clin Pharmacol* (1995) 48, 367–71.
4. Tsai P-L, Tsai T-H. Pharmacokinetics of baicalin in rats and its interactions with cyclosporin A, quinidine and SKF-525A: a microdialysis study. *Planta Med* (2004) 70, 1069–74.

Flavonoids + Rosiglitazone

Quercetin does not appear to affect the pharmacokinetics of rosiglitazone.

Clinical evidence

In a crossover study in 10 healthy subjects, **quercetin** 500 mg daily for 3 weeks had no effect on the pharmacokinetics of a single 4-mg dose of rosiglitazone, or its principal metabolite *N*-desmethylrosiglitazone.[1]

Experimental evidence

No relevant data found.

Mechanism

Rosiglitazone is a specific substrate for the cytochrome P450 isoenzyme CYP2C8, and it therefore appears that multiple-dose quercetin has no clinically relevant effect on this isoenzyme. The rationale that it might was because, *in vitro,* quercetin inhibits the CYP2C8-mediated metabolism of a number of substrates including paclitaxel, see above. However, in the case of paclitaxel (and possibly the other substrates), P-glycoprotein inhibition and CYP3A4 might also be important.

Importance and management

Although evidence appears to be limited to this one study, it is supported by *in vitro* data that suggests the absence of an interaction. No clinically important pharmacokinetic interaction would be expected with long-term use of quercetin supplements in patients taking rosiglitazone, and therefore no dose adjustments would be expected to be needed.

1. Kim K-A, Park P-W, Kim H-K, Ha J-M, Park J-Y. Effect of quercetin on the pharmacokinetics of rosiglitazone, a CYP2C8 substrate, in healthy subjects. *J Clin Pharmacol* (2005) 45, 941–6.

Flavonoids + Saquinavir

Quercetin does not appear to affect the pharmacokinetics of saquinavir.

Clinical evidence

In a study in 10 healthy subjects, the pharmacokinetics of saquinavir 1.2 g three times daily (*Fortovase*; soft capsules) were not affected by the concurrent use of **quercetin** 500 mg three times daily for 8 days. Concurrent use of both products was well tolerated.[1]

Experimental evidence

No relevant data found.

Mechanism

Based on other data for quercetin, it was suggested that this flavonoid might increase saquinavir levels by inhibiting P-glycoprotein, or by effects on the cytochrome P450 isoenzyme CYP3A4.

Importance and management

Although the study appears to be the only published data, the absence of an interaction is fairly well established. Quercetin is unlikely to have a detrimental (or beneficial) pharmacokinetic effect when used with saquinavir, and therefore no dosage adjustments would be expected to be necessary on concurrent use.

1. DiCenzo R, Frerichs V, Larppanichpoonphol P, Predko L, Chen A, Reichman R, Morris M. Effect of quercetin on the plasma and intracellular concentrations of saquinavir in healthy adults. *Pharmacotherapy* (2006) 26, 1255–61.

Flavonoids + Statins

Baicalin decreases the exposure to rosuvastatin in some patients. The interactions between other flavonoids and statins is based on experimental evidence only.

Clinical evidence

In a placebo-controlled study, three groups of 6 healthy subjects, each with different OATP1B1 activity, were given a single 20-mg dose of rosuvastatin after taking baicalin 50 mg three times daily for 14 days. In the group with greatest OATP1B1 activity the AUC of rosuvastatin was decreased by 42%, in the group with intermediate OATP1B1 activity the AUC of rosuvastatin was decreased by about 25%, and in the group with the lowest OATP1B1 activity the AUC of rosuvastatin was unaffected.[1]

Experimental evidence

In *rats,* oral **kaempferol** and **naringenin**, given with **lovastatin**, markedly increased the AUC of lovastatin acid. Increases were 2.7-fold and 3.5-fold with **kaempferol** 2 mg/kg and 10 mg/kg, respectively, and 2.6-fold and 3.9-fold with **naringenin** 2 mg/kg

and 10 mg/kg, respectively.[2] Other *in vitro* studies have shown that **naringenin** inhibits **simvastatin** metabolism.[3,4] *In vitro* studies using atorvastatin and the flavonoids, **apigenin**, **quercetin** and **kaempferol**,[5] have shown that they all have the potential to inhibit OATP1B1, which is involved in the transport of **atorvastatin**, as well as **pravastatin** and **rosuvastatin**.

Mechanism

Kaempferol and naringenin may be esterase inhibitors. In addition, naringenin may inhibit the cytochrome P450 isoenzyme CYP3A4, the main route of metabolism of simvastatin and lovastatin. Esterases hydrolyse lovastatin in the gut to lovastatin acid which is poorly absorbed: esterase inhibition by these flavonoids may be expected to increase the stability of lovastatin, increasing its absorption.[2] Subsequent metabolism then leads to greater levels of lovastatin acid than would have occurred in the absence of the flavonoids. Rosuvastatin is transported into hepatocytes by OATP1B1. Biacalin induces this transporter thereby increasing the uptake and metabolism of rosuvastatin resulting in a decrease in its exposure. The magnitude of the effect depends on the activity of OATP1B1, with rosuvastatin exposure in those with low activity being least affected by biacalin.

Importance and management

There appears to be no clinical evidence to support the experimental findings of an interaction between the flavonoids and statins studied. However, the marked increase in lovastatin levels that occurred with these flavonoids in the *animal* study, and the known important interaction of grapefruit juice (which is a rich source of flavonoids), with lovastatin and simvastatin (leading to rhabdomyolysis and myopathy) suggest that kaempferol and naringenin supplements should generally be avoided in patients taking these statins. This advice should be extended to citrus bioflavonoid supplements. The clinical relevance of the findings with apigenin, quercetin and kaempferol require further study, but raised atorvastatin, pravastatin and rosuvastatin levels are a possibility.

The interaction of biacalin with rosuvastatin would be expected to be of clinical relevance in those with high OATP1B1 activity; however, it is unlikely that this will be known. It would therefore seem prudent to monitor concurrent use for a decrease in rosuvastatin efficacy, stopping the source of biacalin or increasing the dose of rosuvastatin as necessary.

1. Fan L, Zhang W, Guo D, Tan Z-R, Xu P, Li Q, Liu Y-Z, Zhang L, He Y-Y, HU D-L, Wang D, Zhou H-G. The effect of herbal medicine baicalin on pharmacokinetics of rosuvastatin, substrate of organic anion-transporting polypeptide 1B1 *Clin Pharmacol Ther* (2008) 83, 471–6.
2. Li P, Callery PS, Gan L-S, Balani SK. Esterase inhibition by grapefruit juice flavonoids leading to a new drug interaction. *Drug Metab Dispos* (2007) 35, 1203–8.
3. Le Goff N, Koffel JC, Vandenschrieck S, Jung L, Ubeaud G. Comparison of in vitro hepatic models for the prediction of metabolic interaction between simvastatin and naringenin. *Eur J Drug Metab Pharmacokinet* (2002) 27, 233–41.
4. Ubeaud G, Hagenbach J, Vandenschrieck S, Jung L, Koffel JC. In vitro inhibition of simvastatin metabolism in rat and human liver by naringenin. *Life Sci* (1999) 65, 1403–12.
5. Mandery K, Balk B, Bujok K, Schmidt I, Fromm MF, Glaeser H. Inhibition of hepatic uptake transporters by flavonoids *Eur J Pharm Sci* (2012) 46, 79–85.

Flavonoids + Tamoxifen

The interaction between flavonoids and tamoxifen is based on experimental evidence only.

Clinical evidence

No interactions found.

Experimental evidence

(a) Antagonistic effects

Various flavonoids have been investigated *in vitro* for their ability to reduce the proliferation of cancer cells, and *in vivo* some studies have shown synergistic cytotoxicity with tamoxifen (e.g. with **catechins**[1]).

In contrast, and of concern, it has been reported that **tangeretin** abolished the growth inhibitory effects of tamoxifen in *mice,* and shortened the survival time of tamoxifen-treated tumour-bearing mice compared with those receiving tamoxifen alone.[2] This finding was not explained by changes in tamoxifen pharmacokinetics, see below.

(b) Pharmacokinetics

In a study, *mice* receiving **tangeretin** and tamoxifen had higher tamoxifen levels than those receiving tamoxifen alone. In addition, **tangeretin** did not alter the ratio between tamoxifen and its N-desmethyl metabolite.[2]

In a study in *rats,*[3] oral **quercetin** modestly increased the AUC of oral tamoxifen given concurrently. The effect was not dose-dependent; there was a 35% increase with **quercetin** 2.5 mg/kg, a 60% increase with **quercetin** 7.5 mg/kg and a smaller 20% increase with **quercetin** 15 mg/kg. There was also a minor 8 to 29% increase in the AUC of the active 4-hydroxytamoxifen metabolite. When compared with intravenous tamoxifen, **quercetin** 7.5 mg/kg increased the absolute oral bioavailability of tamoxifen by 60% (from 15% to 24%).

Mechanism

These findings suggest that quercetin inhibits both drug transporter proteins and possibly the cytochrome P450 isoenzyme CYP3A4, which decreases the first-pass metabolism of tamoxifen.[3] The authors suggested that the antagonistic effect of tangeretin against tamoxifen was because tangeretin is an inhibitor of natural killer cell activity.[2]

Importance and management

There do not appear to be any clinical data investigating the possible interactions between tamoxifen and flavonoids, and extrapolating the available *animal* findings to the clinical situation is difficult. Nevertheless, some caution is required if patients taking tamoxifen also take products containing tangeretin, because the effect of tamoxifen was abolished in one study, despite an increase in its levels. Studies are clearly needed that assess both efficacy and pharmacokinetic effects of the concurrent use of tangeretin and tamoxifen. The authors of the study with tangeretin suggested that the level of tangeretin used (human equivalent of about 280 mg daily) could not be obtained by eating citrus fruits or drinking juices. However, they advise caution with the use of products containing large amounts of citrus peel oil, and dietary supplements containing large amounts of citrus bioflavonoids as these could provide sufficient amounts of tangeretin to interact. Given the severity of the possible outcome, until more is known, this seems prudent.

1. Rosengren RJ. Catechins and the treatment of breast cancer: possible utility and mechanistic targets. *IDrugs* (2003) 6, 1073–8.
2. Bracke ME, Depypere HT, Boterberg T, Van Marck VL, Vennekens KM, Vanluchene E, Nuytinck M, Serreyn R, Mareel MM. Influence of tangeretin on tamoxifen's therapeutic benefit in mammary cancer. *J Natl Cancer Inst* (1999) 91, 354–9.
3. Shin S-C, Choi J-S, Li X. Enhanced bioavailability of tamoxifen after oral administration of tamoxifen with quercetin in rats. *Int J Pharm* (2006) 313, 144–9.

F

Flaxseed

Linum usitatissimum L. (Linaceae)

Synonym(s) and related species

Flax, Linseed.

Pharmacopoeias

Linseed (*BP 2012, PhEur 7.5*); Linseed Oil, Virgin (*BP 2012, PhEur 7.5*).

Constituents

The seeds contain a fixed oil, composed of glycerides of linoleic and **linolenic acid**. The seeds also contain mucilage; the lignans **secoisolariciresinol** and its diglucoside; and the cyanogenetic glycosides linamarin and lotaustralin.

Use and indications

Flaxseed was formerly used as a demulcent and soothing emollient agent for bronchitis, coughs, and applied externally to burns. More recently, flaxseed oil has been used to lower blood-cholesterol levels, and flaxseed extract is being taken as a form of hormone replacement therapy due to its phytoestrogenic effects, thought to be due to the lignans (although note that the information available on phytoestrogenic lignans is limited).

Pharmacokinetics

Ingested lignans such as secoisolariciresinol have been shown to undergo bacterial hydrolysis and metabolism to produce the mammalian lignans **enterolactone** and enterodiol, which have estrogenic effects.

Interactions overview

Flaxseed lignan supplementation appears to have no significant effect on blood-glucose levels in type 2 diabetic patients also taking oral antidiabetic drugs (not named). Limited evidence suggests that flaxseed oil may increase bleeding times and therefore some caution might therefore be appropriate with aspirin and anticoagulants.

Interactions monographs

- Anticoagulant or Antiplatelet drugs, page 224
- Antidiabetics, page 224
- Food, page 224
- Herbal medicines, page 224

F

223

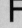

Flaxseed + Anticoagulant or Antiplatelet drugs

Limited evidence suggests that flaxseed oil may have some antiplatelet effects, which could be additive with those of conventional antiplatelet drugs, and increase the risk of bleeding with anticoagulants.

Clinical evidence

Two case reports briefly describe increased bleeding (haematuria and nosebleeds) in patients taking aspirin and flaxseed oil, one of whom was taking low-dose aspirin.[1]

Some studies have investigated the effect of flaxseed oil alone on bleeding time, and one, in 10 healthy subjects, found that a flaxseed oil rich diet (20.5 g daily of α-linolenic acid) for 56 days had no significant effect on bleeding times, prothrombin times or on partial prothrombin times.[2] However, another study in 11 patients with rheumatoid arthritis reported that flaxseed oil 30 g daily for 3 months (9.6 g daily of α-linolenic acid) increased the bleeding time by about one minute when compared with baseline, although this result was not statistically significant.[3]

Experimental evidence

No relevant data found.

Mechanism

Omega-3 fatty acids such as linolenic acid are thought to have some antiplatelet effects and might therefore prolong bleeding time. Theoretically, this effect might be additive with that of other antiplatelet drugs, and increase the risk of bleeding with anticoagulants.

Importance and management

The general significance of these reports is unclear and no interaction is established. Nevertheless, a large epidemiological study would be needed to quantify any excess risk in the order of that seen with antiplatelet doses of aspirin taken with warfarin. As with high doses of fish oils (marine omega-3 fatty acids), it may be prudent to use some caution with the concurrent use of high doses of flaxseed supplements in patients also taking aspirin or anticoagulants.

1. Gruver DI. Does flaxseed interfere with the clotting system? *Plast Reconstr Surg* (2003) 112, 934.
2. Kelley DS, Nelson GJ, Love JE, Branch LB, Taylor PC, Schmidt PC, Mackey BE, Iacono JM. Dietary α-linolenic acid alters tissue fatty acid composition but not blood lipids, lipoproteins or coagulation status in humans. *Lipids* (1993) 28, 533–7.
3. Nordström DCE, Honkanen VEA, Nasu Y, Antila E, Friman C, Konttinen YT. Alpha-linolenic acid in the treatment of rheumatoid arthritis. A double-blind, placebo-controlled and randomized study: flaxseed vs safflower seed. *Rheumatol Int* (1995) 14, 231–4.

Flaxseed + Antidiabetics

Flaxseed lignan supplementation appears to have no significant effect on blood-glucose levels in type 2 diabetic patients also taking oral antidiabetic drugs.

Clinical evidence

In a randomised, crossover study in 68 patients with type 2 diabetes and mild hypercholesterolaemia, taking a supplement containing a total of 360 mg of **flaxseed lignan** daily for 12 weeks had no significant effect on blood-lipid profile, insulin resistance, fasting glucose and insulin concentrations. A minor reduction of glycosylated haemoglobin (HbA$_{1c}$) of about 0.1% occurred, although the clinical significance of this reduction is likely to be minimal. In this particular study, patients continued to take their usual medication, which included oral antidiabetics and lipid-lowering medications, none of which were specifically named in the study. Patients were excluded from the study if they were using insulin.[1] Similarly, in another study, **flaxseed oil** (60 mg/kg α-linolenic acid daily) had no significant effect on blood-glucose control in type 2 diabetics. Patients taking insulin were also excluded from this study; however, information on other concurrent medication was not reported.[2] In another study in 25 menopausal women with hypercholesterolaemia, there was a slight 5.3% reduction in blood-glucose levels (0.1 mmol/L) with **crushed flaxseed**, and this was less than that seen with conventional HRT,[3] which is not considered to have blood-glucose-lowering effects.

Experimental evidence

No relevant data found.

Mechanism

No mechanism expected.

Importance and management

It appears from these studies that flaxseed oil or lignans have minimal effects on glycaemic control in type 2 diabetes, and in one study the lignans had no additive blood-glucose-lowering effects with oral antidiabetic drugs (not named). Flaxseed is therefore unlikely to affect the blood-glucose-lowering efficacy of concurrent antidiabetic medication. However, more detailed information on specific antidiabetic drugs is unavailable.

1. Pan A, Sun J, Chen Y, Ye X, Li H, Yu Z, Wang Y, Gu W, Zhang X, Chen X, Demark-Wahnefried W, Liu Y, Lin X. Effects of a flaxseed-derived lignan supplement in type 2 diabetic patients: a randomised, double-blind, cross-over trial. *PLoS ONE* (2007) 2, e1148.
2. Barre DE, Mizier-Barre KA, Griscti O, Hafez K. High dose flaxseed oil supplementation may affect blood glucose management in human type 2 diabetics. *J Oleo Sci* (2008) 57, 269–73.
3. Lemay A, Dodin S, Kadri N, Jacques H, Forest J-C. Flaxseed dietary supplement versus hormone replacement therapy in hypercholesterolemic menopausal women. *Obstet Gynecol* (2002) 100, 495–504.

Flaxseed + Food

No interactions found.

Flaxseed + Herbal medicines

No interactions found.

Frangula

Frangula alnus Mill. (Rhamnaceae)

Synonym(s) and related species

Alder buckthorn.

Frangula nigra Samp, *Rhamnus cathartica* L., *Rhamnus frangula* L.

Pharmacopoeias

Frangula Bark (*BP 2012, PhEur 7.5*); Standardised Frangula Bark Dry Extract (*BP 12, PhEur 7.5*).

Constituents

The major constituents of frangula are the **anthraquinone glycosides**. The frangulosides are the main components, which include frangulin A and B, emodin derivatives, chrysophanol and physcion glycosides and free aglycones. Frangula also contains **flavonoids** and tannins.

Use and indications

Frangula bark is used as a laxative.

Pharmacokinetics

For information on the pharmacokinetics of an anthraquinone glycoside present in frangula, see under aloes, page 27.

Interactions overview

No interactions with frangula found; however, frangula (by virtue of its anthraquinone content) is expected to share some of the interactions of a number of other anthraquinone-containing laxatives, such as aloes, page 27 and senna, page 423. Of particular relevance are the interactions with corticosteroids, digitalis glycosides, and potassium-depleting diuretics.

F

Fumitory

Fumaria officinalis L. (Papaveraceae)

Synonym(s) and related species

Common fumitory, Earth-smoke.

Pharmacopoeias

Fumitory (*BP 2012, PhEur 7.5*).

Constituents

Fumitory contains **isoquinoline alkaloids** of various structural types, including protopine (fumarine), to which it may be standardised, aurotensine, sanguinarine, fumaritine and fumaritridine. **Flavonoids**, mainly glycosides of quercetin (including isoquercitrin and rutin) and other polyphenols such as chlorogenic, caffeic and fumaric acids are also present.

Use and indications

Fumitory is mainly used as a mild diuretic and laxative, and to increase the flow of bile. Traditionally, it has been used to treat skin conditions such as cutaneous eruptions and chronic eczema, and also for conjunctivitis (as an eye lotion).

Pharmacokinetics

No relevant pharmacokinetic data found. For information on the pharmacokinetics of individual flavonoids present in fumitory, see under flavonoids, page 213.

Interactions overview

No interactions with fumitory found. For information on the interactions of individual flavonoids present in fumitory, see under flavonoids, page 213.

F

Garlic

Allium sativum L. (Alliaceae)

Synonym(s) and related species

Ajo, Allium.

Pharmacopoeias

Garlic (*USP35–NF30 S1*); Garlic Delayed-Release Tablets (*USP35–NF30 S1*); Garlic Fluid extract (*USP35–NF30 S1*); Garlic for homeopathic preparations (*BP 2012, PhEur 7.5*); Garlic Powder (*PhEur 7.5, BP 2012*); Powdered Garlic (*USP35–NF30 S1*); Powdered Garlic Extract (*USP35–NF30 S1*).

Constituents

Garlic products are produced from the bulbs (cloves) of garlic and are usually standardised according to the content of the sulphur-containing compounds, alliin, allicin (produced by the action of the enzyme alliinase on alliin) and/or γ-glutamyl-(*S*)-allyl-L-cysteine.

Other sulphur compounds such as allylmethyltrisulfide, allylpropyldisulfide, diallyldisulfide, diallyltrisulfide, **ajoene** and vinyldithiines, and mercaptan are also present. Garlic also contains various glycosides, monoterpenoids, enzymes, vitamins, minerals and **flavonoids** based on kaempferol and quercetin.

Use and indications

Garlic has been used to treat respiratory infections (such as colds, flu, chronic bronchitis, and nasal and throat catarrh), and cardiovascular disorders. It is believed to possess antihypertensive, antithrombotic, fibrinolytic, antimicrobial, anticancer, expectorant, antidiabetic and lipid-lowering properties.

It is also used extensively as an ingredient in foods.

Pharmacokinetics

There are many active constituents in garlic and their roles have not been fully elucidated. Allicin is subject to a considerable first-pass effect and passes through the liver unmetabolised only at high concentrations,[1] but it is a very unstable compound and, as with ajoene, the vinyldithiins and diallylsulfide, it is not found in blood or urine after oral ingestion.[2]

There have been several experimental studies undertaken to assess the effects garlic and its constituents have on cytochrome P450 isoenzymes. *In vitro* studies suggest that garlic inhibits, to varying degrees; CYP2C9,[3,4] CYP2C19,[3,4] the CYP3A isoenzyme subfamily,[3–6] CYP2A6,[5] CYP1A2,[4] CYP2D6[4] and CYP2E1.[7] Studies

in *rats* suggest that garlic inhibits CYP2E1,[8] and induces CYP2C9*2.[3] However, in clinical studies, garlic and its constituents seem unlikely to affect the cytochrome P450 isoenzymes to a clinically relevant extent, see benzodiazepines, page 229, for CYP3A4, caffeine, page 230, for CYP1A2, and dextromethorphan, page 230, for CYP2D6. The possible exception to the lack of effect of garlic on cytochrome P450 is CYP2E1, which requires further study, see chlorzoxazone, page 230, and paracetamol (acetaminophen), page 232.

Any effect on the drug transporter P-glycoprotein, shown *in vitro*,[3] is also unlikely to be clinically significant, see HIV-protease inhibitors, page 232.

For information on the pharmacokinetics of individual flavonoids present in garlic, see under flavonoids, page 213.

Interactions overview

Case reports suggest that garlic may have additive blood pressure lowering effects with lisinopril, and may cause bleeding in those taking warfarin or fluindione. It has also been suggested that any antiplatelet effects of garlic may be additive with conventional antiplatelet drugs and NSAIDs, and studies suggest that garlic may reduce isoniazid levels. However, no interaction has been proven with any of these drugs.

In general, garlic seems to have no effect, or have only clinically irrelevant effects when it is given with alcohol, benzodiazepines (such as midazolam), caffeine, chlorzoxazone, dextromethorphan, docetaxel, gentamicin, paracetamol (acetaminophen), rifampicin (rifampin), statins (pravastatin and simvastatin studied) or ritonavir. Any interaction between garlic and fish oils may be beneficial.

One study suggested that a high-fat diet did not affect the absorption of some of the active constituents of garlic oil. For information on the interactions of individual flavonoids present in garlic, see under flavonoids, page 213.

Interactions monographs

- ACE inhibitors, page 229
- Alcohol, page 229
- Antiplatelet drugs, page 229
- Benzodiazepines, page 229
- Caffeine, page 230
- Chlorzoxazone, page 230
- Dextromethorphan, page 230
- Docetaxel, page 231
- Food, page 231

G

1. Egen-Schwind C, Eckard R, Kemper FH. Metabolism of garlic constituents in the isolated perfused rat liver. *Planta Med* (1992) 58, 301–5.

2. Amagase H, Petesch BL, Matsuura H, Kasuga S, Itakura Y. Intake of garlic and its bioactive components. *J Nutr* (2001) 131, 955S–962S.

3. Foster BC, Foster MS, Vandenhoek S, Krantis A, Budzinski JW, Arnason JT, Gallicano KD, Choudri S. An *in vitro* evaluation of human cytochrome P450 3A4 and P-glycoprotein inhibition by garlic. *J Pharm Pharm Sci* (2001) 4, 176–84.

4. Zou L, Harkey MR, Henderson GL. Effects of herbal components on cDNA-expressed cytochrome P450 enzyme catalytic activity. *Life Sci* (2002) 71, 1579–89.

5. Fujita K-I, Kamataki T. Screening of organosulfur compounds as inhibitors of human CYP2A6. *Drug Metab Dispos* (2001) 29, 983–9.

6. Greenblatt DJ, Leigh-Pemberton RA, von Moltke LL. In vitro interactions of water-soluble garlic components with human cytochromes P450. *J Nutr* (2006) 136, 806S–809S.

7. Brady JF, Ishizaki H, Fukuto JM, Lin MC, Fadel A, Gapac JM, Yang CS. Inhibition of cytochrome P-450 2E1 by diallyl sulfide and its metabolites. *Chem Res Toxicol* (1991) 4, 642–7.

8. Wargovich MJ. Diallylsulfide and allylmethylsulfide are uniquely effective among organosulfur compounds in inhibiting CYP2E1 protein in animal models. *J Nutr* (2006) 136, 832S–834S.

G

Garlic + ACE inhibitors

In a single report, a patient taking lisinopril developed marked hypotension and became faint after taking garlic capsules.

Evidence, mechanism, importance and management

A man whose blood pressure was 135/90 mmHg while taking **lisinopril** 15 mg daily began to take garlic 4 mg daily (*Boots odourless garlic oil capsules*). After 3 days he became faint on standing and was found to have a blood pressure of 90/60 mmHg. Stopping the garlic restored his blood pressure to 135/90 mmHg within a week. The garlic on its own did not lower his blood pressure. The reasons for this interaction are not known, although garlic has been reported to cause vasodilatation and reduce blood pressure.[1] This seems to be the first and only report of this reaction, so its general importance is small. There seems to be nothing documented about garlic and any of the other ACE inhibitors.

1. McCoubrie M. Doctors as patients: lisinopril and garlic. *Br J Gen Pract* (1996) 46, 107.

Garlic + Alcohol

The interaction between garlic and alcohol is based on experimental evidence only.

Evidence, mechanism, importance and management

Garlic juice, from fresh garlic bulbs, inhibited the metabolism of alcohol in *mice*. Garlic is a common ingredient in food and so it is very unlikely that this interaction is clinically relevant.[1]

1. Kishimoto R, Ueda M, Yoshinaga H, Goda K, Park S-S. Combined effects of ethanol and garlic on hepatic ethanol metabolism in mice. *J Nutr Sci Vitaminol* (1999) 45, 275–86.

Garlic + Antiplatelet drugs

Garlic may have antiplatelet properties. If might therefore be expected to increase the risk of bleeding with conventional antiplatelet drugs and other drugs that have antiplatelet adverse effects.

Clinical evidence

In a study in 23 healthy subjects, liquid aged garlic extract 5 mL (*Kyolic*) given daily for 13 weeks, inhibited both the rate of platelet aggregation and total platelet aggregation.[1] Similar effects were found in another study in 28 healthy subjects given aged garlic extract capsules 2.4 g, 4.8 g and 7.2 g. Each dose was given daily for a 6-week period.[2]

Experimental evidence

Ajoene, a sulphur compound derived from garlic with antiplatelet and antithrombotic properties, was found to synergistically potentiate the antiplatelet actions of **dipyridamole**, **epoprostenol** and **indometacin** *in vitro*.[3]

Mechanism

Uncertain. The authors of an experimental study[3] suggest that ajoene inhibits the binding of fibrinogen to the fibrinogen receptor, which occurs in the final step of the platelet aggregation pathway. Ajoene would therefore be expected to interact synergistically with antiplatelet drugs that act at an earlier step in the pathway.

Importance and management

There is a reasonable body of evidence, which suggests that aged garlic herbal products may have antiplatelet properties. If they do, and are similarly active to low-dose aspirin, they might therefore be expected to increase the risk of bleeding with conventional antiplatelet drugs and other drugs that have antiplatelet adverse effects, such as indometacin. However, considering the widespread use of garlic and garlic products, and the limited information available, it seems unlikely that garlic has any generally important interaction with antiplatelet drugs. Nevertheless, bear the possibility in mind in the event of an unexpected response to treatment.

1. Rahman K, Billington D. Dietary supplementation with aged garlic extract inhibits ADP-induced platelet aggregation in humans. *J Nutr* (2000) 130, 2662–5.
2. Steiner M, Li W. Aged garlic extract, a modulator of cardiovascular risk factors: a dose-finding study on the effects of AGE on platelet functions. *J Nutr* (2001) 131, 980S–984S.
3. Apitz-Castro R, Escalante J, Vargas R, Jain MK. Ajoene, the antiplatelet principle of garlic, synergistically potentiates the antiaggregatory action of prostacyclin, forskolin, indomethacin and dypiridamole [sic] on human platelets. *Thromb Res* (1986) 42, 303–11.

Garlic + Benzodiazepines

Garlic does not appear to affect the pharmacokinetics of alprazolam, midazolam or triazolam to a clinically relevant extent.

Clinical evidence

A study in 14 healthy subjects found that *Kwai* garlic tablets 600 mg twice daily for 14 days did not affect the pharmacokinetics of a single 2-mg dose of **alprazolam**.[1]

Similarly, garlic oil 500 mg three times daily for 28 days did not affect the metabolism of **midazolam** 8 mg in young[2] or elderly[3] healthy subjects.

Experimental evidence

The effect of garlic constituents; alliin, cycloalliin, methylin, *S*-methyl-l-cysteine, *S*-allyl-l-cysteine, N-acetyl-*S*-allyl-l-cysteine, *S*-allomercapto-l-cysteine, and gamma-glutamyl-*S*-allyl-l-cysteine, on the activity of the CYP3A probe substrate, **triazolam**, was investigated using human liver microsomes. Both *S*-methyl-l-cysteine and *S*-allyl-l-cysteine inhibited the activity of CYP3A, with the latter reducing its activity by about 60%. No other significant inhibition was apparent.[4]

Mechanism

The findings of the clinical studies suggest that garlic does not have a clinically relevant effect on CYP3A4 activity. Although some inhibition of CYP3A was seen in the *in vitro* study,[4] it was not considered to be mechanism-based and the concentrations used were an order of magnitude greater than the anticipated *in vivo* concentrations.

Importance and management

The results of the clinical studies suggest that garlic does not affect the metabolism of alprazolam or midazolam, and therefore no dosage adjustments would be expected to be necessary if patients taking these benzodiazepines also take garlic supplements.

Midazolam is used as a probe drug for CYP3A4 activity, and therefore these results also suggest that a pharmacokinetic interaction between garlic and other CYP3A4 substrates is unlikely.

1. Markowitz JS, DeVane CL, Chavin KD, Taylor RM, Ruan Y, Donovan JL. Effects of garlic (*Allium sativum* L.) supplementation on cytochrome P450 2D6 and 3A4 activity in healthy volunteers. *Clin Pharmacol Ther* (2003) 74, 170–177.
2. Gurley BJ, Gardner SF, Hubbard MA, Williams DK, Gentry WB, Cui Y, Ang CYW. Cytochrome P450 phenotypic ratios for predicting herb-drug interactions in humans. *Clin Pharmacol Ther* (2002) 72, 276–87.
3. Gurley BJ, Gardner SF, Hubbard MA, Williams DK, Gentry WB, Cui Y, Ang CYW. Clinical assessment of botanical supplementation on cytochrome P450 phenotypes in the elderly: St John's wort, garlic oil, *Panax ginseng*, and *Ginkgo biloba*. *Drugs Aging* (2005) 22, 525–39.
4. Greenblatt DJ, Leigh-Pemberton RA, von Moltke LL. In vitro interactions of water-soluble garlic components with human cytochromes P450. *J Nutr* (2006) 136, 806S–809S.

G

Garlic + Caffeine

Garlic does not appear to affect the pharmacokinetics of caffeine.

Clinical evidence

Garlic oil 500 mg three times daily for 28 days did not affect the metabolism of a single 100-mg dose of caffeine in young[1] or elderly[2] healthy subjects.

Experimental evidence

No relevant data found.

Mechanism

Garlic does not have a clinically relevant effect on the cytochrome P450 isoenzyme CYP1A2 activity using caffeine as a probe substrate.

Importance and management

Evidence for an interaction between garlic and caffeine appears to come from two well-designed studies in humans. These studies suggest that garlic does not affect the metabolism of caffeine, and therefore an increase in caffeine adverse effects would not be expected in those who also take garlic supplements. Caffeine is used as a probe drug for CYP1A2 activity, and therefore these results also suggest that a pharmacokinetic interaction between garlic and other CYP1A2 substrates is unlikely.

1. Gurley BJ, Gardner SF, Hubbard MA, Williams DK, Gentry WB, Cui Y, Ang CYW. Cytochrome P450 phenotypic ratios for predicting herb-drug interactions in humans. *Clin Pharmacol Ther* (2002) 72, 276–87.
2. Gurley BJ, Gardner SF, Hubbard MA, Williams DK, Gentry WB, Cui Y, Ang CYW. Clinical assessment of botanical supplementation on cytochrome P450 phenotypes in the elderly: St John's wort, garlic oil, *Panax ginseng,* and *Ginkgo biloba. Drugs Aging* (2005) 22, 525–39.

Garlic + Chlorzoxazone

The metabolism of chlorzoxazone is modestly inhibited by garlic but this effect is probably not clinically relevant.

Clinical evidence

Garlic oil 500 mg given to 12 healthy subjects three times daily for 28 days, reduced the conversion of a single 500-mg dose of chlorzoxazone to 6-hydroxychlorzoxazone by about 40%.[1] In a later similar study by the same authors, in 12 *elderly* healthy subjects, a smaller reduction of 22% was seen.[2]

Another study in 8 healthy subjects found that a high dose of the garlic constituent **diallyl sulfide** 200 micrograms/kg (equivalent to 15 cloves of fresh garlic, containing 1 mg/g diallyl sulfide), reduced the conversion of chlorzoxazone to 6-hydroxychlorzoxazone by about 30%.[3]

Experimental evidence

A garlic constituent, **diallyl sulfide** 50 mg/kg and 200 mg/kg, was given to *rats* 12 hours before an intravenous dose of chlorzoxazone 150 micromole/kg. **Diallyl sulfide** increased the AUC of chlorzoxazone by threefold and fivefold, respectively.[4]

Mechanism

Garlic appears to inhibit the activity of the cytochrome P450 isoenzyme CYP2E1, which metabolises chlorzoxazone to 6-hydroxychlorzoxazone.

Importance and management

There appear to be several clinical studies into the potential for an interaction between garlic and chlorzoxazone. Although these studies suggest that metabolism of chlorzoxazone is modestly inhibited

by garlic in healthy subjects, this effect is probably not clinically relevant.

Chlorzoxazone is used as a probe drug for CYP2E1 activity, and therefore these results also suggest that a pharmacokinetic interaction between garlic and other CYP2E1 substrates is unlikely.

1. Gurley BJ, Gardner SF, Hubbard MA, Williams DK, Gentry WB, Cui Y, Ang CYW. Cytochrome P450 phenotypic ratios for predicting herb-drug interactions in humans. *Clin Pharmacol Ther* (2002) 72, 276–87.
2. Gurley BJ, Gardner SF, Hubbard MA, Williams DK, Gentry WB, Cui Y, Ang CYW. Clinical assessment of botanical supplementation on cytochrome P450 phenotypes in the elderly: St John's wort, garlic oil, *Panax ginseng,* and *Ginkgo biloba. Drugs Aging* (2005) 22, 525–39.
3. Loizou GD, Cocker J. The effects of alcohol and diallyl sulphide on CYP2E1 activity in humans: a phenotyping study using chlorzoxazone. *Hum Exp Toxicol* (2001) 20, 321–7.
4. Chen L, Yang CS. Effects of cytochrome P450 2E1 modulators on the pharmacokinetics of chlorzoxazone and 6-hydroxychlorzoxazone in rats. *Life Sci* (1996) 58, 1575–85.

Garlic + Dextromethorphan

Garlic does not appear to affect the pharmacokinetics of dextromethorphan or debrisoquine.

Clinical evidence

A study in 14 healthy subjects found that *Kwai* garlic tablets 600 mg twice daily for 14 days did not affect the pharmacokinetics of a single 30-mg dose of dextromethorphan.[1]

Garlic oil 500 mg three times daily for 28 days did not affect the metabolism of **debrisoquine** 5 mg in young[2] or elderly[3] healthy subjects.

Experimental evidence

The effect of garlic constituents; alliin, cycloalliin, methylin, S-methyl-l-cysteine, S-allyl-l-cysteine, N-acetyl-S-allyl-l-cysteine, S-allomercapto-l-cysteine, and gamma-glutamyl-S-allyl-l-cysteine, on the activity of the CYP2D6 probe substrate, dextromethorphan, was investigated using human liver microsomes. No significant inhibition was apparent.[4]

Mechanism

Garlic does not appear to affect the cytochrome P450 isoenzyme CYP2D6.

Importance and management

There appear to be two clinical studies investigating the potential for an interaction between garlic and dextromethorphan, both of which found that the pharmacokinetics of dextromethorphan were unaffected by garlic and its constituents. Therefore the dosage of dextromethorphan would not need adjusting if patients also wish to take garlic supplements.

Dextromethorphan and debrisoquine are used as probe drugs for CYP2D6 activity, and therefore these results also suggest that a pharmacokinetic interaction between garlic and other CYP2D6 substrates is unlikely.

1. Markowitz JS, DeVane CL, Chavin KD, Taylor RM, Ruan Y, Donovan JL. Effects of garlic (*Allium* sativum L.) supplementation on cytochrome P450 2D6 and 3A4 activity in healthy volunteers. *Clin Pharmacol Ther* (2003) 74, 170–177.
2. Gurley BJ, Gardner SF, Hubbard MA, Williams DK, Gentry WB, Cui Y, Ang CYW. Cytochrome P450 phenotypic ratios for predicting herb-drug interactions in humans. *Clin Pharmacol Ther* (2002) 72, 276–87.
3. Gurley BJ, Gardner SF, Hubbard MA, Williams DK, Gentry WB, Cui Y, Ang CYW. Clinical assessment of botanical supplementation on cytochrome P450 phenotypes in the elderly: St John's wort, garlic oil, *Panax ginseng,* and *Ginkgo biloba. Drugs Aging* (2005) 22, 525–39.
4. Greenblatt DJ, Leigh-Pemberton RA, von Moltke LL. In vitro interactions of water-soluble garlic components with human cytochromes P450. *J Nutr* (2006) 136, 806S–809S.

G

Garlic + Docetaxel

Garlic does not appear to affect the pharmacokinetics of intravenous docetaxel.

Clinical evidence

In a pharmacokinetic study, 10 patients with metastatic, or incurable localised, breast cancer were given 1-hour intravenous infusions of docetaxel 30 mg/m² weekly for 3 weeks (days 1, 8 and 15). Five days after the first infusion, garlic tablets 600 mg were taken twice daily for 13 days (days 5 to 17). The garlic tablets used were *GarliPure Maximum Allicin Formula, Natrol,* containing 3.6 mg of allicin per tablet. Patients were also given a premedication regimen of oral dexamethasone 8 mg 12 hours before each docetaxel infusion and then every 12 hours for two more doses; and ondansetron 8 mg, ranitidine 150 mg and diphenhydramine 25 mg half an hour before each infusion of docetaxel. Garlic tablets had no effect on the pharmacokinetics of docetaxel on the second or third week, when compared with the first week (i.e. after 4 and 12 days use of garlic).[1]

Experimental evidence

No relevant data found.

Mechanism

Docetaxel is metabolised, in part, by the cytochrome P450 isoenzyme CYP3A4. This study suggests that garlic is unlikely to alter the activity of this isoenzyme. See also benzodiazepines, page 229.

Importance and management

Evidence appears to be limited to this one study, but it is supported by the findings of other studies that suggest that garlic does not alter the effects of CYP3A4, the main route of docetaxel metabolism. Therefore what is known suggests that no pharmacokinetic interaction would be expected in patients taking garlic supplements with intravenous docetaxel.

1. Cox MC, Low J, Lee J, Walshe J, Denduluri N, Berman A, Permenter MG, Petros WP, Price DK, Figg WD, Sparreboom A, Swain SM. Influence of garlic (*Allium sativum*) on the pharmacokinetics of docetaxel. *Clin Cancer Res* (2006) 12, 4636–40.

Garlic + Food

The information regarding the use of garlic with food is based on experimental evidence only.

Evidence, mechanism, importance and management

In a study in *rats* that were fed a high-fat or low-fat diet, and also given garlic oil or its constituents diallyl sulfide and diallyl disulfide, there were no biochemical changes between the groups attributable to an interaction between the garlic oil and dietary fat.[1] No clinical interaction is expected; note that garlic is extensively used as a food ingredient.

For the lack of pharmacokinetic interaction of garlic with caffeine, see caffeine, page 230.

1. Sheen L-Y, Chen H-W, Kung Y-L, Cheng-Tzu L, Lii C-K. Effects of garlic oil and its organosulfur compounds on the activities of hepatic drug-metabolizing and antioxidant enzymes in rats fed high- and low-fat diets. *Nutr Cancer* (1999) 35, 160–166.

Garlic + Gentamicin

The information regarding the use of garlic with gentamicin is based on experimental evidence only.

Evidence, mechanism, importance and management

Aged garlic extract or garlic powder extract did not affect the *in vitro* antibacterial activity of gentamicin 2.6 micrograms/L and 2.7 micrograms/L on *Escherichia coli*. The bactericidal effect of gentamicin against *E. coli,* measured by optical density, was increased by *S*-allylcysteine, diallyl sulfide, and diallyl disulfide, at concentrations of 0.25 mg/mL, 0.5 mg/mL and 1 mg/mL but the significance of this is unclear. However, no clinically significant interaction is expected as far as antibacterial activity is concerned.[1]

1. Maldonado PD, Chánez-Cárdenas ME, Pedraza-Chaverrr J. Aged garlic extract, garlic powder extract, S-allylcysteine, diallyl sulfide and diallyl disulfide do not interfere with the antibiotic activity of gentamicin. *Phytother Res* (2005) 19, 252–4.

Garlic + Herbal medicines; Caffeine-containing

Garlic did not interact with caffeine, page 230, and is therefore unlikely to interact with caffeine-containing herbs, as a result of this constituent.

Garlic + Herbal medicines; Fish oil

Garlic supplements and fish oils may have beneficial effects on blood lipids.

Clinical evidence

In a placebo-controlled study in 46 subjects with moderate, untreated hypercholesterolaemia, combined use of garlic pills 300 mg three times daily (*Kwai*) and fish oil capsules 4 g three times daily for 12 weeks was compared with either garlic or fish oil alone. Garlic modestly reduced total cholesterol, and fish oil did not alter this effect. Fish oil reduced triacylglycerol levels, and garlic did not alter this effect. Garlic alone reduced low-density-lipoprotein cholesterol, and combined use with fish oil *reversed* the increase of low-density-lipoprotein cholesterol seen with fish oil alone and produced a reduction similar to that seen with garlic alone. Slight reductions in blood pressure were also reported with all treatments.[1] The fish oil used was 1-g capsules (*Nupulse*) each containing eicosapentaenoic acid 180 mg and docosahexaenoic acid 120 mg.

Experimental evidence

Garlic oil has been found to enhance the antioxidant effects of fish oils in *rats*.[2]

Mechanism

Unclear. In the experimental study, garlic oil synergistically increased the induction of the antioxidant superoxide dismutase by fish oils, and the combination additively increased the protein levels of CYP1A1, CYP2E1 and CYP3A1.

Importance and management

The available clinical evidence appears to come from one study, which suggests that the combined use of garlic supplements and fish oils may have beneficial effects on blood lipids, which are known to be risk factors in coronary artery disease and atherosclerosis. While the clinical importance is inconclusive, any interaction is not expected to be harmful as far as blood lipids are concerned. Further study is needed to establish the benefits of combined use.

1. Adler AJ, Holub BJ. Effect of garlic and fish-oil supplementation on serum lipid and lipoprotein concentrations in hypercholesterolemic men. *Am J Clin Nutr* (1997) 65, 445–50.
2. Chen H-W, Tsai C-W, Yang J-J, Liu C-T, Kuo W-W, Lii C-K. The combined effects of garlic oil and fish oil on the hepatic antioxidant and drug-metabolizing enzymes of rats. *Br J Nutr* (2003) 89, 189–200.

G

Garlic + HIV-protease inhibitors

A garlic supplement reduced the plasma levels of saquinavir in one study, but had little effect in another. Another garlic supplement did not significantly affect the pharmacokinetics of a single dose of ritonavir.

Clinical evidence

In a study in 9 healthy subjects garlic reduced the AUC, and maximum and minimum plasma levels of **saquinavir** by about 50%. The garlic was taken in the form of a dietary supplement (*GarliPure, Maximum Allicin Formula* caplets) twice daily for 20 days. **Saquinavir** 1.2 g three times daily was given for 4-day periods before, during, and after the garlic supplement. Fourteen days after the garlic supplement was stopped the **saquinavir** pharmacokinetics had still not returned to baseline values. Of the 9 subjects, 6 had a substantial drop in the AUC of **saquinavir** while taking garlic, then a rise when garlic was stopped. The remaining 3 had no change in the AUC of **saquinavir** while taking garlic, but had a drop when garlic was stopped.[1] However, in another study, garlic extract (*Garlipure*) 1.2 g daily for 3 weeks had no significant effect on the pharmacokinetics of a single 1.2-g dose of **saquinavir** (a slight decrease in AUC in 7 subjects and a slight increase in 3).[2] A further study in 10 healthy subjects, designed primarily to examine the mechanism of the interaction with garlic, found that garlic extract (*Garlipure* caplets) 600 mg twice daily for 21 days reduced the AUC of a single 1200-mg dose of saquinavir by 10% and increased its half-life by 26%. However, due to the variability in saquinavir pharmacokinetics these findings were not statistically significant.[3]

In a study in 10 healthy subjects the use of a garlic extract (10 mg, equivalent to 1 g of fresh garlic) twice daily for 4 days did not significantly affect the pharmacokinetics of a single 400-mg dose of **ritonavir**. There was a non-significant 17% decrease in the AUC of **ritonavir**. The garlic was given in the form of capsules (*Natural Source Odourless Garlic Life Brand*).[4] Gastrointestinal toxicity was noted in 2 patients taking garlic or garlic supplements when they started to take **ritonavir**-containing regimens.[5]

Experimental evidence

In an experimental study using cell lines, allicin, a major active constituent of garlic, significantly decreased the clearance (efflux) of **ritonavir** from the cells in a dose-dependent manner.[6]

Mechanism

Garlic extract appears to induce P-glycoprotein, which is involved in the intestinal transport of saquinavir and thereby reduces saquinavir bioavailability.[3] Why there was a disparity in the effect of garlic on saquinavir between patients is unclear.

Allicin is thought to have inhibited the activity of P-glycoprotein *in vitro*, which caused the build-up of ritonavir within the cell.[6]

Importance and management

Although information is limited, a reduction in saquinavir plasma levels of the magnitude seen in the first study could diminish its antiviral efficacy. All garlic supplements should probably be avoided in those taking saquinavir as the sole HIV-protease inhibitor, but note that this is no longer generally recommended. The effect of garlic on saquinavir levels in the presence of ritonavir (as a pharmacokinetic enhancer) does not appear to have been studied. The pharmacokinetic effect on single-dose ritonavir was not clinically important, but this requires confirmation in a multiple-dose study.

1. Piscitelli SC, Burstein AH, Welden N, Gallicano KD, Falloon J. The effect of garlic supplements on the pharmacokinetics of saquinavir. *Clin Infect Dis* (2002) 34, 234–8.
2. Jacek H, Rentsch KM, Steinert HC, Pauli-Magnus C, Meier PJ, Fattinger K. No effect of garlic extract on saquinavir kinetics and hepatic CYP3A4 function measured by the erythromycin breath test. *Clin Pharmacol Ther* (2004) 75, P80.
3. Hajida J, Rentsch KM, Gubler C, Steiner H, Steiger B, Fattinger K. Garlic extract induces intestinal P-glycoprotein, but exhibits no effect on intestinal and hepatic CYP3A4 in humans. *Eur J Pharm Sci* (2010) 41, 729–35.

4. Gallicano K, Foster B, Choudhri S. Effect of short-term administration of garlic supplements on single-dose ritonavir pharmacokinetics in healthy volunteers. *Br J Clin Pharmacol* (2003) 55, 199–202.
5. Laroche M, Choudhri S, Gallicano K, Foster B. Severe gastrointestinal toxicity with concomitant ingestion of ritonavir and garlic. *Can J Infect Dis* (1998) 9 (Suppl A), 76A.
6. Patel J, Buddha B, Dey S, Pal D, Mitra AK. *In vitro* interaction of the HIV protease inhibitor ritonavir with herbal constituents: changes in P-gp and CYP3A4 activity. *Am J Ther* (2004) 11, 262–77.

Garlic + Isoniazid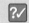

The interaction between garlic and isoniazid is based on experimental evidence only.

Clinical evidence

No interactions found.

Experimental evidence

In a study in *rabbits,* a garlic extract, produced from blended garlic cloves (exact dosage unknown) and given orally over 14 days, reduced the AUC and maximum serum levels of a single 30-mg/kg dose of isoniazid by about 55% and 65%, respectively, when compared with the levels attained after a single 30-mg/kg dose of isoniazid given 7 days before the garlic extract.[1]

Mechanism

Unclear. It was anticipated that garlic might increase isoniazid levels by inhibiting the cytochrome P450 isoenzyme CYP2E1, but *decreased* levels were seen. While the authors speculate that garlic extract may induce enzymes in the intestinal mucosa, which interferes with the absorption of isoniazid, they suggest that the findings cannot be explained solely on this basis.

Importance and management

The evidence is limited to this one study, and because the mechanism is unknown, a crude garlic extract was used, and the data are from *rabbits,* it is difficult to apply these findings to a clinical setting. However, if the reduction was shown to be replicated in humans then isoniazid efficacy might be reduced, so further study is warranted. Until more is known, a conservative approach would be to suggest some caution with the use of garlic supplements in patients taking isoniazid.

1. Dhamija P, Malhotra S, Pandhi P. Effect of oral administration of crude aqueous extract of garlic on pharmacokinetic parameters of isoniazid and rifampicin in rabbits. *Pharmacology* (2006) 77, 100–104.

Garlic + Paracetamol (Acetaminophen)

Studies in healthy subjects found that garlic did not affect the pharmacokinetics of single-dose paracetamol to a clinically relevant extent.

Clinical evidence

A study in 16 healthy subjects found that the use of an aged garlic extract (approximately equivalent to 6 to 7 cloves of garlic daily) for 3 months had little effect on the metabolism of a single 1-g oral dose of paracetamol.[1]

Experimental evidence

Diallyl sulfide, a constituent of garlic, and, to a greater extent, its metabolite diallyl sulfone, protected *mice* from paracetamol-induced hepatotoxicity when given immediately after a toxic dose of paracetamol (200 mg/kg). The effect of diallyl sufone 25 mg/kg was equivalent to that of the known antidote, acetylcysteine.[2]

Mechanism

There was a very slight increase in glucuronidation of a therapeutic dose of paracetamol after the long-term use of garlic in the clinical study, and some evidence that sulfate conjugation was enhanced, but no effect on oxidative metabolism.

It was suggested that diallyl sulfone protected against the hepatotoxicity of paracetamol after a toxic dose in *mice* because it irreversibly inhibited the cytochrome P450 isoenzyme CYP2E1. This isoenzyme is thought to be responsible for the production of a minor but highly reactive paracetamol metabolite, *N*-acetyl-*p*-benzoquinoneimine (NABQI).

Importance and management

The evidence regarding an interaction between paracetamol and garlic is limited, but what is known suggests that no clinically significant interaction would be expected if paracetamol is taken with garlic. The *animal* data suggest that it is possible that some garlic constituents, or substances derived from them, might prove to protect against the hepatotoxicity from higher than therapeutic doses of paracetamol, but this requires further study.

1. Gwilt PR, Lear CL, Tempero MA, Birt DD, Grandjean AC, Ruddon RW, Nagel DL. The effect of garlic extract on human metabolism of acetaminophen. *Cancer Epidemiol Biomarkers Prev* (1994) 3, 155–60.
2. Lin MC, Wang E-J, Patten C, Lee M-J, Xiao F, Reuhl KR, Yang CS. Protective effect of diallyl sulfone against acetaminophen-induced hepatotoxicity in mice. *J Biochem Toxicol* (1996) 11, 11–20.

Garlic + Rifampicin (Rifampin)

The information regarding the use of garlic with rifampicin is based on experimental evidence only.

Clinical evidence

No interactions found.

Experimental evidence

In a study in *rabbits,* a garlic extract, produced from blended garlic cloves (exact dosage unknown) and given orally over 14 days, did not alter the AUC and maximum serum levels of a single 24-mg/kg dose of rifampicin, when compared with the levels attained after a single 24-mg/kg dose of rifampicin given 7 days before the garlic extract.[1]

Mechanism

No mechanism expected.

Importance and management

Evidence appears to be limited to this one study in *animals*. Nevertheless, what is known suggests that no changes in the dose of rifampicin are likely to be needed if it is also taken with garlic.

1. Dhamija P, Malhotra S, Pandhi P. Effect of oral administration of crude aqueous extract of garlic on pharmacokinetic parameters of isoniazid and rifampicin in rabbits. *Pharmacology* (2006) 77, 100–104.

Garlic + Statins

A garlic extract did not affect the pharmacokinetics of single doses of simvastatin or pravastatin in one study.

Clinical evidence

In a randomised, crossover study in 10 healthy subjects, garlic extract (Garlipure caplets) 600 mg twice daily for 21 days had no effect on the pharmacokinetics of single 20-mg doses of pravastatin or simvastatin.[1]

Experimental evidence

No relevant data found.

Mechanism

In this study[1] patients were tested for CYP3A4 activity. Garlic extract was found not to affect CYP3A4 in either the liver or the intestine. Simvastatin is metabolised by CYP3A4 and therefore the concurrent use of garlic extract did not affect simvastatin pharmacokinetics.

Importance and management

Evidence for an interaction between garlic extract and statins appears to be limited to one single dose study using simvastatin and pravastatin, which found no interaction. In addition, from what is known about the metabolism of these statins, and the effects of garlic extract, no interaction would be expected.

1. Hajida J, Rentsch KM, Gubler C, Steinert H, Steiger B, Fattinger K. Garlic extract induces intestinal P-glycoprotein, but exhibits no effect on intestinal and hepatic CYP3A4 in humans. *Eur J Pharm Sci* (2010) 41, 729–35.

Garlic + Warfarin and related drugs

An isolated report described increases in the anticoagulant effects of warfarin in two patients taking garlic supplements. Another report described a decrease in anticoagulant effects of fluindione in a patient taking garlic tablets. Garlic supplements alone have also rarely been associated with bleeding. However, in one study, aged garlic extract did not increase the INR or risk of bleeding in patients taking warfarin.

Clinical evidence

(a) Fluindione

In an 82-year-old man stabilised on fluindione 5 mg (dosage frequency not stated) for chronic atrial fibrillation, the INR dropped to below its usual range (2 to 3) when garlic tablets 600 mg daily were taken, and remained below 2 for 12 consecutive days despite an increase in fluindione dosage to 10 mg. The INR returned to normal, with an associated reduction in fluindione dose, when the garlic tablets were stopped. He was also taking enalapril 20 mg, furosemide 40 mg and pravastatin 20 mg (dosage frequency not stated).[1]

(b) Warfarin

The INR of a patient stabilised on warfarin more than doubled and haematuria occurred 8 weeks after the patient started to take three *Höfels garlic pearles* daily. The situation resolved when the garlic was stopped. The INR rose on a later occasion while the patient was taking two *Kwai* garlic tablets daily. The INR of another patient was also more than doubled by six *Kwai* garlic tablets daily.[2,3]

In contrast, in a placebo-controlled study in 48 patients stabilised on warfarin, there was no change in INR or evidence of increased bleeding in those receiving 5 mL of aged garlic extract (*Kyolic*) twice daily for 12 weeks.[4] Similarly, in a preliminary report of the use of alternative and complementary medicines in 156 patients taking warfarin, there was no apparent increased risk or bleeding or raised INRs in 57 patients taking potentially interacting complementary medicines (garlic in 10%), compared with 84 who did not.[5]

Experimental evidence

No relevant data found.

Mechanism

Garlic has been associated with decreased platelet aggregation. See antiplatelet drugs, page 229 for possible mechanisms. This effect on platelet aggregation has, on at least two documented occasions, led to spontaneous bleeding in the absence of an anticoagulant.[6,7] These effects might therefore increase the risk of bleeding with anticoagulants. However, this would not cause an increase in INR, and the mechanism for this effect in the cases seen is unknown.

G

Importance and management

Information about an adverse interaction between coumarin antico-agulants and garlic seems to be limited to these two reports, with warfarin and fluindione. Bearing in mind the wide-spread use of garlic and garlic products, and the limited information from the review,[5] and the study with aged garlic extract,[4] it seems most unlikely that garlic usually has any generally important interaction with anticoagulants. Nevertheless, bear the possibility in mind in the event of an unexpected response to treatment.

In addition, garlic may have some antiplatelet effects, and although there appear to be no clinical reports of an adverse interaction between garlic and antiplatelet drugs, it may be prudent to consider the potential for an increase in the severity of bleeding if garlic is given with anticoagulants. See Garlic + Antiplatelet drugs, page 229.

1. Pathak A, Léger P, Bagheri H, Senard J-M, Boccalon H, Montastruc J-L. Garlic interaction with fluindione: a case report. *Therapie* (2003) 58, 380–381.
2. Sunter W. Warfarin and garlic. *Pharm J* (1991) 246, 722.
3. Sunter W. Personal communication. July 1991.
4. Macan H, Uykimpang R, Alconcel M, Takasu J, Razon R, Amagase H, Niihara Y. Aged garlic extract may be safe for patients on warfarin therapy. *J Nutr* (2006) 136 (Suppl 3), 793–5.
5. Shalansky S, Neall E, Lo M, Abd-Elmessih E, Vickars L, Lynd L. The impact of complementary and alternative medicine use on warfarin-related adverse outcomes. *Pharmacotherapy* (2002) 22, 1345.
6. German K, Kumar U, Blackford HN. Garlic and the risk of TURP bleeding. *Br J Urol* (1995) 76, 518.
7. Rose KD, Croissant PD, Parliament CF, Levin MP. Spontaneous spinal epidural hematoma with associated platelet dysfunction from excessive garlic ingestion: a case report. *Neurosurgery* (1990) 26, 880–882.

G

Ginger

Zingiber officinale Roscoe (Zingiberaceae)

Synonym(s) and related species

Gan Jiang, Zingiber.

Not to be confused with the wild gingers, which are *Asarum canadense* L. and *Asarum europaeum* L.

Pharmacopoeias

Ginger (*BP 2012, PhEur 7.5, USP35–NF30 S1*); Ginger capsules (*USP35–NF30 S1*); Ginger tincture (*USP35–NF30 S1*); Powdered ginger (*USP35–NF30 S1*); Strong Ginger Tincture (*BP 2012*); Weak Ginger Tincture (*BP 2012*).

Constituents

The constituents of ginger vary depending on whether fresh or dried forms are used. Generally, ginger rhizomes contain volatile oils of which **zingiberene** and **bisabolene** are major components: zingerone, zingiberol, zingiberenol, curcumene, camphene and linalool are minor components.

The rhizomes also contain **gingerols** and their derivatives, gingerdiols, gingerdiones and dihydrogingerdiones. **Shogaols** are formed from **gingerols** during drying, and together, these make up the pungent principles of ginger.

Ginger extracts have been standardised to contain a minimum of 15 mL/kg of essential oil with reference to the dried drug.

Use and indications

Ginger is thought to possess carminative, anti-emetic, anti-inflammatory, antispasmodic and antiplatelet properties. Both fresh and dried ginger are mainly used to settle the stomach, to alleviate the symptoms of motion sickness, and to relieve morning sickness. Ginger has also been used in the treatment of osteoarthritis and rheumatoid arthritis, and for migraines.

Ginger is also an important culinary spice and the pungent properties of ginger have also been exploited for use in cosmetics and soaps.

Ginger is a constituent of *Trikatu,* a medicine used in Ayurvedic medicine in a ratio of 1:1:1 with *Piper nigrum* and *Piper longum,* see pepper, page 372.

Pharmacokinetics

Detailed information on the pharmacokinetics of ginger in humans is scarce but what has been found, in *animals,* is that gingerol, a major constituent of ginger, is rapidly cleared from plasma and elimination by the liver is involved. Gingerol is also a substrate of several UDP-glucuronosyltransferases, which are major phase 2 metabolic enzymes responsible for the metabolism of several drugs. Gut flora also play a part in the metabolism of gingerol.[1]

Interactions overview

There are isolated cases of ginger increasing the response to anticoagulant treatment with warfarin and related drugs, but a controlled study did not confirm an interaction. A small study showed antiplatelet effects for ginger that were synergistic with those of nifedipine, but any effect needs confirming.

For the interactions of ginger as a constituent of *Trikatu,* a medicine used in Ayurvedic medicine, see Pepper + Isoniazid, page 375, Pepper + NSAIDs, page 376, and Pepper + Rifampicin (Rifampin), page 377. For the interactions of ginger as a constituent of Chinese herbal medicines, see under bupleurum, page 98.

Interactions monographs

- Anticoagulants, page 236
- Food, page 236
- Herbal medicines, page 236
- Nifedipine, page 236
- NSAIDs, page 237

1. Ali BH, Blunden G, Tanira MO, Nemmar A. Some phytochemical, pharmacological and toxicological properties of ginger (*Zingiber officinale* Roscoe): a review of recent research. *Food Chem Toxicol* (2008) 46, 409–20.

G

Ginger + Anticoagulants

Evidence from pharmacological studies suggests that ginger does not increase the anticoagulant effect of warfarin, neither does it alter coagulation or platelet aggregation on its own. However, two case reports describe markedly raised INRs with phenprocoumon and warfarin, which were associated with eating dried ginger and drinking ginger tea. A prospective, longitudinal study also reports of an increased risk of self-reported bleeding events in patients taking warfarin and ginger.

Clinical evidence

In a randomised, crossover study in 12 healthy subjects, 3 ginger capsules taken three times daily for 2 weeks did not affect either the pharmacokinetics or pharmacodynamics (INR) of a single 25-mg dose of **warfarin** taken on day 7. The brand of ginger used was *Blackmores Travel Calm Ginger,* each capsule containing an extract equivalent to 400 mg of ginger rhizome powder. Moreover, ginger alone did not affect the INR or platelet aggregation.[1]

However, a case report describes a rise in INR to greater than 10, with epistaxis, in a woman stabilised on **phenprocoumon** several weeks after she started to eat ginger regularly in the form of pieces of dried ginger and tea from ginger powder. She was eventually restabilised on the original dose of **phenprocoumon**, and was advised to stop taking ginger.[2] Another very similar case has been described in a woman taking **warfarin**.[3]

Moreover, in a prospective, longitudinal study of patients taking **warfarin** and a herbal product or dietary supplement, there was a statistically significant increased risk of self-reported bleeding events in patients taking **warfarin** and ginger (7 bleeds in 25 weeks, none of which were major: odds ratio 3.2).[4] No elevated INRs were reported for the combination. Note that the number of patients taking ginger was not reported, except to say it was less than 5% of 171; so it was less than 8 patients. Also, the ginger products used were not mentioned and some patients were taking more than one potentially interacting supplement.

Experimental evidence

See under *Mechanism* below.

Mechanism

Ginger (*Zingiber officinale*) has sometimes been listed as a herb that interacts with warfarin[5,6] on the basis that *in vitro* it inhibits platelet aggregation. However, this antiplatelet effect has generally not been demonstrated in controlled clinical studies (three of which have been reviewed[7]) although in one other study ginger had antiplatelet effects that were synergistic with those of nifedipine,[8] see nifedipine, below.

Importance and management

Evidence from a controlled study suggests that ginger does not increase the anticoagulant effect of warfarin. Despite it being cited as a herb that inhibits platelet aggregation, there is limited evidence that it increases bleeding when given alone or with warfarin, and there are just two case reports of markedly raised INRs with phenprocoumon and warfarin, which were associated with ginger root and ginger tea. Because of the many other factors influencing anticoagulant control, it is not possible to reliably ascribe a change in INR specifically to a drug interaction in a single case report without other supporting evidence. It may be better to advise patients to discuss the use of any herbal products they wish to try, and to increase monitoring if this is thought advisable. Cases of uneventful use should be reported, as they are as useful as possible cases of adverse effects.

1. Jiang X, Williams KM, Liauw WS, Ammit AJ, Roufogalis BD, Duke CC, Day RO, McLachlan AJ. Effect of ginkgo and ginger on the pharmacokinetics and pharmacodynamics of warfarin in healthy subjects. *Br J Clin Pharmacol* (2005) 59, 425–32.
2. Krüth P, Brosi E, Fux R, Mörike K, Gleiter CH. Ginger-associated overanticoagulation by phenprocoumon. *Ann Pharmacother* (2004) 38, 257–60.
3. Lesho EP, Saullo L, Udvari-Nagy S. A 76-year-old woman with erratic anticoagulation. *Cleve Clin J Med* (2004) 71, 651–6.
4. Shalansky S, Lynd L, Richardson K, Ingaszewski A, Kerr C. Risk of warfarin-related bleeding events and supratherapeutic international normalized ratios associated with complementary and alternative medicine: a longitudinal analysis. *Pharmacotherapy* (2007) 27, 1237–47.
5. Argento A, Tiraferri E, Marzaloni M. Anticoagulanti orali e piante medicinali. Una interazione emergente. *Ann Ital Med Int* (2000) 15, 139–43.
6. Braun L. Herb-drug interaction guide. *Aust Fam Physician* (2001) 30, 473–6.
7. Vaes LPJ, Chyka PA. Interactions of warfarin with garlic, ginger, ginkgo, or ginseng: nature of the evidence. *Ann Pharmacother* (2000) 34, 1478–82.
8. Young H-Y, Liao J-C, Chang Y-S, Luo Y-L, Lu M-C, Peng W-H. Synergistic effect of ginger and nifedipine on human platelet aggregation: a study in hypertensive patients and normal volunteers. *Am J Chin Med* (2006) 34, 545–51.

Ginger + Caffeine

For mention that sho-saiko-to (of which ginger is one of 7 constituents) only slightly reduced the metabolism of caffeine in one study, see Bupleurum + Caffeine, page 99.

Ginger + Carbamazepine

For mention that saiko-ka-ryukotsu-borei-to and sho-saiko-to (of which ginger is one of a number of constituents) did not affect the pharmacokinetics of carbamazepine in *animal* studies, see Bupleurum + Carbamazepine, page 99.

Ginger + Food

No interactions found. Ginger is extensively used as a food ingredient.

Ginger + Herbal medicines

No interactions found.

Ginger + Isoniazid

For details of an *animal* study to investigate a possible interaction between isoniazid and *Trikatu,* an Ayurvedic medicine containing ginger, black pepper and long pepper, see Pepper + Isoniazid, page 375.

Ginger + Nifedipine

A small study found that antiplatelet effects for ginger were synergistic with those of nifedipine, but any effect needs confirmation.

Evidence, mechanism, importance and management

In a small study in 10 hypertensive patients and another in 10 healthy subjects, ginger 1 g daily for 7 days given with nifedipine 10 mg twice daily for 7 days inhibited platelet aggregation by up to three times more than nifedipine alone.[1] In these studies, ginger alone had similar antiplatelet effects to aspirin 75 mg (used as a control), either alone, or given with nifedipine. Nifedipine alone also had antiplatelet effects, but these were not as great as aspirin 75 mg alone. The ginger used in this study was dried, but no other details about the preparation were given.

G

Calcium-channel blockers are not generally viewed as antiplatelet drugs, and the finding of synergistic antiplatelet effects between nifedipine and aspirin in this report and its clinical relevance needs further study. Furthermore, this study suggests that ginger alone may have similar antiplatelet effects to low-dose aspirin alone; however, this antiplatelet effect has generally not been demonstrated in other controlled clinical studies of ginger (three of which have been reviewed[2]). Therefore, it is difficult to make any clinical recommendations on the basis of this one small study. Further study is clearly needed.

1. Young H-Y, Liao J-C, Chang Y-S, Luo Y-L, Lu M-C, Peng W-H. Synergistic effect of ginger and nifedipine on human platelet aggregation: a study in hypertensive patients and normal volunteers. *Am J Chin Med* (2006) 34, 545–51.
2. Vaes LPJ, Chyka PA. Interactions of warfarin with garlic, ginger, ginkgo, or ginseng: nature of the evidence. *Ann Pharmacother* (2000) 34, 1478–82.

Ginger + NSAIDs

For details of an *animal* study to investigate a possible interaction between diclofenac and *Trikatu,* an Ayurvedic medicine containing ginger, black pepper and long pepper, see Pepper + NSAIDs, page 376.

Ginger + Ofloxacin

For mention that sairei-to and sho-saiko-to (of which ginger is one of a number of constituents) do not affect the pharmacokinetics of ofloxacin, see Bupleurum + Ofloxacin, page 99.

Ginger + Rifampicin (Rifampin)

For details of an interaction between rifampicin and *Trikatu,* an Ayurvedic medicine containing ginger, black pepper and long pepper, see Pepper + Rifampicin (Rifampin), page 377.

Ginger + Tolbutamide

For conflicting evidence from *animal* studies that sho-saiko-to (of which ginger is one of 7 constituents) might increase or decrease the rate of absorption of tolbutamide, see Bupleurum + Tolbutamide, page 99.

G

Ginkgo

Ginkgo biloba L. (Ginkgoaceae)

Synonym(s) and related species

Fossil tree, Kew tree, Maidenhair tree.

Salisburia adiantifolia Sm., *Salisburia biloba* Hoffmanns.

Pharmacopoeias

Ginkgo (*USP35–NF30 S1*); Ginkgo capsules (*USP35–NF30 S1*); Ginkgo dry extract, refined and quantified (*BP 2012, PhEur 7.5*); Ginkgo leaf (*BP 2012, PhEur 7.5*); Ginkgo tablets (*USP35–NF30 S1*); Powdered ginkgo extract (*USP35–NF30 S1*).

Constituents

Ginkgo leaves contain numerous **flavonoids** including the biflavone glycosides such as ginkgetin, isoginkgetin, bilobetin, sciadopitysin, and also some quercetin and kaempferol derivatives. **Terpene lactones** are the other major component, and these include ginkgolides A, B and C, and bilobalide, Ginkgo extracts may be standardised to contain between 22 and 27% **flavonoids** (flavone glycosides) and between 5 and 12% terpene lactones, both on the dried basis. The leaves contain only minor amounts of ginkgolic acids, and some pharmacopoeias specify a limit for these.

The seeds contain ginkgotoxin (4-*O*-methylpyridoxine) and ginkgolic acids.

Use and indications

The leaves of ginkgo are the part usually used. Ginkgo is often used to improve cognitive function in cases of dementia and memory loss, and it has been investigated for use in the treatment of Alzheimer's disease. The ginkgolides are thought to possess antiplatelet and anti-inflammatory properties and it has been used for cerebrovascular and peripheral vascular disorders, tinnitus, asthma and to relieve the symptoms of altitude sickness.

Ginkgo seeds contain some toxic constituents; nevertheless, they are used in China and Japan, including as a food.

Pharmacokinetics

The two main active components of ginkgo are flavonoids and terpene lactones. For information on the pharmacokinetics of individual flavonoids present in ginkgo, see under flavonoids, page 213. In contrast to the flavonoids, the bioavailability of ginkgolide A and B (but not C) and bilobalide is relatively high and a large proportion of the dose is excreted unchanged in the urine.[1]

The effects of ginkgo on cytochrome P450 isoenzymes appear to have been relatively well studied. It appears that the flavonoid fraction of ginkgo has more of an effect on the cytochrome P450 isoenzymes than the terpene lactones,[2,3] and the effect on these enzymes can be halted relatively quickly when ginkgo is stopped.[4]

In vitro and *rat* studies[2–5] have found that ginkgo may have some modest effects on CYP1A2 (see also theophylline, page 249). However, evidence from clinical studies using the specific probe substrate caffeine suggests that this is not clinically relevant with therapeutic doses of ginkgo. See Ginkgo + Caffeine, page 242.

Similarly, *in vitro* and *rat* studies[2–4,6–8] have suggested that ginkgo affects CYP2C9, CYP2D6, and CYP2E1, but clinical studies using the specific probe substrates tolbutamide, page 249, for CYP2C9; dextromethorphan, page 244, for CYP2D6; and chlorzoxazone, page 244, for CYP2E1 have found no clinically relevant effect.

In contrast, *in vitro* findings suggesting that ginkgo may affect CYP3A4[2–4,6–9] and induce CYP2C9[2–4,6–8] are supported by clinical studies with midazolam, page 241 and omeprazole, page 248, respectively. However, the effect of ginkgo on CYP3A4 is unclear (induction and inhibition reported), but any effect appears weak at best.

In vitro and *rat* studies[4,6,7] also suggest that ginkgo may affect CYP2B6 and CYP2C8, but the effect on CYP2B6 does not appear to be clinically relevant, see bupropion, page 242.

Ginkgo is unlikely to affect the activity of P-glycoprotein to a clinically relevant extent (see digoxin, page 244 and talinolol, page 248).

Interactions overview

Ginkgo appears to decrease the levels of omeprazole; it seems likely that most other proton pump inhibitors will be similarly affected. Some evidence suggests that diltiazem and nifedipine levels may be raised by ginkgo, whereas nicardipine levels may be reduced.

Isolated cases of bleeding have been seen when ginkgo has been taken with conventional antiplatelet drugs, anticoagulants and NSAIDs, and some cases have occurred with ginkgo alone, although a clinically relevant antiplatelet effect for ginkgo alone is not established. Isolated case reports also suggest that ginkgo may cause seizures in patients taking phenytoin and/or valproate and one case had decreased phenytoin and valproate levels. Phenobarbital levels do not appear to be significantly affected, although this is based on experimental data only. Isolated cases also describe coma in a patient taking trazodone with ginkgo, priapism in a patient taking ginkgo with risperidone, virological failure in a patient taking efavirenz and ginkgo, and CNS depression in a patient taking ginkgo with valerian, although this latter case is confused by alcohol consumption.

There are some *animal* data suggesting that ciclosporin levels might be reduced by ginkgo, and it has been suggested that the extrapyramidal adverse effects of haloperidol and the ototoxic effects of amikacin may be enhanced by ginkgo.

G

Ginkgo does not appear to affect the pharmacokinetics/metabolism of alprazolam, bupropion, caffeine, chlorzoxazone, dextromethorphan, diclofenac, digoxin, donepezil, fexofenadine, flurbiprofen, lopinavir boosted with ritonavir, metformin, midazolam, talinolol, propranolol, theophylline, or tolbutamide to a clinically relevant extent.

For a case of anxiety and memory deficits in a woman taking several drugs and herbal medicines, including ginkgo, see St John's wort + Buspirone, page 443.

For information on the interactions of individual flavonoids present in ginkgo, see under flavonoids, page 213.

Interactions monographs

1. Biber A. Pharmacokinetics of Ginkgo biloba extracts. *Pharmacopsychiatry* (2003) 36, S32–S37.
2. Gaudineau C, Beckerman R, Welbourn S, Auclair K. Inhibition of human P450 enzymes by multiple constituents of the *Ginkgo biloba* extract. *Biochem Biophys Res Commun* (2004) 318, 1072–8.
3. von Moltke LL, Weemhoff JL, Bedir E, Khan IA, Harmatz JS, Goldman P, Greenblatt DJ. Inhibition of human cytochromes P450 by components of *Ginkgo biloba*. *J Pharm Pharmacol* (2004) 56, 1039–44.
4. Sugiyama T, Kubota Y, Shinozuka K, Yamada S, Yamada K, Umegaki K. Induction and recovery of hepatic drug metabolizing enzymes in rats treated with *Ginkgo biloba* extract. *Food Chem Toxicol* (2004) 42, 953–7.
5. Hellum BH, Hu Z, Nilsen OG. The induction of CYP1A2, CYP2D6 and CYP3A4 by six trade herbal products in cultured primary human hepatocytes. *Basic Clin Pharmacol Toxicol* (2007) 100, 23–30.
6. Etheridge AS, Black SR, Patel PR, So J, Mathews JM. An *in vitro* evaluation of cytochrome P450 inhibition and P-glycoprotein interaction with goldenseal, *Ginkgo biloba*, grape seed, milk thistle, and ginseng extracts and their constituents. *Planta Med* (2007) 73, 731–41.
7. Sugiyama T, Shinozuka K, Sano A, Yamada S, Endoh K, Yamada K, Umegaki K. Effects of various *Ginkgo biloba* extracts and proanthocyanidin on hepatic cytochrome P450 activity in rats. *Shokuhin Eiseigaku Zasshi* (2004) 45, 295–301.
8. Yale SH, Glurich I. Analysis of the inhibitory potential of *Ginkgo biloba, Echinacea purpurea,* and *Serenoa repens* on the metabolic activity of cytochrome P450 3A4, 2D6, and 2C9. *J Altern Complement Med* (2005) 11, 433–9.
9. Hellum BH, Nilsen OG. *In vitro* inhibition of CYP3A4 metabolism and P-glycoprotein-mediated transport by trade herbal products. *Basic Clin Pharmacol Toxicol* (2008) 102, 466–75.

G

Ginkgo + Aminoglycosides

The interaction between ginkgo and amikacin is based on experimental evidence only.

Clinical evidence

No interactions found.

Experimental evidence

Ginkgo 100 mg/kg (EGb 761) daily for 20 days and amikacin 600 mg/kg daily for the first 14 days were given to *rats*. Amikacin-induced ototoxicity developed earlier and to a greater level than that caused by amikacin given alone. Ginkgo alone did not induce ototoxicity.[1]

Mechanism

Unknown.

Importance and management

Ginkgo appears to accelerate the appearance of amikacin-induced ototoxicity and to increase its ototoxic effects in *rats*. Because the development of ototoxicity is cumulative, if ginkgo accelerates this process, there is potential for ototoxicity to develop at a lower cumulative dose. The available evidence is weak, but until more is known it may be prudent to carefully consider the risks and benefits of continuing ginkgo during treatment with drugs such as the aminoglycosides.

1. Miman MC, Ozturan O, Iraz M, Erdem T, Olmez E. Amikacin ototoxicity enhanced by *Ginkgo biloba* extract (EGb 761). *Hear Res* (2002) 169, 121–9.

Ginkgo + Antiepileptics

Case reports describe seizures in three patients taking valproate, or valproate and phenytoin, when ginkgo was also taken.

Clinical evidence

A 55-year-old man taking **valproate** and **phenytoin** for a seizure disorder that developed following coronary artery bypass surgery, suffered a fatal breakthrough seizure while swimming a year later. Analysis of his medical history showed that he had unexplained subtherapeutic serum levels of **valproate** and **phenytoin** on three occasions over the previous year. It was later found that the patient had also been taking numerous vitamins, supplements and herbal medicines without the knowledge of his physician, of which a ginkgo extract was stated to be the most common ingredient.[1] The only other herbal medicines named in the report were ginseng and saw palmetto.

In another case, a 78-year-old man, whose epileptic seizures had been well controlled by **valproate** 1.2 g daily for 7 years, suffered a cluster of seizures after taking a ginkgo extract 120 mg daily for 2 weeks for the management of mild cognitive impairment. The ginkgo was stopped and the patient was reportedly seizure-free 8 months later. All other medications taken by the patient remained unchanged.[2]

An 84-year-old epileptic woman with severe dementia taking **valproate** 1.2 g daily had been seizure-free for 2 years. After taking a ginkgo extract 120 mg daily for 12 days prescribed by her psychiatrist, she suffered a cluster of seizures, which were treated with intravenous diazepam in the emergency department. The ginkgo extract was stopped on admission and the patient remained free of seizures 4 months later. All other medications taken by the patient were unchanged.[2]

Experimental evidence

No relevant data found.

Mechanism

Unknown. Ginkgo *seeds* (nuts) contain the neurotoxin 4-*O*-methoxypyridoxine (ginkgotoxin), which indirectly inhibits the activity of glutamate decarboxylase, which in turn results in seizure induction by lowering the levels of γ-amino-butyric acid (GABA). A large quantity of ginkgo nuts (about 70 to 80) alone have been reported to be the cause of seizures in a healthy 36-year-old woman.[3] However, leaf extracts would not generally be expected to contain sufficient levels of this neurotoxin to be a problem.

Another possible mechanism is induction of the cytochrome P450 isoenzyme CYP2C19 by ginkgo. Phenytoin is a substrate of CYP2C19 and therefore, in theory, ginkgo may increase the metabolism of phenytoin and thereby reduce its levels. Ginkgo has been seen to induce CYP2C19 in clinical studies. See Ginkgo + Proton pump inhibitors, page 248.

Importance and management

Evidence for an interaction between ginkgo and valproate and phenytoin appears to be limited to case reports. The only case that measured serum levels of these antiepileptics is complicated by the use of numerous other supplements. An interaction is therefore by no means established. Nevertheless, it may be prudent to consider the possibility of reduced effects if a patients taking phenytoin and/or valproate wishes to also take ginkgo.

For details of a possible interaction between ginkgo and phenobarbital in *animals* see Ginkgo + Phenobarbital, page 247.

1. Kupiec T, Raj V. Fatal seizures due to potential herb-drug interactions with Ginkgo biloba. *J Anal Toxicol* (2005) 29, 755–8.
2. Granger AS. *Ginkgo biloba* precipitating epileptic seizures. *Age Ageing* (2001) 30, 523–5.
3. Miwa H, Iijima M, Tanaka S, Mizuno Y. Generalised convulsions after consuming a large amount of ginkgo nuts. *Epilepsia* (2001) 42, 280–281.

Ginkgo + Antiplatelet drugs

Ginkgo biloba has been associated with platelet, bleeding, and clotting disorders, and there are isolated reports of serious adverse reactions after its concurrent use with antiplatelet drugs such as aspirin, clopidogrel, and ticlopidine.

Clinical evidence

A study in 10 healthy subjects found no significant increase in the antiplatelet effects of single doses of **clopidogrel** 75 mg or **cilostazol** 100 mg when a single dose of ginkgo 120 mg was added. However, the bleeding time was significantly increased when **cilostazol** was combined with ginkgo, although none of the subjects developed any significant adverse effects.[1] Another study[2] in 8 healthy subjects found that ginkgo 40 mg three times daily had no significant effect on the pharmacokinetics of a single 250-mg dose of **ticlopidine** taken on day 4.

A randomised, double-blind study in 55 patients with established peripheral artery disease (PAD) or with risk factors for developing PAD, found that the addition of ginkgo 300 mg (standardised extract EGb 761) in divided doses to **aspirin** 325 mg daily did not have a significant effect on platelet aggregation. Five of the patients taking combined therapy reported nosebleeds or minor bleeding; however, 4 patients from the **aspirin**-only group also reported minor bleeding.[3] Similarly, a study in 41 healthy subjects found that 120-mg ginkgo-coated tablets (EGb 761) twice daily had no effect on the antiplatelet activity of **aspirin** 500 mg daily given for seven days. Minor bleeding was seen in a few subjects but this was attributed to the use of **aspirin**.[4] In an analysis of supplement use, 23% of 123 patients were currently taking supplements, and 4 patients were found to be taking ginkgo and **aspirin**. However, no problems from this use were found on review of the patients' notes.[5]

Nevertheless, a number of cases of clinically significant bleeding have been reported. A 70-year-old man developed spontaneous bleeding from the iris into the anterior chamber of his eye within one week of starting to take a ginkgo supplement (*Ginkoba*) tablet twice daily. He experienced recurrent episodes of blurred vision in one eye lasting about 15 minutes, during which he could see a red discoloration through his cornea. Each tablet contained 40 mg of concentrated (50:1) extract of ginkgo. He was also taking **aspirin** 325 mg daily, which he had taken uneventfully for 3 years since having coronary bypass surgery. He stopped taking the ginkgo but continued with the **aspirin**, and 3 months later had experienced no recurrence of the bleeding.[6] Another case reports persistent post-operative bleeding from a hip arthroplasty wound, which continued despite stopping **aspirin**. On closer questioning, the patient had continued to take ginkgo extract 120 mg daily postoperatively. The oozing from the wound gradually reduced when the ginkgo was stopped.

A search of Health Canada's database of spontaneous adverse reactions for the period January 1999 to June 2003 found 21 reports of suspected adverse reactions associated with ginkgo. Most of these involved platelet, bleeding, and clotting disorders. One report of a fatal gastrointestinal haemorrhage was associated with ticlopidine and ginkgo, both taken over 2 years along with other medications. Another report was of a stroke in a patient taking multiple drugs, including **clopidogrel**, **aspirin**, and a herbal product containing ginkgo.[7]

Experimental evidence

Ginkgo (EGb 761) 40 mg/kg daily had no effect on the antiplatelet activity of **ticlopidine** 50 mg/kg daily when given to *rats* for 3 days. However, when both were given for 5 days, the inhibition of platelet aggregation was double that of **ticlopidine** given alone and the bleeding time was increased by about 60%. Also, when given for 9 days, the combination was twice as effective at inhibiting thrombus formation when compared to the same dose of **ticlopidine** alone.[8]

Mechanism

The reason for the bleeding is not known, but ginkgo extract contains ginkgolide B, which is a potent inhibitor of platelet-activating factor *in vitro*, which is needed for arachidonate-independent platelet aggregation. However, in one controlled study in healthy subjects, taking a ginkgo preparation alone for two weeks had no effect on platelet function.[9] Nevertheless, there are case reports of ginkgo supplements, on their own, being associated with prolonged bleeding times,[10–12] left and bilateral subdural haematomas,[10,13] a right parietal haematoma,[14] a retrobulbar haemorrhage,[15] post-laparoscopic cholecystectomy bleeding,[16] and subarachnoid haemorrhage.[11] It seems that the effects of ginkgo and conventional antiplatelet drugs can be additive, leading to bleeding complications on rare occasions.

Importance and management

The evidence from these case reports is too slim to advise patients taking aspirin, clopidogrel, or ticlopidine to avoid ginkgo, but some do recommend caution,[7] which seems prudent, especially as this is generally advised with most combinations of conventional antiplatelet drugs. There may also be a theoretical risk of increased bleeding if ginkgo is taken with other antiplatelet drugs and anticoagulants; interactions have been reported with NSAIDs, some of which have antiplatelet effects, and with warfarin.

Consider also Ginkgo + NSAIDs, page 247 and Ginkgo + Warfarin and related drugs, page 250.

1. Aruna D, Naidu MUR. Pharmacodynamic interaction studies of *Ginkgo biloba* with cilostazol and clopidogrel in healthy human subjects. *Br J Clin Pharmacol* (2007) 63, 333–8.
2. Lu W-J, Huang J-d, Lai M-L. The effects of ergoloid mesylates and Ginkgo biloba on the pharmacokinetics of ticlopidine. *J Clin Pharmacol* (2006) 46, 628–34.
3. Gardner CD, Zehnder JL, Rigby AJ, Nicholus JR, Farquhar JW. Effect of Ginkgo biloba (EGb 761) and aspirin on platelet aggregation and platelet function analysis among older adults at risk of cardiovascular disease: a randomized clinical trial. *Blood Coagul Fibrinolysis* (2007) 18, 787–93.
4. Wolf HRD. Does *Ginkgo biloba* special extract EGb 761® provide additional effects on coagulation and bleeding when added to acetylsalicylic acid 500 mg daily? *Drugs R D* (2006) 7, 163–72.
5. Ly J, Percy L, Dhanani S. Use of dietary supplements and their interactions with prescription drugs in the elderly. *Am J Health-Syst Pharm* (2002) 59, 1759–62.
6. Rosenblatt M, Mindel J. Spontaneous hyphema associated with ingestion of *Ginkgo biloba* extract. *N Engl J Med* (1997) 336, 1108.
7. Griffiths J, Jordan S, Pilon S. Natural health products and adverse reactions. *Can Adverse React News* (2004) 14, 2–3.

8. Kim YS, Pyo MK, Park KM, Park PH, Hahn BS, Wu SJ, Yun-Choi HS. Antiplatelet and antithrombotic effects of a combination of ticlopidine and *Ginkgo biloba* ext (EGb 761). *Thromb Res* (1998) 91, 33–8.
9. Beckert BW, Concannon MJ, Henry SL, Smith DS, Puckett CL. The effect of herbal medicines on platelet function: an in vivo experiment and review of the literature. *Plast Reconstr Surg* (2007) 120, 2044–50.
10. Rowin J, Lewis SL. Spontaneous bilateral subdural hematomas associated with chronic *Ginkgo biloba* ingestion. *Neurology* (1996) 46, 1775–6.
11. Vale S. Subarachnoid haemorrhage associated with *Ginkgo biloba*. *Lancet* (1998) 352, 36.
12. Bebbington A, Kulkarni R, Roberts P. Ginkgo biloba: persistent bleeding after total hip arthroplasty caused by herbal self-medication. *J Arthroplasty* (2005) 20, 125–6.
13. Gilbert GJ. *Ginkgo biloba*. *Neurology* (1997) 48, 1137.
14. Benjamin J, Muir T, Briggs K, Pentland B. A case of cerebral haemorrhage - can *Ginkgo biloba* be implicated? *Postgrad Med J* (2001) 77, 112–13.
15. Fong KCS, Kinnear PE. Retrobulbar haemorrhage associated with chronic *Gingko* [*sic*] *biloba* ingestion. *Postgrad Med J* (2003) 79, 531–2.
16. Fessenden JM, Wittenborn W, Clarke L. Gingko biloba: a case report of herbal medicine and bleeding postoperatively from a laparoscopic cholecystectomy. *Am Surg* (2001) 67, 33–5.

Ginkgo + Benzodiazepines

Ginkgo does not significantly affect the pharmacokinetics of alprazolam or diazepam. Studies with midazolam suggest that ginkgo may increase, decrease, or have no effect on its metabolism.

Clinical evidence

(a) Alprazolam

Ginkgo leaf extract 120 mg twice daily for 16 days was given to 12 healthy subjects before and with a single 2-mg dose of **alprazolam** on day 14. The ginkgo preparation (*Ginkgold*) was standardised to ginkgo flavonol glycosides 24% and terpene lactones 6%. The **alprazolam** AUC was reduced by 17%, and the maximum concentration was not significantly affected.[1]

(b) Diazepam

In a study in 12 healthy subjects, ginkgo 40 mg four times daily for 28 days did not affect the metabolism of a single 10-mg dose of **diazepam**, or its *N*-desmethyl metabolite. The ginkgo preparation used was stated to contain 24% flavone glycosides and 6% terpene lactones.[2]

(c) Midazolam

In 12 healthy subjects, ginkgo 60 mg four times daily for 28 days did not affect the metabolism of **midazolam** 8 mg. The ginkgo preparation used was stated to contain 24% flavone glycosides and 6% terpene lactones.[3] These findings were repeated in a later study using the same criteria in 12 elderly healthy subjects,[4] and a further study in 17 healthy subjects given another ginkgo extract, EGb 761, for 8 days.[5] In contrast, in another similar study, ginkgo 120 mg twice daily modestly *reduced* the AUC and maximum serum levels of a single 8-mg dose of **midazolam** by about one-third. The ginkgo preparation was assayed, and contained 29% flavonol glycosides and 5% terpene lactones.[6] Furthermore, in yet another study in 10 healthy subjects, ginkgo 360 mg daily for 28 days *increased* the AUC of a single 8-mg dose of oral **midazolam** by about one-quarter. The ginkgo preparation used was *Ginkgold*, which was stated to contain 24% flavone glycosides and 6% terpene lactones.[7]

Experimental evidence

In an experimental study, unfamiliar pairs of *rats* were placed together in a novel arena for 10 minutes to determine the effects of combined administration of ginkgo and **diazepam** on social behaviour. Social contact between *rats* given ginkgo 96 mg/kg (EGb 761) daily for 8 days and then a single injection of **diazepam** 1 mg/kg 30 minutes before testing, was significantly higher than those given ginkgo or **diazepam** alone.[8]

Mechanism

Alprazolam and midazolam are probe substrates for the cytochrome P450 isoenzyme CYP3A4. The studies here show that ginkgo has minimal effects on this isoenzyme, the maximum effect on midazolam being about a 33% reduction in AUC. However, it is unusual

G

for studies to show opposite effects (one of the studies found a minor increase in midazolam AUC), and the reasons for this are unclear, but may be to do with the methodology (use of midazolam metabolic ratios rather than midazolam exposure, and length of sampling time[6] and the fact that in one study the subjects had previously received lopinavir boosted with ritonavir for 30 days, concurrently with the ginkgo for 2 weeks, just 2 weeks before the midazolam[6]).

The experimental findings suggested that ginkgo may interact with diazepam through its effects on the gamma-aminobutyric acid (GABA) receptor. The reasons for this are unclear. The clinical study suggests that there is no pharmacokinetic component to any interaction.

Importance and management

The pharmacokinetic evidence here shows that alprazolam and midazolam levels are not significantly affected by ginkgo, and no clinically relevant interaction would be expected. The conflicting finding of the metabolism of midazolam being slightly inhibited in one study *and* slightly induced in another is, however, unexplained, but either effect would be modest at the most. Alprazolam and midazolam are used as a probe drugs for CYP3A4 activity, and therefore these results also suggest that a clinically relevant pharmacokinetic interaction as a result of this mechanism between ginkgo and other CYP3A4 substrates is unlikely.

The clinical relevance of the possible interaction of ginkgo with diazepam in *rats* is unknown; however, no clinically relevant pharmacokinetic interaction is expected, suggesting that diazepam dose alterations would not be expected to be necessary in patients taking ginkgo.

1. Markowitz JS, Donovan JL, DeVane CL, Sipkes L, Chavin KD. Multiple-dose administration of *Ginkgo biloba* did not affect cytochrome P-450 2D6 or 3A4 activity in normal volunteers. *J Clin Psychopharmacol* (2003) 23, 576–81.
2. Zuo X-C, Zhang B-K, Jia S-J, Liu S-K, Zhou L-Y, Li J, Zhang J, Dai L-L, Chen B-M, Yang G-P, Yuan H. Effects of *ginkgo biloba* extracts on diazepam metabolism: a pharmacokinetic study in healthy Chinese male subjects *Eur J Clin Pharmacol* (2010) 66, 503–9.
3. Gurley BJ, Gardner SF, Hubbard MA, Williams DK, Gentry WB, Cui Y, Ang CYW. Cytochrome P450 phenotypic ratios for predicting herb-drug interactions in humans. *Clin Pharmacol Ther* (2002) 72, 276–87.
4. Gurley BJ, Gardner SF, Hubbard MA, Williams DK, Gentry WB, Cui Y, Ang CYW. Clinical assessment of botanical supplementation on cytochrome P450 phenotypes in the elderly: St John's wort, garlic oil, *Panax ginseng*, and *Ginkgo biloba*. *Drugs Aging* (2005) 22, 525–39.
5. Zadoyan G, Rokitta D, Klement S, Dienel A, Hoerr R, Gramatté T, Fuhr U. Effect of *Ginkgo biloba* special extract EGb 761® on human cytochrome P450 activity: a cocktail interaction study in healthy volunteers *Eur J Clin Pharmacol* (2012) 68, 553–60.
6. Robertson SM, Davey RT, Voell J, Formentini E, Alfaro RM, Penzak SR. Effect of *Ginkgo biloba* extract on lopinavir, midazolam and fexofenadine pharmacokinetics in healthy subjects. *Curr Med Res Opin* (2008) 24, 591–9.
7. Uchida S, Yamada H, Li DX, Maruyama S, Ohmori Y, Oki T, Watanabe H, Umegaki K, Ohashi K, Yamada T. Effects of Ginkgo biloba extract on pharmacokinetics and pharmacodynamics of tolbutamide and midazolam in healthy volunteers. *J Clin Pharmacol* (2006) 46, 1290–1298.
8. Chermat R, Brochet D, DeFeudis FV, Drieu K. Interactions of *Ginkgo biloba* extract (EGb 761), diazepam and ethyl β-carboline-3-carboxylate on social behaviour of the rat. *Pharmacol Biochem Behav* (1997) 56, 333–9.

Ginkgo + Bupropion

Ginkgo does not appear to affect the pharmacokinetics of bupropion to a clinically relevant extent.

Clinical evidence

In a study, 14 healthy subjects were given a single 150-mg dose of sustained-release bupropion before and after taking ginkgo 120 mg twice daily for 14 days. Gingko had no effect on the pharmacokinetics of bupropion or its metabolite, hydroxybupropion, aside from a small increase in the maximum concentrations of hydroxybupropion. In this study the ginkgo preparation used was stated to contain 24% flavone glycosides and 6% terpene lactones.[1]

Experimental evidence

An *in vitro* study examining the effect of ginkgo and its terpene and flavonol constituents on bupropion metabolism found that flavonol aglycones and ginkgo biloba extract were inhibitors of the cytochrome P450 isoenzyme CYP2B6.[2] See also, *Pharmacokinetics,* under Gingko, page 238.

Mechanism

Ginkgo appears to inhibit CYP2B6 but the effects in clinical use appear weak.

Importance and management

Although *in vitro* data suggested that gingko might increase bupropion exposure, studies in healthy subjects have found no clinically relevant effect on bupropion pharmacokinetics. It would therefore appear that the dose of bupropion would not be expected to need adjusting in patients who also take ginkgo.

1. Lei H-P, Ji W, Lin J, Chen H, Tan Z-R, Hu D-L, Liu L-J, Zhou H-H. Effects of *Ginkgo biloba* extract on the pharmacokinetics of bupropion in healthy volunteers *Br J Clin Pharmacol* (2009) 68, 201–6.
2. Lau AJ, Chang TKH. Inhibition of human CYP2B6-catalyzed bupropion hydroxylation by *Ginkgo biloba* extract: effect of terpene trilactones and flavonols *Drug Metab Dispos* (2009) 37, 1931–7.

Ginkgo + Buspirone

For a case of anxiety, with episodes of over-sleeping and memory deficits in a woman taking fluoxetine and buspirone with St John's wort, ginkgo and melatonin, see St John's wort + Buspirone, page 443.

Ginkgo + Caffeine

Ginkgo does not appear to affect the pharmacokinetics of caffeine.

Clinical evidence

In 12 healthy subjects, ginkgo 60 mg four times daily for 28 days did not affect the metabolism of caffeine 100 mg. The ginkgo preparation used was standardised to 24% flavone glycosides and 6% terpene lactones.[1] These findings were repeated in a later study using the same criteria in 12 elderly healthy subjects,[2] and a further study in 18 healthy subjects given another extract of ginkgo, EGb 761, at a dose of either 120 mg twice daily or 240 mg daily for 8 days.[3]

Experimental evidence

No relevant data found.

Mechanism

This study shows that ginkgo has no clinically relevant effect on the cytochrome P450 isoenzyme CYP1A2.

Importance and management

Evidence from studies in healthy subjects suggests that ginkgo does not affect the metabolism of caffeine and is therefore unlikely to increase its adverse effects. Caffeine is used as a probe drug for CYP1A2 activity, and therefore these results also suggest that a pharmacokinetic interaction as a result of this mechanism between ginkgo and other CYP1A2 substrates is unlikely.

1. Gurley BJ, Gardner SF, Hubbard MA, Williams DK, Gentry WB, Cui Y, Ang CYW. Cytochrome P450 phenotypic ratios for predicting herb-drug interactions in humans. *Clin Pharmacol Ther* (2002) 72, 276–87.
2. Gurley BJ, Gardner SF, Hubbard MA, Williams DK, Gentry WB, Cui Y, Ang CYW. Clinical assessment of botanical supplementation on cytochrome P450 phenotypes in the elderly: St John's wort, garlic oil, *Panax ginseng*, and *Ginkgo biloba*. *Drugs Aging* (2005) 22, 525–39.
3. Zadoyan G, Rokitta D, Klement S, Dienel A, Hoerr R, Gramatté T, Fuhr U. Effect of *Ginkgo biloba* special extract EGb 761® on human cytochrome P450 activity: a cocktail interaction study in healthy volunteers *Eur J Clin Pharmacol* (2012) 68, 553–60.

Ginkgo + Calcium-channel blockers; Diltiazem

The interaction between ginkgo and diltiazem is based on experimental evidence only.

Clinical evidence

No interactions found.

Experimental evidence

Ginkgo 20 mg/kg approximately doubled the AUC and maximum serum levels of oral diltiazem 30 mg/kg when given to *rats* one hour before diltiazem. Ginkgo 20 mg/kg had no significant effect on the levels of intravenous diltiazem 3 mg/kg.[1]

Mechanism

The authors suggest that ginkgo may inhibit the activity of the cytochrome P450 isoenzyme CYP3A4 or P-glycoprotein, both of which would raise diltiazem levels by inhibiting its metabolism or increasing its absorption, respectively.[1] However, in clinical studies, ginkgo had no clinically relevant effect on the P-glycoprotein substrate digoxin, page 244, or on the conventional CYP3A4 probe substrate, midazolam, page 241.

Importance and management

An interaction between ginkgo and diltiazem has only been demonstrated in one study in *rats,* and ginkgo does not appear to have clinically relevant effects on the activity of P-glycoprotein or on the metabolism of other CYP3A4 substrates such as the benzodiazepines. Because the findings of *animal* studies cannot be directly extrapolated to humans, further study is needed before any specific recommendations can be made. Until more is known, bear the possibility of an interaction in mind in the event of an unexpected response to treatment.

1. Ohnishi N, Kusuhara M, Yoshioka M, Kuroda K, Soga A, Nishikawa F, Koishi T, Nakagawa M, Hori S, Matsumoto T, Yamashita M, Ohta S, Takara K, Yokoyama T. Studies on interactions between functional foods or dietary supplements and medicines. I. Effects of *Ginkgo biloba* leaf extract on the pharmacokinetics of diltiazem in rats. *Biol Pharm Bull* (2003) 26, 1315–20.

Ginkgo + Calcium-channel blockers; Nicardipine

The interaction between ginkgo and nicardipine is based on experimental evidence only.

Clinical evidence

No interactions found.

Experimental evidence

In an experimental study in *rats,* ginkgo extract 0.5% daily for 4 weeks significantly reduced the hypotensive effects of both oral nicardipine 30 mg/kg and intravenous nicardipine 30 micrograms/kg.[1] These findings were repeated in a later study in *rats*: ginkgo extract 0.5% daily for 2 weeks reduced the maximum serum levels and AUC of oral nicardipine 30 mg/kg by about 65%.[2] The ginkgo extract contained 24% flavonoids (12% quercetin) and 9% terpene lactones.

Mechanism

The authors suggested that ginkgo may induce the cytochrome P450 subfamily CYP3A, which would increase the metabolism of nicardipine, a CYP3A4 substrate, and reduce its levels. However, in contrast, studies with diltiazem, above and nifedipine, below have shown *inhibition* of CYP3A4 and increased levels. Moreover, note also that clinically relevant CYP3A4 inhibition has not been

see with the conventional CYP3A4 probe substrate, midazolam, page 241.

Importance and management

These experiments in *rats* suggest that ginkgo can significantly reduce the levels of nicardipine by inducing CYP3A, but note that there is experimental evidence of ginkgo increasing nifedipine and diltiazem levels. Moreover, clinical studies with CYP3A4 substrates such as the benzodiazepines, page 241, have not shown any clinically relevant pharmacokinetic interaction. Because of this, and because the doses used were higher than those used in humans, the *animal* data here are unlikely to be of general clinical importance.

1. Shinozuka K, Umegaki K, Kubota Y, Tanaka N, Mizuno H, Yamauchi J, Nakamura K, Kunitomo M. Feeding of *Ginkgo biloba* extract (GBE) enhances gene expression of hepatic cytochrome P-450 and attenuates the hypotensive effect of nicardipine in rats. *Life Sci* (2002) 70, 2783–92.
2. Kubota Y, Kobayashi K, Tanaka N, Nakamura K, Kunitomo M, Umegaki K, Shinozuka K. Interaction of *Ginkgo biloba* extract (GBE) with hypotensive agent, nicardipine, in rats. *In Vivo* (2003) 17, 409–12.

Ginkgo + Calcium-channel blockers; Nifedipine

Ginkgo may increase the levels and some of the effects of nifedipine.

Clinical evidence

In the preliminary report of a clinical study, 22 healthy subjects were given ginkgo 120 mg daily for 18 days before a single 10-mg oral dose of nifedipine. Ginkgo increased the levels of nifedipine by about 50%.[1]

In another study, a single 240-mg dose of ginkgo extract did not significantly affect the pharmacokinetics of a single 10-mg oral dose of nifedipine when they were given at the same time to 8 healthy subjects. However, the maximum level tended to increase (30% increase), and two subjects experienced a doubling of nifedipine maximum serum levels. In addition, the incidence and severity of headaches, hot flushes and dizziness tended to be higher with the combination when compared with nifedipine alone. Subjects also experienced increased heart rate with the combination although the decrease in blood pressure was unaffected.[2] The ginkgo extract used in this study contained 24% flavonoids and 6% terpene lactones.

Experimental evidence

In a study in *rats,* ginkgo extract 20 mg/kg increased the maximum serum levels and AUC of an oral dose of nifedipine 5 mg/kg by about 60% when they were given at the same time.[3] Ginkgo extract had no effect on the pharmacokinetics of intravenous nifedipine.

Mechanism

Experimental data[3] has found that ginkgo has no significant effect on the pharmacokinetics of intravenous nifedipine, suggesting that ginkgo reduces the first-pass metabolism of nifedipine. Ginkgo may therefore inhibit the cytochrome P450 isoenzyme CYP3A4, which would reduce the pre-systemic metabolism of nifedipine, a CYP3A4 substrate, and increase its levels. Note that simultaneous administration of single doses is probably insufficient to completely evaluate CYP3A4 inhibition. Note also that clinically relevant CYP3A4 inhibition has not been seen with the conventional CYP3A4 probe substrates such as midazolam. See Ginkgo + Benzodiazepines, page 241.

Importance and management

Limited clinical data suggest that ginkgo may raise the levels of nifedipine and increase its effects. Until more is known, some caution might be warranted when they are used together. Monitor for signs of nifedipine adverse effects such as headaches, hot flushes, dizziness and palpitations. If they become apparent, advise the patient to stop taking ginkgo.

G

1. Smith M, Lin KM, Zheng YP. An open trial of nifedipine-herb interactions: nifedipine with St. John's wort, ginseng or Ginko [sic] biloba. *Clin Pharmacol Ther* (2001) 69, P86.
2. Yoshioka M, Ohnishi N, Koishi T, Obata Y, Nakagawa M, Matsumoto T, Tagagi K, Takara K, Ohkuni T, Yokoyama T, Kuroda K. Studies on interactions between functional foods or dietary supplements and medicines. IV. Effects of *Ginkgo biloba* leaf extract on the pharmacokinetics and pharmacodynamics of nifedipine in healthy volunteers. *Biol Pharm Bull* (2004) 27, 2006–9.
3. Yoshioka M, Ohnishi N, Sone N, Egami S, Takara K, Yokoyama T, Kuroda K. Studies on interactions between functional foods or dietary supplements and medicines. III. Effects of *Ginkgo biloba* leaf extract on the pharmacokinetics of nifedipine in rats. *Biol Pharm Bull* (2004) 27, 2042–5.

Ginkgo + Chlorzoxazone

Ginkgo does not appear to affect the pharmacokinetics of chlorzoxazone.

Evidence, mechanism, importance and management

In a study in 12 healthy subjects, ginkgo 60 mg four times daily for 28 days did not significantly affect the metabolism of chlorzoxazone 500 mg. The ginkgo preparation used was standardised to 24% flavone glycosides and 6% terpene lactones.[1] These findings were repeated in a later study using the same criteria in 12 elderly healthy subjects.[2]

Chlorzoxazone is used a probe substrate for the cytochrome P450 isoenzyme CYP2E1, and this study shows that ginkgo has no clinically relevant effect on this isoenzyme. No action is necessary with combined use, and no pharmacokinetic interaction would be expected with other substrates of CYP2E1.

1. Gurley BJ, Gardner SF, Hubbard MA, Williams DK, Gentry WB, Cui Y, Ang CYW. Cytochrome P450 phenotypic ratios for predicting herb-drug interactions in humans. *Clin Pharmacol Ther* (2002) 72, 276–87.
2. Gurley BJ, Gardner SF, Hubbard MA, Williams DK, Gentry WB, Cui Y, Ang CYW. Clinical assessment of botanical supplementation on cytochrome P450 phenotypes in the elderly: St John's wort, garlic oil, *Panax ginseng*, and *Ginkgo biloba*. *Drugs Aging* (2005) 22, 525–39.

Ginkgo + Ciclosporin

The interaction between ginkgo and ciclosporin is based on experimental evidence only.

Clinical evidence

No interactions found.

Experimental evidence

In a study in *rats,* ginkgo extract 8 mL/kg (containing the flavonoid quercetin 775 nanomol/kg) reduced the maximum serum levels and AUC of oral ciclosporin by about 60% and 50% respectively, but had no effect on the pharmacokinetics of intravenous ciclosporin.[1]

Mechanism

The authors suggest the flavonoid component of ginkgo, quercetin, might affect ciclosporin levels via its effects on P-glycoprotein or cytochrome P450 isoenzyme CYP3A4. However, in clinical studies, ginkgo had no clinically relevant effect on the P-glycoprotein substrate digoxin, page 244, or on midazolam, page 241, a CYP3A4 substrate.

Importance and management

The evidence for an interaction between ginkgo and ciclosporin is limited to one study in *rats*. However, ginkgo contains flavonoids, and of these quercetin has been implicated in modest interactions with ciclosporin in other studies (see Flavonoids + Ciclosporin, page 217 for more information). On this basis, while there is insufficient evidence to suggest that concurrent use should be avoided, there is the possibility that ginkgo may make ciclosporin levels less stable as the quercetin content of different preparations is likely to vary. Some caution might therefore be prudent on concurrent use.

1. Yang CY, Chao PDL, Hou YC, Tsai SY, Wen KC, Hsiu SL. Marked decrease of cyclosporin bioavailability caused by coadministration of ginkgo and onion in rats. *Food Chem Toxicol* (2006) 44, 1572–8.

Ginkgo + Dextromethorphan

Ginkgo does not appear to affect the metabolism of dextromethorphan.

Clinical evidence

Ginkgo leaf extract 120 mg twice daily for 16 days was given to 12 healthy subjects with a single 30-mg dose of dextromethorphan on day 14. The ginkgo preparation (*Ginkgold*) contained ginkgo flavonol glycosides 24% and terpene lactones 6%. There was no change in the metabolism of dextromethorphan when it was taken after the ginkgo.[1] Similarly, in 14 healthy subjects, the use of a ginkgo extract, EGb 761, 120 mg twice daily for 8 days had no effect on the metabolism of dextromethorphan given on day 8. The use of the same extract of ginkgo in a dose of 240 mg daily had a borderline effect, but this was not considered clinically relevant.[2]

In 12 healthy subjects, ginkgo 60 mg four times daily for 28 days did not significantly affect the metabolism of **debrisoquine** 5 mg. The ginkgo preparation used was standardised to 24% flavone glycosides and 6% terpene lactones.[3] These findings were repeated in a later study using the same criteria in 12 elderly healthy subjects.[4]

Experimental evidence

In *in vitro* experiments, low-dose and high-dose ginkgo modestly decreased and increased the metabolism of dextromethorphan, respectively.[5,6]

Mechanism

Dextromethorphan is used as a probe substrate for the cytochrome P450 isoenzyme CYP2D6, and the study shows that ginkgo has no clinically relevant effect on this isoenzyme. Studies with debrisoquine, another CYP2D6 substrate, also suggest that ginkgo does not affect CYP2D6.

Importance and management

The available evidence seems to reliably suggest that ginkgo does not affect the pharmacokinetics of dextromethorphan. No action is therefore needed on concurrent use.

Dextromethorphan is used as a probe drug for CYP2D6 activity, and therefore these results (along with those for debrisoquine) also suggest that a clinically relevant pharmacokinetic interaction between ginkgo and other CYP2D6 substrates is unlikely.

1. Markowitz JS, Donovan JL, DeVane CL, Sipkes L, Chavin KD. Multiple-dose administration of *Ginkgo biloba* did not affect cytochrome P-450 2D6 or 3A4 activity in normal volunteers. *J Clin Psychopharmacol* (2003) 23, 576–81.
2. Zadoyan G, Rokitta D, Klement S, Dienel A, Hoerr R, Gramatté T, Fuhr U. Effect of *Ginkgo biloba* special extract EGb 761® on human cytochrome P450 activity: a cocktail interaction study in healthy volunteers *Eur J Clin Pharmacol* (2012) 68, 553–60.
3. Gurley BJ, Gardner SF, Hubbard MA, Williams DK, Gentry WB, Cui Y, Ang CYW. Cytochrome P450 phenotypic ratios for predicting herb-drug interactions in humans. *Clin Pharmacol Ther* (2002) 72, 276–87.
4. Gurley BJ, Gardner SF, Hubbard MA, Williams DK, Gentry WB, Cui Y, Ang CYW. Clinical assessment of botanical supplementation on cytochrome P450 phenotypes in the elderly: St John's wort, garlic oil, *Panax ginseng*, and *Ginkgo biloba*. *Drugs Aging* (2005) 22, 525–39.
5. Hellum BH, Nilsen OG. The *in vitro* inhibitory potential of trade herbal products on human CYP2D6-mediated metabolism and the influence of ethanol. *Basic Clin Pharmacol Toxicol* (2007) 101, 350–358.
6. Hellum BH, Hu Z, Nilsen OG. The induction of CYP1A2, CYP2D6 and CYP3A4 by six trade herbal products in cultured primary human hepatocytes. *Basic Clin Pharmacol Toxicol* (2007) 100, 23–30.

Ginkgo + Digoxin

Ginkgo does not appear to affect the pharmacokinetics of digoxin.

Clinical evidence

A study in 8 healthy subjects found that ginkgo biloba leaf extract 80 mg three times daily had no effect on the pharmacokinetics of a single 500-microgram dose of digoxin.[1]

Experimental evidence

In *in vitro* experiments, ginkgo modestly inhibited the cellular transport of digoxin resulting in the intracellular accumulation of digoxin.[2]

Mechanism

Digoxin is a P-glycoprotein substrate and *in vitro* studies[2] suggest that ginkgo might inhibit the activity of this drug transporter protein, which could lead to increased digoxin levels. However, any effect does not appear to be clinically relevant. Studies with other P-glycoprotein substrates (see Talinolol, page 248) support this suggestion.

Importance and management

The clinical study suggests that ginkgo is unlikely to alter digoxin levels in clinical use. Therefore no dose adjustment would be expected to be necessary if patients taking digoxin also wish to take ginkgo. As digoxin is used as a probe substrate for P-glycoprotein, this study also suggests that ginkgo is unlikely to interact with other drugs that are substrates of P-glycoprotein. No action is necessary with combined use.

1. Mauro VF, Mauro LS, Kleshinski JF, Khuder SA, Wang Y, Erhardt PW. Impact of Ginkgo biloba on the pharmacokinetics of digoxin. *Am J Ther* (2003) 10, 247–51.
2. Hellum BH, Nilsen OG. *In vitro* inhibition of CYP3A4 metabolism and P-glycoprotein-mediated transport by trade herbal products. *Basic Clin Pharmacol Toxicol* (2008) 102, 466–75.

Ginkgo + Donepezil

Ginkgo does not appear to alter the pharmacokinetics or effects of donepezil.

Evidence, mechanism, importance and management

In a pharmacokinetic study, 14 elderly patients with Alzheimer's disease were given donepezil 5 mg daily for at least 20 weeks, after which ginkgo extract 90 mg daily was also given for a further 30 days. Concurrent use did not affect the pharmacokinetics or cholinesterase activity of donepezil, and cognitive function appeared to be unchanged.[1] Therefore, over the course of 30 days, concurrent use appears neither beneficial nor detrimental. No action is necessary with combined use.

1. Yasui-Furukori N, Furukori H, Kaneda A, Kaneko S, Tateishi T. The effects of *Ginkgo biloba* extracts on the pharmacokinetics and pharmacodynamics of donepezil. *J Clin Pharmacol* (2004) 44, 538–42.

Ginkgo + Efavirenz

A case report suggests that ginkgo may reduce efavirenz levels.

Clinical evidence

A case report describes a 47-year-old HIV-positive man who had been taking efavirenz, emtricitabine and tenofovir for 2 years, when he developed virological failure. Plasma efavirenz levels, taken from stored plasma samples, suggested that his efavirenz levels had decreased over a period of 2 years (from 1.26 mg/L to 0.48 mg/L): this coincided with an increase in viral load. On questioning, it was established that the patient had been taking ginkgo for a period of several months, and so the decrease in efavirenz levels was attributed to an interaction with ginkgo. The patient was subsequently successfully switched to alternative antiretrovirals.[1]

Experimental evidence

No relevant data found.

Mechanism

Not established. The authors suggest that ginkgo may have reduced efavirenz metabolism by inducing the cytochrome P450 isoenzyme CYP3A4 and the drug transporter, P-glycoprotein.[1] However, the available evidence suggests that an effect on P-glycoprotein is unlikely, see Ginkgo + Digoxin, page 244, as is a clinically relevant effect on CYP3A4, see Ginkgo + Benzodiazepines, page 241.

Importance and management

Evidence for an interaction between ginkgo and efavirenz is limited to this isolated case and is by no means established. Nevertheless, the case gives cause for some concern about concurrent use, and consideration should therefore be given to the possibility of reduced antiviral efficacy if a patient taking efavirenz wishes to take ginkgo. Until more is known, if concurrent use is considered desirable it would be prudent to be alert for reduced efavirenz levels.

1. Wiegman D-J, Brinkman K, Franssen EJF. Interaction of *Ginkgo biloba* with efavirenz. *AIDS* (2009) 23, 1184–5.

Ginkgo + Fexofenadine

Ginkgo does not appear to affect the pharmacokinetics of fexofenadine.

Evidence, mechanism, importance and management

In a clinical study, 13 healthy subjects took a single oral dose of fexofenadine 120 mg after 4 weeks of twice-daily doses of ginkgo 120 mg containing 29% flavonol glycosides and 5% terpene lactones. The pharmacokinetics of fexofenadine were not significantly affected.[1]

Fexofenadine is a P-glycoprotein substrate and the findings of this study therefore suggest that ginkgo does not affect P-glycoprotein activity. No action is necessary with combined use.

1. Robertson SM, Davey RT, Voell J, Formentini E, Alfaro RM, Penzak SR. Effect of *Ginkgo biloba* extract on lopinavir, midazolam and fexofenadine pharmacokinetics in healthy subjects. *Curr Med Res Opin* (2008) 24, 591–9.

Ginkgo + Food

No interactions found.

Ginkgo + Haloperidol

Animal studies suggest that ginkgo may increase extrapyramidal effects in response to haloperidol, but clinical studies do not appear to have reported this effect.

Clinical evidence

Ginkgo has been tried in schizophrenia as an addition to standard antipsychotics such as haloperidol. For example, in one clinical study, an improvement in positive symptoms was seen in 43 schizophrenic patients given ginkgo extract 360 mg daily with haloperidol 250 micrograms/kg daily for 12 weeks.[1] This study did not report any adverse events.

Experimental evidence

High-dose ginkgo extract, (EGb 761, *Tebonin*®) 80 mg/kg daily for 5 days, significantly potentiated the cataleptic adverse effects of

G

haloperidol 2 mg/kg given to *rats* on the first and last day.[2] The cataleptic response to haloperidol is used as an *animal* model of extrapyramidal adverse effects.

Mechanism

Unknown. Haloperidol is a dopamine D_2 antagonist. It is thought that ginkgo may interfere with dopamine neurotransmission by scavenging nitric oxide, which in turn reduces locomotor activity.

Importance and management

The authors of the experimental study caution that there is a possibility of an increase in extrapyramidal effects when ginkgo is used with haloperidol.[2] However, their study in *rats* used high doses, and there are clinical studies investigating the addition of ginkgo to haloperidol that do not mention this adverse effect. Nevertheless, a clinical study specifically of extrapyramidal effects would be required to investigate this further. It may be prudent to be aware of this possible interaction in case there is an unexpected outcome in patients taking haloperidol and ginkgo.

1. Zhang XY, Zhou DF, Su JM, Zhang PY. The effect of extract of Ginkgo biloba added to haloperidol on superoxide dismutase in inpatients with chronic schizophrenia. *J Clin Psychopharmacol* (2001) 21, 85–8.
2. Fontana L, Souza AS, Del Bel EA, de Oliveira RMW. *Ginkgo biloba* leaf extract (EGb 761) enhances catalepsy induced by haloperidol and L-nitroarginine in mice. *Braz J Med Biol Res* (2005) 38, 1649–54.

Ginkgo + Herbal medicines; Valerian

A case report describes psychotic symptoms in a woman who took ginkgo with valerian, but an interaction was not established as the cause.

Clinical evidence

A 51-year-old woman taking valerian 1 to 2 g daily and an unknown amount of ginkgo daily, and who regularly consumed over 1 L of wine daily, was admitted to hospital after a fainting episode and changes in mental status. Over the next couple of days she exhibited a variety of psychotic symptoms including paranoid delusions, disorganised behaviour, anxiety, and auditory hallucinations. Her blood alcohol level was zero on admission and there was no evidence of alcohol withdrawal during her stay in hospital.[1]

Experimental evidence

No relevant data found.

Mechanism

Unclear. Valerian has been associated with CNS depressant effects when given alone and ginkgo is used primarily to improve cognitive function and memory loss. Alcohol, valerian and ginkgo were also all being withdrawn at the same time. These factors make it difficult to find the exact cause of the psychotic symptoms.

Importance and management

This appears to be the only case report in the literature and, because of the multiple factors involved, such as a history of alcohol abuse, it is difficult to assess its general importance. Bear this interaction in mind in case of an adverse response to the combination of ginkgo and valerian.

1. Chen D, Klesmer J, Giovanniello A, Katz J. Mental status changes in an alcohol abuser taking valerian and Ginkgo biloba. *Am J Addict* (2002) 11, 75–7.

Ginkgo + HIV-protease inhibitors

Ginkgo does not appear to affect the pharmacokinetics of lopinavir boosted with ritonavir.

Clinical evidence

In a study in 14 healthy subjects, ginkgo 120 mg twice daily for 2 weeks had no significant effect on the pharmacokinetics of **lopinavir** boosted with ritonavir 400/100 mg twice daily (given for 2 weeks alone before adding the ginkgo). The ginkgo extract was assayed and contained 29% flavonol glycosides and 5% terpene lactones.[1]

Experimental evidence

No relevant data found.

Mechanism

The authors suggest that without ritonavir, the levels of lopinavir would have been reduced by ginkgo because they also found that ginkgo modestly reduced the levels of midazolam, probably by inducing the cytochrome P450 isoenzyme CYP3A4. As ritonavir is an inhibitor of CYP3A4, they suggest that it attenuates the action of ginkgo on lopinavir metabolism. However, note that all HIV-protease inhibitors are inhibitors of CYP3A4, and note also that in other studies with midazolam, ginkgo had no effect on midazolam levels, or even caused a minor increase in levels, which suggests that ginkgo does not have a clinically relevant effect on CYP3A4 activity. Consider also Ginkgo + Benzodiazepines, page 241.

Importance and management

The study here shows that ginkgo does not alter the pharmacokinetics of lopinavir boosted with ritonavir, and no special precautions are required on concurrent use. This would be expected to apply to all other HIV-protease inhibitors boosted with ritonavir. As regards HIV-protease inhibitors that are not boosted by ritonavir, the authors of this study recommend avoiding ginkgo.[1] This seems an over-cautious approach, given that the sum of studies available show that ginkgo does not have a clinically relevant effect on the probe CYP3A4 substrate midazolam.

1. Robertson SM, Davey RT, Voell J, Formentini E, Alfaro RM, Penzak SR. Effect of *Ginkgo biloba* extract on lopinavir, midazolam and fexofenadine pharmacokinetics in healthy subjects. *Curr Med Res Opin* (2008) 24, 591–9.

Ginkgo + Metformin

Ginkgo did not appear to alter the pharmacokinetics of metformin, and appeared to have a slight beneficial effect on glycaemic control.

Evidence, mechanism, importance and management

In a small crossover study that included 10 patients with type 2 diabetes taking metformin, ginkgo (EGb 761) 120 mg daily for 3 months slightly improved HbA_{1c} when compared with placebo (HbA_{1c} 7.2% versus 7.7%). The pharmacokinetics of metformin were assessed on one day at the end of the study, when the usual daily dose of metformin was taken with the daily dose of ginkgo. Ginkgo did not appear to have any effects on metformin pharmacokinetics.[1] In a further 10 healthy subjects, ginkgo 120 mg daily had no effect on the pharmacokinetics of a single 500-mg dose of metformin, except for a reduction in the time to reach the maximum plasma level.[1]

This study indicates that ginkgo is unlikely to alter the pharmacokinetics of metformin. In addition, it provides some limited evidence that it may have a slight beneficial effect on glycaemic control, although this requires confirmation in a larger study.

1. Kudolo GB, Weng W, Javors M, Blodgett J. The effect of the ingestion of *Ginkgo biloba* extract (EGb 761) on the pharmacokinetics of metformin in non-diabetic and type 2 diabetic subjects–a double blind placebo-controlled, crossover study *Clin Nutr* (2006) 25, 606–16.

G

Ginkgo + NSAIDs

An isolated case describes fatal intracerebral bleeding in a patient taking ginkgo with ibuprofen, and another case describes prolonged bleeding and subdural haematomas in another patient taking gingko and rofecoxib. Studies with diclofenac and flurbiprofen showed that ginkgo had no effect on the pharmacokinetics of these drugs.

Clinical evidence

A case of fatal intracerebral bleeding has been reported in a 71-year-old patient taking a ginkgo supplement (*Gingium*) 4 weeks after he started to take **ibuprofen** 600 mg daily.[1] A 69-year-old man taking a ginkgo supplement and **rofecoxib** had a subdural haematoma after a head injury, then recurrent small spontaneous haematomas. He was subsequently found to have a prolonged bleeding time, which returned to normal one week after stopping the ginkgo supplement and **rofecoxib**, and remained normal after restarting low-dose **rofecoxib**.[2]

A placebo-controlled study in 11 healthy subjects who were given ginkgo leaf (*Ginkgold*) 120 mg twice daily for three doses, followed by a single 100-mg dose of **flurbiprofen**, found that the pharmacokinetics of **flurbiprofen** were unchanged.[3]

A study in 12 healthy subjects who were given **diclofenac** 50 mg twice daily for 14 days, with ginkgo extract (*Ginkgold*) 120 mg twice daily on days 8 to 15, found no alteration in the AUC or oral clearance of **diclofenac**.[4]

Experimental evidence

See *Mechanism*, below.

Mechanism

The reason for the bleeding is not known, but ginkgo extract contains ginkgolide B, which is a potent inhibitor of platelet-activating factor *in vitro*, which is needed for arachidonate-independent platelet aggregation. However, in one controlled study in healthy subjects, taking a ginkgo preparation alone for two weeks had no effect on platelet function.[5] Nevertheless, there are case reports of ginkgo supplements, on their own, being associated with prolonged bleeding times,[6,7] left and bilateral subdural haematomas,[6,8] a right parietal haematoma,[9] a retrobulbar haemorrhage,[10] post-laparoscopic cholecystectomy bleeding,[11] and subarachnoid haemorrhage.[7] Ibuprofen is an inhibitor of platelet aggregation, but selective inhibitors of COX-2 such as rofecoxib have no effect on platelets and would not be expected to potentiate any bleeding effect of ginkgo.

The pharmacokinetic studies involving diclofenac and flurbiprofen were designed to identify whether ginkgo exerted an inhibitory effect on cytochrome P450 isoenzyme CYP2C9, and confirm that ginkgo has no effect on this isoenzyme.

Importance and management

The evidence from these reports is too slim to forbid patients to take NSAIDs and ginkgo concurrently, but some do recommend caution.[12] Medical professionals should be aware of the possibility of increased bleeding tendency with ginkgo, and report any suspected cases.[9]

For other reports of bleeding events with ginkgo see Ginkgo + Antiplatelet drugs, page 240, and Ginkgo + Warfarin and related drugs, page 250.

1. Meisel C, Johne A, Roots I. Fatal intracerebral mass bleeding associated with *Ginkgo biloba* and ibuprofen. *Atherosclerosis* (2003) 167, 367.
2. Hoffman T. Ginko, Vioxx and excessive bleeding - possible drug-herb interactions: case report. *Hawaii Med J* (2001) 60, 290.
3. Greenblatt DJ, von Moltke LL, Luo Y, Perloff ES, Horan KA, Bruce A, Reynolds RC, Harmatz JS, Avula B, Khan IA, Goldman P. Ginkgo biloba does not alter clearance of flurbiprofen, a cytochrome P450-2C9 substrate. *J Clin Pharmacol* (2006) 46, 214–21.
4. Mohutsky MA, Anderson GD, Miller JW, Elmer GW. *Ginkgo biloba*: evaluation of CYP2C9 drug interactions in vitro and in vivo. *Am J Ther* (2006) 13, 24–31.
5. Beckert BW, Concannon MJ, Henry SL, Smith DS, Puckett CL. The effect of herbal medicines on platelet function: an in vivo experiment and review of the literature. *Plast Reconstr Surg* (2007) 120, 2044–50.

6. Rowin J, Lewis SL. Spontaneous bilateral subdural hematomas associated with chronic *Ginkgo biloba* ingestion. *Neurology* (1996) 46, 1775–6.
7. Vale S. Subarachnoid haemorrhage associated with *Ginkgo biloba*. *Lancet* (1998) 352, 36.
8. Gilbert GJ. *Ginkgo biloba*. *Neurology* (1997) 48, 1137.
9. Benjamin J, Muir T, Briggs K, Pentland B. A case of cerebral haemorrhage - can *Ginkgo biloba* be implicated? *Postgrad Med J* (2001) 77, 112–13.
10. Fong KCS, Kinnear PE. Retrobulbar haemorrhage associated with chronic *Gingko biloba* ingestion. *Postgrad Med J* (2003) 79, 531–2.
11. Fessenden JM, Wittenborn W, Clarke L. Gingko biloba: a case report of herbal medicine and bleeding postoperatively from a laparoscopic cholecystectomy. *Am Surg* (2001) 67, 33–5.
12. Griffiths J, Jordan S, Pilon S. Natural health products and adverse reactions. *Can Adverse React News* (2004) 14, 2–3.

Ginkgo + Phenobarbital

The interaction between ginkgo and phenobarbital is based on experimental evidence only.

Clinical evidence

No interactions found.

Experimental evidence

In an experimental study in *rats,* ginkgo extract 0.5% daily (equating to about 1.3 g/kg) for 2 weeks modestly reduced the maximum serum levels of a single 90-mg/kg dose of phenobarbital by about 35%, and reduced the AUC by about 18% (not statistically significant). Conversely, the phenobarbital-induced sleeping time was reduced markedly from about 8 hours to about 3 hours. The ginkgo extract used was standardised to 24% flavonoids and 9% terpenes.[1]

Mechanism

Ginkgo may induce the cytochrome P450 isoenzyme CYP2B subfamily, which would increase the metabolism of phenobarbital, a CYP2B6 substrate, and reduce its levels. However, the modest reduction in levels seen with high-dose ginkgo does not explain the marked reduction in sleeping time.

Importance and management

The evidence for this interaction is limited to an *animal* study and the doses used are far higher than those used in humans. It is therefore difficult to assess the clinical relevance of this interaction. If anything, it would appear that the interaction may be beneficial (reduced sedation), but this is far from established.

For details of possible interactions with other antiepileptics, see Ginkgo + Antiepileptics, page 240.

1. Kubota Y, Kobayashi K, Tanaka N, Nakamura K, Kunitomo M, Umegaki K, Shinozuka K. Pretreatment with *Ginkgo biloba* extract weakens the hypnosis action of phenobarbital and its plasma concentration in rats. *J Pharm Pharmacol* (2004) 56, 401–5.

Ginkgo + Propranolol

The interaction between ginkgo and propranolol is based on experimental evidence only.

Clinical evidence

No interactions found.

Experimental evidence

The maximum serum levels and AUC of propranolol 10 mg/kg given to *rats* pretreated with ginkgo extract 100 mg/kg (EGb 761) for 10 days, were reduced by about 40% and 45% respectively when compared with propranolol alone. The serum levels and AUC of its metabolite, *N*-desisopropylpropranolol were increased by about 70% and 55%. Ginkgo extract 10 mg/kg had no effect.[1]

Mechanism

The authors suggested that ginkgo may induce the activity of the cytochrome P450 isoenzyme CYP1A2, which is one of the

G

major enzymes involved in the metabolism of propranolol. Ginkgo would therefore reduce the levels of propranolol by inducing its metabolism. However, compare caffeine, page 242.

Importance and management

This experiment in *rats* suggests that high-dose ginkgo might significantly reduce the levels of propranolol by inducing CYP1A2. However, a human study using caffeine as a CYP1A2 probe substrate, found that ginkgo does not affect CYP1A2 to a clinically relevant extent (see Ginkgo + Caffeine, page 242). Therefore an interaction with propranolol based on this mechanism is unlikely to be clinically important.

1. Zhao L-Z, Huang M, Chen J, Ee PLR, Chan E, Duan W, Guan Y-Y, Hong Y-H, Chen X, Zhou S. Induction of propranolol metabolism by *Ginkgo biloba* extract EGb 761 in rats. *Curr Drug Metab* (2006) 7, 577–87.

Ginkgo + Proton pump inhibitors

Ginkgo induces the metabolism of omeprazole. Most other proton pump inhibitors are likely to be similarly affected.

Clinical evidence

In one study, 18 healthy Chinese subjects were given a single 40-mg dose of **omeprazole** before and after a 12-day course of a standardised extract of ginkgo 140 mg twice daily. The subjects were divided into three groups: homozygous extensive CYP2C19 metabolisers (6 subjects), heterozygous extensive CYP2C19 metabolisers (5) and poor CYP2C19 metabolisers (7). The AUC of **omeprazole** was modestly decreased by 42%, 27% and 40%, respectively, and the plasma levels of the inactive metabolite, hydroxyomeprazole, were increased by 38%, 100%, and 232% in the three groups, respectively. Renal clearance of hydroxyomeprazole was also reduced by ginkgo.[1] In another study, in 18 healthy subjects, the use of a ginkgo extract, EGb 761, 240 mg daily for 8 days had no effect on the metabolism of **omeprazole** given on day 8. The use of the same extract of ginkgo in a dose of 120 mg twice daily had a borderline effect, but this was not considered clinically relevant.[2]

Experimental evidence

No relevant data found.

Mechanism

In the first study,[1] it was concluded that ginkgo increases the metabolism (hydroxylation) of omeprazole by inducing the cytochrome P450 isoenzyme CYP2C19.

Importance and management

There appear to be only two studies examining the effects of ginkgo on proton pump inhibitors. In one study,[1] the reduction seen in the AUC of omeprazole (about 40%) suggests that there might be a possibility that omeprazole could be slightly less effective in patients taking ginkgo. As all PPIs are metabolised by CYP2C19 to varying extents, it is likely that the effects of ginkgo seen in these studies will be similar with other PPIs, although note that **rabeprazole** is much less dependent on this route of metabolism than other PPIs. However, the second study,[2] designed primarily to investigate the effect of ginkgo on CYP2C19, suggested that ginkgo does not have a clinically relevant effect on omeprazole metabolism.

Taken together, there is insufficient evidence to generally recommend that ginkgo should be avoided in patients taking PPIs. However, the potential reduction in the efficacy of the PPI should be borne in mind, particular where the consequences may be serious, such as in patients with healing ulcers.

1. Yin OQP, Tomlinson B, Waye MMY, Chow AHL, Chow MSS. Pharmacogenetics and herb-drug interactions: experience with Ginkgo biloba and omeprazole. *Pharmacogenetics* (2004) 14, 841–50.

2. Zadoyan G, Rokitta D, Klement S, Dienel A, Hoerr R, Gramatté T, Fuhr U. Effect of *Ginkgo biloba* special extract EGb 761® on human cytochrome P450 activity: a cocktail interaction study in healthy volunteers *Eur J Clin Pharmacol* (2012) 68, 553–60.

Ginkgo + Risperidone

An isolated case describes priapism in a patient taking risperidone and ginkgo.

Clinical evidence

A 26-year-old patient with paranoid schizophrenia who had been taking risperidone 3 mg daily for the past 3 years developed priapism that had lasted for 4 hours, two weeks after starting ginkgo 160 mg daily for occasional tinnitus. The priapism required treatment, and both ginkgo and risperidone were stopped. Risperidone was then restarted and the patient reported no further episodes of priapism at follow-up 6 months later.[1]

Experimental evidence

No relevant data found.

Mechanism

Unclear. Risperidone alone does rarely cause priapism, probably because of its alpha-adrenergic properties, and ginkgo might have vascular effects that could be additive with the effects of risperidone. Ginkgo is unlikely to affect the metabolism of risperidone by inhibiting CYP2D6 because it has no clinical effect on other CYP2D6 substrates. See Ginkgo + Dextromethorphan, page 244.

Importance and management

Evidence for an interaction between ginkgo and risperidone appears to be limited to this isolated case. Its general relevance is therefore unclear. Bear it in mind in the event of an unexpected response to treatment.

1. Lin Y-Y, Chu S-J, Tsai S-H. Association between priapism and concurrent use of risperidone and *Ginkgo biloba*. *Mayo Clin Proc* (2007) 82, 1288–91.

Ginkgo + Talinolol

Ginkgo slightly increases the exposure to talinolol.

Clinical evidence

In a study in 10 healthy subjects, ginkgo 120 mg three times daily for 14 days increased the AUC of a single 100-mg dose of talinolol given on day 14 by 22%, and increased its maximum plasma concentration by 36%. In this study ginkgo was given as a tablet containing a standardised *Ginkgo biloba* extract.[1] The same or very similar data has been reported elsewhere.[2]

Experimental evidence

No relevant data found.

Mechanism

Talinolol is a substrate of P-glycoprotein and possibly also multidrug resistance-protein 2 (MRP2) and the uptake transporter, organic anion transporting protein (OATP).[2] *In vitro* studies[3] suggest that ginkgo might inhibit the activity of P-glycoprotein, which could lead to increased talinolol exposure. However, this effect seems to be very slight.

Importance and management

The studies of the effects of ginkgo on talinolol disposition were conducted to assess drug interaction mechanisms. Nevertheless, the clinical data shows that it causes a very slight reduction in the AUC

G

of talinolol, which is considered to be of little or no clinically relevance.

1. Fan L, Tao G-Y, Wang G, Chen Y, He Y-J, Li Q, Lei H-P, Jiang F, Hu D-L, Huang Y-F, Zhou H-H. Effects of ginkgo biloba extract ingestion on the pharmacokinetics of talinolol in healthy Chinese volunteers *Ann Pharmacother* (2009) 43, 944–9.
2. Fan L, Mao X-Q, Tao G-Y, Wang G, Jiang F, Chen Y, Li Q, Zhang W, Lei H-P, Hu D-L, Huang Y-F, Wang D, Zhou H-H. Effect of *Schisandra chinensis* extract and *Ginkgo biloba* extract on the pharmacokinetics of talinolol in healthy volunteers. *Xenobiotica* (2009) 39, 249–54.
3. Hellum BH, Nilsen OG. *In vitro* inhibition of CYP3A4 metabolism and P-glycoprotein-mediated transport by trade herbal products. *Basic Clin Pharmacol Toxicol* (2008) 102, 466–75.

Ginkgo + Theophylline

The interaction between ginkgo and theophylline is based on experimental evidence only.

Clinical evidence

No interactions found.

Experimental evidence

In an experimental study in *rats* pretreated with oral ginkgo extract 100 mg/kg daily for 5 days, the serum levels and AUC of a single 10 mg/kg oral dose of theophylline given on day 6 were reduced by about 20% and 40%, respectively. The clearance was increased by 70%. A less marked effect was seen with ginkgo 10 mg/kg (30% increase in clearance). Similar results were seen with intravenous theophylline 10 mg/kg.[1]

Mechanism

This interaction is thought to be due to the induction of the cytochrome P450 isoenzyme CYP1A2 by ginkgo. Theophylline is a substrate of CYP1A2 and by inducing the activity of this isoenzyme, theophylline is more readily metabolised and cleared from the body. However, ginkgo had no relevant effect on another CYP1A2 substrate, caffeine, in humans. See Ginkgo + Caffeine, page 242.

Importance and management

The evidence for this interaction is limited to experimental data and the dose of ginkgo used is far higher than the most common clinical dose. A human study using caffeine as a CYP1A2 probe substrate, found that ginkgo does not affect CYP1A2 to a clinically relevant extent. Therefore an interaction with theophylline based on this mechanism is unlikely to be clinically important.

1. Tang J, Sun J, Zhang Y, Li L, Cui F, He Z. Herb-drug interactions: Effect of *Ginkgo biloba* extract on the pharmacokinetics of theophylline in rats. *Food Chem Toxicol* (2007) 45, 2441–5.

Ginkgo + Tolbutamide

Gingko does not appear to have a clinically relevant effect on the metabolism or blood-glucose-lowering effects of tolbutamide.

Clinical evidence

In healthy subjects, ginkgo extract (*Ginkgold*) 120 mg twice daily for 7 days had no effect on the urinary metabolic ratio of tolbutamide.[1] Similarly, in another 18 healthy subjects, another ginkgo extract, EGb 761, at a dose of 120 mg twice daily or 240 mg daily for 8 days, had no effect on the metabolism of a single 125-mg dose of tolbutamide.[2]

In another study in 10 healthy subjects, ginkgo 360 mg daily for 28 days slightly reduced the AUC of a single 125-mg oral dose of tolbutamide by about 16%, with no significant changes in other pharmacokinetic parameters. The ginkgo product used was *Ginkgold,* which contained 24% flavone glycosides and 6% terpene

lactones. The pharmacodynamics of tolbutamide were not significantly altered although there was a tendency towards the attenuation of its hypoglycaemic effects by ginkgo (14% reduction).[3]

Experimental evidence

In an experimental study, ginkgo 32 mg/kg given daily for 5 days before a single 40-mg/kg dose of tolbutamide significantly reduced its blood-glucose-lowering effects in aged *rats*. However, when a single 100-mg/kg dose of ginkgo was given with a single 40-mg/kg dose of tolbutamide, the blood-glucose levels were significantly lower, when compared with tolbutamide alone, suggesting that ginkgo potentiated the blood-glucose-lowering effects of tolbutamide.[4]

Mechanism

It was suggested that ginkgo might induce the cytochrome P450 isoenzyme CYP2C9, by which tolbutamide is metabolised. However, the clinical study shows that ginkgo has little or no clinically relevant effect on CYP2C9. The disparate effects between single and multiple dose administration in the *animal* study are not understood.

Importance and management

From the clinical evidence, it is clear that ginkgo has little, if any, effect on the metabolism and blood-glucose-lowering effects of tolbutamide. A clinically relevant interaction therefore seems unlikely.

Tolbutamide is used as a probe drug for CYP2C9 activity, and therefore these results also suggest that a clinically relevant pharmacokinetic interaction between ginkgo and other CYP2C9 substrates is unlikely.

1. Mohutsky MA, Anderson GA, Miller JW, Elmer GW. *Ginkgo biloba:* evaluation of CYP2C9 drug interactions in vitro and in vivo. *Am J Ther* (2006) 13, 24–31.
2. Zadoyan G, Rokitta D, Klement S, Dienel A, Hoerr R, Gramatté T, Fuhr U. Effect of *Ginkgo biloba* special extract EGb 761® on human cytochrome P450 activity: a cocktail interaction study in healthy volunteers *Eur J Clin Pharmacol* (2012) 68, 553–60.
3. Uchida S, Yamada H, Li DX, Maruyama S, Ohmori Y, Oki T, Watanabe H, Umegaki K, Ohashi K, Yamada S. Effects of Ginkgo biloba extract on pharmacokinetics and pharmacodynamics of tolbutamide and midazolam in healthy volunteers. *J Clin Pharmacol* (2006) 46, 1290–1298.
4. Sugiyama T, Kubota Y, Shinozuka K, Yamada S, Wu J, Umegaki K. Ginkgo biloba extract modifies hypoglycemic action of tolbutamide via hepatic cytochrome P450 mediated mechanism in aged rats. *Life Sci* (2004) 75, 1113–22.

Ginkgo + Trazodone

Coma developed in an elderly patient with Alzheimer's disease after she took trazodone and ginkgo.

Clinical evidence

An 80-year-old woman with Alzheimer's disease became comatose a few days after starting to take low-dose trazodone 20 mg twice daily and ginkgo. The patient woke immediately after being given flumazenil 1 mg intravenously.[1]

Experimental evidence

No relevant data found.

Mechanism

It was suggested that the flavonoids in the ginkgo had a subclinical direct effect on the benzodiazepine receptor. In addition, it was suggested that ginkgo increased the metabolism of trazodone to its active metabolite, 1-(m-chlorophenyl)piperazine (mCPP) by the cytochrome P450 isoenzyme CYP3A4. The increased levels of the metabolite were thought to have enhanced the release of GABA (gamma-amino butyric acid). Flumazenil may have blocked the direct effect of the flavonoids, thus causing the GABA activity to fall below the level required to have a clinical effect. However, note that clinically relevant CYP3A4 induction has not been seen

G

with the conventional CYP3A4 probe substrate midazolam. See Ginkgo + Benzodiazepines, page 241.

Importance and management

Evidence for an interaction between ginkgo and trazodone appears to be limited to this isolated case, from which no general conclusions can be drawn. Bear this interaction in mind in case of an unexpected response to concurrent use.

1. Galluzzi S, Zanetti O, Binetti G, Trabucchi M, Frisoni GB. Coma in a patient with Alzheimer's disease taking low dose trazodone and ginkgo biloba. *J Neurol Neurosurg Psychiatry* (2000) 68, 679–80.

Ginkgo + Warfarin and related drugs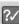

Evidence from pharmacological studies in patients and healthy subjects suggests that ginkgo does not usually interact with warfarin. However, an isolated report describes intracerebral haemorrhage associated with the use of ginkgo and warfarin, and there are a few reports of bleeding associated with the use of ginkgo alone.

Clinical evidence

In a randomised, crossover study in 21 patients stabilised on **warfarin**, ginkgo extract 100 mg daily (*Bio-Biloba*) for 4 weeks did not alter the INR or the required dose of **warfarin**, when compared with placebo.[1] Similarly, in another study in healthy subjects,[2] *Tavonin* (containing standardised dry extract EGb 761 of ginkgo equivalent to 2 g of leaf) two tablets three times daily for 2 weeks did not affect either the pharmacokinetics or pharmacodynamics (INR) of a single dose of **warfarin** given on day 7. Moreover, a retrospective review of 21 clinical cases involving the concurrent use of ginkgo and **warfarin** also found no evidence of altered INRs.[3]

Conversely, a report describes an intracerebral haemorrhage, which occurred in an elderly woman within 2 months of her starting to take ginkgo. Her prothrombin time was found to be 16.9 seconds and her partial thromboplastin time was 35.5 seconds. She had been taking **warfarin** uneventfully for 5 years.[4] The author of the report speculated that ginkgo may have contributed towards the haemorrhage.

Experimental evidence

In *animal* studies it was found that the AUC of **warfarin** was decreased by 23.4% when the ginkgo extract EGb 761 was given, and the prothrombin time was also reduced by EGb 761, which would suggest that ginkgo should *reduce* the effects of **warfarin**.[3]

Mechanism

Uncertain. Isolated cases of bleeding have been reported with ginkgo alone (which have been the subject of a review[5]). In pharmacological studies, ginkgo extract alone did not alter coagulation parameters or platelet aggregation.[2,3] Moreover, the experimental study suggests that ginkgo might reduce the effects of warfarin. Ginkgo extracts also do not appear to affect the metabolism of a number of substrates of the cytochrome P450 isoenzyme CYP2C9, suggesting that a pharmacokinetic interaction with warfarin, which is metabolised by this route, is unlikely. Consider also Ginkgo + NSAIDs, page 247, and Ginkgo + Tolbutamide, page 249.

Importance and management

There is good evidence from pharmacological studies in patients and healthy subjects that ginkgo extract would not be expected to interact with warfarin. However, there is one case report of over-anticoagulation, and a few reports of bleeding with ginkgo alone. This is insufficient evidence to justify advising patients taking warfarin to avoid ginkgo, but they should be warned to monitor for early signs of bruising or bleeding and seek informed professional advice if any bleeding problems arise.

Consider also Ginkgo + Antiplatelet drugs, page 240, and Ginkgo + NSAIDs, page 247 for other reports of bleeding events.

1. Engelsen J, Nielsen JD, Winther K. Effect of coenzyme Q_{10} and ginkgo biloba on warfarin dosage in stable, long-term warfarin treated outpatients. A randomised, double blind, placebo-crossover trial. *Thromb Haemost* (2002) 87, 1075–6.
2. Jiang X, Williams KM, Liauw WS, Ammit AJ, Roufogalis BD, Duke CC, Day RO, McLachlan AJ. Effect of ginkgo and ginger on the pharmacokinetics and pharmacodynamics of warfarin in healthy subjects. *Br J Clin Pharmacol* (2005) 59, 425–32.
3. Lai C-F, Chang C-C, Fu C-H, Chen C-M. Evaluation of the interaction between warfarin and ginkgo biloba extract. *Pharmacotherapy* (2002) 22, 1326.
4. Matthews MK. Association of *Ginkgo biloba* with intracerebral hemorrhage. *Neurology* (1998) 50, 1933.
5. Vaes LPJ, Chyka PA. Interactions of warfarin with garlic, ginger, ginkgo, or ginseng: nature of the evidence. *Ann Pharmacother* (2000) 34, 1478–82.

G

Ginseng

Panax ginseng C.A.Mey. (Araliaceae)

Synonym(s) and related species

Many species and varieties of ginseng are used.

Panax ginseng C.A.Mey is also known as Asian ginseng, Chinese ginseng, Korean ginseng, Oriental ginseng, Renshen.

Panax quinquefolius L. is also known as American ginseng.

Other species used include: *Panax notoginseng* (Burkill) F.H.Chen ex C.Y.Wu & K.M.Feng known as Sanchi ginseng, Tienchi ginseng and *Panax pseudo-ginseng* Wall. also known as Himalayan ginseng.

It is important to note that Siberian ginseng (*Eleutherococcus senticosus* Maxim.) is often used and marketed as a ginseng, but it is from an entirely different plant of the Araliaceae family and possesses constituents that are chemically different. It will be covered in this monograph with distinctions made throughout.

Not to be confused with ashwagandha, page 45, which is *Withania somnifera*. This is sometimes referred to as Indian ginseng.

Not to be confused with Brazilian ginseng, which is *Pfaffia paniculata*.

Pharmacopoeias

American Ginseng (*USP35–NF30 S1*); American Ginseng Capsules (*USP35–NF30 S1*); American Ginseng Tablets (*USP35–NF30 S1*); Asian Ginseng (*USP35–NF30 S1*); Asian Ginseng Tablets (*USP35–NF30 S1*); Eleuthero (*USP35–NF30 S1*); Eleutherococcus (*BP 2012, PhEur 7.5*); Ginseng [*Panax ginseng* C.A.Mey] (*BP 2012, PhEur 7.5*); Powdered American Ginseng (*USP35–NF30 S1*); Notoginseng Root (*BP 2012, PhEur 7.5*); Powdered American Ginseng Extract (*USP35–NF30 S1*); Powdered Asian Ginseng (*USP35–NF30 S1*); Powdered Asian Ginseng Extract (*USP35–NF30 S1*); Powdered Eleuthero (*USP35–NF30 S1*); Powdered Eleuthero Extract (*USP35–NF30 S1*).

Constituents

The actual composition of ginseng extracts used varies depending on the species used and the way the root is prepared. The main constituents are the **saponin glycosides** such as the **ginsenosides** or the **panaxosides** in *Panax* species, or the **eleutherosides** in *Eleutherococcus senticosus,* which are chemically different. Also present are volatile oils containing mainly sesquiterpenes.

Use and indications

Ginseng is used to enhance the body's resistance to stress and to improve mental and physical performance. It has also been used for diabetes, insomnia, sexual inadequacy, for degenerative conditions associated with ageing, to improve healing, and as a stimulant.

Pharmacokinetics

In vitro studies of various extracts and individual ginsenosides from *Panax ginseng* (Asian ginseng) and *Panax quinquefolius* (American ginseng) have generally found little to suggest that they interfere with the activity of cytochrome P450 isoenzymes.[1–5] This also seems to be the case for *Eleutherococcus senticosus* (Siberian ginseng) and the eleutherosides.[3,5]

The ginsenosides have been reported to inhibit CYP1A2 to some extent,[6] and various ginsenoside metabolites have been found to exert an inhibitory effect on CYP3A4.[1–4] However, the clinical relevance of these *in vitro* findings appears to be small, as clinical studies have found that *Panax ginseng* and *Eleutherococcus senticosus* have, at worst, weak effects on CYP3A4 (see benzodiazepines, page 254) or CYP2D6 (see dextromethorphan, page 255), and *Panax ginseng* also does not affect CYP1A2 (see caffeine, page 254) or CYP2E1 (see chlorzoxazone, page 254).

Some ginsenosides have been shown to be substrates for P-glycoprotein *in vitro,* and may actually inhibit its activity.[4,7] Whether this is clinically relevant is uncertain. Consider also fexofenadine, page 255.

Interactions overview

Panax ginseng (Asian ginseng), *Panax quinquefolius* (American ginseng) and *Eleutherococcus senticosus* (Siberian ginseng) appear to modestly lower blood-glucose levels and may therefore potentiate the blood-glucose-lowering effects of conventional oral antidiabetics, although this was not demonstrated in one study. *Panax ginseng* and *Panax quinquefolius* may *reduce* the effects of warfarin. As both ginsengs also contain antiplatelet components, *excessive* bleeding also cannot be ruled out. *Panax ginseng, Panax quinquefolius* and *Eleutherococcus senticosus* may also interfere with digoxin assays and although the evidence is limited, the psychoactive effects of ginseng may be additive with those of MAOIs. Some data suggests that *Panax ginseng* may increase the clearance of midazolam, albendazole and alcohol, but the clinical significance of this is either not clear or of limited general importance. *Panax ginseng* is a constituent of some Chinese herbal medicines. For interactions relating to these products, see under bupleurum, page 98.

Interactions monographs

- Albendazole, page 253
- Alcohol, page 253
- Antidiabetics, page 253
- Benzodiazepines, page 254
- Caffeine, page 254

G

1. Liu Y, Li W, Li P, Deng M-C, Yang S-L, Yang L. The inhibitory effect of intestinal bacterial metabolite of ginsenosides on CYP3A activity. *Biol Pharm Bull* (2004) 27, 1555–60.

2. Liu Y, Zhang J-W, Li W, Ma H, Sun J, Deng M-C, Yang L. Ginsenoside metabolites, rather than naturally occurring ginsenosides, lead to inhibition of human cytochrome P450 enzymes. *Toxicol Sci* (2006) 91, 356–64.
3. Henderson GL, Harkey MR, Gershwin ME, Hackman RM, Stern JS, Stresser DM. Effects of ginseng components on c-DNA-expressed cytochrome P450 enzyme catalytic activity. *Life Sci* (1999) 65, 209–14.
4. Etheridge AS, Black SR, Patel PR, So J, Mathews JM. An *in vitro* evaluation of cytochrome P450 inhibition and P-glycoprotein interaction with Goldenseal, *Ginkgo biloba*, grape seed, milk thistle, and ginseng extracts and their constituents. *Planta Med* (2007) 73, 731–41.
5. Budzinski JW, Foster BC, Vandenhoek S, Arnason JT. An *in vitro* evaluation of human cytochrome P450 3A4 inhibition by selected commercial herbal extracts and tinctures. *Phytomedicine* (2000) 7, 273–82.
6. Chang TKH, Chen J, Benetton SA. In vitro effect of standardized ginseng extracts and individual ginsenosides on the catalytic activity of human CYP1A1, CYP1A2, and CYP1B1. *Drug Metab Dispos* (2002) 30, 378–84.
7. Kim S-W, Kwon H-Y, Chi D-W, Shim J-H, Park J-D, Lee Y-H, Pyo S, Rhee D-K. Reversal of P-glycoprotein-mediated multidrug resistance by ginsenoside Rg$_3$. *Biochem Pharmacol* (2003) 65, 75–82.

G

Ginseng + Albendazole

The interaction between *Panax ginseng* (Asian ginseng) and albendazole is based on experimental evidence only.

Clinical evidence

No interactions found.

Experimental evidence

Panax ginseng (**Asian ginseng**) 10 mg/kg given intravenously to *rats,* increased the intestinal clearance of intravenous albendazole sulfoxide 10 mg/kg, the active metabolite of albendazole, by about 25%. The AUC was not significantly affected.[1]

Mechanism

Uncertain. *Panax ginseng* may interfere with the metabolism of albendazole.

Importance and management

The findings of this study using intravenous *Panax ginseng* (Asian ginseng) may not apply to oral use, as is used clinically. However, even if replicated in humans, the minor changes seen in the clearance of albendazole would be unlikely to be clinically relevant. Based on this study, no action is needed if patients taking albendazole also wish to take *Panax ginseng*.

1. Merino G, Molina AJ, Garcıa JL, Pulido MM, Prieto JG, Álvarez AI. Ginseng increases intestinal elimination of albendazole sulfoxide in the rat. *Comp Biochem Physiol C Toxicol Pharmacol* (2003) 136, 9–15.

Ginseng + Alcohol

Panax ginseng (Asian ginseng) increases the clearance of alcohol and lowers blood-alcohol levels.

Clinical evidence

Fourteen healthy subjects, each acting as their own control, were given alcohol (72 g/65 kg as a 25% solution) with and without a *Panax ginseng* (**Asian ginseng**) extract (3 g/65 kg) mixed in with it. They drank the alcohol or the alcohol/ginseng mixture over a 45-minute period in 7 portions, the first four at 5-minute intervals and the next three at 10-minute intervals. Measurements taken 40 minutes later showed that the presence of the ginseng lowered blood-alcohol levels by an average of about 39%. The alcohol levels of 10 subjects were lowered by 32 to 51% by the ginseng, 3 showed reductions of 14 to 18% and one showed no changes at all.[1]

Experimental evidence

In one study in *rats,* oral *Panax ginseng* (**Asian ginseng**) reduced the AUC of alcohol after oral, but not after intraperitoneal, administration;[2] however, in another study, it increased the clearance of intravenous alcohol.[3]

Mechanism

The reasons for this interaction are uncertain, but it is suggested that *Panax ginseng* possibly increases the activity of the enzymes (alcohol and aldehyde dehydrogenase)[4] that are concerned with the metabolism of the alcohol, thereby increasing the clearance of the alcohol.

Importance and management

Evidence for an interaction between *Panax ginseng* (Asian ginseng) and alcohol comes from a clinical study, which confirms the initial findings of some experimental studies.[2,3] What the reduction in blood-alcohol levels means in practical terms is not clear but the authors of the clinical report suggest the possibility of using *Panax*

ginseng to treat alcoholic patients and those with acute alcohol intoxication;[1] however, this suggestion needs confirmation in further clinical studies. The available data does however suggest that the concurrent use of alcohol and *Panax ginseng* is unlikely to be detrimental.

1. Lee FC, Ko JH, Park KJ, Lee JS. Effect of *Panax ginseng* on blood alcohol clearance in man. *Clin Exp Pharmacol Physiol* (1987) 14, 543–6.
2. Lee YJ, Pantuck CB, Pantuck EJ. Effect of ginseng on plasma levels of ethanol in the rat. *Planta Med* (1993) 59, 17–19.
3. Petkov V, Koushev V, Panova Y. Accelerated ethanol elimination under the effect of ginseng (experiments on rats). *Acta Physiol Pharmacol Bulg* (1977) 3, 46–50.
4. Choi CW, Lee SI, Huh K. Effect of ginseng on the hepatic alcohol metabolizing enzyme system activity in chronic alcohol-treated mice. *Korean J Pharmacol* (1984) 20, 13–21.

Ginseng + Antidiabetics

In patients with diabetes taking various oral antidiabetics, *Panax quinquefolius* (American ginseng) and *Panax ginseng* (Asian ginseng) have both shown modest reductions in postprandial glucose levels after a glucose tolerance test, but *Panax ginseng* did not result in any improvement in diabetes control when given for 12 weeks.

Clinical evidence

In a placebo-controlled crossover study, 19 patients with well-controlled type 2 diabetes were treated with oral *Panax ginseng* (**Asian ginseng**) 2 g three times daily 40 minutes before meals in addition to their usual treatment (antidiabetics and/or diet) for 12 weeks. The ginseng had no effect on glycosylated blood-glucose, which remained at about 6.5%, but it did slightly decrease the blood-glucose levels after a 75 g oral glucose tolerance test. All patients in the study were diet controlled: 5 patients received no additional treatment; 3 patients were taking a **sulfonylurea**; 3 patients were taking **metformin**; 5 patients were taking a **sulfonylurea** with **metformin**; 1 patient was taking a **sulfonylurea** with **metformin** and **rosiglitazone**; 1 patient was taking a **sulfonylurea** and **rosiglitazone**; and 1 patient was taking **acarbose**.[1]

In earlier studies by the same research group, single dose *Panax quinquefolius* (**American ginseng**) 3 to 9 g slightly reduced the post-prandial blood-glucose concentrations by about 20 to 24% in patients with type 2 diabetes when given 40 minutes before or at the same time as a 25 g oral glucose challenge. These patients were being treated with diet alone, **sulfonylureas**, or **sulfonylureas** plus **metformin**.[2,3] When comparing the effect between those receiving antidiabetics and those not, there was no difference, suggesting no specific drug interaction.[4]

Experimental evidence

The blood-glucose-lowering effects of *Panax quinquefolius* (**American ginseng**) and *Panax ginseng* (**Asian ginseng**) has been demonstrated in various *animal* models, and is not covered here because there is adequate clinical information. In an experimental study, *Eleutherococcus senticosus* (**Siberian ginseng**) also showed significant blood-glucose-lowering activity in *mice*.[5]

Mechanism

Additive blood-glucose-lowering effects are theoretically possible when ginseng is given with antidiabetics. However, very limited data suggest no specific interactions with conventional antidiabetics.

Importance and management

These studies show that *Panax ginseng* (Asian ginseng) and *Panax quinquefolius* (American ginseng) might possess blood-glucose-lowering activity, but the multiple-dose study showed this was not clinically relevant in patients with well-controlled diabetes. The available data suggest that it is very unlikely a dramatic hypoglycaemic effect will occur in patients with diabetes.

Eleutherococcus senticosus (Siberian ginseng) may also have blood-glucose-lowering properties.

1. Vuksan V, Sung M-K, Sievenpiper JL, Stavro PM, Jenkins AL, Di-Buono M, Lee K-S, Leiter LA, Nam KY, Arnason JT, Choi M, Naeem A. Korean red ginseng (*Panax ginseng*) improves glucose and insulin regulation in well-controlled, type 2 diabetes: results of a randomized, double-blind, placebo-controlled study of efficacy and safety. *Nutr Metab Cardiovasc Dis* (2008) 18, 46–56.
2. Vuksan V, Sievenpiper JL, Koo VYY, Francis T, Beljan-Zdravkovic U, Xu Z, Vidgen E. American ginseng (*Panax quinquefolius* L) reduces postprandial glycemia in non-diabetic subjects and subjects with type 2 diabetes mellitus. *Arch Intern Med* (2000) 160, 1009–13.
3. Vuksan V, Stavro MP, Sievenpiper JL, Beljan-Zdravkovic U, Leiter LA, Josse RG, Xu Z. Similar postprandial glycemic reductions with escalation of dose and administration time of American Ginseng in type 2 diabetes. *Diabetes Care* (2000) 23, 1221–6.
4. Vuksan V, Sievenpiper JL. Panax (ginseng) is not a panacea. Author reply. *Arch Intern Med* (2000) 160, 3330–3331.
5. Hikino H, Takahashi M, Otake K, Konno C. Isolation and hypoglycemic activity of eleutherans A, B, C, D, E, F, and G: glycans of *Eleutherococcus senticosus* roots. *J Nat Prod* (1986) 49, 293–7.

Ginseng + Benzodiazepines

Eleutherococcus senticosus (Siberian ginseng) did not alter the pharmacokinetics of alprazolam, and *Panax ginseng* (Asian ginseng) did not alter midazolam metabolism in two studies, but slightly reduced midazolam exposure in another.

Clinical evidence

A study in 12 healthy subjects found that *Eleutherococcus senticosus* (Siberian ginseng), 485 mg twice daily for 15 days, did not significantly affect the pharmacokinetics of a single 2-mg dose of **alprazolam** given with the morning dose on day 14.[1]

Similarly, in 12 healthy subjects, *Panax ginseng* (Asian ginseng), 500 mg three times daily for 28 days, did not significantly affect the metabolism of oral **midazolam** 8 mg. The ginseng preparation used was standardised to 5% ginsenosides.[2] These findings were repeated in a later study using the same criteria in 12 elderly healthy subjects.[3] In contrast, in a study in 12 healthy subjects given a single 8-mg oral dose of midazolam before and after ginseng 500 mg twice daily for 28 days, ginseng reduced the exposure to midazolam by 34%. In this study ginseng was given as *Panax ginseng* root powder, *Vitamer Laboratories*.[4]

Experimental evidence

No relevant data found.

Mechanism

Eleutherococcus senticosus does not appear to affect the cytochrome P450 isoenzyme CYP3A4, by which alprazolam is, in part, metabolised. Panax ginseng might induce the metabolism of midazolam by CYP3A4, but evidence is conflicting.

Importance and management

Evidence for an interaction between ginseng and the benzodiazepines is limited. The study with *Eleutherococcus senticosus* (Siberian ginseng) and alprazolam found no effect on alprazolam pharmacokinetics suggesting that no dose adjustments are likely to be needed on their concurrent use. The studies with *Panax ginseng* (Asian ginseng) are somewhat conflicting, with two studies finding no effect on midazolam pharmacokinetics and one study finding a slight decrease in midazolam exposure. Although a clinically relevant interaction seems generally unlikely it might be prudent to consider the possibility of an interaction if midazolam seems less effective.

Midazolam is used as a probe drug for CYP3A4 activity, and therefore these results also suggest that *Panax ginseng* might be a weak inducer of CYP3A4.

1. Donovan JL, DeVane CL, Chavin KD, Taylor RM, Markowitz JS. Siberian ginseng (*Eleutheroccus* [sic] *senticosus*) effects on CYP2D6 and CYP3A4 activity in normal volunteers. *Drug Metab Dispos* (2003) 31, 519–22.
2. Gurley BJ, Gardner SF, Hubbard MA, Williams DK, Gentry WB, Cui Y, Ang CYW. Cytochrome P450 phenotypic ratios for predicting herb-drug interactions in humans. *Clin Pharmacol Ther* (2002) 72, 276–87.
3. Gurley BJ, Gardner SF, Hubbard MA, Williams DK, Gentry WB, Cui Y, Ang CYW. Clinical assessment of botanical supplementation on cytochrome P450 phenotypes in the elderly: St John's wort, garlic oil, *Panax ginseng*, and *Ginkgo biloba*. *Drugs Aging* (2005) 22, 525–39.

4. Malati CY, Robertson SM, Hunt JD, Chairez C, Alfaro RM, Kovacs JA, Penzak SR. Influence of *Panax ginseng* on cytochrome P450 (CYP)3A and P-glycoprotein (P-gp) activity in healthy participants *J Clin Pharmacol* (2012) 52, 932–9.

Ginseng + Caffeine

Panax ginseng (Asian ginseng) did not alter caffeine metabolism in one study. Note that both ginseng and caffeine have stimulant effects.

Clinical evidence

In a study in 12 healthy subjects *Panax ginseng* (Asian ginseng), 500 mg three times daily for 28 days, did not significantly affect the pharmacokinetics of caffeine 100 mg. The ginseng preparation used was standardised to 5% ginsenosides.[1] These findings were repeated in a later study using the same criteria in 12 elderly healthy subjects.[2]

Experimental evidence

No relevant data found.

Mechanism

These studies show that *Panax ginseng* does not have a clinically significant effect on the cytochrome P450 isoenzyme CYP1A2 by which caffeine is metabolised.

Importance and management

These studies suggest that *Panax ginseng* (Asian ginseng) is unlikely to affect the metabolism of caffeine. Therefore it would not be expected to reduce the effects or increase the adverse effects of caffeine. Nevertheless, ginseng is considered to be a stimulant, and it is possible that additive stimulant effects might occur with caffeine, although there do not appear to be much data on this. However, if both substances are given, bear the possibility of increased stimulant effects in mind.

Caffeine is used as a probe substrate for CYP1A2 activity, and therefore these results also suggest that a pharmacokinetic interaction as a result of this mechanism between *Panax ginseng* and other CYP1A2 substrates is unlikely.

For information on one study where the stimulant effects of a caffeine-containing herb appeared to be additive with those of *Panax ginseng*, see Ginseng + Herbal medicines; Guarana, page 255.

1. Gurley BJ, Gardner SF, Hubbard MA, Williams DK, Gentry WB, Cui Y, Ang CYW. Cytochrome P450 phenotypic ratios for predicting herb-drug interactions in humans. *Clin Pharmacol Ther* (2002) 72, 276–87.
2. Gurley BJ, Gardner SF, Hubbard MA, Williams DK, Gentry WB, Cui Y, Ang CYW. Clinical assessment of botanical supplementation on cytochrome P450 phenotypes in the elderly: St John's wort, garlic oil, *Panax ginseng*, and *Ginkgo biloba*. *Drugs Aging* (2005) 22, 525–39.

Ginseng + Carbamazepine

For mention that saiko-ka-ryukotsu-borei-to and sho-saiko-to (of which ginseng is one of a number of constituents) did not affect the pharmacokinetics of carbamazepine in *animal* studies, see Bupleurum + Carbamazepine, page 99.

Ginseng + Chlorzoxazone

Panax ginseng (Asian ginseng) did not alter chlorzoxazone metabolism in one study.

G

Clinical evidence

In a study in 12 healthy subjects, *Panax ginseng* (**Asian ginseng**) 500 mg three times daily for 28 days did not significantly affect the pharmacokinetics of chlorzoxazone 500 mg. The ginseng preparation used was standardised to 5% ginsenosides.[1] These findings were repeated in a later study using the same criteria in 12 elderly healthy subjects.[2]

Experimental evidence

No relevant data found.

Mechanism

These studies show that *Panax ginseng* does not have a clinically significant effect on the cytochrome P450 isoenzyme CYP2E1 by which chlorzoxazone is metabolised.

Importance and management

These studies suggest that *Panax ginseng* (Asian ginseng) is unlikely to affect the pharmacokinetics of chlorzoxazone. Chlorzoxazone is used as a probe drug for CYP2E1 activity, and therefore these results also suggest that a pharmacokinetic interaction as a result of this mechanism between *Panax ginseng* and other CYP2E1 substrates is unlikely.

1. Gurley BJ, Gardner SF, Hubbard MA, Williams DK, Gentry WB, Cui Y, Ang CYW. Cytochrome P450 phenotypic ratios for predicting herb-drug interactions in humans. *Clin Pharmacol Ther* (2002) 72, 276–87.
2. Gurley BJ, Gardner SF, Hubbard MA, Williams DK, Gentry WB, Cui Y, Ang CYW. Clinical assessment of botanical supplementation on cytochrome P450 phenotypes in the elderly: St John's wort, garlic oil, *Panax ginseng*, and *Ginkgo biloba*. *Drugs Aging* (2005) 22, 525–39.

Ginseng + Dextromethorphan

Eleutherococcus senticosus (**Siberian ginseng**) does not appear to affect the metabolism of dextromethorphan.

Clinical evidence

A study in 12 healthy subjects found that *Eleutherococcus senticosus* (**Siberian ginseng**), 485 mg twice daily for 14 days, did not significantly affect the metabolism of a single 30-mg dose of dextromethorphan.[1]

Experimental evidence

No relevant data found.

Mechanism

This study shows that *Eleutherococcus senticosus* does not have a clinically significant effect on the cytochrome P450 isoenzyme CYP2D6 by which dextromethorphan is metabolised. Note also that *Panax ginseng* (**Asian ginseng**) had no effect on the metabolism of debrisoquine, another CYP2D6 probe substrate, in clinical pharmacokinetic interaction studies.[2,3]

Importance and management

This study suggests that *Eleutherococcus senticosus* (Siberian ginseng) is unlikely to interact with dextromethorphan. Dextromethorphan and debrisoquine are used as probe drugs for CYP2D6 activity, and therefore these results also suggest that a pharmacokinetic interaction as a result of this mechanism between *Panax ginseng* (Asian ginseng) or *Eleutherococcus senticosus* and other CYP2D6 substrates is unlikely.

1. Donovan JL, DeVane CL, Chavin KD, Taylor RM, Markowitz JS. Siberian ginseng (*Eleutheroccus* [sic] *senticosus*) effects on CYP2D6 and CYP3A4 activity in normal volunteers. *Drug Metab Dispos* (2003) 31, 519–22.
2. Gurley BJ, Gardner SF, Hubbard MA, Williams DK, Gentry WB, Cui Y, Ang CYW. Cytochrome P450 phenotypic ratios for predicting herb-drug interactions in humans. *Clin Pharmacol Ther* (2002) 72, 276–87.
3. Gurley BJ, Gardner SF, Hubbard MA, Williams DK, Gentry WB, Cui Y, Ang CYW. Clinical assessment of botanical supplementation on cytochrome P450 phenotypes in the elderly: St John's wort, garlic oil, *Panax ginseng*, and *Ginkgo biloba*. *Drugs Aging* (2005) 22, 525–39.

Ginseng + Digoxin

Ginseng has been shown to interfere with some methods of measuring serum digoxin, see Ginseng + Laboratory tests, page 256

Ginseng + Fexofenadine

Panax ginseng (**Asian ginseng**) **does not appear to affect the absorption of fexofenadine.**

Clinical evidence

In a study in 12 healthy subjects given a single 120-mg oral dose of fexofenadine before and after ginseng 500 mg twice daily for 28 days, ginseng had no effect on the pharmacokinetics of fexofenadine. In this study ginseng was given as Panax ginseng root powder, Vitamer Laboratories.[1]

Experimental evidence

In a study in rats, ginseng (given as a suspension of *Panax ginseng*) reduced the bioavailability of fexofenadine by 16% and decreased the ratio of brain to plasma fexofenadine concentrations.[2]

Mechanism

Fexofenadine can be used to study the effects of other drugs on P-glycoprotein. These studies suggest that *Panax ginseng* is unlikely to have a clinically relevant effect on intestinal P-glycoprotein, but might induce P-glycoprotein in the brain.

Importance and management

Evidence for an interaction between fexofenadine and ginseng appears to be limited to one study and in vitro data relating to the use of *Panax ginseng* (Asian ginseng). What is known suggests that ginseng is unlikely to have a clinically relevant effect on fexofenadine absorption, but that the distribution of fexofenadine might be affected. The clinical relevance of this latter finding is unclear; nevertheless, the available data suggests that a dose adjustment of fexofenadine is unlikely to be needed in the presence of ginseng.

1. Malati CY, Robertson SM, Hunt JD, Chairez C, Alfaro RM, Kovacs JA, Penzak SR. Influence of *Panax ginseng* on cytochrome P450 (CYP)3A and P-glycoprotein (P-gp) activity in healthy participants *J Clin Pharmacol* (2012) 52, 932–9.
2. Zhang R, Jie J, Zhou Y, Cao Z, Li W. Long-term effects of panax ginseng on disposition of fexofenadine in rats in vivo *Am J Chin Med* (2009) 37, 657–67.

Ginseng + Food

No interactions found.

Ginseng + Herbal medicines; Guarana

The stimulant effects of guarana, a caffeine-containing herb, appear to be additive with those of *Panax ginseng* (Asian ginseng).

Clinical evidence

In a well-controlled single-dose study in healthy subjects, guarana extract 75 mg improved cognitive performance in 'attention' tasks and *Panax ginseng* (Asian ginseng) 200 mg improved 'memory' tasks. The combination improved both attention and memory tasks, with no clear evidence for synergistic effects, except for better performance in the increased serial sevens subtractions compared with

G

either drug alone. In this study, the ginseng extract was standardised to 4% of ginsenosides, and the guarana extract to 11 to 13% of xanthines (caffeine and theobromine), or a maximum of about 10 mg of caffeine per dose.[1]

Experimental evidence

Because of the quality of the clinical data available, experimental evidence has not been sought.

Mechanism

Both guarana and ginseng are used for their putative stimulative effects. In this study, they affected different tasks, and in combination, their effects were generally additive. The effect of guarana was not considered to be solely attributable to the caffeine content, since the dose of caffeine was low.[1]

Importance and management

Caffeine-containing herbs such as guarana are often combined with ginseng for their stimulant and cognitive effects. This study provides some evidence that they do not appear to have synergistic effects, but that the combination is the sum of the different effects of the two herbs. Note that the guarana dose used in this study provided only a low dose of caffeine.

1. Kennedy DO, Haskell CF, Wesnes KA, Scholey AB. Improved cognitive performance in human volunteers following administration of guarana (*Paullinia cupana*) extract: comparison and interaction with *Panax ginseng*. Pharmacol Biochem Behav (2004) 79, 401–11.

Ginseng + Laboratory tests

Panax ginseng (Asian ginseng), *Panax quinquefolius* (American ginseng) and *Eleutherococcus senticosus* (Siberian ginseng) may interfere with the results of digoxin assays.

Clinical evidence

A 74-year-old man who had been taking **digoxin** for many years (serum levels normally in the range 0.9 to 2.2 nanograms/mL) was found, during a routine check, to have **digoxin** levels of 5.2 nanograms/mL, but without evidence of toxicity or bradycardia or any other ECG changes.[1] The levels remained high even when the **digoxin** was stopped. It turned out he had also been taking *Eleutherococcus senticosus* (**Siberian ginseng**) capsules. When the ginseng was stopped, the **digoxin** levels returned to the usual range, and **digoxin** was resumed. Later rechallenge with the ginseng caused a rise in his serum **digoxin** levels. No **digoxin** or **digitoxin** contamination was found in the capsules, and the authors of the report also rejected the idea that the eleutherosides (chemically related to cardiac glycosides) in ginseng might have been converted *in vivo* into **digoxin**, or that the renal elimination of **digoxin** might have been impaired, since the patient showed no signs of toxicity.[1]

Experimental evidence

Panax ginseng (**Asian ginseng**), *Panax quinquefolius* (**American ginseng**) and *Eleutherococcus senticosus* (**Siberian ginseng**) have been found to interfere with some **digoxin** assays including fluorescence polarisation immunoassay (FPIA, Abbott Laboratories)[2–4] and microparticle enzyme immunoassay (MEIA, Abbott Laboratories).[2,3] The more specific monoclonal antibody-based **digoxin** immunoassay, Tina-quant (Roche), was unaffected by all the ginsengs,[3,4] and the Beckman (Synchron LX system) monoclonal assay was unaffected by *Panax ginseng* (**Asian ginseng**).[4]

Mechanism

Uncertain. One possible explanation is that the ginsengs affected the accuracy of the digoxin assays so that they gave false results.

Importance and management

The interference in the digoxin measurements described in the assays was not as high as that reported in the elderly patient and there is some doubt as to whether the herbal medicine taken by the patient was actually *Eleutherococcus senticosus* (Siberian ginseng).[3,5] So, whether this is clinically important, and measurement of serum digoxin levels is actually affected, is uncertain. Nevertheless it may be sensible to ask about ginseng use when interpreting unexpected digoxin levels and consider using a more specific monoclonal immunoassay.

1. McRae S. Elevated serum digoxin levels in a patient taking digoxin and Siberian ginseng. *Can Med Assoc J* (1996) 155, 293–5.
2. Dasgupta A, Wu S, Actor J, Olsen M, Wells A, Datta P. Effect of Asian and Siberian ginseng on serum digoxin measurement by five digoxin immunoassays. Significant variation in digoxin-like immunoreactivity among commercial ginsengs. *Am J Clin Pathol* (2003) 119, 298–303.
3. Dasgupta A, Reyes MA. Effect of Brazilian, Indian, Siberian, Asian, and North American ginseng on serum digoxin measurement by immunoassays and binding of digoxin-like immunoreactive components of ginseng with Fab fragment of antidigoxin antibody (Digibind). *Am J Clin Pathol* (2005) 124, 229–36.
4. Chow L, Johnson M, Wells A, Dasgupta A. Effect of the traditional Chinese medicines Chan Su, Lu-Shen-Wan, Dan Shen, and Asian ginseng on serum digoxin measurement by Tina-quant (Roche) and Synchron LX System (Beckman) digoxin immunoassays. *J Clin Lab Anal* (2003) 17, 22–7.
5. Awang DVC. Siberian ginseng toxicity may be case of mistaken identity. *CMAJ* (1996) 155, 1237.

Ginseng + MAOIs

Case reports describe headache, insomnia and tremulousness, which was attributed to the concurrent use of ginseng and phenelzine.

Clinical evidence

A 64-year-old woman taking **phenelzine** [60 mg daily] developed headache, insomnia, and tremulousness after taking *Natrol High*, a product containing ginseng,[1,2] probably *Eleutherococcus senticosus* (**Siberian ginseng**). She had the same symptoms on another occasion after drinking a ginseng tea (type not stated), which she had used without problem before starting **phenelzine**.[1] Three years later, while taking **phenelzine** 45 mg daily, she experienced the same symptoms and an increase in depression 72 hours after starting to take ginseng capsules (type not stated) and a herbal tea.[2]

Another depressed woman taking ginseng (type not stated) and bee pollen experienced relief of her depression and became active and extremely optimistic when she started to take **phenelzine** 45 mg daily, but this was accompanied by insomnia, irritability, headaches and vague visual hallucinations. When the **phenelzine** was stopped and then re-started in the absence of the ginseng and bee pollen, her depression was not relieved.[3]

Experimental evidence

No relevant data found.

Mechanism

Uncertain. It seems unlikely that the bee pollen had any part to play. Note that the ginsengs have stimulant effects, and adverse effects include insomnia, nervousness, hypertension and euphoria.

Importance and management

Evidence is limited to three case reports, and the general importance of these poorly documented early cases is unclear. It may be that these cases could just represent idiosyncratic reactions, and not be due to an interaction. The data is therefore too limited to suggest any particular caution. Nevertheless, consider the possibility of an interaction in case of an unexpected response to treatment with phenelzine (or potentially any MAOI) in a patient taking any type of ginseng.

1. Shader RI, Greenblatt DJ. Phenelzine and the dream machine – ramblings and reflections. *J Clin Psychopharmacol* (1985) 5, 65.
2. Shader RI, Greenblatt DJ. Bees, ginseng and MAOIs revisited. *J Clin Psychopharmacol* (1988) 8, 235.
3. Jones BD, Runikis AM. Interaction of ginseng with phenelzine. *J Clin Psychopharmacol* (1987) 7, 201–2.

Ginseng + Ofloxacin

For mention that sairei-to and sho-saiko-to (of which ginseng is one of a number of constituents) do not affect the pharmacokinetics of ofloxacin, see Bupleurum + Ofloxacin, page 99.

Ginseng + Tamoxifen and other oestrogen antagonists

Ginseng may contain oestrogenic compounds that might directly stimulate breast cancer growth and oppose the actions of competitive oestrogen receptor antagonists such as tamoxifen. However, there is some evidence that ginseng use before diagnosis might not adversely affect breast cancer survival.

Evidence, mechanism, importance and management

In one report ginseng root was listed as an example of a herbal medicine with oestrogenic activity that might directly stimulate breast cancer growth and oppose the actions of competitive oestrogen receptor antagonists such as tamoxifen, see Chinese angelica + Oestrogens or Oestrogen antagonists, page 146.

However, there is some evidence that ginseng use before diagnosis might not adversely affect breast cancer survival. In the Shanghai breast cancer study, 398 women who regularly used ginseng before diagnosis actually had better disease-free and overall survival over 5 years than 1057 women who had never used ginseng. Data on ginseng use had been obtained within 66 days of diagnosis of breast cancer. Most of the ginseng used was *Panax quinquefolius* (**American ginseng**) or white *Panax ginseng* (**Asian ginseng**), the average daily dose was 1.3 g of ginseng root, and the average cumulative duration of use was 4.3 months per year. It should be noted that ginseng users were of higher educational achievement and were more likely to have used tamoxifen (69% versus 61%), both factors that might contribute to increased survival. Although ginseng use post-diagnosis was assessed at follow-up interview, it was not possible to examine the effect of this on survival since there were no data on post-diagnosis use of ginseng in patients who had already died.[1] While not conclusive, this study does provide some reassurance about the use of ginseng in breast cancer. However, a prospective randomised study is required to fully ascertain this.

1. Cui Y, Shu X-O, Gao Y-T, Cai H, Tao M-H, Zheng W. Association of ginseng use with survival and quality of life among breast cancer patients. *Am J Epidemiol* (2006) 163, 645–53.

Ginseng + Tolbutamide

For conflicting evidence that sho-saiko-to (of which ginseng is one of 7 constituents) might increase or decrease the rate of absorption of tolbutamide in *animal* studies, see Bupleurum + Tolbutamide, page 99.

Ginseng + Warfarin and related drugs

One pharmacological study found that *Panax quinquefolius* (American ginseng) modestly decreased the effect of warfarin, whereas another study found that *Panax ginseng* (Asian ginseng) did not alter the effect of warfarin. Two case reports describe decreased warfarin effects, one with thrombosis, attributed to the use of ginseng (probably *Panax ginseng*).

Clinical evidence

In a placebo-controlled study, 20 healthy subjects were given warfarin 5 mg daily for 3 days alone then again on days 15 to 17 of a 3-week course of *Panax quinquefolius* (**American ginseng**) 1 g twice daily. In the 12 subjects given ginseng, the peak INR was modesty reduced by 0.16, compared with a non-significant reduction of 0.02 in the 8 subjects given placebo. There was also a modest reduction in the AUC of warfarin. In this study, *Panax quinquefolius* root was ground and capsulated.[1]

Evidence from two earlier case reports supports a reduction in warfarin effect. A man taking warfarin long-term, and also diltiazem, glyceryl trinitrate and salsalate, had a fall in his INR from 3.1 to 1.5 within 2 weeks of starting to take ginseng capsules (*Ginsana*) three times daily. This preparation contains 100 mg of standardised concentrated ginseng [probably *Panax ginseng* (**Asian ginseng**)] in each capsule. Within 2 weeks of stopping the ginseng his INR had risen again to 3.3.[2] Another patient taking warfarin was found to have thrombosis of a prosthetic aortic valve, with a subtherapeutic INR of 1.4. Three months prior to this episode his INR had become persistently subtherapeutic, requiring a progressive increment in his warfarin dose. It was suggested that this might have been because he had begun using a ginseng product (not identified).[3]

In contrast, in a randomised, crossover study in 12 healthy subjects, ginseng capsules 1 g three times daily for 2 weeks did not affect either the pharmacokinetics or pharmacodynamics (INR) of a single 25-mg dose of warfarin taken on day 7. The brand of ginseng used was *Golden Glow,* each capsule containing an extract equivalent to 0.5 g of *Panax ginseng* (**Asian ginseng**) root.[4]

Experimental evidence

A study in *rats* failed to find any evidence of an interaction between warfarin and an extract from *Panax ginseng* (**Asian ginseng**).[5] See also Andrographis + Anticoagulants, page 34, for details of a lack of an interaction between Kan Jang, a standardised fixed combination of extracts from *Andrographis paniculata* and *Eleutherococcus senticosus* (**Siberian ginseng**), and warfarin.

Mechanism

It is unclear why ginseng might reduce the efficacy of warfarin, particularly as no pharmacokinetic interaction occurs. *In vitro* experiments have found that *Panax ginseng* contains antiplatelet components that inhibit platelet aggregation and thromboxane formation,[6] although antiplatelet activity was not demonstrated in a study in healthy subjects.[7] If an antiplatelet effect were confirmed, this might suggest the possibility of an *increased* risk of bleeding with the combination of ginseng and warfarin. There are a few reports of vaginal bleeding in women using ginseng preparations (unspecified) in the absence of an anticoagulant,[8–10] but these are probably due to a possible hormonal effect of ginseng.

Importance and management

The available evidence suggests that ginseng might *decrease* the effect of warfarin. It is possible that the effect is greater with, or specific to, *Panax quinquefolius* (American ginseng), since this interacted in one study whereas *Panax ginseng* (Asian ginseng) did not. Although the ginseng dose was higher in the *Panax ginseng* study, the treatment duration was not as long, which may have obscured an effect. Moreover, the two case reports of decreased warfarin effects attributed to the use of ginseng were probably *Panax ginseng*.

Until further information becomes available it would seem prudent to be alert for decreased effects of warfarin and related drugs in patients using ginseng, particularly *Panax quinquefolius*. However, the possibility of an *increased* risk of bleeding due to the antiplatelet component of *Panax ginseng* cannot entirely be ruled out, although the clinical study suggests that this is unlikely.

1. Yuan C-S, Wei G, Dey L, Karrison T, Nahlik L, Maleckar S, Kasza K, Ang-Lee M, Moss J. Brief communication: American ginseng reduces warfarin's effect in healthy patients. *Ann Intern Med* (2004) 141, 23–7.
2. Janetzky K, Morreale AP. Probable interaction between warfarin and ginseng. *Am J Health-Syst Pharm* (1997) 54, 692–3.

G

3. Rosado MF. Thrombosis of a prosthetic aortic valve disclosing a hazardous interaction between warfarin and a commercial ginseng product. *Cardiology* (2003) 99, 111.

4. Jiang X, Williams KM, Liauw WS, Ammit AJ, Roufogalis BD, Duke CC, Day RO, McLachlan AJ. Effect of St John's wort and ginseng on the pharmacokinetics and pharmacodynamics of warfarin in healthy subjects. *Br J Clin Pharmacol* (2004) 57, 592–9.

5. Zhu M, Chan KW, Ng LS, Chang Q, Chang S, Li RC. Possible influences of ginseng on the pharmacokinetics and pharmacodynamics of warfarin in rats. *J Pharm Pharmacol* (1999) 51, 175–80.

6. Kuo S-C, Teng C-M, Leed J-C, Ko F-N, Chen S-C, Wu T-S. Antiplatelet components in Panax ginseng. *Planta Med* (1990) 56, 164–7.

7. Beckert BW, Concannon MJ, Henry SL, Smith DS, Puckett CL. The effect of herbal medicines on platelet function: an in vivo experiment and review of the literature. *Plast Reconstr Surg* (2007) 120, 2044–50.

8. Hopkins MP, Androff L, Benninghoff AS. Ginseng face cream and unexplained vaginal bleeding. *Am J Obstet Gynecol* (1988) 159, 1121–2.

9. Greenspan EM. Ginseng and vaginal bleeding. *JAMA* (1983) 249, 2018.

10. Kabalak AA, Soyal OB, Urfalioglu A, Saracoglu F, Gogus N. Menometrorrhagia and tachyarrhythmia after using oral and topical ginseng. *J Womens Health (Larchmt)* (2004) 13, 830–833.

G

Glossy privet

Ligustrum lucidum W.T.Aiton (Oleaceae)

Synonym(s) and related species

Chinese privet, Nepal privet, Tree privet, Wax-leaf privet, White wax-tree.

Constituents

The main constituents of glossy privet are the dammarane triterpenes (mainly acetyl derivatives) and oleanolic acid; the secoiridoid glucosides nuezhenide, neonuezhenide, isonuezhenide, ligustroside, lucidomoside, oleuropein and oleoside dimethyl ester; and **flavonoids**[1] including quercetin, apigenin, luteolin and their derivatives.

Use and indications

Glossy privet is used in the treatment of a wide variety of ailments including pain, atherosclerosis, diabetes, liver disorders, and as a general tonic.

Pharmacokinetics

No relevant pharmacokinetic data found. For information on the pharmacokinetics of individual flavonoids present in glossy privet, see under flavonoids, page 213.

Interactions overview

No interactions with glossy privet found. For information on the interactions of individual flavonoids present in glossy privet, see under flavonoids, page 213.

1. Xu X-H, Yang N-Y, Qian S-H, Xie N, Yu M-Y, Duan J-A. Stduy [sic] on flavonoids in *Ligustrum lucidum*. *Zhong Yao Cai* (2007) 30, 538–40.

G

Glucosamine

2-Amino-2-deoxy-β-D-glucopyranose

Types, sources and related compounds

Chitosamine, Glucosamine hydrochloride, Glucosamine sulfate potassium chloride, Glucosamine sulfate sodium chloride.

Pharmacopoeias

Glucosamine hydrochloride (*PhEur 7.5, USP35–NF30 S1*); Glucosamine sulfate potassium chloride (*USP35–NF30 S1*); Glucosamine sulfate sodium chloride (*PhEur 7.5, USP35–NF30 S1*); Glucosamine tablets (*USP35–NF30 S1*).

Use and indications

Glucosamine is a natural substance found in chitin, mucoproteins, and mucopolysaccharides. It can be made by the body, and is found in relatively high concentrations in cartilage, tendons and ligaments. The primary use of supplemental glucosamine is for the treatment of osteoarthritis and other joint disorders. It is sometimes given with chondroitin, page 152. Glucosamine in supplements may be prepared synthetically, or extracted from chitin.

Pharmacokinetics

The oral bioavailability of glucosamine has been estimated to be about 25 to 50%, probably due to first-pass metabolism in the liver. Glucosamine is rapidly absorbed and distributed into numerous tissues, with a particular affinity for articular cartilage.[1,2]

Interactions overview

Glucosamine supplements have modestly increased the INR in a few patients taking warfarin. Increased blood-glucose has been recorded in patients with diabetes, but no interaction was found in a controlled study. Glucosamine might modestly increase tetracycline or oxytetracycline levels, and very limited evidence suggests that glucosamine may possibly decrease the efficacy of paracetamol and some cytotoxic antineoplastics. Unnamed diuretics may slightly reduce the efficacy of glucosamine.

Interactions monographs

- Antidiabetics, page 261
- Antineoplastics, page 261
- Diuretics, page 261
- Food, page 261
- Herbal medicines, page 261
- Paracetamol (Acetaminophen), page 261
- Tetracyclines, page 262
- Warfarin and related drugs, page 262

1. Setnikar I, Palumbo R, Canali S, Zanolo G. Pharmacokinetics of glucosamine in man. *Arzneimittelforschung* (1993) 43, 1109–13.
2. Setnikar I, Rovati LC. Absorption, distribution, metabolism and excretion of glucosamine sulfate. A review. *Arzneimittelforschung* (2001) 51, 699–725.

G

Glucosamine + Antidiabetics

In a controlled study, glucosamine supplements with chondroitin had no effect on glycaemic control in patients taking oral antidiabetic drugs but one report notes that unexpected increases in blood-glucose levels have occurred.

Evidence, mechanism, importance and management

In 2000, the Canadian Adverse Drug Reaction Monitoring Programme (CADRMP) briefly reported that unexpected increases in blood-glucose levels had occurred in diabetic patients taking glucosamine sulfate, or glucosamine with chondroitin.[1] However, in a well controlled study, *Cosamin DS* (glucosamine hydrochloride 1.5 g daily with chondroitin sulfate sodium 1.2 g) daily for 90 days had no effect on the control of diabetes (glycosylated haemoglobin) in 22 patients with type 2 diabetes, 4 who were diet-controlled and 18 who were receiving oral antidiabetics (specific drugs not named).[2]

Endogenous glucosamine has a role in glucose metabolism, and may increase insulin resistance. In one case, glucosamine also reduced hypoglycaemic episodes in a patient with metastatic insulinoma.[3]

The interaction is not established, and the results of the controlled study suggest that glucosamine supplements are generally unlikely to affect the control of diabetes. However, it has been suggested that the results of this study may not be applicable to patients in the later stages of diabetes[4] (i.e. those with type 2 diabetes who require, or are expected to require, insulin). Therefore it may be prudent to increase monitoring of blood-glucose in these patients if glucosamine supplements are taken. Also, if glucose control unexpectedly deteriorates, bear the possibility of self-medication with supplements such as glucosamine in mind.

1. Canadian Adverse Drug Reaction Monitoring Programme (CADRMP). Communiqué. Glucosamine sulfate: hyperglycemia. *Can Adverse Drug React News* (2000) 10, 7.
2. Scroggie DA, Albright A, Harris MD. The effect of glucosamine-chondroitin supplementation on glycosylated hemoglobin levels in patients with type 2 diabetes mellitus: a placebo-controlled, double-blinded, randomized clinical trial. *Arch Intern Med* (2003) 163, 1587–90.
3. Chan NN, Baldeweg SE, Tan TMM, Hurel SJ. Glucosamine sulphate and osteoarthritis. *Lancet* (2001) 357, 1618–19.
4. Jain RK, McCormick JC. Can glucosamine supplements be applied for all patients with type 2 diabetes with osteoarthritis? *Arch Intern Med* (2004) 164, 807.

Glucosamine + Antineoplastics

The interaction between glucosamine and antineoplastics is based on experimental evidence only.

Clinical evidence

No interactions found

Experimental evidence

An *in vitro* study found that colon and ovary cancer cell lines showed resistance to **doxorubicin** and **etoposide** after exposure to glucosamine at a concentration of 10 mmol. Only a weak effect of glucosamine was found in the responsiveness of breast cancer cell lines to **etoposide**.[1]

Mechanism

It is suggested that the expression of topoisomerase II was reduced by the presence of glucosamine. Topoisomerase II is required for doxorubicin and etoposide to exert their antineoplastic effects, therefore decreasing the levels of this enzyme increased the resistance to these antineoplastics.

Importance and management

This possible interaction appears not to have been studied *in vivo*, and, until more data are available, the clinical significance of the

findings is unclear. However, the implication is that glucosamine could reduce the efficacy of these antineoplastics. Bear this possibility in mind should an unexpected response to treatment with topoisomerase inhibitors occur.

1. Yun J, Tomida A, Nagata K Tsuruo. Glucose-regulated stresses confer resistance to VP-16 in human cancer cells through decreased expression of DNA topoisomerase II. *Oncol Res* (1995) 7, 583–90.

Glucosamine + Diuretics

Limited evidence from a large open study suggests that unnamed diuretics may slightly reduce the efficacy of glucosamine.

Clinical evidence

In a large open study, 1183 evaluable patients with osteoarthritis were given glucosamine 1.5 g taken daily for an average of 50 days. The overall assessment of efficacy was 'good' in about 59% of patients and 'sufficient' in 36%. When response was analysed by concurrent treatment, in the 64 patients also taking diuretics (none specifically named), there was a slightly lower incidence of good efficacy (44%) and a slightly higher incidence of sufficient efficacy (52%), which reached statistical significance.[1] However, note that this study was non-randomised, and other patient factors might therefore have accounted for these differences.

Experimental evidence

No relevant data found.

Mechanism

Unknown.

Importance and management

The concurrent use of glucosamine and diuretics is probably quite common, and the fact that this old study appears to be the only report in the literature of a possible interaction, and in itself is inconclusive, suggests that any interaction is, in the main, unlikely to be clinically important.

1. Tapadinhas MJ, Rivera IC, Bignamini AA. Oral glucosamine sulphate in the management of arthrosis: report on a multi-centre open investigation in Portugal. *Pharmatherapeutica* (1982) 3, 157–68.

Glucosamine + Food

No interactions found.

Glucosamine + Herbal medicines

No interactions found.

Glucosamine + Paracetamol (Acetaminophen)

Limited evidence suggests that glucosamine may reduce the efficacy of paracetamol (acetaminophen).

Evidence, mechanism, importance and management

In a survey of herbal medicine use in 122 patients from 6 outpatient clinics, 2 patients with osteoarthritis (a 66-year-old man

G

and a 74-year-old woman), had complained of reduced paracetamol (acetaminophen) efficacy when starting glucosamine. The salt of glucosamine used was not mentioned.[1]

It has been suggested that increased serum sulfate levels arising from glucosamine sulfate might lead to increased metabolism of paracetamol by sulfate conjugation.[2] However, there are no studies assessing this. Note that this would only occur with glucosamine sulfate salts and would not occur with glucosamine hydrochloride.

The combined use of glucosamine and paracetamol to alleviate the symptoms of osteoarthritis is common, and the limited evidence here does not provide any reason to suggest any changes to this practice.

1. Bush TM, Rayburn KS, Holloway SW, Sanchez-Yamamoto DS, Allen BL, Lam T, So BK, Tran DH, Greyber ER, Kantor S, Roth LW. Adverse interactions between herbal and dietary substances and prescription medications: a clinical survey. *Altern Ther Health Med* (2007) 13, 30–35.
2. Hoffer LJ, Kaplan LN, Hamadeh MJ, Grigoriu AC, Baron M. Sulfate could mediate the therapeutic effect of glucosamine sulfate. *Metabolism* (2001) 50, 767–70.

Glucosamine + Tetracyclines

Glucosamine modestly increases tetracycline levels.

Clinical evidence

A single-dose study in healthy subjects given **tetracycline** 250 mg alone or with glucosamine 250 mg found that the serum **tetracycline** levels were 105%, 50% and 25% higher at 2, 3, and 6 hours after administration, respectively, in those patients who had received the combined treatment. Similar results were found when **oxytetracycline** was given with glucosamine, with the corresponding increases being 36%, 44% and 30% at 2, 3 and 6 hours after administration, respectively.[1] The AUC of the antibacterials was not reported.

In contrast, in another single-dose study in 12 healthy subjects given **tetracycline** 250 mg alone, and then with glucosamine 125 mg and 250 mg at one-week intervals, the addition of glucosamine slightly increased serum **tetracycline** levels at 2, 3, 6 and 8 hours, but this was not statistically significant.[2]

Experimental evidence

A study in *dogs* and *mice* found that giving glucosamine hydrochloride with radioactive **oxytetracycline** increased the serum radioactivity, suggesting an increase in serum **oxytetracycline** levels. In the *dogs,* the increase in radioactivity was over twofold at 30 minutes, 1 hour and 24 hours after drug administration, whereas in the *mice* the increase was only greater than twofold at 15 minutes after drug administration.[3]

Mechanism

Unknown.

Importance and management

These very early studies from the 1950s suggest that glucosamine might cause a modest increase in tetracycline levels. As a result of these studies, it appears that a preparation of oxytetracycline formulated with glucosamine was tried. A modest increase in tetracycline or oxytetracycline levels is unlikely to have adverse consequences, and, if anything, might be slightly beneficial.

1. Welch H, Wright WW, Staffa AW. The effect of glucosamine on the absorption of tetracycline and oxytetracycline administered orally. *Antibiotic Med Clin Ther* (1958) 5, 52–8.
2. Anderson K, Keynes R. Studies with glucosamine on the absorption of tetracycline. *Med J Aust* (1959) 46, 246–7.
3. Snell JF, Garkuscha R. Radioactive oxytetracycline (Terramycin). III. Effect of glucosamine HCl on serum concentrations. *Proc Soc Exp Biol Med* (1958) 98, 148–50.

Glucosamine + Warfarin and related drugs

A few reports suggest that glucosamine with or without chondroitin may increase the INR in patients taking warfarin. In contrast, one case of a decreased INR has been reported when glucosamine was given with acenocoumarol.

Clinical evidence

The first indication of a possible interaction was in 2001, when the Canadian Adverse Drug Reaction Monitoring Program briefly reported that an increase in INR had been noted when glucosamine was given to patients taking warfarin, and that INR values decreased when glucosamine was stopped.[1] In 2004, a full case report was published. In this case, a 69-year-old man stabilised on warfarin 47.5 mg weekly had an increase in his INR from 2.58 to 4.52 four weeks after starting to take 6 capsules of *Cosamin DS* (glucosamine hydrochloride 500 mg, sodium chondroitin sulfate 400 mg, manganese ascorbate per capsule) daily. His warfarin dose was reduced to 40 mg weekly, and his INR returned to the target range of 2 to 3 (INR 2.15) with continued *Cosamin DS* therapy.[2] A comment on this report noted that this is twice the usual dose of glucosamine.[3] Since then, one other similar case of a modest rise in INR has been published. A man taking warfarin and glucosamine hydrochloride 500 mg with chondroitin sulfate 400 mg twice daily had a gradual increase in his INR (from 2.3 to 4.7 over 5 weeks) when he trebled the dose of the glucosamine supplement.[4]

Analysis of regulatory authority data has revealed other unpublished reports. In 2006 the CHM in the UK reported that they had received 7 reports of an increase in INR in patients taking warfarin after they started taking glucosamine supplements.[5] In 2007, a search of the FDA database identified 20 possible cases,[4] and a search of the WHO database identified 22 possible case reports of an increase in warfarin effect with glucosamine, which originated from Australia, Canada, Denmark, Sweden, the UK and USA.[6] In two of the WHO cases, chondroitin was used, but the other cases were with glucosamine alone. Of 15 reports giving details of time to onset, the increased INR was noted within 3 days (in a 99-year-old) and up to 6 months; most commonly the interaction took several weeks to manifest.[6]

In contrast, a 71-year-old man stabilised on **acenocoumarol** 15 mg weekly had a *decrease* in his INR to 1.6 after taking glucosamine sulfate (*Xicil*) 1.5 g daily for 10 days. The glucosamine was stopped and the INR reached 2.1. When the glucosamine was restarted, with an increase in **acenocoumarol** dose to 17 mg weekly, the INR only reached 1.9. The glucosamine was eventually stopped.[7] Similarly, the WHO database contained one report of a decreased effect of warfarin with glucosamine.[6] The Australian Adverse Drug Reactions Advisory Committee have also identified 12 cases of alterations in INR in patients taking warfarin. Nine of these cases are included in the WHO report.[8]

There do not appear to have been any controlled studies of the effects of glucosamine supplements on the pharmacodynamics or pharmacokinetics of oral anticoagulants.

Experimental evidence

No relevant data found.

Mechanism

Unknown.

Importance and management

Glucosamine is a widely used supplement, particularly in the middle-aged and elderly, who are also the group most likely to be using warfarin or similar anticoagulants. Despite this, there are just three published reports of a possible interaction, two describing moderate rises in INR and one a decrease. Even taking into account the possible cases reported to regulatory authorities, the interaction would seem to be quite rare. Nevertheless, the cases described suggest it would be prudent to monitor the INR more closely if glucosamine is started or stopped. Also, if a patient shows an unexpected change in INR, bear in mind the possibility of self-medication with supplements such as glucosamine.

Note that in 2006 the CHM in the UK recommend that patients taking warfarin do not take glucosamine,[5] but the subsequent 2007 UK-approved labelling for the prescription-only glucosamine product *Alateris* recommends close monitoring when a patient taking a coumarins anticoagulant starts or stops glucosamine.[9]

1. Canadian Adverse Drug Reaction Monitoring Programme (CADRMP). Communiqué. Warfarin and glucosamine: interaction. *Can Adverse Drug React News* (2001) 11, 8.
2. Rozenfeld V, Crain JL, Callahan AK. Possible augmentation of warfarin effect by glucosamine-chondroitin. *Am J Health-Syst Pharm* (2004) 61, 306–7.
3. Scott GN. Interaction of warfarin with glucosamine – chondroitin. *Am J Health-Syst Pharm* (2004) 61, 1186.
4. Knudsen JF, Sokol GH. Potential glucosamine-warfarin interaction resulting in increased international normalized ratio: case report and review of the literature and MedWatch database. *Pharmacotherapy* (2008) 28, 540–548.
5. Commission on Human Medicines/Medicines and Healthcare Products Regulatory Agency. Glucosamine adverse reactions and interactions. *Current Problems* (2006) 31, 8.
6. Yue Q-Y, Strandell J, Myrberg O. Concomitant use of glucosamine may potentiate the effect of warfarin. The Uppsala Monitoring Centre. http://www.who-umc.org/graphics/9722.pdf (accessed 17/11/2008).
7. Garrote Garcra M, Iglesias Piñeiro MJ, Martrn Álvarez R, Pérez González J. Interacción farmacológica del sulfato de glucosamina con acenocumarol. *Aten Primaria* (2004) 33, 162–4.
8. Adverse Drug Reactions Advisory Committee (ADRAC). Interaction between glucosamine and warfarin. *Aust Adverse Drug React Bull* (2008) 27, 3.
9. Alateris (Glucosamine hydrochloride). Ransom UK Summary of product characteristics, June 2007.

Goat's rue

Galega officinalis L. (Fabaceae)

Synonym(s) and related species

French lilac, Italian fitch, Professor-weed.

Constituents

The main active constituents are **guanidine derivatives**, including guanidine and galegine; **flavonoids** such as those based on kaempferol and quercetin; and unspecified saponins and lectins.

Use and indications

Goat's rue is used in traditional medicine for the treatment of diabetes and to increase lactation. It is also being investigated for a potential anti-obesity effect. Guanidines isolated from goat's rue led to the development of the biguanide drugs (such as metformin), which are now in clinical use.

Pharmacokinetics

No relevant pharmacokinetic data found. For information on the pharmacokinetics of individual flavonoids present in goat's rue, see under flavonoids, page 213.

Interactions overview

No interactions with goat's rue found. For information on the interactions of individual flavonoids present in goat's rue, see under flavonoids, page 213.

G

Goldenseal

Hydrastis canadensis L. (Ranunculaceae)

Synonym(s) and related species

Hidrastis, Hydrastis, Orange root, Yellow root.
Xanthorhiza simplicissima Marsh.

Pharmacopoeias

Goldenseal (*USP35–NF30 S1*); Goldenseal rhizome (*PhEur 7.5*); Goldenseal root (*BP 2012*); Powdered goldenseal (*USP35–NF30 S1*); Powdered goldenseal extract (*USP35–NF30 S1*).

Constituents

The rhizome of goldenseal contains the isoquinoline alkaloids **hydrastine** and **berberine**, to which it may be standardised, and also berberastine, hydrastinine, canadine (tetrahydroberberine), canalidine and others.

Use and indications

Used for inflammatory and infective conditions, such as amoebic dysentery and diarrhoea; gastric and liver disease. The alkaloids are antibacterial, amoebicidal and fungicidal. For details on the uses of berberine, a major constituent of goldenseal, see berberine, page 63.

Pharmacokinetics

In several *in vitro* studies, goldenseal root has been identified as a potent inhibitor of the cytochrome P450 isoenzyme CYP3A4,[1–4] but more modest inhibitory effects were seen clinically with the CYP3A4 probe substrate, midazolam, page 266. Two studies in healthy subjects, found that goldenseal, given for 14 to 28 days reduced the metabolism or urinary clearance of debrisoquine, a probe substrate of CYP2D6, by 36% and 47%, respectively.[5,6] *In vitro* studies using another CYP2D6 probe, dextromethorphan, also found that goldenseal inhibits CYP2D6, and suggested that this may be, at least in part, due to berberine; hydrastine had no effects on CYP2D6.[4]

Goldenseal has also been reported to possibly have some inhibitory effect on CYP2C8[4] (see paclitaxel, page 267) and CYP2C9[3] (see diclofenac, page 266). Another study[4] suggested that goldenseal had no significant effect on CYP2E1 (see chlorzoxazone, page 266), CYP1A2 (see caffeine, page 266), or CYP2C19. In addition, there is some *in vitro* evidence of P-glycoprotein inhibition,[4] but no effect was seen on the levels of digoxin, page 267, which is used as a probe substrate of this transporter.

For information on the pharmacokinetics of the constituent berberine, see under berberine, page 63.

Interactions overview

Goldenseal appears to modestly decrease the metabolism of midazolam, but has no significant effects on the pharmacokinetics of indinavir or digoxin.

Goldenseal does not appear to affect the metabolism of caffeine or chlorzoxazone. The interaction between goldenseal and diclofenac, paclitaxel or tolbutamide is based on experimental evidence only.

For a possible interaction with ciclosporin, occurring as a result of the constituent berberine, see Berberine + Ciclosporin, page 64.

Interactions monographs

- Benzodiazepines, page 266
- Caffeine, page 266
- Chlorzoxazone, page 266
- Diclofenac, page 266
- Digoxin, page 267
- Food, page 267
- Herbal medicines, page 267
- Indinavir, page 267
- Paclitaxel, page 267
- Tolbutamide, page 268

G

1. Budzinski JW, Foster BC, Vandenhoek S, Arnason JT. An *in vitro* evaluation of human cytochrome P450 3A4 inhibition by selected commercial herbal extracts and tinctures. *Phytomedicine* (2000) 7, 273–82.
2. Budzinski JW, Trudeau VL, Drouin CE, Panahi M, Arnason JT, Foster BC. Modulation of human cytochrome P450 3A4 (CYP3A4) and P-glycoprotein (P-gp) in Caco-2 cell monolayers by selected commercial-source milk thistle and goldenseal products. *Can J Physiol Pharmacol* (2007) 85, 966–78.
3. Chatterjee P, Franklin MR. Human cytochrome P450 inhibition and metabolic-intermediate complex formation by goldenseal extract and its methylenedioxyphenyl components. *Drug Metab Dispos* (2003) 31, 1391–7.
4. Etheridge AS, Black SR, Patel PR, So J, Mathews JM. An *in vitro* evaluation of cytochrome P450 inhibition and p-glycoprotein interaction with goldenseal, *Ginkgo biloba*, grape seed, milk thistle, and ginseng extracts and their constituents. *Planta Med* (2007) 73, 731–41.
5. Gurley BJ, Gardner SF, Hubbard MA, Williams DK, Gentry WB, Khan IA, Shah A. In vivo effects of goldenseal, kava kava, black cohosh, and valerian on human cytochrome P450 1A2, 2D6, 2E1, and 3A4/5 phenotypes. *Clin Pharmacol Ther* (2005) 77, 415–26.
6. Gurley BJ, Swain A, Hubbard MA, Williams DK, Barone G, Hartsfield F, Tong Y, Carrier DJ, Cheboyina S, Battu SK. Clinical assessment of CYP2D6-mediated herb-drug interactions in humans: Effects of milk thistle, black cohosh, goldenseal, kava kava, St John's wort, and *Echinacea*. *Mol Nutr Food Res* (2008) 52, 755–63.

Goldenseal + Benzodiazepines

Goldenseal appears to modestly decrease the metabolism of midazolam.

Clinical evidence

A study in 12 healthy subjects investigated the effects of goldenseal 900 mg three times daily taken for 28 days on a single 8-mg dose of oral midazolam. Goldenseal reduced the metabolism of midazolam to hydroxymidazolam by about 40%. The supplement used had no standardisation information.[1] Similarly, in a study in 16 healthy subjects given a single 8-mg dose of midazolam after goldenseal 1323 mg three times daily for 14 days, there was a significant increase in the maximum concentration and AUC of midazolam of 41% and 62%, respectively, and a reduction in the clearance of about 36%. These increases were considered moderate when compared with the effects of clarithromycin and rifampicin in the study, which produced a 448% increase and 93% decrease in the AUC of midazolam, respectively. The goldenseal product used gave an estimated daily dose of berberine of about 77 mg and of hydrastine of 132 mg.[2]

Experimental evidence

Goldenseal appears to be a potent inhibitor of the cytochrome P450 isoenzyme CYP3A4 *in vitro*. See *pharmacokinetics*, page 265.

Mechanism

A standardised goldenseal extract appears to modestly inhibit the cytochrome P450 isoenzyme CYP3A4, which is the major route of midazolam metabolism. Concurrent use therefore raises midazolam levels.

Importance and management

Evidence for an interaction between goldenseal and midazolam is based on clinical studies in healthy subjects. They suggest that some caution might be appropriate if patients taking goldenseal supplements are given oral midazolam; however, the effects were modest. Nevertheless, the clinical effects of this interaction do not appear to have been studied and so it may be prudent to be aware of the small possibility of increased sedation if midazolam is given to patients taking goldenseal supplements. Any interaction is unlikely to be significant in patients given a single dose of intravenous or oral midazolam pre-operatively.

Midazolam is used as a probe drug for CYP3A4 activity, and therefore these results also suggest that a modest pharmacokinetic interaction between goldenseal and other CYP3A4 substrates is possible. See the table Drugs and herbs affecting or metabolised by the cytochrome P450 isoenzyme CYP3A4, page 7, for a list of known CYP3A4 substrates.

For mention of an *animal* study of the possible anxiolytic effect of high-dose berberine and its interaction with diazepam, see Berberine + Anxiolytics, page 64.

1. Gurley BJ, Gardner SF, Hubbard MA, Williams DK, Gentry WB, Khan IA, Shah A. In vivo effects of goldenseal, kava kava, black cohosh, and valerian on human cytochrome P450 1A2, 2D6, 2E1, and 3A4/5 phenotypes. *Clin Pharmacol Ther* (2005) 77, 415–26.
2. Gurley BJ, Swain A, Hubbard MA, Hartsfield F, Thaden J, Williams DK, Gentry WB, Tong Y. Supplementation with goldenseal (*Hydrastis canadensis*) but not kava kava (*Piper methysticum*), inhibits human CYP3A activity *in vivo*. *Clin Pharmacol Ther* (2008) 83, 61–9.

Goldenseal + Caffeine

Goldenseal did not affect caffeine metabolism in one study.

Clinical evidence

A study in 12 healthy subjects found that a goldenseal supplement 900 mg three times daily taken for 28 days had no significant effects

on the metabolism of a single 100-mg oral dose of caffeine.[1] The supplement used had no standardisation information.

Experimental evidence

See under *Mechanism,* below.

Mechanism

A standardised goldenseal extract did not inhibit CYP1A2 *in vitro*,[2] nor did goldenseal have a clinically relevant effect on the cytochrome P450 isoenzyme CYP1A2 activity using caffeine as a probe substrate.

Importance and management

This study suggests that goldenseal does not have any clinically relevant effect on caffeine metabolism in healthy subjects.

Caffeine is used as a probe substrate for CYP1A2 activity, and therefore these results also suggest that a pharmacokinetic interaction as a result of this mechanism between goldenseal and other CYP1A2 substrates is unlikely.

1. Gurley BJ, Gardner SF, Hubbard MA, Williams DK, Gentry WB, Khan IA, Shah A. In vivo effects of goldenseal, kava kava, black cohosh, and valerian on human cytochrome P450 1A2, 2D6, 2E1, and 3A4/5 phenotypes. *Clin Pharmacol Ther* (2005) 77, 415–26.
2. Etheridge AS, Black SR, Patel PR, So J, Mathews JM. An *in vitro* evaluation of cytochrome P450 inhibition and p-glycoprotein interaction with goldenseal, *Ginkgo biloba*, grape seed, milk thistle, and ginseng extracts and their constituents. *Planta Med* (2007) 73, 731–41.

Goldenseal + Chlorzoxazone

Goldenseal did not affect chlorzoxazone metabolism in one study.

Clinical evidence

In a study in 12 healthy subjects, a goldenseal supplement 900 mg three times daily taken for 28 days had no significant effects on the metabolism of a single oral dose of chlorzoxazone 250 mg.[1] The supplement used had no standardisation information.

Experimental evidence

See under *Mechanism,* below.

Mechanism

A standardised goldenseal extract did not inhibit CYP2E1 *in vitro*,[2] nor did goldenseal have a clinically relevant effect on the cytochrome P450 isoenzyme CYP2E1 activity using chlorzoxazone as a probe substrate.

Importance and management

Evidence from the clinical study suggests that goldenseal is unlikely to affect the metabolism of chlorzoxazone. Chlorzoxazone is used as a probe substrate for CYP2E1 activity, and therefore these results also suggest that a pharmacokinetic interaction as a result of this mechanism between goldenseal and other CYP2E1 substrates is unlikely.

1. Gurley BJ, Gardner SF, Hubbard MA, Williams DK, Gentry WB, Khan IA, Shah A. In vivo effects of goldenseal, kava kava, black cohosh, and valerian on human cytochrome P450 1A2, 2D6, 2E1, and 3A4/5 phenotypes. *Clin Pharmacol Ther* (2005) 77, 415–26.
2. Etheridge AS, Black SR, Patel PR, So J, Mathews JM. An *in vitro* evaluation of cytochrome P450 inhibition and p-glycoprotein interaction with goldenseal, *Ginkgo biloba*, grape seed, milk thistle, and ginseng extracts and their constituents. *Planta Med* (2007) 73, 731–41.

Goldenseal + Diclofenac

The interaction between goldenseal and diclofenac is based on experimental evidence only.

Evidence, mechanism, importance and management

An *in vitro* study investigated the effects of a goldenseal extract, (containing equal amounts of the active constituents hydrastine and berberine) on the activity of the cytochrome P450 isoenzyme CYP2C9 in human liver microsomes, using diclofenac as a probe drug. Goldenseal 0.98% inhibited the hydroxylation of diclofenac by about 50%. When berberine and hydrastine were tested separately, hydrastine inhibited CYP2C9 to a greater extent than berberine.[1] However, note that another *in vitro* study found that goldenseal had little effect on the metabolism of tolbutamide, page 268, another probe drug for CYP2C9 activity.

The general relevance of this is unknown as there are no clinical studies reporting the effects of goldenseal on CYP2C9. However, note that in the study cited here, goldenseal was about five times more potent as an inhibitor of CYP3A4 than CYP2C9, and clinically, goldenseal has only a modest effect on the CYP3A4 substrate midazolam, page 266. This provides some indication that CYP2C9 inhibition by goldenseal might not be clinically relevant. However, a clinical study is needed to confirm this.

1. Chatterjee P, Franklin MR. Human cytochrome P450 inhibition and metabolic-intermediate complex formation by goldenseal extract and its methylenedioxyphenyl components. *Drug Metab Dispos* (2003) 31, 1391–7.

Goldenseal + Digoxin

Goldenseal has only very small effects on the pharmacokinetics of digoxin.

Clinical evidence

A study in 20 healthy subjects given a single 500-microgram dose of digoxin before and on the last day of treatment with standardised goldenseal root extract 1070 mg three times daily for 14 days, found a 14% increase in the maximum digoxin plasma levels, but no other changes in the pharmacokinetics of digoxin. The product gave an estimated daily dose of berberine of about 77 mg and of hydrastine of about 132 mg.[1]

Experimental evidence

See under *Mechanism*, below.

Mechanism

It was suggested that constituents of goldenseal may alter digoxin pharmacokinetics by affecting P-glycoprotein, since goldenseal alkaloids are modulators of P-glycoprotein *in vitro*.[2] However, the clinical study showed that goldenseal does not cause clinically relevant changes in digoxin pharmacokinetics.[1]

Importance and management

Evidence from the clinical study suggests that goldenseal has only very modest effects on the pharmacokinetics of digoxin, which would not be expected to be clinically relevant. No dosage adjustment would be expected to be necessary if patients taking digoxin also wish to take goldenseal.

Digoxin is used as a probe substrate for P-glycoprotein activity and therefore this study also suggests that goldenseal is unlikely to have a clinically relevant effect on the transport of other drugs by P-glycoprotein.

1. Gurley BJ, Swain A, Barone GW, Williams DK, Breen P, Yates CR, Stuart LB, Hubbard MA, Tong Y, Cheboyina S. Effect of goldenseal (*Hydrastis Canadensis*) and kava kava (*Piper methysticum*) supplementation on digoxin pharmacokinetics in humans. *Drug Metab Dispos* (2007) 35, 240–245.
2. Etheridge AS, Black SR, Patel PR, So J, Mathews JM. An *in vitro* evaluation of cytochrome P450 inhibition and p-glycoprotein interaction with goldenseal, *Ginkgo biloba*, grape seed, milk thistle, and ginseng extracts and their constituents. *Planta Med* (2007) 73, 731–41.

Goldenseal + Food

No interactions found.

Goldenseal + Herbal medicines

No interactions found.

Goldenseal + Indinavir

Goldenseal root had no clinically relevant effect on the pharmacokinetics of a single dose of indinavir in one study.

Clinical evidence

In a study in 10 healthy subjects, goldenseal root (*Nature's Way*) 1.14 g twice daily for 2 weeks did not alter the mean peak plasma level, half-life or oral clearance of a single 800-mg dose of indinavir. Eight of the subjects had less than a 20% increase or decrease in oral clearance, but one subject had a 46% increase and one a 46% decrease.[1]

Experimental evidence

No relevant data found.

Mechanism

Goldenseal was found to be an inhibitor of CYP3A4 *in vitro*.[2] This was confirmed in a clinical study using oral midazolam as a probe substrate for CYP3A4, which found a decrease of about 40% in the metabolism of midazolam to hydroxymidazolam.[3] Goldenseal root might therefore have been expected to inhibit the metabolism of indinavir.

Importance and management

The study suggests that goldenseal root has no effect on indinavir exposure, and that no clinically relevant pharmacokinetic interaction would therefore be expected on the concurrent use of this HIV-protease inhibitor.

1. Sandhu RS, Prescilla RP, Simonelli TM, Edwards DJ. Influence of goldenseal root on the pharmacokinetics of indinavir. *J Clin Pharmacol* (2003) 43, 1283–8.
2. Budzinski JW, Foster BC, Vandenhoek S, Arnason JT. An in vitro evaluation of human cytochrome P450 3A4 inhibition by selected commercial herbal extracts and tinctures. *Phytomedicine* (2000) 7, 273–82.
3. Gurley BJ, Gardner SF, Hubbard MA, Williams DK, Gentry WB, Khan IA, Shah A. In vivo effects of goldenseal, kava kava, black cohosh, and valerian on human cytochrome P450 1A2, 2D6, 2E1, and 3A4/5 phenotypes. *Clin Pharmacol Ther* (2005) 77, 415–26.

Goldenseal + Paclitaxel

The interaction between goldenseal and paclitaxel is based on experimental evidence only.

Evidence, mechanism, importance and management

In an *in vitro* study using human liver microsomes, an aqueous and ethanolic goldenseal extract inhibited CYP2C8 activity by about 50 to 60% when used at a concentration of 20 micromol alkaloids (sum of hydrastine and berberine), and had a lesser effect at 1 micromol (40%). However, because of wide confidence intervals, only the 60% decrease with the ethanolic extract was statistically significant. Paclitaxel was used as a probe cytochrome P450 isoenzyme CYP2C8 substrate, and therefore this study also suggests that goldenseal has the potential to inhibit the metabolism of other CYP2C8 substrates. When studied individually, both berberine and hydrastine had some CYP2C8 inhibitory activity (also not statistically significant).[1]

The general relevance of the effect of goldenseal on paclitaxel metabolism is unknown as there are no clinical studies reporting the effects of goldenseal on CYP2C8 substrates. Note that high-dose berberine blocked the anticancer effects of paclitaxel in one *in vitro* study, see Berberine + Paclitaxel, page 65, and therefore, until more data is available, some caution may be prudent.

1. Etheridge AS, Black SR, Patel PR, So J, Mathews JM. An *in vitro* evaluation of cytochrome P450 inhibition and p-glycoprotein interaction with goldenseal, *Ginkgo biloba*, grape seed, milk thistle, and ginseng extracts and their constituents. *Planta Med* (2007) 73, 731–41.

Goldenseal + Tolbutamide

The interaction between goldenseal and tolbutamide is based on experimental evidence only.

Evidence, mechanism, importance and management

An *in vitro* study investigated the effects of aqueous and alcoholic extracts of goldenseal on the cytochrome P450 isoenzyme CYP2C9 as measured by the activity of tolbutamide hydroxylase. The activity of CYP2C9 was increased by about 35% when incubated with the extract with an alkaloid concentration of 1 micromol, but this was only statistically significant for the ethanolic extract. Moreover, the higher alkaloid concentration of 20 micromol had no effect.[1] Note that another *in vitro* study found that goldenseal *inhibited* the metabolism of diclofenac, page 266, a probe drug for CYP2C9.

The clinical relevance of these results is unknown, and the disparate findings of goldenseal on CYP2C9 are not easily explained, but any effect was modest. Therefore goldenseal would be expected to have only modest, if any, effects on the response to tolbutamide. Further study is needed to assess these effects.

1. Etheridge AS, Black SR, Patel PR, So J, Mathews JM. An *in vitro* evaluation of cytochrome P450 inhibition and p-glycoprotein interaction with goldenseal, *Ginkgo biloba*, grape seed, milk thistle, and ginseng extracts and their constituents. *Planta Med* (2007) 73, 731–41.

G

Gotu kola

Centella asiatica (L.) Urb. (Apiaceae)

Synonym(s) and related species

Asiatic pennywort, Centella, Gota kola, Gotu cola, Hydrocotyle, Indian pennywort, Indian water navelwort.

Hydrocotyle asiatica L., *Hydrocotyle lurida* Hance.

Pharmacopoeias

Centella (*BP 2012, PhEur 7.5*); *Centella asiatica* (*USP35–NF30 S1*); *Centella asiatica* Triterpenes (*USP35–NF30 S1*); Powdered *Centella asiatica* (*USP35–NF30 S1*); Powdered *Centella asiatica* Extract (*USP35–NF30 S1*).

Constituents

Gotu kola contains a wide range of triterpene saponin glycosides such as **asiaticoside** (to which it may be standardised), centelloside, madecassoside, brahmoside, brahminoside, and others. Free asiatic, centellic, centoic betulinic and **madecassic acids** are also present and these are considered to be the main active constituents. **Flavonoids** based on quercetin and kaempferol, and a small amount of volatile oil containing farnesene, germacrene-D, elemene and other terpenes are also present.

Use and indications

Gotu kola is widely used, mainly for inflammatory dermatological disorders and to aid the healing of ulcers and wounds. It is applied externally and taken internally for venous insufficiency and as an immunomodulator and antioxidant, and for many other conditions including memory enhancement, circulatory disorders and anxiety. A number of pharmacological and clinical studies support some of these activities.

Pharmacokinetics

No relevant pharmacokinetic data found. For information on the pharmacokinetics of the individual flavonoids present in gotu kola, see under flavonoids, page 213.

Interactions overview

No interactions with gotu kola found. For information on the interactions of the individual flavonoids present in gotu kola, see under flavonoids, page 213.

G

Grapefruit

Citrus × paradisi Macfad. (Rutaceae)

Synonym(s) and related species

Citrus paradisi Macfad.

Grapefruit is a hybrid of the Pummelo or Pomelo (*Citrus maxima* (Burm.) Merr) with the sweet orange (*Citrus sinensis* (L.) Osbeck).

Constituents

Grapefruit contains **furanocoumarins** including bergamottin, 6',7'-dihydroxybergamottin, bergapten, bergaptol, geranylcoumarin and paradisin A; **flavonoid glycosides** such as naringin and **flavonoid** aglycones galangin, kaempferol, morin, naringenin, quercetin and others.

The peel contains a volatile oil, mostly composed of limonene.

Note that some **grapefruit seed extracts** have been found to contain preservatives such as benzethonium chloride, triclosan and methyl-p-hydroxybenzoate, which might be present because of the methods of production.

Use and indications

Grapefruit is used as a source of flavonoids (citrus bioflavonoids), which are widely used for their supposed antioxidant effects, and are covered under flavonoids, page 213.

Grapefruit seed extracts are used for their antimicrobial properties, but there is some controversy that this might be due to preservative content rather than natural constituents. Grapefruit and grapefruit juice are commonly ingested as part of the diet, and the oil is used as a fragrance.

Pharmacokinetics

Most of the data on the pharmacokinetics of grapefruit relate to the juice, which are summarised below. Note that it should not be directly extrapolated to herbal medicines containing grapefruit, because some differences in interaction potential have been seen. For information on the pharmacokinetics of the flavonoid constituents of grapefruit, see under flavonoids, page 213, and for information on the furanocoumarin constituents of grapefruit, see under natural coumarins, page 356.

(a) Cytochrome P450 isoenzymes

Grapefruit juice has been found to irreversibly inhibit the cytochrome P450 isoenzyme CYP3A4, and to cause drug interactions in quantities as low as 200 mL.[1] Several compounds present are known to have inhibitory effects on CYP3A4, CYP2D6, and CYP2C9 *in vitro,* with the most potent thought to be the furanocoumarins, particularly dihydroxybergamottin, and the flavonoids naringenin and quercetin.[2] However, the exact constituents that are responsible for the well-established clinical interactions of grapefruit juice are still uncertain. Naringin is present in grapefruit, but absent from other citrus fruits which led to the suggestion that naringin is the active principle, but this was later refuted.[3] Quercetin has been reported to inhibit CYP3A4 *in vitro*; however, a clinical study found that, unlike grapefruit juice, quercetin alone, given at a concentration 40 times that found in the grapefruit juice, had no significant effect on the metabolism of nifedipine by CYP3A4.[4] Furanocoumarins may also contribute to the interactions of grapefruit juice, because furanocoumarin-free grapefruit juice did not interact with felodipine, page 272, in one study.[5] Nevertheless, none of the furanocoumarins individually appear to have much effect, and it appears that the net effect of all the furanocoumarins present determines the clinical effect.[3,6] The effect of grapefruit juice on CYP3A is thought to be mainly exerted on intestinal CYP3A rather than hepatic CYP3A, because drugs given intravenously tend to be affected only to a small extent.

(b) P-glycoprotein

Based on the results of *in vitro* and interaction studies, it is thought that some component of grapefruit juice inhibits the activity of P-glycoprotein. However, note that there is no significant interaction with digoxin, a substrate of P-glycoprotein.

(c) Organic anion-transporting polypeptide (OATP)

In vitro, grapefruit juice has been shown to inhibit the organic anion-transporting protein (OATP), as have the individual ingredients bergamottin, 6',7'-dihydroxybergamottin, quercetin, naringin, naringenin and tangeretin. The inhibitory effect of naringin on OATP1A2, has also been confirmed in another *in vitro* study.[7] Inhibition of this transporter protein results in a modest reduction in the bioavailability of drugs that are substrates for this transporter, such as fexofenadine, page 272.

Interactions overview

The vast majority of known drug interactions of grapefruit have been reported with grapefruit *juice,* which is not used as a medicine or dietary supplement. For this reason, these interactions are not included here in detail, but they are summarised in the table Summary of established drug interactions of grapefruit juice, page 271. While most clinically important interactions of grapefruit juice result in an increase in drug exposure, note that modest *decreased* exposure occurs with the beta blockers celiprolol and talinolol, and with the antihistamine, fexofenadine.

The interactions of grapefruit juice are probably also applicable to the consumption of the fresh fruit, as reported with carbamazepine and some calcium-channel blockers, such as felodipine. An interaction has also been reported with grapefruit marmalade and tacrolimus. However, grapefruit juice interactions cannot be directly extrapolated

Summary of established drug interactions of grapefruit juice[1]

Drug	Effect on AUC	Recommendation
Avoid grapefruit juice with these drugs		
Ciclosporin	Increase of 15 to 85% (trough level)	Because of the likely adverse consequences of these
Dronedarone[†]	Threefold increase	interactions, it is probably best to avoid concurrent grapefruit
Felodipine*	Increase of two to threefold	juice altogether.
Halofantrine	2.8-fold increase	
Lovastatin	Up to 15-fold increase	
Nisoldipine*	Two- to fourfold increase	
Primaquine	Up to twofold increase	
Simvastatin	Up to 16-fold increase	
Tacrolimus**	Increase of 300% (trough level)	
Drugs requiring caution with grapefruit juice intake		
Amiodarone	Increase of 50%	Monitor the effects of concurrent use. Consider advising
Atorvastatin	2.5-fold increase	limiting the intake of grapefruit juice and/or reducing the dose
Budesonide[†]	Twofold increase in bioavailability	of the drug. Bear in mind that variability in the constituents of
Buspirone	9-fold increase	grapefruit juice and variability in timing and amount of the juice
Carbamazepine*	Increase of 40%	consumed complicate management of these interactions.
Celiprolol	Decrease of 87%	
Ivabradine	Twofold increase	
Nicardipine, nifedipine,* nimodipine	Up to twofold increase	
Tolvaptan[†]	Increase of 80%	
Verapamil[†]	Increase of 30 to 50%	
Drugs for which the interaction with grapefruit juice is usually of little practical importance		
Dextromethorphan	Fivefold increase	These interactions are generally unlikely to be clinically
Diazepam	3.2-fold increase	relevant. Bear them in mind in the event of an unexpected
Digoxin	Increase of 10%	response to treatment.
Erythromycin	Increase of 49%	
Fexofenadine	Decrease of up to 67%	
Fluvoxamine	Increase of 60%	
Methylprednisolone	Increase of 75%	
Oral Midazolam	Increase of 52 to 65%	
Praziquantel	Increase of 90%	
Saquinavir	Increase of 50%	
Sertraline	Increase of 50% (trough level)	
Sildenafil[†]	Increase of 23%	
Talinolol	Decrease of 44%	
Triazolam	Increase of 50 to 150%	

1. Compiled from Baxter K (ed), Stockley's Drug Interactions. [online] London: Pharmaceutical Press <http://www.medicinescomplete.com> (accessed on 14/09/2010). This table does not include drugs that are predicted to interact, and for which there is no evidence, or drugs for which no interaction occurs.

* Effect also seen with the fruit (grapefruit segments or grapefruit pulp).

** Effect also seen with excessive consumption of grapefruit marmalade.

[†] Manufacturers generally advise avoidance of grapefruit juice with these drugs.

G

to other grapefruit products such as the citrus bioflavonoids. In general, bioflavonoids are unlikely to interact to the same extent as grapefruit juice, because usually the furanocoumarins are required for a significant interaction to occur. However, there is evidence that citrus bioflavonoids alone might have an important interaction with lovastatin and simvastatin. For interactions of individual bioflavonoids present in grapefruit supplements, see under flavonoids, page 213, and for the interaction of individual furanocoumarins, see under natural coumarins, page 356.

There is one report of grapefruit seed extract interacting with warfarin; however, this was shown be due to the preservative content rather than the grapefruit extract.

Interactions monographs

1. Bailey DG, Dresser GK. Interactions between grapefruit juice and cardiovascular drugs. *Am J Cardiovasc Drugs* (2004) 4, 281–97.
2. Girennavar B, Jayaprakasha GK, Patil BS. Potent inhibition of human cytochrome P450 3A4, 2D6, and 2C9 isoenzymes by grapefruit juice and its furocoumarins. *J Food Sci* (2007) 72, C417–C421.
3. Guo L-Q, Yamazoe Y. Inhibition of cytochrome P450 by furanocoumarins in grapefruit juice and herbal medicines. *Acta Pharmacol Sin* (2004) 25, 129–36.
4. Rashid J, McKinstry C, Renwick AG, Dirnhuber M, Waller DG, George CF. Quercetin, an *in vitro* inhibitor of CYP3A, does not contribute to the interaction between nifedipine and grapefruit juice. *Br J Clin Pharmacol* (1993) 36, 460–463.
5. Paine MF, Widmer WW, Hart HL, Pusek SN, Beavers KL, Criss AB, Brown SS, Thomas BF, Watkins PB. A furanocoumarin-free grapefruit establishes furanocoumarins as the mediators of the grapefruit juice-felodipine interaction. *Am J Clin Nutr* (2006) 83, 1097–2105.
6. Bailey DG, Dresser GK, Bend JR. Bergamottin, lime juice, and red wine as inhibitors of cytochrome P450 3A4 activity: comparison with grapefruit juice. *Clin Pharmacol Ther* (2003) 73, 529–37.
7. Bailey DG, Dresser GK, Leake BF, Kim RB. Naringin is a major and selective clinical inhibitor of organic anion-transporting polypeptide 1A2 (OATP1A2) in grapefruit juice. *Clin Pharmacol Ther* (2007) 81, 495–502.

Grapefruit + Caffeine

For mention that grapefruit *juice* and one of its constituents naringin, a grapefruit flavonoid, had no effect on the metabolism of caffeine, see Flavonoids + Caffeine, page 216.

Grapefruit + Calcium-channel blockers

Grapefruit segments increase the exposure to nifedipine, nisoldipine and felodipine.

Clinical evidence

In a single-dose pharmacokinetic study in 12 healthy subjects, homogenised grapefruit segments or an extract from the segment-free parts increased the AUC of **felodipine** by 3.2-fold and 3.6-fold, respectively.[1] This increase was the same or slightly greater than the increase seen with 250 mL of grapefruit juice.[1] In another single-dose study in 8 healthy subjects, grapefruit pulp from one grapefruit increased the AUC of both **nifedipine** and **nisoldipine** by about 30%, and increased the maximum concentration of **nifedipine** and **nisoldipine** by about 40% and 50%, respectively, when the grapefruit was eaten one hour before taking the calcium-channel blocker. The authors noted that these increases were smaller than those previously seen with grapefruit juice.[2]

Experimental evidence

Because these interactions are established, experimental data have not been sought.

Mechanism

Grapefruit appears to inhibit the activity of the cytochrome P450 isoenzymes CYP3A subfamily in the intestinal wall so that the first-pass metabolism of these calcium-channel blockers is reduced, thereby increasing their bioavailability and therefore their effects. Grapefruit juice is well-established to have this effect.

One small clinical study suggests that quercetin is not involved in the interaction between grapefruit juice and nifedipine.[3]

Importance and management

These interactions are established. It has been suggested that **whole grapefruit** should be avoided in patients taking felodipine.[1] Given the data here, this would appear to be prudent advice. It has also been suggested that other products made from whole grapefruit such as **marmalade** should be avoided,[1] although there is no published evidence that grapefruit marmalade may interact with calcium-channel blockers. However, an isolated case describes raised tacrolimus levels and toxicity associated with the excessive consumption of grapefruit marmalade. See Grapefruit + Tacrolimus, page 273.

For mention that furanocoumarin-free grapefruit juice had no consistent effect on felodipine pharmacokinetics, but also that no individual furanocoumarin tested had an effect as great as grapefruit juice, see Natural coumarins + Felodipine, page 359.

Some caution would also be appropriate with nifedipine and nisoldipine. There appears to be no specific information on a potential interaction between whole grapefruit and other calcium-channel blockers. However, it may be worth considering an interaction with grapefruit in any patient who complains of an otherwise unexplained increase in adverse effects with any of the calcium-channel blockers.

1. Bailey DG, Dresser GK, Kreeft JH, Munoz C, Freeman DJ, Bend JR. Grapefruit-felodipine interaction: effect of unprocessed fruit and probable active ingredients. *Clin Pharmacol Ther* (2000) 68, 468–77.

2. Ohtani M, Kawabata S, Kariya S, Uchino K, Itou K, Kotaki H, Kasuyama K, Morikawa A, Seo I, Nishida N. Effect of grapefruit pulp on the pharmacokinetics of the dihydropyridine calcium antagonists nifedipine and nisoldipine. *Yakugaku Zasshi* (2002) 122, 323–9.
3. Rashid J, McKinstry C, Renwick AG, Dirnhuber M, Waller DG, George CF. Quercetin, an *in vitro* inhibitor of CYP3A, does not contribute to the interaction between nifedipine and grapefruit juice. *Br J Clin Pharmacol* (1993) 36, 460–463.

Grapefruit + Carbamazepine

A case of possible carbamazepine toxicity has been seen when a man taking carbamazepine started to eat grapefruit.

Clinical evidence

A 58-year-old man, taking carbamazepine 1 g daily for epilepsy developed visual disturbances with diplopia, and was found to have a carbamazepine level of 11 micrograms/mL (therapeutic range 4 to 10 micrograms/mL). Previous levels had not exceeded 5.4 micrograms/mL. The patient said that one month previously he had started to eat one whole grapefruit each day. The levels restabilised at 5.1 micrograms/mL after the carbamazepine dose was reduced to 800 mg daily.[1]

Experimental evidence

No relevant data found.

Mechanism

The cytochrome P450 isoenzyme CYP3A4 is the main isoenzyme involved in the metabolism of carbamazepine. Components of grapefruit juice are known to inhibit CYP3A4, which in this case would lead to a reduction in the metabolism of carbamazepine, and therefore an increase in levels.[1,2]

Importance and management

Evidence for an interaction between grapefruit and carbamazepine appears to be limited to one isolated case. In this report, the patient continued to eat grapefruit, and this was successfully managed by a reduction in the carbamazepine dose. However, it should be noted that intake of a set amount of grapefruit would need to be maintained for this approach to work, and carbamazepine dosage adjustment and monitoring of levels should be undertaken as appropriate. If monitoring is not practical, or regular intake of grapefruit is not desired, it may be prudent to avoid grapefruit.

1. Bonin B, Vandel P, Vandel S, Kantelip JP. Effect of grapefruit intake on carbamazepine bioavailability: a case report. *Therapie* (2001) 56, 69–71.
2. Garg SK, Kumar N, Bhargava VK, Prabhakar SK. Effect of grapefruit juice on carbamazepine bioavailability in patients with epilepsy. *Clin Pharmacol Ther* (1998) 64, 286–8.

Grapefruit + Fexofenadine

For mention that grapefruit *juice* and, to a lesser extent, naringin, a grapefruit flavonoid, modestly decrease the AUC of fexofenadine, see Flavonoids + Fexofenadine, page 219.

Grapefruit + Food

No interactions found. For mention that grapefruit *juice* and one of its constituents naringin, a grapefruit flavonoid, had no effect on the metabolism of caffeine, see Flavonoids + Caffeine, page 216. Note that grapefruit is commonly consumed as part of the diet.

Grapefruit + Herbal medicines

No interactions found. Note that naringin, a grapefruit flavonoid, and grapefruit juice do not alter the metabolism of caffeine, see Flavonoids + Caffeine, page 216, and so would be unlikely to interact with caffeine in caffeine-containing herbs, page 106.

Grapefruit + Tacrolimus

A case of tacrolimus toxicity has been seen when a man ate more than 1.5 kg of grapefruit marmalade during one week.

Clinical evidence

A 52-year-old man with a liver transplant, stabilised on tacrolimus 3 mg twice daily, began to feel anxious and febrile with continued trembling and blurred vision. Within 5 days he deteriorated and developed severe left chest pain. His tacrolimus whole blood level was found to be markedly raised to 55.4 micrograms/L from a previous therapeutic level (between 8 and 13 micrograms/L), and he had renal impairment (serum creatinine of 174 micromols/L). It transpired that during the week preceding the onset of symptoms he had eaten more than 1.5 kg of a home-made marmalade, which was made with more than 50% grapefruit.[1]

Experimental evidence

No relevant data found.

Mechanism

It is well established that grapefruit *juice* increases levels of tacrolimus, and this case appears to show that this can occur with grapefruit marmalade. The process of making marmalade uses the whole fruit, and it appears that whatever the active interacting constituents are, these are not destroyed by the long boiling.[1]

Importance and management

This is the first case to show that a drug interaction can occur with grapefruit marmalade. As such, it requires confirmation by further study. Note that in this case, the patient consumed an unusually large amount of marmalade (estimated 14 dessert spoonfuls (15 g) daily). More modest consumption (a spoonful of about 15 g daily) would appear unlikely to interact. Note that grapefruit *juice* is well established to interact with tacrolimus and combined use should be avoided.

1. Peynaud D, Charpiat B, Vial T, Gallavardin M, Ducerf C. Tacrolimus severe overdosage after intake of masked grapefruit in orange marmalade. *Eur J Clin Pharmacol* (2007) 63, 721–2.

Grapefruit + Warfarin

A rise in INR occurred in a couple taking warfarin who took a grapefruit seed extract product containing considerable amounts of the preservative benzethonium chloride for three days. One of them developed a minor haematoma.

Clinical evidence

A couple, both well stabilised on warfarin, took some drops of a grapefruit seed extract product (*Estratto di Semillas di Pompelmo,* Lakshmi, Italy) for 3 days. No more was taken, but after a further 3 days the woman developed a minor subcutaneous haematoma, and her INR was found to be 7.9. The man was found to have an INR of 5.1, with no evidence of bleeding.[1]

Experimental evidence

See under *Mechanism,* below.

Mechanism

The product used was stated to contain grapefruit seed extract, glycerol and water. However, chemical analysis of this product revealed that it also contained considerable amounts (77 mg/mL) of the preservative, benzethonium chloride, and did not contain any significant amount of natural substances from grapefruit seeds. The constituents of two other commercial grapefruit seed products were similar on analysis (*Citroseed* and *Citricidal*).

Further, *in vitro* analysis showed that benzethonium chloride, and the three products, were potent inhibitors of the cytochrome P450 isoenzyme CYP2C9, suggesting that they could inhibit the metabolism of warfarin.

Importance and management

Data presented in this report, and other papers (one of which is cited as an example[2]), suggests that the primary constituent of many grapefruit seed extract products appears to be the preservative benzethonium chloride. The evidence from the two cases, backed by *in vitro* data, suggests that this has the potential to interact with warfarin. On this basis, it would probably be prudent for patients taking warfarin to avoid grapefruit seed extract products, or for concurrent use to be monitored closely. Some caution might also be appropriate with other pharmaceutical preparations containing benzethonium chloride.

1. Brandin H, Myrberg O, Rundlöf T, Arvidsson AK, Brenning G. Adverse effects by artificial grapefruit seed extract products in patients on warfarin therapy. *Eur J Clin Pharmacol* (2007) 63, 565–70.
2. Takeoka G, Dao L, Wong RY, Lundin R, Mahoney N. Identification of benzethonium chloride in commercial grapefruit seed extracts. *J Agric Food Chem* (2001) 49, 3316–20.

G

Grapeseed

Vitis vinifera L. (Vitaceae)

Synonym(s) and related species

Vitis vinifera is the Grape vine, of which there are many cultivars.

Constituents

Grapeseed extract contains **flavonoids**, which include gallic acid, catechin, (-)-epicatechin, and their galloylated derivatives, and proanthocyanidins. **Resveratrol**, a polyphenolic stilbene derivative, and tocopherols and tocotrienols are also present.

Use and indications

Grapeseed extract is promoted as an antioxidant supplement for preventing degenerative disorders in particular, in the same way as other flavonoid-containing products. The *in vitro* antioxidant properties are well-documented and there is some clinical evidence to suggest it can promote general cardiovascular health.

Pharmacokinetics

An *in vitro* study found that grapeseed extract potently *inhibits* CYP3A4, but only when the catechin content is high.[1] In contrast, another *in vitro* study found that grapeseed extract is a weak *inducer* of the cytochrome P450 isoenzyme CYP3A4. The author suggests that grapeseed therefore has the potential to cause interactions.[2] However, the effect of grapeseed extract was less than that of omeprazole, which does not commonly interact by this mechanism, suggesting that any effect is unlikely to be clinically relevant. Furthermore, a study in *rats* suggests that grapeseed extract does not significantly alter the pharmacokinetics of midazolam, page 275, a probe substrate for CYP3A4.

Another *in vitro* study found that grapeseed extract does not affect the activity of CYP1A2, CYP2C8, CYP2C19, and CYP2E1, and only moderately inhibits CYP2C9 and CYP2D6 at high concentrations of catechins.[1] In addition, it has no significant effect on P-glycoprotein.[1]

Grapeseed extracts appear to moderately inhibit the transporter protein OATP-B, but the clinical implications of this have not been established.[3]

See under flavonoids, page 213, for information on the individual flavonoids present in grapeseed, and see under resveratrol, page 401, for the pharmacokinetics of resveratrol.

Interactions overview

Contrary to expectation, the concurrent use of grapeseed extracts and ascorbic acid may have detrimental cardiovascular effects. Evidence for other clinically relevant interactions appears to be generally lacking. For information on the interactions of flavonoids, see under flavonoids, page 213, and for the interactions of resveratrol, see under resveratrol, page 401.

Interactions monographs

- Ascorbic acid (Vitamin C), page 275
- Food, page 275
- Herbal medicines, page 275
- Midazolam, page 275

1. Etheridge AS, Black SR, Patel PR, So J, Mathews JM. An in vitro evaluation of cytochrome P450 inhibition and P-glycoprotein interaction with goldenseal, Ginkgo biloba, grape seed, milk thistle, and ginseng extracts and their constituents. *Planta Med* (2007) 73, 731–41.
2. Raucy JL. Regulation of CYP3A4 expression in human hepatocytes by pharmaceuticals and natural products. *Drug Metab Dispos* (2003) 31, 533–9.
3. Fuchikami H, Satoh H, Tsujimoto M, Ohdo S, Ohtani H, Sawada Y. Effects of herbal extracts on the function of human organic anion-transporting polypeptide OATP-B. *Drug Metab Dispos* (2006) 34, 577–82.

G

Grapeseed + Ascorbic acid (Vitamin C)

The concurrent use of grapeseed and ascorbic acid (vitamin C) appears to increase systolic and diastolic blood pressure.

Clinical evidence

A placebo-controlled study in 69 hypertensive patients taking one or more antihypertensive medications, investigated the effects on cardiovascular parameters of vitamin C 250 mg twice daily, grapeseed polyphenols 500 mg twice daily, or a combination of the two, for 6 weeks. There was a 3-week washout period between treatments. Vitamin C alone *reduced* systolic blood pressure by about 1.8 mmHg, but the grapeseed polyphenols had no effect on blood pressure. However, treatment with the combination of vitamin C and polyphenols *increased* systolic blood pressure by 4.8 and 6.6 mmHg and diastolic blood pressure by between 1.5 and 3.2 mmHg. Endothelium-dependent and -independent vasodilation, and markers of oxidative damage were not significantly altered.[1]

Experimental evidence

No relevant data found.

Mechanism

Unknown.

Importance and management

Evidence is limited to one study, with no supporting mechanism to explain the effects seen, and so an interaction between vitamin C and grapeseed extract is not established. The authors of this study suggest that caution should be used when advising patients with hypertension on taking a combination of vitamin C and grapeseed. However, the general importance of any interaction is difficult to assess as the effect of taking these two supplements together is likely to vary depending on the patient and the degree to which their hypertension is controlled. It may be prudent to question a patient with poorly controlled blood pressure to establish if they are taking supplements containing both vitamin C and grapeseed, and discuss the option of stopping them to see if this improves their blood pressure control.

1. Ward NC, Hodgson JM, Croft KD, Burke V, Beilin LJ, Puddey IB. The combination of vitamin C and grape-seed polyphenols increases blood pressure: a randomized, double-blind, placebo-controlled trial. *J Hypertens* (2005) 23, 427–34.

Grapeseed + Food

No interactions found.

Grapeseed + Herbal medicines

No interactions found.

Grapeseed + Midazolam

The interaction between grapeseed and midazolam is based on experimental evidence only.

Clinical evidence

No interactions found.

Experimental evidence

In a study in *rats*, a single dose of an aqueous grapeseed extract had no significant effects on the pharmacokinetics of midazolam. However, after one week of treatment, grapeseed extract increased the elimination rate of midazolam by about 30%, and reduced its half-life by 28%. However, these effects were modest, and the AUC of midazolam was not significantly altered.[1]

Mechanism

The study in *rats* suggests that grapeseed weakly induces the cytochrome P450 isoenzyme CYP3A4, the main route of midazolam metabolism. Some *in vitro* studies support this suggestion, although stronger effects may occur if the catechin content is high, see pharmacokinetics, page 274.

Importance and management

Clinical evidence regarding an interaction between grapeseed and midazolam appears to be lacking. However, evidence from *rat* studies suggests that a clinically relevant interaction is unlikely and therefore no dose adjustments of midazolam are likely to be needed if grapeseed extract is also taken.

1. Nishikawa M, Ariyoshi N, Kotani A, Ishii I, Nakamura H, Nakasa H, Ida M, Nakamura H, Kimura N, Kimura M, Hasegawa A, Kusu F, Ohmori S, Nakazawa K, Kitada M. Effects of continuous ingestion of green tea or grape seed extracts on the pharmacokinetics of midazolam. *Drug Metab Pharmacokinet* (2004) 19, 280–289.

G

Gravel root

Eupatorium purpureum L. (Asteraceae)

Synonym(s) and related species

Gravelweed, Joe-Pye weed, Kidney root, Purple boneset, Queen of the meadow.

Eupatorium trifoliatum L.

Constituents

Gravel root is the root and rhizome of *Eupatorium purpureum* and contains the **benzofurans** euparin, euparone, cistifolin and others. A **flavonoid**, eupatorin, and a volatile oil are also present. Unsaturated pyrrolizidine alkaloids are found in other species of Eupatorium, for example in the aerial parts of E. cannabinum L. but have not been found in gravel root.

Use and indications

Gravel root is used for the treatment of renal and urinary stones, urinary-tract infections, urethritis and prostatitis. It is also used as a diuretic and for rheumatism and gout.

Pharmacokinetics

No relevant pharmacokinetic data found.

Interactions overview

No interactions with gravel root found.

G

Greater celandine

Chelidonium majus L. (Papaveraceae)

Synonym(s) and related species

Celandine, Common celandine, Garden celandine, Swallow wort.

Not to be confused with Lesser celandine, which is *Ranunculus ficaria* L.

Note that the synonym Tetterwort has been used for both Greater celandine and the unrelated Bloodroot, page 84 (*Sanguinaria canadensis*), and care should be taken to avoid any confusion between the two.

Pharmacopoeias

Greater Celandine (*BP 2012, PhEur 7.5*).

Constituents

All parts of the plant contain benzylisoquinoline alkaloids, including **berberine**, chelerythrine, chelidonine, coptisine, cryptopine, protopine, and sanguinarine.

Use and indications

Greater celandine has been traditionally used in the treatment of jaundice, gall bladder and biliary diseases; and eczema and other skin disorders. In Chinese medicine it has been used as an antitussive, anti-inflammatory and detoxicant. However, information on the safety and toxicity of greater celandine is limited: hepatotoxic effects, including severe hepatitis, severe cholestasis and fibrosis, have been reported with long-term use (one month or more).

Pharmacokinetics

No relevant pharmacokinetic data for greater celandine found, but see berberine, page 63, for details on this constituent of greater celandine.

Interactions overview

No interactions with greater celandine found. However, for the interactions of one of its constituents, berberine, see under berberine, page 63.

G

Ground ivy

Glechoma hederacea L. (Lamiaceae)

Synonym(s) and related species

Ale-hoof, Gundelrebe, Gundermann.

Nepeta glechoma Benth., *Nepeta hederacea* (L.) Trevis.

Constituents

Ground ivy contains **flavonoids** including isoquercitrin, luteolin diglucoside, and rutin, and other polyphenolic compounds such as glycosides of icariol, cistanoside E and rosmarinic acid. Other compounds present include β-sitosterol, the triterpenes oleanolic acid and α- and β-ursolic acids, and a volatile oil containing the monoterpenes *p*-cymene, linalool, limonene, and terpineol, among others. The sesquiterpene glechomafuran, and the diterpene marrubiin are also present. Two alkaloids, hederacine A and B, which may have cytotoxic activity, have been found in very small amounts in the plant.

Use and indications

Ground ivy is used as a mild expectorant for chronic bronchial catarrh. It is also said to be astringent, and therefore used for wound healing, haemorrhoids, gastritis and diarrhoea.

Pharmacokinetics

No relevant pharmacokinetic data found. For information on the pharmacokinetics of individual flavonoids present in ground ivy, see under flavonoids, page 213.

Interactions overview

No interactions with ground ivy found. For information on the interactions of individual flavonoids present in ground ivy, see under flavonoids, page 213.

G

Guarana

Paullinia cupana Kunth (Sapindaceae)

Synonym(s) and related species

Brazilian cocoa.
   Paullinia sorbilis.

Constituents

Guarana seeds contain xanthine derivatives; principally
caffeine (also known as guaranine, up to 7%), with
theobromine, theophylline and others and small amounts
of flavonoids, from the flavanol group, such as catechin.
Other constituents include saponins and an essential oil
containing estragole and anethole.

Use and indications

The main use is as a tonic or stimulant for tiredness and to
promote alertness, which can be attributed to the caffeine
content.

Pharmacokinetics

The pharmacokinetics of caffeine are discussed under caffeine, page 106.

Interactions overview

Guarana contains significant amounts of caffeine, therefore
the interactions of caffeine, page 106 are relevant to
guarana. Two case reports describe muscular disorders,
which were related to the use of guarana-containing herbal
supplements. For mention of a study in which a herbal
supplement containing guarana and black tea, among other
ingredients, slightly increased blood pressure, see Tea +
Antihypertensives, page 464.

Interactions monographs

- Food, page 280
- Herbal medicines, page 280

G

Guarana + Antihypertensives

For mention of a study in which a herbal supplement containing guarana and black tea, among other ingredients, slightly increased blood pressure, see Tea + Antihypertensives, page 464.

Guarana + Food

No interactions found; however, the effects of caffeine from herbal medicines or supplements containing guarana and caffeine-containing foods or beverages, will be additive.

Guarana + Herbal medicines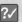

Two case reports describe muscular disorders in patients who took supplements containing guarana and ephedra, and guarana and kava.

Evidence, mechanism, importance and management

A case report describes a 54-year-old woman, with no signif-icant medical history, who developed rhabdomyolysis after she started to take guarana 190 mg and **ephedra** 150 mg (containing ephedrine 12 mg), with other dietary supplements. The creatine kinase elevations resolved within 3 weeks of stopping the herbal weight-loss supplement. The authors of this report suggest that as guarana contains caffeine alkaloids, this and the combination of ephedrine effects may have contributed to the myopathy.[1] Another case describes myoglobinuria in a patient taking a supplement containing guarana, **ginkgo** and **kava**.[2] Again, this was thought to be related to the combined effects of guarana and other herbal medicines, in this case, **kava**.

The general importance of these cases is unclear, and many patients taking drugs that are known to cause muscle damage such as the statins, frequently take caffeine, which is found in guarana, food or beverages.

The caffeine content of guarana suggests that it may interact with other herbal medicines in the same way as caffeine, see Caffeine + Herbal medicines; Bitter orange, page 111, and Ephedra + Caffeine, page 202.

The stimulant effects of guarana and **ginseng** appear to be additive, see Ginseng + Herbal medicines; Guarana, page 255.

1. Mansi IA, Huang J. Rhabdomyolysis in response to weight-loss herbal medicine. *Am J Med Sci* (2004) 327, 356–7.
2. Donadio V, Bonsi P, Zele I, Monari L, Liguori R, Vetrugno R, Albani F, Montagna P. Myoglobinuria after ingestion of extracts of guarana, *Ginkgo biloba* and kava. *Neurol Sci* (2000) 21, 124.

G

Guggul

Commiphora wightii (Arn.) Bhandari (Burseraceae)

Synonym(s) and related species

Mukul myrrh.

Commiphora mukul Engl., *Balsamodendrum mukul* , *Balsamodendrum wightii* .

Pharmacopoeias

Guggul (*USP35–NF30 S1*); Guggul Tablets (*USP35–NF30 S1*); Purified Guggul Extract (*USP35–NF30 S1*); Native Guggul Extract (*USP35–NF30 S1*).

Constituents

The resinous sap, harvested from the tree bark by tapping, is extracted to produce guggul. **Gugulipid** is the purified standardised extract of crude gum guggul, and contains the active **guggulsterone** components Z-guggulsterone and E-guggulsterone, with cembrenoids, myrrhanone and myrrhanol derivatives.

Use and indications

Guggul is used mainly in Ayurvedic medicine and has been traditionally used to treat hypertension, osteoporosis, epilepsy, ulcers, cancer, obesity, and rheumatoid arthritis. It is now often used for hyperlipidaemia, but clinical studies have found conflicting results for its lipid-lowering effects.

Pharmacokinetics

An *in vitro* study reported that gugulipid extract and purified guggulsterones may induce the expression of the cytochrome P450 isoenzyme CYP3A4. However, the clinical significance of this is unclear and further study is needed.[1]

Interactions overview

In healthy subjects, the absorption of diltiazem and propranolol was modestly reduced by gugulipid. If the mechanism is confirmed, guggul might interact with a wide range of other drugs. A case of rhabdomyolysis has been attributed to the use of guggul alone, which should be borne in mind if it is combined with the statins, which also, rarely, cause this adverse effect.

Interactions monographs

- Diltiazem, page 282
- Food, page 282
- Herbal medicines, page 282
- Propranolol, page 282
- Statins, page 282

G

1. Brobst DE, Ding X, Creech KL, Goodwin B, Kelley B, Staudinger JL. Guggulsterone activates multiple nuclear receptors and induces CYP3A gene expression through the pregnane X receptor. *J Pharmacol Exp Ther* (2004) 310, 528–35.

Guggul + Diltiazem

Limited evidence suggests that guggul modestly reduces the absorption of single-dose diltiazem.

Clinical evidence

A crossover study in 7 fasting healthy subjects found that a single 1-g dose of **gugulipid** reduced the AUC and maximum concentration of a single 60-mg dose of diltiazem by 35% and 41%, respectively. This single dose of diltiazem did not have any effect on blood pressure or heart rate in these particular subjects,[1] so it was not possible to assess the effect of the reduction in levels of diltiazem on its pharmacological effects. No details were given of the **gugulipid** or diltiazem preparations used.

Experimental evidence

No relevant data found.

Mechanism

Gugulipid is an oleoresin extracted from guggul. The authors of this study suggest that it might bind with drugs in the gut and reduce their absorption in a similar way to colestyramine and colestipol.[1]

Importance and management

Gugulipid modestly reduced the absorption of diltiazem in this study, and this degree of reduction is probably unlikely to be clinically relevant. However, the formulation of diltiazem given was not stated and the effects of multiple dosing, or of larger doses of diltiazem, is unknown. Further study is needed. Bear in mind the potential for an interaction should a patient taking guggul have a reduced response to diltiazem.

1. Dalvi SS, Nayak VK, Pohujani SM, Desai NK, Kshirsagar NA, Gupta KC. Effect of gugulipid on bioavailability of diltiazem and propranolol. *J Assoc Physicians India* (1994) 42, 454–5.

Guggul + Food

No interactions found.

Guggul + Herbal medicines

No interactions found.

Guggul + Propranolol

Limited evidence suggests that guggul modestly reduces the absorption of single-dose propranolol.

Clinical evidence

A crossover study in 10 fasting healthy subjects found that a single 1-g dose of **gugulipid** reduced the AUC and maximum concentration of a single 40-mg dose of propranolol by 34% and 43%, respectively. This single dose of propranolol did not have any effect on blood pressure or heart rate in these particular subjects,[1] so it was not possible to assess the effect of the reduction in levels of

propranolol on its pharmacological effects. No details were given of the **gugulipid** or propranolol preparations used.

Experimental evidence

No relevant data found.

Mechanism

Gugulipid is an oleoresin extracted from guggul. The authors of this study suggest that it might bind with drugs in the gut and reduce their absorption in a similar way to colestyramine and colestipol.[1]

Importance and management

Gugulipid modestly reduced the absorption of propranolol in this study. The clinical relevance of this reduction is not certain, but it is likely to be minor. Bear in mind the potential for an interaction should a patient taking guggul have a reduced response to propranolol.

1. Dalvi SS, Nayak VK, Pohujani SM, Desai NK, Kshirsagar NA, Gupta KC. Effect of gugulipid on bioavailability of diltiazem and propranolol. *J Assoc Physicians India* (1994) 42, 454–5.

Guggul + Statins

An isolated case suggests that guggul alone can cause rhabdomyolysis. If statins are also taken, the risk could be additive.

Clinical evidence

A case of rhabdomyolysis has been reported in a patient, 2 weeks after an extract of guggul 300 mg three times daily was started. The rhabdomyolysis resolved when the guggul preparation was stopped. The patient was not reported to be taking any other medication known to cause rhabdomyolysis and simvastatin had been stopped one year previously because of an increase in creatine kinase. The herbal product used was prepared by a local chemist using a standardised drug extract of the oleo gum resin without excipients.[1]

Experimental evidence

No relevant data found.

Mechanism

Not known. The possibility that the resin used was adulterated was not investigated.

Importance and management

This appears to be the only case report of rhabdomyolysis occurring with a guggul-containing preparation. Guggul is widely used for cholesterol-lowering, and the most commonly used conventional drugs for this condition are the statins, which are well recognised, rarely, to cause rhabdomyolysis. It is quite likely that guggul and statins are being used together, and the concern generated by this case report is that, if guggul alone can cause rhabdomyolysis, then combined use might increase the risk of rhabdomyolysis. However, this is only one case, and the mechanism (which could include adulteration) is uncertain. Bear the possibility of an additive effect in mind if myositis occurs with concurrent use. All patients taking statins should be warned about the symptoms of myopathy and told to report muscle pain or weakness. It would be prudent to reinforce this advice if they are known to be taking guggul.

1. Bianchi A, Cantù P, Firenzuoli F, Mazzanti G, Menniti-Ippolito F, Raschetti R. Rhabdomyolysis caused by *Commiphora mukul*, a natural lipid-lowering agent. *Ann Pharmacother* (2004) 38, 1222–5.

G

Hawthorn

Crataegus laevigata DC., *Crataegus monogyna* Jacq. (Rosaceae)

Synonym(s) and related species

Crataegus, Haw, May, Weissdorn, Whitethorn.

Crataegus oxyacantha auct., *Crataegus oxyacanthoides* Thuill.

Pharmacopoeias

Hawthorn Berries (*BP 2012, PhEur 7.5*); Hawthorn Leaf and Flower (*BP 2012, PhEur 7.5*); Hawthorn Leaf and Flower Dry Extract (*BP 2012, PhEur 7.5*); Hawthorn Leaf with Flower (*USP35–NF30 S1*); Powdered Hawthorn Leaf with Flower (*USP35–NF30 S1*); Quantified Hawthorn Leaf and Flower Liquid Extract (*BP 2012, PhEur 7.5*).

Constituents

The leaves and flowers of hawthorn are usually standardised to their **flavonoid** content, and the berries may be standardised to their **procyanidin** content. Other **flavonoids** present include quercetin, isoquercetin and their glycosides, and rutin. Other constituents include catechins and epicatechin dimers, polyphenolic acid derivatives including chlorogenic and caffeic acids, phenethylamine, dopamine, and ursolic and oleanolic acid triterpenenoid derivatives.

Use and indications

Hawthorn extracts are used as a cardiotonic, mild antihypertensive and antisclerotic.

Pharmacokinetics

No relevant pharmacokinetic data found. For information on the pharmacokinetics of individual flavonoids present in hawthorn, see under flavonoids, page 213.

Interactions overview

The safety of hawthorn extracts was investigated in a comprehensive systematic review,[1] which included data up to January 2005 from the WHO, relevant medical journals and conference proceedings. The investigators found that 166 adverse events were reported in 5577 patients from 24 clinical studies, and 18 cases of adverse events were reported via the WHO spontaneous reporting scheme. None of these involved drug interactions. In the clinical studies assessed, the daily dose and duration of treatment with hawthorn preparations ranged from 160 to 1800 mg and from 3 to 24 weeks, and the extracts most used contained leaves and flowers and were WS 1442 (standardised to 18.75% oligomeric procyanidins) and LI 132 (standardised to 2.25% flavonoids). Other studies do not appear to have identified any clinically significant drug interactions.

For information on the interactions of individual flavonoids present in hawthorn, see under flavonoids, page 213.

Interactions monographs

- Antidiabetics, page 284
- Antihypertensives, page 284
- Digoxin, page 284
- Food, page 284
- Herbal medicines, page 284

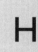

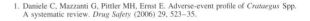

1. Daniele C, Mazzanti G, Pittler MH, Ernst E. Adverse-event profile of *Crataegus* Spp. A systematic review. *Drug Safety* (2006) 29, 523–35.

Hawthorn + Antidiabetics

Hawthorn does not appear to affect the glycaemic control in patients taking conventional antidiabetic drugs.

Clinical evidence

In a randomised study, 80 patients with type 2 diabetes taking antidiabetics (including **metformin, gliclazide** and/or low-dose **insulin**) with or without antihypertensives were given hawthorn extract 600 mg twice daily, or placebo, for 16 weeks. There was no difference between the two groups in measures of glycaemic control (fasting glucose, glycosylated haemoglobin and fructosamine) at 16 weeks. The hawthorn extract used in this study, LI 132, contained dried flowering tops and was standardised to 2.2% flavonoids.[1]

Experimental evidence

No relevant data found.

Mechanism

No mechanism expected.

Importance and management

Evidence is limited to this one study. However, as no alteration in glycaemic control was reported, no interventions are deemed necessary in patients taking antidiabetics and hawthorn extract.

1. Walker AF, Marakis G, Simpson E, Hope JL, Robinson PA, Hassanein M, Simpson HCR. Hypotensive effects of hawthorn for patients with diabetes taking prescription drugs: a randomised controlled trial. *Br J Gen Pract* (2006) 56, 437–43.

Hawthorn + Antihypertensives

Limited evidence suggests that there may be additive blood pressure-lowering effects if hawthorn is taken with conventional antihypertensives, but the effects are small.

Clinical evidence

In a randomised study, 80 patients with type 2 diabetes, of whom 71% were taking antihypertensives (including **ACE inhibitors, calcium-channel blockers, beta blockers** and/or **diuretics**), were given hawthorn extract 600 mg twice daily or placebo for 16 weeks. The group given hawthorn extract (39 of 40 patients assessed) had a small additional 2.6 mmHg reduction in diastolic blood pressure compared with no change in the placebo group. The 3.6 mmHg decline in systolic blood pressure in the hawthorn group was not statistically significant. The hawthorn extract used in this study, LI 132, contained dried flowering tops and was standardised to 2.2% flavonoids.[1]

Experimental evidence

No relevant data found.

Mechanism

Little known. Additive blood pressure-lowering effects might occur.

Importance and management

Evidence appears to be limited to this one clinical study. Although hawthorn extract caused a reduction in diastolic blood pressure in patients, many of whom were taking antihypertensives, the effect was small. As such, it is unlikely that clinically important hypotension would occur if hawthorn is added to existing antihypertensive treatment.

1. Walker AF, Marakis G, Simpson E, Hope JL, Robinson PA, Hassanein M, Simpson HCR. Hypotensive effects of hawthorn for patients with diabetes taking prescription drugs: a randomised controlled trial. *Br J Gen Pract* (2006) 56, 437–43.

Hawthorn + Digoxin

Hawthorn does not appear to affect digoxin levels.

Clinical evidence

In a randomised, crossover study, 8 healthy subjects were given hawthorn extract 450 mg twice daily with digoxin 250 micrograms daily for 21 days, or digoxin 250 micrograms alone daily for 10 days. While digoxin levels tended to be lower when hawthorn was given (the biggest difference being a 23% reduction in the trough level), these reductions were not statistically significant. There was no change in ECG effects or heart rate, and the combination was well tolerated. The hawthorn extract used in this study, WS 1442, contained an extract of leaves with flowers standardised to 84.3 mg of oligomeric procyanidins.[1]

Experimental evidence

No relevant data found.

Mechanism

Little known. It was thought that flavonoids in hawthorn might have an effect on P-glycoprotein, of which digoxin is a substrate. In addition, it is possible that the cardioactive constituents of hawthorn might increase the effect of digoxin on cardiac contractility.[1]

Importance and management

This study appears to be the only evidence reported. It suggests that, despite theoretical concerns that hawthorn may affect treatment with digoxin, in practice there appears to be no clinically relevant alteration in digoxin levels or effects. It therefore appears that hawthorn can be given to patients taking digoxin without the need for further monitoring.

1. Tankanow R, Tamer HR, Streetman DS, Smith SG, Welton JL, Annesley T, Aaronson KD, Bleske BE. Interaction study between digoxin and a preparation of hawthorn (*Crataegus oxyacantha*). *J Clin Pharmacol* (2003) 43, 637–42.

Hawthorn + Food

No interactions found.

Hawthorn + Herbal medicines

No interactions found.

H

Henbane

Hyoscyamus niger L. (Solanaceae)

Synonym(s) and related species

Black henbane, Hog's-bean, Stinking nightshade, *Hyoscyamus agrestis* Kit, *Hyoscyamus bohemicus* F.W.Schmidt.

Pharmacopoeias

Hyoscyamus for Homeopathic Preparations (*BP 2012, PhEur 7.5*).

Constituents

The active constituents of henbane are the tropane alkaloids **hyoscyamine** and **hyoscine** (scopolamine).

Use and indications

Henbane is used as an antispasmodic for the digestive and urinary tracts, and as a sedative. Hyoscine is widely used in conventional medicine as an antiemetic in pre- and post-operative medication and to treat travel sickness.

Pharmacokinetics

No relevant pharmacokinetic data found. The pharmacokinetics of the hyoscine (scopolamine) constituent are well described. It is readily absorbed from the gastrointestinal tract and is also well absorbed after application to the skin.

Interactions overview

No interactions with henbane found. Note however, that henbane could be consumed from herbal preparations in quantities sufficient to produce levels of alkaloids equivalent to therapeutic doses of hyoscyamine or hyoscine and so it might be expected to interact similarly. Therefore, it would be prudent to be alert for evidence of additive antimuscarinic effects if henbane is given with other drugs that are known to have antimuscarinic effects.

H

Hibiscus

Hibiscus sabdariffa L. (Malvaceae)

Synonym(s) and related species

Jamaica sorrel, Karkadé, Red sorrel, Roselle.

Pharmacopoeias

Roselle (*BP 2012, PhEur 7.5*).

Constituents

Hibiscus flowers contain **anthocyanins** based on delphinidin and cyanidin, and include delphinidin-3-glucoxyloside (delphinidin-3-sambubioside or hibiscin), delphinidin, cyanidin-3-sambubioside, cyanidin-3, 5-diglucoside and others; other **flavonoid** glycosides including hibiscitrin (hibiscetin 3-glucoside), sabdaritrin, gossypitrin, gossytrin and other gossypetin glucosides; other **polyphenolic compounds** such as protocatechuic acid; organic acids including citric and malic acid; mucilage (about 65% dry weight of petals) based on galactose, galacturonic acid and rhamnose; and volatile compounds.

Use and indications

Hibiscus flowers have traditionally been used for loss of appetite, colds and other upper respiratory tract disorders, as a gentle laxative and as a diuretic. It has also been used for the treatment of high blood pressure. There is some clinical evidence that it does possess antihypertensive and hypolipidaemic effects, but a recent systematic review did not find reliable evidence to support its use for the treatment of primary hypertension.[1]

Pharmacokinetics

In a study in healthy subjects given a single dose of hibiscus containing a total of 147 mg of anthocyanins calculated as cyanidin equivalents, oral absorption of the anthocyanin glycosides appeared to be very low, with just 0.018% of the administered dose excreted in urine. It was suggested that human glycosidases in the intestine are not able to deglycosylate anthocyanins.[2] See also flavonoids, page 213 for the general pharmacokinetics of other flavonoids.

Interactions overview

Taking hibiscus extract as a beverage appears to modestly reduce the bioavailability of chloroquine, but does not appear to affect the pharmacokinetics of paracetamol (acetaminophen). It is unclear if any interaction occurs between hibiscus extract and diclofenac. Experimental evidence suggests that hydrochlorothiazide exposure and diuretic efficacy might be potentiated by hibiscus.

Interactions monographs

- Chloroquine, page 287
- Diclofenac, page 287
- Food, page 287
- Herbal medicines, page 287
- Hydrochlorothiazide, page 287
- Paracetamol (Acetaminophen), page 287

1. Wahabi HA, Alansary LA, Al-Sabban AH, Glasziuo P. The effectiveness of *Hibiscus sabdariffa* in the treatment of hypertension: a systematic review. *Phytomedicine* (2010) 17, 83–6.
2. Frank T, Janßen M, Netzel M, Straß G, Kler A, Kriesl E, Bitsch I. Pharmacokinetics of anthocyanidin-3-glycosides following consumption of *Hibiscus sabdariffa* L. extract. *J Clin Pharmacol* (2005) 45, 203–10.

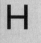

H

Hibiscus + Chloroquine

An hibiscus drink appeared to cause a modest decrease in the bioavailability of chloroquine.

Clinical evidence

In a study in 6 healthy fasting subjects, administration of a single 600-mg dose of chloroquine with karkadi (an hibiscus drink) resulted in a 71% and 73% reduction in the chloroquine AUC and maximum plasma concentration, respectively, when compared with administration with water. The drink had a low pH (2.7). Similar findings were seen with two other acidic drinks.[1]

Experimental evidence

No interactions found.

Mechanism

The hibiscus drink was acidic, and might therefore lead to greater ionisation of the basic drug chloroquine, and thereby reduce its absorption.[1] Note that the presence of food might attenuate this effect.

Importance and management

The general clinical importance of this finding is unclear, but if similar reductions in chloroquine levels were seen in practice, treatment failure or reduced response is possible. Bear this potential interaction in mind if a reduced or unexpectedly low response to chloroquine is seen in patients also drinking hibiscus extracts. Separating administration should reduce any effect. If the mechanism is correct, solid oral dose forms of hibiscus extracts might not have the same effect.

1. Mahmoud BM, Ali HM, Homeida MM, Bennett JL. Significant reduction in chloroquine bioavailability following coadministration with the Sudanese beverages Aradaib, Karkadi and Lemon. *J Antimicrob Chemother* (1994) 33, 1005–9.

Hibiscus + Diclofenac

An hibiscus tea appeared to slightly reduce the amount of unchanged diclofenac excreted in the urine.

Evidence, mechanism, importance and management

In a study in 12 healthy fasting subjects, administration of a single 25-mg dose of diclofenac with 300 mL of a water extract of hibiscus reduced the amount of unchanged diclofenac excreted in the urine over 8 hours by 38%, when compared with administration with water.[1] It is not possible to interpret this finding in the absence of any data on plasma levels of diclofenac, especially since very little diclofenac is excreted unchanged in the urine anyway. Nevertheless, the slight reduction of itself appears unlikely to be of any clinical relevance.

1. Fakeye TO, Adegoke AO, Omoyeni OC, Famakinde AA. Effects of water extract of *Hibiscus sabdariffa*, Linn (Malvaceae) 'Roselle' on excretion of a diclofenac formulation. *Phytother Res* (2007) 21, 96–8.

Hibiscus + Food

No interactions found.

Hibiscus + Herbal medicines

No interactions found.

Hibiscus + Hydrochlorothiazide

The information regarding the use of hibiscus with hydrochlorothiazide is based on experimental evidence only.

Clinical evidence

No interactions found.

Experimental evidence

Concurrent administration of hibiscus 20 to 40 mg/kg and hydrochlorothiazide 10 mg/kg increased hydrochlorothiazide exposure by about 70% in an *animal* study.[1] In addition, concurrent administration increased urine volume after 24 hours by about 50% and decreased urine pH from pH 9.28 to pH 8.6. The extract also decreased urine sodium, bicarbonate, and chloride concentrations by about 40%, 50%, and 80% respectively.

Mechanism

Not understood.

Importance and management

Evidence appears to be limited to the experimental study cited, which suggests that hydrochlorothiazide exposure and diuretic efficacy might be potentiated by hibiscus. Hibiscus has been reported to reduce blood pressure in some (but not all) studies, and, if the experimental data above were confirmed, this might indicate that in patients taking hydrochlorothiazide, any antihypertensive effect could be, at least in part, due to a pharmacokinetic interaction. Furthermore, it seems possible, that patients might have an enhanced response to hydrochlorothiazide if they take hibiscus concurrently, which, unless they take hibiscus regularly, could lead to fluctuations in blood pressure control. However, further study is needed to establish the extent of any effect and its clinical relevance.

1. Ndu OO, Nworu CS, Ehiemere CO, Ndukwe NC, Ochiogu IS. Herb-drug interaction between the extract of *Hibiscus sabdariffa* L. and hydrochlorothiazide in experimental animals. *J Med Food* (2011) 14, 640–644.

Hibiscus + Paracetamol (Acetaminophen)

Hibiscus extract does not appear to affect the pharmacokinetics of single-dose paracetamol to a clinically relevant extent.

Evidence, mechanism, importance and management

A study in 6 healthy subjects found that Zobo drink (*Hibiscus sabdariffa* water extract) given 78 minutes before a single 1-g dose of paracetamol did not affect the absorption or AUC of paracetamol, but the total body clearance increased by 12%.[1] This is not expected to be clinically relevant.

1. Kolawole JA, Maduenyi A. Effect of Zobo drink (Hibiscus sabdariffa water extract) on the pharmacokinetics of acetaminophen in human volunteers. *Eur J Drug Metab Pharmacokinet* (2004) 29, 25–9.

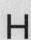

Holy basil

Ocimum sanctum L. (Lamiaceae)

Synonym(s) and related species

Sacred basil, Tulsi.

Ocimum tenuiflorum L.

Constituents

Holy basil leaves contain an essential oil composed of **eugenol**, eugenal, caryophyllene, linalool, and others; **triterpenoids** such as **ursolic acid**; together with the **flavonoids** cirsimaritin, apigenin and its glycosides, luteolin and its glycosides and many others.

Holy basil seeds contain a fixed oil containing fatty acids such as linolenic acid.

Use and indications

Holy basil is widely used in Ayurvedic medicine to treat asthma, bronchitis, coughs and colds, pain and inflammation, and for its insecticidal and vermicidal properties. It is particularly valued as a tonic for stress-induced disorders.

Pharmacokinetics

No relevant pharmacokinetic data found. For information on the pharmacokinetics of individual flavonoids present in holy basil, see under flavonoids, page 213.

Interactions overview

Holy basil leaves might have modest blood-glucose-lowering activity, which could be additive with that of antidiabetics. Animal studies have found that the seed oil potentiated the sedative effect of pentobarbital and prolonged bleeding time, which might, in theory, increase the risk of bleeding when used with other antiplatelet drugs or anticoagulants. Other animal studies found that oil extracted from holy basil (part used not stipulated) increased the absorption of flurbiprofen and labetalol applied to the skin. For information on the interactions of individual flavonoids present in holy basil, see under flavonoids, page 213.

Interactions monographs

- Anticoagulant or antiplatelet drugs, page 289
- Antidiabetics, page 289
- Antihypertensives, page 289
- Food, page 289
- Herbal medicines, page 289
- Miscellaneous, page 289
- Pentobarbital, page 290

H

Holy basil + Anticoagulant or Antiplatelet drugs

The interaction between holy basil seed oil and anticoagulant or antiplatelet drugs is based on experimental evidence only.

Evidence, mechanism, importance and management

No interactions found. In a study in *rats*, intraperitoneal administration of the fixed oil from holy basil seed (3 mL/kg) prolonged blood clotting time to a similar extent as aspirin 100 mg/kg.[1] Omega-3 fatty acids such as linolenic acid are thought to have some antiplatelet effects and might therefore prolong bleeding time. Theoretically, this effect might be additive with that of other antiplatelet drugs, and increase the risk of bleeding with anticoagulants. The clinical relevance of this study of holy basil seed oil is not known, and requires confirmation in human studies. Note that these interactions would not be expected with holy basil leaves or extracts, since the constituents of the leaf are different to the seed oil.

1. Singh S, Rehan HM, Majumdar DK. Effect of Ocimum sanctum fixed oil on blood pressure, blood clotting time and pentobarbitone-induced sleeping time. *J Ethnopharmacol* (2001) 78, 139–43.

Holy basil + Antidiabetics

Limited evidence suggests holy basil leaf can modestly decrease blood-glucose levels in patients with diabetes, and theoretically, this might be additive with the effect of antidiabetic drugs.

Clinical evidence

No interactions found. In a placebo-controlled crossover study in 40 patients with established or newly diagnosed type 2 diabetes, taking holy basil leaves daily for 4 weeks reduced fasting blood-glucose by a mean of 21 mg/dL (17.6%) compared with placebo. There was a smaller (7.3%) decrease in postprandial blood-glucose and a 6.5% reduction in total cholesterol. In this study, patients stopped taking antidiabetic drugs at least 7 days before the study, and holy basil was taken daily as a dried leaf powder (equivalent to 2.5 g of fresh leaves) mixed with 200 mL of water first thing in the morning on an empty stomach.[1]

Experimental evidence

In various *animal* models of diabetes, holy basil leaf extracts have shown hypoglycaemic activity. For example, decreased blood-glucose and glycosylated haemoglobin levels,[2] increased insulin secretion,[3] and prevention of insulin resistance[4] has been shown. In one of these studies, the stimulatory effect of holy basil leaf extract on insulin secretion was potentiated by tolbutamide.[3]

Mechanism

The mechanism for the blood-glucose-lowering activity of holy basil is uncertain. Any effect might be additive with that of conventional antidiabetics.

Importance and management

The limited data from humans suggest that holy basil leaves may have a modest blood-glucose-lowering effect and it is possible that this could be additive with that of antidiabetics. Whether this might increase the risk of hypoglycaemia is unknown and so it might be prudent to bear this possibility in mind.

1. Agrawal P, Rai V, Singh RB. Randomized placebo-controlled, single blind trial of holy basil leaves in patients with noninsulin-dependent diabetes mellitus. *Int J Clin Pharmacol Ther* (1996) 34, 406–9.
2. Narendhirakannan RT, Subramanian S, Kandaswamy M. Biochemical evaluation of antidiabetogenic properties of some commonly used Indian plants on streptozotocin-induced diabetes in experimental rats. *Clin Exp Pharmacol Physiol* (2006) 33, 1150–1157.

3. Hannan JM, Marenah L, Ali L, Rokeya B, Flatt PR, Abdel-Wahab YH. Ocimum sanctum leaf extracts stimulate insulin secretion from perfused pancreas, isolated islets and clonal pancreatic beta-cells. *J Endocrinol* (2006) 189, 127–36.
4. Reddy SS, Karuna R, Baskar R, Saralakumari D. Prevention of insulin resistance by ingesting aqueous extract of Ocimum sanctum to fructose-fed rats. *Horm Metab Res* (2008) 40, 44–9.

Holy basil + Antihypertensives

The interaction between holy basil seed oil and antihypertensives is based on experimental evidence only.

Evidence, mechanism, importance and management

No interactions found. In a study in *dogs*, intravenous administration of the fixed oil from holy basil seed (0.3 mL) reduced blood pressure. It was suggested that this was due to omega-3 fatty acids in the oil.[1] Theoretically, the effect might be additive with that of antihypertensive drugs and increase the risk of hypotension. The clinical relevance of this study of holy basil seed oil is not known, and requires confirmation in human studies. Note, that these interactions would not be expected with holy basil leaves or extracts, since the constituents of the leaf are different to the seed oil.

1. Singh S, Rehan HM, Majumdar DK. Effect of Ocimum sanctum fixed oil on blood pressure, blood clotting time and pentobarbitone-induced sleeping time. *J Ethnopharmacol* (2001) 78, 139–43.

Holy basil + Food

No interactions found.

Holy basil + Herbal medicines

No interactions found.

Holy basil + Miscellaneous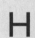

The interaction between holy basil oil and topical flurbiprofen is based on experimental evidence only.

Evidence, mechanism, importance and management

The fixed oil from holy basil enhanced the absorption of **flurbiprofen** across the skin in a study in *rats,* but to less of an extent than turpentine oil.[1] In another study in *rats,* holy basil oil 5% promoted the transdermal penetration of **labetalol**.[2] Essential oils are known to have skin permeation-enhancing effects, which could increase the absorption of topically applied drugs if used at the same time. Bear in mind that if holy basil oil and topical formulations of drugs are applied to the skin at the same time, there may be an increase in the absorption of the drug. The clinical effects of this may not necessarily be adverse.

1. Charoo NA, Shamsher AA, Kohli K, Pillai K, Rahman Z. Improvement in bioavailability of transdermally applied flurbiprofen using tulsi (Ocimum sanctum) and turpentine oil. *Colloids Surf B Biointerfaces* (2008) 65, 300–307.
2. Jain R, Aqil M, Ahad A, Ali A, Khar RK. Basil oil is a promising skin penetration enhancer for transdermal delivery of labetalol hydrochloride. *Drug Dev Ind Pharm* (2008) 34, 384–9.

Holy basil + Pentobarbital

The interaction between holy basil seed oil and pentobarbital is based on experimental evidence only.

Evidence, mechanism, importance and management

In a study in *mice,* intraperitoneal administration of the fixed oil from holy basil seed (2 or 3 mL/kg) potentiated pentobarbital-induced sleeping time by two to threefold. It was suggested that this was due to omega-3 fatty acids in the oil causing inhibition of metabolism,[1] but note that these fatty acids are not known to inhibit hepatic metabolism. The clinical relevance of this study of holy basil seed oil is not known and requires confirmation in human studies. Note, that these interactions would not be expected with holy basil leaves or extracts, since the constituents of the leaf are different to the seed oil.

1. Singh S, Rehan HM, Majumdar DK. Effect of *Ocimum sanctum* fixed oil on blood pressure, blood clotting time and pentobarbitone-induced sleeping time. *J Ethnopharmacol* (2001) 78, 139–43.

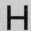

Honeybush

Cyclopia species (Fabaceae)

Synonym(s) and related species

Bergtee, Boertee, Bossiestee, Bush tea, Heuingbos, Heuningtee.

Cyclopia intermedia E. Mey, *Cyclopia genistoides* (L.) Vent, *Cyclopia subternata* Vogel and other species are all referred to as Honeybush.

Constituents

The leaves of honeybush contain the xanthones mangiferin and isomangiferin and **flavonoids** including hesperidin, hesperitin, isokuranetin and kaempferols. The leaves also contain **isoflavones** such as formonometin and afrormosin, and coumestans such as medicagol. The quantity of **flavonoids** is reduced when honeybush is fermented, however the non-flavonoid components increase. Honeybush does not contain caffeine.[1]

Use and indications

Honeybush has been traditionally used in South Africa for a variety of ailments including digestive problems, skin problems and to promote lactation.[1] Honeybush is principally used to produce a tea-like beverage. There is experimental evidence of various activities including antioxidant, chemopreventative, antidiabetic, and immunomodulating effects.[1]

Pharmacokinetics

No relevant pharmacokinetic data found. For the pharmacokinetics of individual flavonoids and isoflavones present in honeybush, see flavonoids, page 213, and isoflavones, page 300.

Interactions overview

No interactions with honeybush found. For information on the interactions of individual flavonoids and isoflavones present in honeybush, see under flavonoids, page 213, and isoflavones, page 300.

1. McKay , DL, Blumberg , JB. A review of the bioactivity of South African Herbal Teas: Rooibos (*Aspalathus Linearis*) and Honeybush (*Cyclopia intermedia*). *Phytother Res* (2007) 21, 1–16.

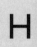

Hoodia

Hoodia gordonii Sweet (Asclepiadaceae)

Synonym(s) and related species

Hoodia barklyi Dyer, *Hoodia burkei* N.E.Br., *Hoodia longispina* Plowes, *Stapelia gordoni* Masson. Other species of *Hoodia* are also used, but are less well investigated.

Constituents

The succulent flesh of hoodia contains a large number of oxypregnane glycosides known as the hoodigosides, and steroidal glycosides, the gordonosides. The active constituent (an oxypregnane glycoside of hoodigogenin) is often referred to as P57AS3, or more commonly, P57.

Use and indications

Hoodia is used to suppress appetite and thirst. The active constituent, P57, is reported to have a CNS effects.

Pharmacokinetics

An *in vitro* study has shown that P57, an active constituent isolated from *Hoodia gordonii,* weakly inhibited the action of the cytochrome P450 isoenzyme CYP3A4 in a dose-dependent manner. CYP1A2, CYP2C9 and CYP2D6 were unaffected by P57. These results suggest that pharmacokinetic interactions with substrates of these isoenzymes are unlikely. This study also indicated that P57 may be a substrate of P-glycoprotein.[1]

Interactions overview

No interactions with hoodia found.

1. Magdula VLM, Avula B, Pawar RS, Shukla YJ, Khan IA, Walker LA, Khan SI. *In vitro* metabolic stability and intestinal transport of P57AS3 (P57) from *Hoodia gordonii* and its interaction with drug metabolizing enzymes. *Planta Med* (2008) 74, 1269–75.

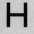
H

Hops

Humulus lupulus L. (Cannabaceae)

Synonym(s) and related species

Humulus, Lupulus.

Pharmacopoeias

Hop Strobile (*BP 2012, PhEur 7.5*).

Constituents

The flowers (strobiles) of hops contain a volatile oil composed mainly of humulene (alpha-caryophyllene), with beta-caryophyllene, myrcene, farnesene and others. There is also an oleo-resin fraction composed of bitter acids. **Flavonoids** present include glycosides of kaempferol and quercetin, and a series of prenylated **flavonoids** (including 6-prenylnaringenin) and prenylated chalcones. A number of hop proanthocyanidins, based on gallocatechin, afzelechin and epicatechin derivatives, and the trans isomer of the stilbenoid **resveratrol** and its glucoside, piceid, have also been isolated. Note that a large variety of hops genotypes exist, and the relative content of these constituents may vary between genotype.

Use and indications

Hops are used mainly as a sedative, anxiolytic, hypnotic and tranquillizer. These properties have been demonstrated pharmacologically but there is little clinical evidence to date. Hops also contain a number of compounds with oestrogenic activity such as 6-prenylnaringenin. Many products include hops as one of several ingredients rather than as a single extract. There are also many varieties of hops, normally produced for their flavour and other characteristics useful for beer production. The variety used medicinally is usually not stated.

Pharmacokinetics

Most of the investigations carried out into the metabolism of hops have concerned the metabolism of isoxanthohumol to the more potent phytoestrogen 8-prenylnaringenin by human liver microsomes,[1] and by intestinal microflora, particularly in the colon.[2,3] These studies suggest that the levels of active constituents vary between individuals, and may be altered by antibacterial treatment, which suggests that the activity (particularly the oestrogenic activity[4]) of hops, and its potential to interact, is also likely to vary between individuals. The cytochrome P450 isoenzymes CYP1A2, CYP2C19 and CYP2C8 may be involved,[4] but information is too sparse to be able to comment further on the potential for conventional drugs to diminish the effects of hops.

See under flavonoids, page 213, for information on the individual flavonoids present in hops, and see under resveratrol, page 401, for the pharmacokinetics of resveratrol.

Interactions overview

Animal studies suggest that hops extracts potentiate the analgesic effects of paracetamol, suppress the stimulant effects of cocaine, suppress the effects of diazepam and potentially alter the sedative effects of pentobarbital. For information on the interactions of flavonoids, see under flavonoids, page 213, and for the interactions of resveratrol, see under resveratrol, page 401.

Interactions monographs

- Cocaine, page 294
- Diazepam, page 294
- Food, page 294
- Herbal medicines, page 294
- Oestrogens or Oestrogen antagonists, page 294
- Paracetamol, page 294
- Pentobarbital, page 295

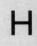

H

1. Nikolic D, Li Y, Chadwick LR, Pauli GF, van Breemen RB. Metabolism of xanthohumol and isoxanthohumol, prenylated flavonoids from hops (*Humulus lupulus* L.) by human liver microsomes. *J Mass Spectrom* (2005) 40, 289–99.
2. Possemiers S, Bolca S, Grootaert C, Heyerick A, Decroos K, Dhooge W, De Keukeleire D, Rabot S, Verstraete W, Van de, Wiele T. The prenylflavonoid isoxanthohumol from hops (*Humulus lupulus* L.) is activated into the potent phytoestrogen 8-prenylnaringenin in vitro and in the human intestine. *J Nutr* (2006) 136, 1862–7.
3. Bolca S, Possemiers S, Maervoet V, Huybrechts I, Heyerick A, Vervarcke S, Depypere H, De Keukeleire D, Bracke M, De Henauw S, Verstraete W, Van de, Wiele T. Microbial and dietary factors associated with the 8-prenylnaringenin producer phenotype: a dietary intervention trial with fifty healthy post-menopausal Caucasian women. *Br J Nutr* (2007) 98, 950–959.
4. Guo J, Nikolic D, Chadwick LR, Pauli GF, van Breemen RB. Identification of human hepatic cytochrome P450 enzymes involved in the metabolism of 8-prenylnaringenin and isoxanthohumol from hops (*Humulus lupulus* L.). *Drug Metab Dispos* (2006) 34, 1152–9.

Hops + Cocaine

The interaction between hops and cocaine is based on experimental evidence only.

Clinical evidence

No interactions found.

Experimental evidence

In a study of the interactions of various genotypes of hops, *mice* were given cocaine 25 mg/kg after they had received four intraperitoneal doses of a 0.5% alcoholic extract of hops. Three hops genotypes were used; Aroma, Magnum and wild hops. The study found that the Magnum hops extracts almost completely suppressed the excitatory effects of cocaine (measured by spontaneous motility), when compared with controls. Extracts of the wild genotype also decreased the excitatory effects of cocaine, but to a lesser extent than the Magnum genotype, whereas the Aroma genotype did not alter the effects of cocaine.[1]

Mechanism

It has been suggested that hops may alter the effects of cocaine on the central nervous system, but it is not known how this occurs.

Importance and management

Evidence appears to be limited to this one study in *mice,* the clinical relevance of which is unclear. What is known suggests that any interaction may be advantageous, or more likely, not clinically important. Of more interest is the variability in the interaction between the different hops genotypes, which suggests that the exact source of the hops used in any preparation is likely to be of importance in establishing their potential for interactions.

1. Horvat O, Raskovic A, Jakovljevic V, Sabo J, Berenji J. Interaction of alcoholic extracts of hops with cocaine and paracetamol in mice. *Eur J Drug Metab Pharmacokinet* (2007) 32, 39–44.

Hops + Diazepam

The interaction between hops and diazepam is based on experimental evidence only.

Clinical evidence

No interactions found.

Experimental evidence

In study of the interactions of various genotypes of hops, *mice* were given diazepam 3 mg/kg after they had received four intraperitoneal doses of a 0.5% alcoholic extract of hops. Three hops genotypes were used; Aroma, Magnum and wild hops. The study found that the hops extracts suppressed the effects of diazepam (assessed by co-ordination of movements). The most pronounced effect occurred with the extracts of Magnum and Aroma genotypes whereas the wild genotype had no significant effect.[1]

Mechanism

It has been suggested that hops may prevent diazepam exerting its effect on GABA receptors in the central nervous system, thereby diminishing its effects.

Importance and management

Evidence appears to be limited to this one study in *mice,* the clinical relevance of which is unclear. What is known suggests that hops may diminish the effects of diazepam, which is in contrast to what would be expected, given that hops is given for similar reasons to diazepam. It is difficult to extrapolate these findings to humans,

but there appears to be no good reason to avoid concurrent use. Of more interest is the variability in the interaction between the different hops genotypes, which suggests that the exact source of the hops used in any preparation is likely to be of importance in establishing their potential for interactions.

1. Raskovic A, Horvat O, Jakovljevic V, Sabo J, Vasic R. Interaction of alcoholic extracts of hops with pentobarbital and diazepam in mice. *Eur J Drug Metab Pharmacokinet* (2007) 32, 45–9.

Hops + Food

No interactions found.

Hops + Herbal medicines

No interactions found.

Hops + Oestrogens or Oestrogen antagonists

Hops contains oestrogenic compounds. This may result in additive effects with oestrogens or it may oppose the effects of oestrogens. Similarly, hops may have additive effects with oestrogen antagonists or oppose the effects of oestrogen antagonists (e.g. tamoxifen). See Chinese angelica + Oestrogens or Oestrogen antagonists, page 146 for more information.

Hops + Paracetamol (Acetaminophen)

The interaction between hops and paracetamol is based on experimental evidence only.

Clinical evidence

No interactions found.

Experimental evidence

In a study of the interactions of various genotypes of hops, *mice* were given paracetamol 80 mg/kg after they had received four intraperitoneal doses of a 0.5% alcoholic extract of hops. Three hops genotypes were used; Aroma, Magnum and wild hops. The study found that the hops extracts alone did not possess an analgesic effect, but each of the extracts increased the analgesic effect of paracetamol 80 mg/kg, with the most pronounced effect occurring with the extracts of Aroma and wild genotypes hops.[1]

Mechanism
Unknown.

Importance and management

Evidence appears to be limited to this one study in *mice,* the clinical relevance of which is unclear. What is known suggests that any interaction may be advantageous. Of more interest is the variability in the interaction between the different hops genotypes, which suggests that the exact source of the hops used in any preparation is likely to be of importance in establishing their potential for interactions.

1. Horvat O, Raskovic A, Jakovljevic V, Sabo J, Berenji J. Interaction of alcoholic extracts of hops with cocaine and paracetamol in mice. *Eur J Drug Metab Pharmacokinet* (2007) 32, 39–44.

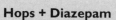

Hops + Pentobarbital

The interaction between hops and pentobarbital is based on experimental evidence only.

Clinical evidence
No interactions found.

Experimental evidence
In a study of the interactions of various genotypes of hops, *mice* were given pentobarbital 40 mg/kg after they had received four intraperitoneal doses of 0.5% alcoholic extract of hops. Three hops genotypes were used; Aroma, Magnum and wild hops. The study found that the hops extracts suppressed the hypnotic effects of pentobarbital (measured by a decrease in the sleeping time of the *mice*). The most pronounced effect occurred with the extracts of Magnum and Aroma genotypes whereas the wild genotype had no significant effect. However, the effects varied greatly between individual *mice*, with some sleeping for a longer time.[1]

Mechanism
It has been suggested that hops may alter the effects of phenobarbital on the central nervous system, but it is not known how this occurs.

Importance and management
Evidence appears to be limited to this one study in *mice,* the clinical relevance of which is unclear. What is known suggests that hops may slightly decrease the sedative effects of pentobarbital in some individuals, or increase them in others. It is difficult to extrapolate these findings to humans, but there appears to be no good reason to avoid concurrent use, although patients should be aware that there is a possibility that they may be more or less sedated than with either medicine alone. Of more interest is the variability in the interaction between the different hops genotypes, which suggests that the exact source of the hops used in any preparation is likely to be of importance in establishing their potential for interactions.

1. Raskovic A, Horvat O, Jakovljevic V, Sabo J, Vasic R. Interaction of alcoholic extracts of hops with pentobarbital and diazepam in mice. *Eur J Drug Metab Pharmacokinet* (2007) 32, 45–9.

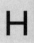

Horse chestnut

Aesculus hippocastanum L. (Hippocastanaceae)

Synonym(s) and related species

Aesculus.

Hippocastanum vulgare Gaertn.

Pharmacopoeias

Horse Chestnut (*USP35–NF30 S1*); Powdered Horse Chestnut (*USP35–NF30 S1*); Powdered Horse Chestnut Extract (*USP35–NF30 S1*).

Constituents

Horse chestnut seeds contain more than 30 saponins, a complex mixture known as '**aescin**' or '**escin**' (to which it may be standardised), based on the aglycones protoescigenin and barringtogenol-C. Other compounds including sterols and triterpenes such as friedelin, taraxerol and spinasterol, and **flavonoids**, based on quercetin and kaempferol are also present. The natural coumarins found in horse chestnut (such as aesculin (esculin) and fraxin) do not possess the minimum structural requirements for anticoagulant activity.

Use and indications

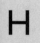

Horse chestnut extracts (aescin) are used to treat vascular insufficiency, especially varicose veins, venous ulcers, haemorrhoids, and inflammation. They are usually applied as topical preparations, particularly gel formulations, but a licensed oral dosage form is also available.[1] There is a considerable body of clinical and pharmacological evidence to support their use.

Pharmacokinetics

An isolated *in vitro* study suggests that horse chestnut may inhibit P-glycoprotein-mediated transport, assessed using digoxin, page 297 as a substrate. In this study, horse chestnut did not inhibit cytochrome P450 isoenzyme CYP3A4.[2] Similarly, in a previous study, the authors briefly noted that, *in vitro,* horse chestnut had little inhibitory effect on CYP1A2, CYP2D6 and CYP3A4.[3] For information on the pharmacokinetics of individual flavonoids present in horse chestnut, see under flavonoids, page 213.

Interactions overview

One *in vitro* study suggests that horse chestnut may affect P-glycoprotein, and could therefore affect the pharmacokinetics of drugs such as digoxin, although the clinical significance of this is unknown. Some have suggested that horse chestnut may interact with anticoagulants, presumably based on its natural coumarin content, but the coumarins present are not known to possess the structural requirements necessary for anticoagulant activity. For more information, see Natural coumarins + Warfarin and related drugs, page 360. For information on the interactions of individual flavonoids present in horse chestnut, see under flavonoids, page 213.

Interactions monographs

- Digoxin, page 297
- Food, page 297
- Herbal medicines, page 297

1. Venaforce (Horse chestnut). Bioforce (UK) Ltd. UK Summary of product characteristics, February 2008.
2. Hellum BH, Nilsen OG. *In vitro* inhibition of CYP3A4 metabolism and P-glycoprotein-mediated transport by trade herbal products. *Basic Clin Pharmacol Toxicol* (2008) 102, 466–75.
3. Hellum BH, Hu Z, Nilsen OG. The induction of CYP1A2, CYP2D6 and CYP3A4 by six trade herbal products in cultured primary human hepatocytes. *Basic Clin Pharmacol Toxicol* (2007) 100, 23–30.

H

Horse chestnut + Digoxin

The interaction between horse chestnut and digoxin is based on experimental evidence only.

Evidence, mechanism, importance and management

An *in vitro* study to investigate the effects of a horse chestnut product (*Venostat*) on P-glycoprotein transport found that the extract inhibited the transport of digoxin by P-glycoprotein to a minor extent. Nevertheless, the authors predicted that inhibitory levels might easily be reached in the small intestine with usual therapeutic doses of horse chestnut.[1]

Since this appears to be the only available study, this inhibition of digoxin transport needs confirming, and then an *in vivo* clinical study would be required to assess whether horse chestnut does alter digoxin absorption on concurrent use, and whether any changes are clinically relevant. No specific recommendations can be made on the basis of this single *in vitro* study.

1. Hellum BH, Nilsen OG. *In vitro* inhibition of CYP3A4 metabolism and P-glycoprotein-mediated transport by trade herbal products. *Basic Clin Pharmacol Toxicol* (2008) 102, 466–75.

Horse chestnut + Food

No relevant interactions found.

Horse chestnut + Herbal medicines

No interactions found.

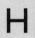

Horsetail

Equisetum arvense (Equisetaceae)

Synonym(s) and related species

Equisetum.

The related species *Equisetum hyemale* L. has also been used, but note that standardised pharmacopoeial preparations of horsetail should contain no more than 5% of other *Equisetum* species.

Pharmacopoeias

Horsetail (*BP 2012*); Equisetum Stem (*PhEur 7.5*).

Constituents

Horsetail contains high concentrations of **silicic acid**, up to 8%, and is sometimes used as an organic source of silicon. It also contains **flavonoids** such as apigenin, kaempferol, luteolin and quercetin and their derivatives, and may be standardised to the total **flavonoid** content expressed as **isoquercitroside**. Other polyphenolic compounds such as caffeic acid derivatives, and trace amounts of the alkaloid nicotine, and sterols including cholesterol, isofucosterol and campesterol are also present. Horsetail also contains thiaminase (an enzyme that breaks down thiamine), and this is inactivated in some supplements.

Use and indications

Horsetail is used mainly as an astringent, haemostatic, and anti-inflammatory agent, and for urinary tract complaints such as cystitis, prostatitis, urethritis and enuresis. There is little pharmacological, and no clinical evidence, to support the main uses.

Pharmacokinetics

An *in vitro* study using alcoholic extracts of horsetail found that it had only weak inhibitory effects on the cytochrome P450 isoenzyme CYP3A4.[1] For information on the pharmacokinetics of individual flavonoids present in horsetail, see under flavonoids, page 213.

Interactions overview

An isolated case of lithium toxicity has been reported in a patient who took a herbal diuretic containing horsetail among other ingredients, see under Parsley + Lithium, page 364. For information on the interactions of individual flavonoids present in horsetail, see under flavonoids, page 213.

Interactions monographs

- Food, page 299
- Herbal medicines, page 299

1. Scott IM, Leduc RI, Burt AJ, Marles RJ, Arnason JT, Foster BC. The inhibition of human cytochrome P450 by ethanol extracts of North American botanicals. *Pharm Biol* (2006) 44, 315–27.

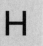

Horsetail + Food

No interactions found.

Horsetail + Herbal medicines

No interactions found.

Horsetail + Lithium

For mention of a case of lithium toxicity in a woman who had been taking a non-prescription herbal diuretic containing corn silk, *Equisetum hyemale,* juniper, buchu, parsley and bearberry, all of which are believed to have diuretic actions, see under Parsley + Lithium, page 364. Note that this case was with *Equisetum hyemale,* which is not the species more commonly used (*Equisetum arvense*).

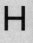

H

Isoflavones

Isoflavonoids

This is a large group of related compounds with similar structures and biological properties in common, which are widely available as additives in dietary supplements as well as the herbs or foods they were originally derived from. Isoflavones are the subject of intensive investigations and new information is constantly being published.

You may have come to this monograph via a herb that contains isoflavones. The information in this monograph relates to the individual isoflavones, and the reader is referred back to the herb (and vice versa) where appropriate. It is very difficult to confidently predict whether a herb that contains one of the isoflavones mentioned, will interact in the same way. The levels of the isoflavone in the particular herb can vary a great deal between specimens, related species, extracts and brands and it is important to take this into account when viewing the interactions described below.

Types, sources and related compounds

Isoflavones are plant-derived polyphenolic compounds that are a distinct group of flavonoids, page 213. They can exert oestrogen-like effects, and therefore belong to the family of 'phytoestrogens'. Most occur as simple isoflavones, but there are other derivatives such as the **coumestans**, the **pterocarpans** and the **rotenoids**, some of which also have oestrogenic properties.

The isoflavones are found in small amounts in many legumes, seeds, grains and vegetables, but soya, page 430, is by far the most concentrated dietary source; it contains principally **genistein** and **daidzein**. There are various other isoflavone-rich supplements, including those derived from alfalfa, page 21 and red clover, page 398 (both of which are rich in **biochanin A** and **formononetin**), and kudzu, page 321, which contains **puerarin**. In addition, some popular herbal medicines, such as astragalus, page 50 and shatavari, page 427 contain isoflavones as well as other types of active constituents.

In plants, isoflavones are usually found in the glycoside form, i.e. bound to a sugar molecule, but digestion results in the release of the sugar molecule leaving the aglycone. The most important isoflavones are **genistein** and **daidzein**, which are hydrolysed from their glycosides genistin, daidzin and **puerarin** (daidzein 8-C-glucoside); **glycetein** and its glycoside glycitin; **formononetin**, **biochanin A**, isoformononetin, prunetin, calycosin, ononin, orobol; and others.

Use and indications

Epidemiological studies show that a high dietary intake of isoflavones from foods such as soya, page 430 might be protective against certain cancers (breast, endometrium, prostate) and degenerative diseases, in the same way as the flavonoids, page 213. Although isoflavone supplements are used for these possible benefits, it remains to be seen whether they are effective. Many of their biological effects, as with the flavonoids, appear to be related to their ability to modulate cell signalling pathways, and genistein in particular has been widely investigated for its tyrosine kinase-inhibiting properties, and it is now also considered by some to be a SERM (selective oestrogen receptor modulator). Some biologically active constituents of genistein have given cause for concern, as it can be genotoxic and cause cell damage, and it is a topoisomerase II inhibitor.

Isoflavones have weak oestrogenic effects, but under certain conditions (for example in premenopausal women) they can also act as oestrogen antagonists by preventing the more potent natural compounds, such as estriol, from binding to receptor sites. In some cases the activities are tissue-selective. Isoflavones also inhibit the synthesis and activity of enzymes involved in oestrogen and testosterone metabolism, such as aromatase.

Because of their oestrogenic effects, isoflavone supplements have been investigated for treating menopausal symptoms such as hot flushes (hot flashes)[1,2] and for prevention of menopausal osteoporosis,[3] with generally modest to no benefits when compared with placebo in randomised controlled studies. Isoflavones have also been extensively studied for lipid-lowering,[4] and there are a few studies on other cardiovascular benefits, and effects on cognitive function. In a 2006 analysis, the American Heart Advisory Committee concluded that the efficacy and safety of soya isoflavones was not established for any indication, and for this reason, they recommended against the use of isoflavone supplements in food or pills.[4]

Pharmacokinetics

The uptake, metabolism and disposition of the isoflavones is highly complex and has not yet been fully elucidated. Isoflavone glycosides are probably hydrolysed in the gut wall by intestinal beta-glucosidases to release the aglycones (genistein, daidzein, etc.), which can then be absorbed.[5] Intestinal bacteria may also hydrolyse the glycosides, and, in some people, they metabolise daidzein to the more active oestrogen equol.[6] After absorption, the aglycones are conjugated, predominantly to glucuronic acid. Gut bacteria also extensively metabolise isoflavones: for example, daidzein may be metabolised to equol, a metabolite with greater oestrogenic activity than daidzein, but also to other compounds that are less oestrogenic.[7] Because of differences in gut flora, there are individual differences in the metabolism of isoflavones, which might have important implications for their effects: for example, studies measuring urinary equol excretion after soya consumption indicate that only about one-third of Western individuals metabolise daidzein to equol.[8]

In a study in 9 healthy subjects the isoflavone puerarin, given orally, was rapidly absorbed and reached peak levels at 2 hours, and had a half-life of about 4.5 hours. The elimination half-life was not significantly altered after repeated administration. The authors concluded that three times a day dosing is recommended, as accumulation will not occur, and plasma levels remain at levels that are biologically active, even 8 hours after the last steady-state dose.[9] For mention that colonic bacteria hydrolyse puerarin to the more active aglycone daidzein, see Isoflavones + Antibacterials, page 302.

In an *in vitro* study in human liver microsomes, fluvoxamine was a potent inhibitor of genistein and tangeretin metabolism.[10] This finding suggests that these isoflavones are principally metabolised by CYP1A2, of which fluvoxamine is a potent inhibitor. The relevance of this to the activity of these isoflavones is unknown, since the relative activity of the metabolites to the parent isoflavone is unknown.

The isoflavones genistein and equol were found to inhibit the cytochrome P450 isoenzymes CYP2E1 and CYP1A2,[11] see also theophylline, page 305, but note also that infant formulas, including soya-based formulas, appear to induce CYP1A2, see Soya + Caffeine, page 432.

In vitro, the soya isoflavones daidzein and genistein and a hydrolysed soya extract inhibited CYP3A4,[12,13] and CYP2C9.[13] However, in one of these studies,[12] St John's wort also inhibited CYP3A4, but clinically this herb is known to be an inducer of CYP3A4. This highlights the problems of extrapolating the findings of *in vitro* studies to the clinical situation.[13]

Genistein and biochanin A inhibit P-glycoprotein-mediated drug transport, for example, see paclitaxel, page 303 and digoxin, page 302.

Interactions overview

The interactions covered in the following sections relate to individual isoflavones. Some of these may be directly applicable to isoflavone supplements; however, caution must be taken when extrapolating these interactions to herbs or foods known to contain the isoflavone in question. This is because the amount of the isoflavone found in the herb or food can be highly variable, and might not be known, and other constituents present in the herb or food might affect the bioavailability or activity of the isoflavone. Therefore, although data on isolated isoflavones is useful, it is no substitute for direct studies of the herb or food in question.

Interactions monographs

1. Krebs EE, Ensrud KE, MacDonald R, Wilt TJ. Phytoestrogens for treatment of menopausal symptoms: a systematic review. *Obstet Gynecol* (2004) 104, 824–36.
2. Lethaby AE, Brown J, Marjoribanks J, Kronenberg F, Roberts H, Eden J. Phytoestrogens for vasomotor menopausal symptoms (review). Available in The Cochrane Database of Systematic Reviews; Issue 4. Chichester: John Wiley; 2007..
3. Kreijkamp-Kaspers S, Kok L, Grobbee DE, de Haan EHF, Aleman A, Lampe JW, van der Schouw YT. Effect of soy protein containing isoflavones on cognitive function, bone mineral density, and plasma lipids in postmenopausal women: a randomized controlled trial. *JAMA* (2004) 292, 65–74.
4. Sacks FM, Lichtenstein A, Van Horn L, Harris W, Kris-Etherton P, Winston M. Soy protein, isoflavones, and cardiovascular health: an American Heart Association Science Advisory for professionals from the Nutrition Committee. *Circulation* (2006) 113, 1034–44.
5. Setchell KDR, Brown NM, Zimmer-Nechemias L, Brashear WT, Wolfe BE, Kirschner AS, Heubi JE. Evidence for lack of absorption of soy isoflavone glycosides in humans, supporting the crucial role of intestinal metabolism for bioavailability. *Am J Clin Nutr* (2002) 76, 447–53.
6. Setchell KD, Clerici C, Lephart ED, Cole SJ, Heenan C, Castellani D, Wolfe BE, Nechemias-Zimmer L, Brown NM, Lund TD, Handa RJ, Heubi JE. S-equol, a potent ligand for estrogen receptor β, is the exclusive enantiomeric form of the soy isoflavone metabolite produced by human intestinal bacterial flora. *Am J Clin Nutr* (2005) 81, 1072–9.
7. Rowland I, Faughnan M, Hoey L, Wahala K, Williamson G, Cassidy A. Bioavailability of phyto-oestrogens. *Br J Nutr* (2003) 89 (Suppl 1), S45–S58.
8. Setchell KD, Brown NM, Lydeking-Olsen E. The clinical importance of the metabolite equol-a clue to the effectiveness of soy and its isoflavones. *J Nutr* (2002) 132, 3577–84.
9. Penetar DM, Teter CJ, Ma Z, Tracy M, Lee DY, Lukas SE. Pharmacokinetic profile of the isoflavone puerarin after acute and repeated administration of a novel kudzu extract to human volunteers. *J Altern Complement Med* (2006) 12, 543–8.
10. Breinholt VM, Rasmussen SE, Brøsen K, Friedberg TH. *In vitro* metabolism of genistein and tangeretin by human and murine cytochrome P450s. *Pharmacol Toxicol* (2003) 93, 14–22.
11. Helsby NA, Chipman JK, Gescher A, Kerr D. Inhibition of mouse and human CYP 1A- and 2E1-dependent substrate metabolism by the isoflavonoids genistein and equol. *Food Chem Toxicol* (1998) 36, 375–82.
12. Foster BC, Vandenhoek S, Hana J, Krantis A, Akhtar MH, Bryan M, Budzinski JW, Ramputh A, Arnason JT. *In vitro* inhibition of human cytochrome P450-mediated metabolism of marker substrates by natural products. *Phytomedicine* (2003) 10, 334–42.
13. Anderson GD, Rosito G, Mohustsy MA, Elmer GW. Drug interaction potential of soy extract and Panax ginseng. *J Clin Pharmacol* (2003) 43, 643–8.

Isoflavones + Antibacterials

The interaction between isoflavones and antibacterials is based on a prediction only.

Clinical evidence

No interactions found.

Experimental evidence

It is well known that colonic bacteria are involved in the metabolism of isoflavones. For example, it has been shown that equol is exclusively formed from **daidzin** by colonic bacteria, but that only about one-third of people are equol producers.[1] In another study, the isoflavone glycosides **puerarin** and **daidzin** were incubated with human intestinal bacteria. All bacteria hydrolysed **daidzin** to the aglycone **daidzein**, and a few bacteria also transformed puerarin to **daidzein**. Human faecal specimens hydrolysed **puerarin** and **daidzin** to **daidzein**, but their hydrolysing activities varied between individual specimens. When the oestrogenic effects of the glycosides **puerarin** and **daidzin** were compared with those of the aglycone **daidzein**, the aglycone metabolite was more potent.[2] Intestinal bacteria have also been reported to metabolise **daidzein** to the more active oestrogen equol.[3]

However, it is also now established that beta-glucosidases in the intestinal wall are also important for the hydrolysis of glycosides to form the aglycones (see pharmacokinetics, page 300).

Mechanism

Colonic bacteria appear to play an important role in the metabolism of soya isoflavones, therefore, it is possible that antibacterials that decimate colonic bacteria could alter isoflavone metabolism and biological activity.

Importance and management

Evidence is limited to experimental studies that were not designed to study drug interactions; however, what is known suggests that the concurrent use of antibacterials active against gut flora might theoretically alter or reduce the efficacy of some isoflavones. However, there is no clinical evidence to support this supposition, and in any case, the effect is likely to be temporary. No action is therefore needed.

1. Setchell KDR, Brown NM, Lydeking-Olsen E. The clinical importance of the metabolite equol-a clue to the effectiveness of soy and its isoflavones. *J Nutr* (2002) 132, 3577–84.
2. Park E-K, Shin J, Bae E-A, Lee Y-C, Kim D-H. Intestinal bacteria activate estrogenic effect of main constituents puerarin and daidzin of *Pueraria thunbergiana*. *Biol Pharm Bull* (2006) 29, 2432–5.
3. Setchell KDR, Clerici C, Lephart ED, Cole SJ, Heenan C, Castellani D, Wolfe BE, Nechemias-Zimmer L, Brown NM, Lund TD, Handa RJ, Heubi JE. S-equol, a potent ligand for estrogen receptor β, is the exclusive enantiomeric form of the soy isoflavone metabolite produced by human intestinal bacterial flora. *Am J Clin Nutr* (2005) 81, 1072–9.

Isoflavones + Antidiabetics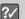

The interaction between isoflavones and antidiabetics is based on experimental evidence only.

Evidence, mechanism, importance and management

In various studies in *animal* models of diabetes, a couple of which are cited for information,[1,2] **puerarin**, an isoflavone found in kudzu, page 321, has demonstrated blood glucose-lowering effects.

Some have interpreted these studies to indicate that kudzu might have additive effects with antidiabetic drugs, and that the dose of antidiabetic medications might need to be adjusted. Given the nature of the evidence, and the fact that it relates to isolated isoflavone constituents, this appears to be a very cautious approach.

1. Chen W-C, Hayakawa S, Yamamoto T, Su H-C, Liu I-M, Cheng J-T. Mediation of β-endorphin by the isoflavone puerarin to lower plasma glucose in streptozotocin-induced diabetic rats. *Planta Med* (2004) 70, 113–16.
2. Hsu F-L, Liu I-M, Kuo D-H, Chen W-C, Su H-C, Cheng J-T. Antihyperglycemic effect of puerarin in streptozotocin-induced diabetic rats. *J Nat Prod* (2003) 66, 788–92.

Isoflavones + Benzodiazepines

The interaction between isoflavones and benzodiazepines is based on experimental evidence only.

Evidence, mechanism, importance and management

In two experimental studies,[1,2] the isoflavone **puerarin** has been shown to be a weak benzodiazepine antagonist. It is therefore theoretically possible that **puerarin** might reduce the effects of benzodiazepines if given concurrently. However, there is no clinical evidence to support this supposition. The fact that the information relates to an isolated isoflavone, and the effect was only weak, suggests that a clinically important interaction between isoflavones and benzodiazepines is unlikely.

1. Overstreet DH, Kralic JE, Morrow AL, Ma ZZ, Zhang YW, Lee DYW. NPI-031G (puerarin) reduces anxiogenic effects of alcohol withdrawal or benzodiazepine inverse or 5-HT$_{2C}$ agonists. *Pharmacol Biochem Behav* (2003) 75, 619–25.
2. Shen XL, Witt MR, Nielsen M, Sterner O. Inhibition of [^{3}H] flunitrazepam binding to rat brain membranes *in vitro* by puerarin and daidzein. *Yao Xue Xue Bao* (1996) 31, 59–62.

Isoflavones + Cardiovascular drugs; Miscellaneous

The interaction between isoflavones and miscellaneous cardiovascular drugs is based on experimental evidence only.

Evidence, mechanism, importance and management

Some experimental studies have shown that isoflavones from kudzu, page 321, may inhibit of platelet aggregation.[1] In one small study in patients with angina,[2] treatment with the isoflavone **puerarin** reduced the activation of platelet surface activity protein.

Some have interpreted these studies to indicate that theoretically, kudzu might increase the risk of bleeding when used with antiplatelet drugs or anticoagulants, and that caution is warranted on concurrent use. Given the nature of the evidence, and the fact that it relates to isolated isoflavone constituents of kudzu, this appears to be a very cautious approach.

Note that **puerarin** injection is used in China to treat angina and cardiovascular disease. Clinical studies comparing standard Western treatment (**nitrates**, **beta blockers**, **calcium-channel blockers**, **aspirin**, **anticoagulants** etc.) with or without **puerarin** injection have been reviewed. It was concluded that although adverse events were inadequately reported, treatment including the injection tended to result in more adverse effects.[3]

1. Choo M-K, Park E-K, Yoon H-K, Kim D-H. Antithrombotic and antiallergic activities of daidzein, a metabolite of puerarin and daidzin produced by human intestinal microflora. *Biol Pharm Bull* (2002) 25, 1328–32.
2. Luo ZR, Zheng B. Effect of puerarin on platelet activating factors CD63 and CD62P, plasminogen activator inhibitor and C-reactive protein in patients with unstable angina pectoris [In Chinese]. *Zhongguo Zhong Xi Yi Jie He Za Zhi* (2001) 21, 31–3.
3. Wang Q, Wu T, Chen X, Ni J, Duan X, Zheng J, Qiao J, Zhou L, Wei J. Puerarin injection for unstable angina pectoris. Available in The Cochrane Database of Systematic Reviews; Issue 3. Chichester: John Wiley; 2007..

Isoflavones + Digoxin

The interaction between isoflavones and digoxin is based on experimental evidence only.

Clinical evidence

No interactions found.

Experimental evidence

In a study in *rats,* **biochanin A** 100 mg/kg increased the AUC and maximum serum levels of an oral 20-mg/kg dose of digoxin by 75% and 71%, respectively.[1] No significant changes in mean residence time and terminal half-life of digoxin were observed, suggesting a negligible effect of **biochanin A** on renal elimination.

Mechanism

Digoxin is a substrate for P-glycoprotein. Biochanin A may modestly inhibit P-glycoprotein, resulting in a moderate increase in oral bioavailability of digoxin.

Importance and management

There appears to be no clinical data regarding an interaction between biochanin A and digoxin, and the clinical relevance of the experimental data needs to be determined. However, until more is known, because of the narrow therapeutic index of digoxin, it may be prudent to be cautious if patients taking digoxin also wish to take supplements containing high doses of biochanin A. Patients should be alert for any evidence of adverse effects, such as bradycardia, and if these occur it may be prudent to monitor digoxin levels.

1. Peng SX, Ritchie DM, Cousineau M, Danser E, Dewire R, Floden J. Altered oral bioavailability and pharmacokinetics of P-glycoprotein substrates by coadministration of biochanin A. *J Pharm Sci* (2006) 95, 1984–93.

Isoflavones + Fexofenadine

The interaction between isoflavones and fexofenadine is based on experimental evidence only.

Clinical evidence

No interactions found.

Experimental evidence

The effects of **biochanin A** on the pharmacokinetics of fexofenadine was investigated in *rats*. **Biochanin A** 100 mg/kg decreased the oral bioavailability and peak plasma concentration of fexofenadine 20 mg/kg by about 30% and 57%, respectively. No significant changes in mean residence time and terminal half-life were observed, suggesting a negligible effect of **biochanin A** on fexofenadine hepatic or renal elimination.[1]

Mechanism

Fexofenadine is a substrate for P-glycoprotein and OATP, both of which affect fexofenadine uptake. Biochanin A appears to preferentially inhibit OATP over P-glycoprotein in the intestine, leading to the decreased oral absorption of fexofenadine.

Importance and management

There appears to be no clinical data regarding an interaction between biochanin A and fexofenadine, and therefore the clinical relevance of the experimental data needs to be determined. However, the modest reduction in bioavailability of fexofenadine suggests that a clinically important interaction is unlikely. No action is therefore required.

1. Peng SX, Ritchie DM, Cousineau M, Danser E, Dewire R, Floden J. Altered oral bioavailability and pharmacokinetics of P-glycoprotein substrates by coadministration of biochanin A. *J Pharm Sci* (2006) 95, 1984–93.

Isoflavones + Food

No interactions found

Isoflavones + Herbal medicines

No interactions found. Isoflavones are regularly ingested as part of the diet.

Isoflavones + Nicotine

Soya isoflavones slightly decrease the metabolism of nicotine.

Clinical evidence

The effects of soya isoflavones on nicotine metabolism were investigated in a study in 7 healthy Japanese subjects who were nonsmokers. Taking an isoflavone tablet (containing **daidzein** 4.2 mg, **genistein** 5.2 mg and **glycitein** 600 micrograms) six times daily for 5 days, in addition to their usual diet, slightly reduced nicotine metabolism by about 24% (measured 2 hours after chewing a piece of nicotine gum). This was when compared with nicotine metabolism after abstaining from soya foods for one week.[1]

Experimental evidence

In vitro, these isoflavones decreased nicotine metabolism, by inhibiting the cytochrome P450 isoenzyme CYP2A6.[1]

Mechanism

Isoflavones slightly decrease the metabolism of nicotine by the inhibition of CYP2A6.

Importance and management

Although evidence is limited to one study, it is a well-designed clinical study. The minor change in nicotine metabolism when the subjects were taking isoflavones suggests that isoflavone supplements are unlikely to have a clinically relevant effect on the efficacy of nicotine replacement therapy. No action is therefore needed.

1. Nakajima M, Itoh M, Yamanaka H, Fukami T, Tokudome S, Yamamoto Y, Yamamoto H, Yokoi T. Isoflavones inhibit nicotine C-oxidation catalyzed by human CYP2A6. *J Clin Pharmacol* (2006) 46, 337–44.

Isoflavones + Paclitaxel

The interaction between isoflavones and paclitaxel is based on experimental evidence only.

Clinical evidence

No interactions found.

Experimental evidence

In a study in *rats,* **genistein** 10 mg/kg given orally 30 minutes before a single dose of oral or intravenous paclitaxel modestly increased the AUC of paclitaxel by 55% and 43%, respectively. The increase in AUC with a lower dose of **genistein** 3.3 mg/kg was not significant, although it did increase the peak concentration of paclitaxel by 67%.[1]

In another similar study, **biochanin A** 100 mg/kg caused a marked 3.8-fold increase in the oral bioavailability of paclitaxel 20 mg/kg.[2]

Mechanism

It seems that these isoflavones increase the systemic exposure of oral paclitaxel by inhibiting P-glycoprotein. In addition, isoflavones might reduce paclitaxel drug resistance via their effects on P-glycoprotein.

Importance and management

The available evidence for an interaction between isoflavones and paclitaxel is from experimental studies, the clinical relevance of which needs to be determined. Furthermore, paclitaxel is given intravenously, and the effect of biochanin A has only been assessed with oral paclitaxel. However, genistein modestly increased the AUC of intravenous paclitaxel, and therefore, until more is known, some caution might be appropriate with high doses of these individual isoflavones, in view of the possibility of increased exposure and increased toxicity of paclitaxel.

1. Li X, Choi JS. Effect of genistein on the pharmacokinetics of paclitaxel administered orally or intravenously in rats. *Int J Pharm* (2007) 337, 188–93.
2. Peng SX, Ritchie DM, Cousineau M, Danser E, Dewire R, Floden J. Altered oral bioavailability and pharmacokinetics of P-glycoprotein substrates by coadministration of biochanin A. *J Pharm Sci* (2006) 95, 1984–93.

Isoflavones + Tamoxifen

The available evidence on the effect of isoflavone supplements on the efficacy of tamoxifen in breast cancer is inconclusive, and the effect of isoflavones on breast tissue appears to be complex. It is possible that whether the effect is beneficial or antagonistic might be related to the dose of isoflavones used, and also the oestrogen status of the patient (pre- or postmenopausal).

Evidence and mechanism

(a) Breast cancer

In various *animal* studies, soya isoflavones have either inhibited or enhanced the preventative effect of tamoxifen on the development of breast cancer. Note that the body of evidence is vast, and only a selection of representative papers have therefore been cited. For example, in a study in *rats* given tamoxifen, a diet supplemented with **daidzein** increased protection against chemically-induced breast cancer, whereas a diet supplemented with **genistein** reduced protection, when compared with tamoxifen alone.[1] In another study, a 'low-dose' isoflavone enriched diet (**genistein** plus **daidzein**) halved the protective effect of tamoxifen against the development of breast tumours, whereas a soy meal or 'high-dose' isoflavones did not have any effect.[2] In yet another study, **genistein** and tamoxifen had a synergistic effect on delaying the growth of oestrogen-dependent breast tumours in *mice,* especially at lower levels of tamoxifen.[3]

Note that disparate findings (both prevention and stimulation) have been found for **genistein** alone on induction of mammary tumours in *animals.* It has been suggested that the effect might depend on age, with a preventative effect seen at a young age, and a stimulatory effect seen when oestrogen levels are low, as occurs postmenopausally. Note also that there is a large body of epidemiological data on the effect of dietary soya products on the risk of breast cancer, which suggest a possible reduction in risk.[4]

Some *animal* studies have clearly shown that **genistein** can antagonise the inhibitory effect of tamoxifen on growth of oestrogen-dependent human breast cancer.[5] In an *in vitro* study, this effect was shown to be biphasic, with low levels of **genistein** simulating cancer cell growth, and high levels of **genistein** inhibiting cancer cell growth.[2] Similarly, *in vitro* studies have shown that **genistein** has a synergistic or additive inhibitory effect on the growth of breast cancer cells exposed to tamoxifen,[6] or antagonises the response of breast cancer cells to tamoxifen.[7]

Note that, in one study in 17 women with biopsy-confirmed breast cancer, supplementation with soya isoflavones 200 mg daily for 2 weeks did not increase tumour growth over the 2 to 6 weeks before surgery. There was a trend towards cancer growth inhibition in the isoflavone treatment group, manifested as an increase in the apoptosis/mitosis ratio, when compared with those from a historical control group, although this was not statistically significant.[8] However, in another study in women requiring surgery for a benign or malignant breast tumour, supplementation with dietary soy, containing isoflavones 45 mg daily for 2 weeks, increased proliferation

markers in a healthy zone of the breast.[9] Similarly, another study of dietary supplementation with soya protein (providing 37.4 mg of **genistein** daily) for 6 months found an increase in breast secretion (an assessment of breast gland function) in pre-menopausal women, but a small or lack of an increase, in postmenopausal women and epithelial hyperplasia in about one-third of the women, which was suggestive of oestrogenic breast tissue stimulation in response to **genistein**.[10]

(b) Menopausal symptoms

In a placebo-controlled crossover study in 149 women with a history of breast cancer, about two-thirds of whom were taking tamoxifen, soya isoflavones (**genistein**, **daidzein** and **glycitein**) 50 mg three times daily for 4 weeks had no effect on the incidence of hot flushes.[11] Another similar study also reported a lack of efficacy for hot flushes in 157 women breast cancer survivors given a soya beverage (90 mg isoflavones daily) or placebo beverage for 12 weeks, of whom about one-third were taking tamoxifen. Vaginal spotting was reported by 4 women who drank the soya beverage and one woman who drank the placebo beverage, but this was not thought to be due to the soya.[12] In a third study, in 72 women with breast cancer, 78% of whom were taking tamoxifen, a soya supplement (35 mg of isoflavones twice daily; *Phytosoya*) for 12 weeks had no effect on menopausal symptoms when compared with placebo.[13]

These studies are probably too short, and too small, to detect any possible effect of the isoflavones on the efficacy of tamoxifen. Nevertheless, they show that isoflavones are probably no more effective than placebo for one of the most common reasons they are used in this patient group.

(c) Tamoxifen metabolism

In a cross-sectional study in 380 Asian-American women (including Chinese and Japanese Americans) with breast cancer the serum levels of tamoxifen and its major metabolites were unrelated to serum levels of isoflavones (**genistein**, **daidzein**, **equol**) or reported dietary soya intake.[14]

In an *in vitro* study using female rat liver microsomes, **genistein** inhibited α-hydroxylation of tamoxifen (a minor metabolic route), but did not affect 4-hydroxylation, *N*-demethylation, or *N*-oxidation (major metabolic routes). A combination of three to five isoflavones (**genistein**, **daidzein**, and **glycitein**, or these three isoflavones plus **biochanin A** and **formononetin**) inhibited tamoxifen α-hydroxylation to a greater extent, but did not decrease the formation of other metabolites. Studies using selective chemical inhibitors showed that tamoxifen α-hydroxylation was mainly mediated by CYP1A2 and CYP3A1/2 in *rats.* Although α-hydroxytamoxifen is a minor metabolite of tamoxifen, it is thought to be responsible for DNA adduct formation and increased risk of endometrial cancer with tamoxifen. The authors concluded that using **genistein** and its isoflavone analogs with tamoxifen might potentially be beneficial because of the inhibition of the formation of α-hydroxytamoxifen.[15] However, this requires confirmation in humans. Also, note that isoflavones themselves may not be free of endometrial adverse effects, for example, in one study, long-term clinical use of isoflavones (**genistein**, **daidzein**, **glycitein**) induced endometrial hyperplasia in some women.[16]

Importance and management

The available evidence on the effect of isoflavone supplements on the efficacy of tamoxifen in breast cancer is inconclusive, and the effect of isoflavones on breast tissue appears to be complex. It is possible that whether the effect is beneficial or antagonistic might be related to the dose of isoflavones used, and also the oestrogen status of the patient (pre- or postmenopausal). Because of differences in gut flora, there are individual differences in the metabolism of isoflavones, which might have important implications for their effects: for example, studies measuring urinary equol (which has more potent oestrogenic effects than daidzein) excretion after soya consumption indicate that only about one-third of Western individuals metabolise daidzein to equol.[17]

Most authorities recommend that patients taking oestrogen antagonists (that is, drugs such as tamoxifen and the aromatase inhibitors) for breast cancer should avoid isoflavone supplements. Given the available evidence, this seems a sensible precaution, particularly because there is no clear clinical evidence that isoflavones are beneficial for menopausal symptoms in these women. The advice to avoid isoflavone supplements is not usually extended to soya foods, although some have argued that available data does not appear to warrant making this distinction.[18] Further study is needed.

1. Constantinou AI, White BEP, Tonetti D, Yang Y, Liang W, Li W, van Breemen RB. The soy isoflavone daidzein improves the capacity of tamoxifen to prevent mammary tumours. *Eur J Cancer* (2005) 41, 647–54.
2. Liu B, Edgerton S, Yang X, Kim A, Ordonez-Ercan D, Mason T, Alvarez K, McKimmey C, Liu N, Thor A. Low-dose dietary phytoestrogen abrogates tamoxifen-associated mammary tumor prevention. *Cancer Res* (2005) 65, 879–86.
3. Mai Z, Blackburn GL, Zhou JR. Soy phytochemicals synergistically enhance the preventive effect of tamoxifen on the growth of estrogen-dependent human breast carcinoma in mice. *Carcinogenesis* (2007) 28, 1217–23.
4. Qin L-Q, Xu J-Y, Wang P-Y, Hoshi K. Soyfood intake in the prevention of breast cancer risk in women: a meta-analysis of observational epidemiological studies. *J Nutr Sci Vitaminol* (2006) 52, 428–36.
5. Ju YH, Doerge DR, Allred KF, Allred CD, Helferich WG. Dietary genistein negates the inhibitory effect of tamoxifen on growth of estrogen-dependent human breast cancer (MCF-7) cells implanted in athymic mice. *Cancer Res* (2002) 62, 2474–7.
6. Tanos V, Brzezinski A, Drize O, Strauss N, Peretz T. Synergistic inhibitory effects of genistein and tamoxifen on human dysplastic and malignant epithelial breast cells in vitro. *Eur J Obstet Gynecol Reprod Biol* (2002) 102, 188–94.
7. Jones JL, Daley BJ, Enderson BL, Zhou J-R, Karlstad MD. Genistein inhibits tamoxifen effects on cell proliferation and cell cycle arrest in T47D breast cancer cells. *Am Surg* (2002) 68, 575–9.
8. Sartippour MR, Rao JY, Apple S, Wu D, Henning S, Wang H, Elashoff R, Rubio R, Heber D, Brooks MN. A pilot clinical study of short-term isoflavone supplements in breast cancer patients. *Nutr Cancer* (2004) 49, 59–65.
9. McMichael-Phillips DF, Harding C, Morton M, Roberts SA, Howell A, Potten CS, Bundred NJ. Effects of soy-protein supplementation on epithelial proliferation in the histologically normal human breast. *Am J Clin Nutr* (1998) 68 (Suppl 6), S1431–S1436.
10. Petrakis NL, Barnes S, King EB, Lowenstein J, Wiencke J, Lee MM, Miike R, Kirk M, Coward L. Stimulatory influence of soy protein isolate on breast secretion in pre- and postmenopausal women. *Cancer Epidemiol Biomarkers Prev* (1996) 5, 785–94.
11. Quella SK, Loprinzi CL, Barton DL, Knost JA, Sloan JA, LaVasseur BI, Swan D, Krupp KR, Miller KD, Novotny PJ. Evaluation of soy phytoestrogens for the treatment of hot flashes in breast cancer survivors: a North Central Cancer Treatment Group Trial. *J Clin Oncol* (2000) 18, 1068–74.
12. Van Patten CL, Olivotto IA, Chambers GK, Gelmon KA, Hislop TG, Templeton E, Wattie A, Prior JC. Effect of soy phytoestrogens on hot flashes in postmenopausal women with breast cancer: a randomized, controlled clinical trial. *J Clin Oncol* (2002) 20, 1449–55.
13. MacGregor CA, Canney PA, Patterson G, McDonald R, Paul J. A randomised double-blind controlled trial of oral soy supplements *versus* placebo for treatment of menopausal symptoms in patients with early breast cancer. *Eur J Cancer* (2005) 41, 708–14.
14. Wu AH, Pike MC, Williams LD, Spicer D, Tseng C-C, Churchwell MI, Doerge DR. Tamoxifen, soy, and lifestyle factors in Asian American women with breast cancer. *J Clin Oncol* (2007) 25, 3024–30.
15. Chen J, Halls SC, Alfaro JF, Zhou Z, Hu M. Potential beneficial metabolic interactions between tamoxifen and isoflavones via cytochrome P450-mediated pathways in female rat liver microsomes. *Pharm Res* (2004) 21, 2095–2104.
16. Unfer V, Casini ML, Costabile L, Mignosa M, Gerli S, Di Renzo GC. Endometrial effects of long-term treatment with phytoestrogens: a randomized, double-blind, placebo-controlled study. *Fertil Steril* (2004) 82, 145–8.
17. Setchell KD, Brown NM, Lydeking-Olsen E. The clinical importance of the metabolite equol-a clue to the effectiveness of soy and its isoflavones. *J Nutr* (2002) 132, 3577–84.
18. Messina MJ, Loprinzi CL. Soy for breast cancer survivors: a critical review of the literature. *J Nutr* (2001) 131 (Suppl 11), S3095–S3108.

Isoflavones + Theophylline

High doses of isoflavones might modestly increase theophylline levels.

Clinical evidence

In a placebo-controlled study in 20 healthy non-smoking subjects, pre-treatment with **daidzein** 200 mg twice daily for 10 days increased the AUC and maximum level of a single 100-mg dose of theophylline by about 34% and 24%, respectively, and increased the elimination half-life from about 9 hours to about 12 hours.[1]

Experimental evidence

The isoflavones **genistein** and **equol** were found to inhibit the cytochrome P450 isoenzyme CYP1A2.[2] Conversely, note that soya-based infant formula *induced* CYP1A2 *in vitro*, see Soya + Caffeine, page 432.

Mechanism

Daidzein, and some other isoflavones, appear to be moderate inhibitors of cytochrome P450 isoenzyme CYP1A2, of which theophylline is a substrate.

Importance and management

The dose of daidzein used in this study was higher than that usually taken in isoflavone supplements, or as part of the diet, and the effects on theophylline pharmacokinetics were modest. Nevertheless, bear in mind that high doses of isoflavones might modestly increase theophylline levels and that this could be clinically important in patients with theophylline levels already at the higher end of the therapeutic range. Note that an increase in theophylline levels has been seen in a patient given the synthetic isoflavone, ipriflavone.[3] **Aminophylline** would be expected to interact similarly.

Note also that, conversely, there is evidence that infants receiving formula feeds, (which may include soya-based formula) require higher doses of caffeine (which, like theophylline, is a substrate of CYP1A2) than those that are breastfed, see Soya + Caffeine, page 432.

1. Peng W-X, Li H-D, Zhou H-H. Effect of daidzein on CYP1A2 activity and pharmacokinetics of theophylline in healthy volunteers. *Eur J Clin Pharmacol* (2003) 59, 237–41.
2. Helsby NA, Chipman JK, Gescher A, Kerr D. Inhibition of mouse and human CYP 1A- and 2E1-dependent substrate metabolism by the isoflavonoids genistein and equol. *Food Chem Toxicol* (1998) 36, 375–82.
3. Takahashi J, Kawakatsu K, Wakayama T, Sawaoka H. Elevation of serum theophylline levels by ipriflavone in a patient with chronic obstructive pulmonary disease. *Eur J Clin Pharmacol* (1992) 43, 207–8.

I

Ispaghula

Plantago ovata Forssk (Plantaginaceae)

Synonym(s) and related species

Blond psyllium, Indian plantago, Pale psyllium, *Plantago ispaghula*, Psyllium, Spogel.

Note that the term ispaghula is used only for *P. ovata*, whereas the term psyllium is applied to a number of Plantago species (*Plantago psyllium, Plantago indica* and *Plantago ovata*). Psyllium is sometimes obtained from other Plantago species.

Pharmacopoeias

PhEur 7.5 (Ispaghula husk) *P. ovata*

PhEur 7.5 (Ispaghula seed) *P. ovata*

USP 35-NF30 S1 (Plantago seed) *P. psyllium, P. indica,* or *P. ovata*

USP 35-NF30 S1 (Psyllium husk) *P. ovata* or *P. psyllium*

USP 35-NF30 S1 (Psyllium hemicellulose) *P. ovata*

Constituents

The main active constituent of ispaghula seed is the mucilage, composed mainly of arabinoxylan mucopolysaccharides, which is localised in the husk. The monoterpene alkaloids (+)-boschniakine (indicaine) and (+)-boschniakinic acid (plantagonine); the phenylethanoids forsythoside and acteoside; sterols including campesterol, β-sitosterol, and stigmasterol; and the triterpenes α- and β-amyrin are also present.

Use and indications

Ispaghula seeds and seed husks are used as a demulcent and bulk laxative.

Pharmacokinetics

No pharmacokinetic data. Ispaghula is not absorbed into the systemic circulation.

Interactions overview

Theoretically, ispaghula should not be given with mesalazine (mesalamine) but no interaction was seen in one study. Ispaghula may reduce the bioavailability of carbamazepine and lithium, but does not appear to affect the absorption of digoxin, ethinylestradiol, gemfibrozil or warfarin and related drugs.

Interactions monographs

- Carbamazepine, page 307
- Digoxin, page 307
- Ethinylestradiol, page 307
- Food, page 307
- Gemfibrozil, page 307
- Herbal Medicines, page 308
- Lithium, page 308
- Mesalazine (Mesalamine), page 308
- Warfarin and related drugs, page 308

Ispaghula + Carbamazepine

In a very small study, the bioavailability of carbamazepine was reduced by ispaghula.

Clinical evidence

In a study in 4 healthy subjects, 3.5 g of ispaghula husk given with a single 200-mg dose of carbamazepine reduced the AUC and maximum plasma concentration of carbamazepine by 45% and 52% respectively. The time to reach maximum plasma concentration was increased 4-fold.[1]

Experimental evidence

No relevant data found.

Mechanism

Not established. The author suggests a number of mechanisms related to the gastrointestinal actions of bulk laxatives ranging from formation of the viscous gel retarding dissolution of the dissolved drug to reduction in transit time and stimulation of peristalsis reducing the time available for absorption.[1]

Importance and management

Evidence is limited to this one very small study. In general, ispaghula is not considered to interact with carbamazepine. However, if the reductions in carbamazepine bioavailability that occurred in the study were replicated in clinical practice, then it is possible that symptom control (most seriously when carbamazepine is given for seizures), may be affected. It would seem prudent to bear this in mind in the event that a patient stabilised on carbamazepine suddenly experiences an otherwise unexplained reduction in symptom control after starting a preparation containing ispaghula.

1. Etman MA. Effect of a bulk forming laxative on the bioavailability of carbamazepine in man. *Drug Dev Ind Pharm* (1995) 21, 1901–6.

Ispaghula + Digoxin

Bulk-forming laxatives containing ispaghula appear to have no significant effect on the absorption of digoxin.

Clinical evidence

An ispaghula preparation (*Vi-Siblin S*) was found to have no significant effect on the serum digoxin levels of 16 elderly patients.[1] The same lack of effect was seen in another study in 6 healthy subjects and 10 patients also given ispaghula (*Visiblin*)[2] and in a further 15 patients given 3.6 g of an ispaghula preparation (*Metamucil*) three times daily.[3]

Experimental evidence

No interactions found.

Mechanism

Not established. Digoxin can bind to some extent to fibre within the gut.[4] However, *in vitro* studies (with bran, carrageenan, pectin, sodium pectinate, xylan and carboxymethylcellulose) have shown that most of the binding is reversible.[5]

Importance and management

Ispaghula (as *Vi-Siblin* or *Metamucil*) does not appear to have a clinically important effect on serum digoxin levels. No special precautions would appear to be necessary.

1. Nordström M, Melander A, Robertsson E, Steen B. Influence of wheat bran and of a bulk-forming ispaghula cathartic on the bioavailability of digoxin in geriatric in-patients. *Drug Nutr Interact* (1987) 5, 67–9.

2. Reissell P, Manninen V. Effect of administration of activated charcoal and fibre on absorption, excretion and steady state blood levels of digoxin and digitoxin. Evidence for intestinal secretion of glycosides. *Acta Med Scand Suppl* (1982) 668, 88–90.
3. Walan A, Bergdahl B, Skoog M-L. Study of digoxin bioavailability during treatment with a bulk forming laxative (*Metamucil*). *Scand J Gastroenterol* (1977) 12 (Suppl 45), 111.
4. Floyd RA. Digoxin interaction with bran and high fiber foods. *Am J Hosp Pharm* (1978) 35, 660.
5. Hamamura J, Burros BC, Clemens RA, Smith CH. Dietary fiber and digoxin. *Fedn Proc* (1985) 44, 759.

Ispaghula + Ethinylestradiol

The interaction between psyllium and ethinylestradiol is based on experimental evidence only.

Clinical evidence

No interactions found.

Experimental evidence

In an *animal* study, the administration of 3.5 g of ispaghula husk with 1 mg/kg of ethinylestradiol resulted in a minor increase in the extent of absorption of the ethinylestradiol, a minor decrease in its maximum plasma concentration and a slower rate of absorption compared with ethinylestradiol alone.[1]

Mechanism

No mechanism expected.

Importance and management

Evidence is limited to one *animal* study, which suggests that the effects of ispaghula on ethintlestradiol pharmacokinetics are unlikely to be of any clinical importance.

1. Garcra JJ, Fernández N, Diez MJ, Sahagún A, González A, Alonso ML, Prieto C, Calle AP, Sierra M. Influence of two dietary fibers in the oral bioavailability and other pharmacokinetic parameters of ethinyloestradiol *Contraception* (2000) 62, 253–7.

Ispaghula + Food

Ispaghula does not affect the absorption of calcium from food.

Evidence, mechanism, importance and management

A controlled study in 15 healthy subjects found that ispaghula 3.4 g (as *Metamucil*) reduced the absorption of **calcium** from a fortified orange juice drink (Citrus Hill Plus Calcium) providing 219 mg calcium, by 2.4% when administered together, compared with the orange juice alone.[1] The reduction in calcium absorption seen in this study is unlikely to be clinically important and there would seem to be no need to separate ispaghula administration and food or calcium consumption.

1. Heaney RP, Weaver CM. Effect of psyllium on absorption of co-ingested calcium. *J Am Geriatr Soc* (1995) 43, 261–3.

Ispaghula + Gemfibrozil

In a small study, psyllium caused a minor reduction in gemfibrozil exposure.

Evidence, mechanism, importance and management

In a study in 10 healthy subjects given gemfibrozil 600 mg with, or 2 hours after, ispaghula 3 g in 240 mL of water, the AUC of gemfibrozil was reduced by about 10%.[1] This reduction is almost certainly too small to be clinically significant.

1. Forland FC, Cutler RE. The effect of psyllium on the pharmacokinetics of gemfibrozil. *Clin Res* (1990) 38, 94A.

I

Ispaghula + Herbal medicines

No interactions found.

Ispaghula + Lithium

In an isolated case, the withdrawal of ispaghula resulted in an increase in lithium levels. Ispaghula slightly reduced the absorption of lithium in a study in healthy subjects.

Clinical evidence

A 47-year-old woman who had recently started taking lithium was found to have a blood lithium level of 0.4 mmol/L five days after an increment in her lithium dose and whilst also taking one teaspoonful of ispaghula husk twice daily. The ispaghula husk was stopped 3 days later and lithium levels measured 4 days later were found to be 0.76 mmol/L.[1] A study in 6 healthy subjects similarly found that the absorption of lithium (as measured by the urinary excretion) was reduced by about 14% by ispaghula.[2]

Experimental evidence

No interactions found.

Mechanism

Not understood. One idea is that the absorption of the lithium from the gut is reduced by ispaghula.[1,2]

Importance and management

Information is very limited and the general importance of this interaction is uncertain, but it would seem prudent to bear this interaction in mind in patients taking lithium who are given ispaghula preparations. If an interaction is suspected consider monitoring lithium levels and separating the administration of the two drugs by at least an hour, or use an alternative laxative.

1. Perlman BB. Interaction between lithium salts and ispaghula husk. *Lancet* (1990) 335, 416.
2. Toutoungi M, Schulz P, Widmer J, Tissot R. Probable interaction entre le psyllium et le lithium. *Therapie* (1990) 45, 358–60.

Ispaghula + Mesalazine (Mesalamine)

On theoretical grounds, formulations designed to release mesalazine in response to the higher pH in the colon should not be given with ispaghula. However, a study suggests that ispaghula does not affect the bioavailability of mesalazine.

Clinical evidence and mechanism

Asacol is a preparation of mesalazine coated with an acrylic based resin (*Eudragit S*) that disintegrates above pH 7 and thereby releases the mesalazine into the terminal ileum and colon.[1] Ispaghula can lower colonic pH (from 6.5 to 5.8 in the right colon,

and from 7.3 to 6.6 in the left colon).[2] However, a study in patients given mesalazine found that despite this colonic acidification by ispaghula husk (*Fybogel*), the release of mesalazine appeared not to be affected, as 24-hour faecal and urinary excretion of mesalazine metabolites were unchanged.[3]

Experimental evidence

No interactions found.

Importance and management

Although on theoretical grounds ispaghula husk might be expected to reduce the effects of mesalazine, from the above study no interaction of clinical importance seems to occur, and there have been no reports as yet that a clinically important interaction occurs in practice. However, the UK manufacturers of *Asacol* recommend avoiding concurrent use of preparations that can lower the pH of the gut as they may reduce the efficacy of mesalazine.[1] Also note that this interaction is not mentioned by the US manufacturers of *Asacol*.[4] Furthermore, Salofalk is another preparation of mesalazine with a pH-dependent enteric coating.[5] This preparation disintegrates above pH 6, but no warning regarding drugs that affect the pH in the lower part of the gut is given.

1. Asacol 800 mg MR Tablets Mesalazine. Warner Chilcott UK Limited UK Summary of product characteristics, November 2010.
2. Evans DF, Crompton J, Pye G, Hardcastle JD. The role of dietary fibre on acidification of the colon in man. *Gastroenterology* (1988) 94, A118.
3. Riley SA, Tavares IA, Bishai PM, Bennett A, Mani V. Mesalazine release from coated tablets: effect of dietary fibre. *Br J Clin Pharmacol* (1991) 32, 248–50.
4. Asacol HD Mesalamine. Procter & Gamble Pharmaceuticals US Prescribing information, October 2010.
5. Salofalk Tablets Mesalazine. Dr Falk Pharma UK Ltd. UK Summary of product characteristics, March 2012.

Ispaghula + Warfarin and related drugs

Ispaghula did not affect either the absorption or the anticoagulant effects of warfarin in one study. A cohort study also found no evidence of an interaction in patients taking acenocoumarol or phenprocoumon and ispaghula.

Evidence, mechanism, importance and management

In a study in 6 healthy subjects, ispaghula (given as a 14-g dose of colloid (*Metamucil*) in a small amount of water with a single 40-mg dose of **warfarin**, and three further doses of ispaghula every 2 hours thereafter) did not affect either the absorption or the anticoagulant effects of the **warfarin**.[1] Similarly, in a population-based cohort study in patients taking **acenocoumarol** or **phenprocoumon**, there was no increased risk of over-anticoagulation (INR greater than 6) associated with the use of ispaghula (psyllium seeds), although the number of people treated was small.[2] No alteration of the anticoagulant response would therefore be expected on concurrent use.

1. Robinson DS, Benjamin DM, McCormack JJ. Interaction of warfarin and nonsystemic gastrointestinal drugs. *Clin Pharmacol Ther* (1971) 12, 491–5.
2. Visser LE, Penning-van Beest FJA, Wilson JHP, Vulto AG, Kasbergen AAH, De Smet PAGM, Hofman A, Stricker BHC. Overanticoagulation associated with combined use of lactulose and acenocoumarol or phenprocoumon. *Br J Clin Pharmacol* (2003) 57, 522–4.

Jamaica dogwood

Piscidia piscipula (L.) Sarg. (Fabaceae)

Synonym(s) and related species

Fish poison, West Indian dogwood.

Erythrina piscipula L., *Ichthyomethia communis* S.F.Blake, *Ichthyomethia piscipula* (L.) Hitchc., *Piscidia erythrina* L., *Piscidia inebrians* Medik., *Piscidia toxicaria* Salisb., *Robinia alata* Mill.

Not to be confused with American dogwood (*Cornus florida* L.), which is unrelated.

Constituents

The major constituents of the bark are **isoflavones** and **rotenoids**, which include ichthynone, jamaicin, piscerythrone, piscidone, lisetin, milletone, isomillettone, dehydromillettone, **rotenone** and sumatrol. Piscidic acid and other acids are also present.

Use and indications

Jamaica dogwood is used as a sedative, mainly in compound preparations, and as an antispasmodic for various conditions including asthma, dysmennorhoea, insomnia, migraine and whooping cough. Although some *animal* studies support the sedative and antispasmodic properties, there is no clinical evidence. The rotenoids (**rotenone** in particular) are toxic to fish, hence the traditional use of Jamaica dogwood as a fish poison, and although they appear to be relatively harmless to *mammals* when ingested orally, Jamaica dogwood is irritant and toxic to humans in large doses.

Pharmacokinetics

No relevant pharmacokinetic data found. For information on the pharmacokinetics of individual isoflavones present in Jamaica dogwood, see under isoflavones, page 300.

Interactions overview

No interactions with Jamaica dogwood found. However, if the sedative effect of Jamaica dogwood is proven clinically, these effects might reasonably be expected to be additive with those of other CNS depressant drugs. For information on the interactions of individual isoflavones present in Jamaica dogwood, see under isoflavones, page 300.

Java tea

Orthosiphon stamineus Benth. (Lamiaceae)

Synonym(s) and related species

Clerodendranthus spicatus (Thunb.) C.Y. Wu ex H.W. Li, *Clerodendranthus stamineus*, *Orthosiphon aristatus* Miq., *Orthosiphon aristatus* var. *aristatus*, *Orthosiphon spicatus* Benth, *Catoferia spicata*,

Pharmacopoeias

Java Tea (*BP 2012, PhEur 7.5*)

Constituents

The leaf contains **pimarane diterpenes**, including the orthosiphols, orthosiphonones and related compounds; **triterpenes**; **benzochromenes** including orthochromene A, methylripariochromene A and acetovanillochromene; **flavonoids** such as sinensetin (to which it may be standardised), eupatorin, salvigenin, trimethylapigenin, methylated and hydroxylated derivatives of scutellarein, luteolin and methoxyflavone, and quercetin and kaempferol glycosides; **phenylpropanoids** including rosmarinic acid and caffeic acid derivatives; and potassium salts. The **essential oil** (0.02–0.7%) is composed mainly of β-elemene, β-caryophyllene, α-humulene, and β-caryophyllene oxide.

Use and indications

Java tea is traditionally used to treat hypertension, diabetes, bladder and kidney disorders, gallstones, gout and rheumatism. It is reported to have diuretic and hypoglycaemic properties.

Pharmacokinetics

In *in vitro* studies, none of four extracts of Java tea, or the constituents sinensetin, eupatorin or rosmarinic acid, showed inhibitory effects on CYP2C9. Of the extracts and constituents, the activity of CYP2D6 was inhibited by just eupatorin. Moderate inhibition of CYP3A4 activity was also shown by the dichloromethane and petroleum ether extracts, but not by the aqueous or methanol extracts, and strong inhibition was shown by eupatorin.[1] In another similar set of *in vitro* studies, the activity of CYP2C19 was inhibited by just the petroleum ether extract of Java tea, and eupatorin.[2] These studies provide some reassurance that aqueous and ethanol extracts of Java tea (i.e. the extracts in general use in herbal medicine) are unlikely to cause clinically relevant inhibition of CYP3A4, CYP2D6, CYP2C9 or CYP2C19. For information on the pharmacokinetics of individual flavonoids present in java tea, see under flavonoids, page 213.

Interactions overview

No interactions with java tea found. For information on the interactions of individual flavonoids present in java tea, see under flavonoids, page 213.

1. Yan P, Abd-Rashid BA, Ismail Z, Ismail R, Mak JW, Pook PC, Er HM, Ong CE. In vitro effects of active constituents and extracts of *Orthosiphon stamineus* on the activities of three major human cDNA-expressed cytochrome P450 enzymes. *Chem Biol Interact* (2011) 190, 1–8.
2. Yan P, Abd-Rashid BA, Ismail Z, Ismail R, Mak JW, Pook PC, Er HM, Ong CE. *In vitro* modulatory effects of *Andrographis paniculata*, *Centella asiatica* and *Orthosiphon stamineus* on cytochrome P450 2C19 (CYP2C19). *J Ethnopharmacol* (2011) 133, 881–7.

J

Juniper

Juniperus communis L. (Cupressaceae)

Synonym(s) and related species

Common juniper, Juniper berry, Mountain juniper.

Pharmacopoeias

Juniper (*BP 2012, PhEur 7.5*); Juniper Oil (*BP 2012, PhEur 7.5*).

Constituents

Juniper berries contain a volatile oil consisting primarily of **monoterpenes** including sabinene, α-pinene, myrcene, limonene and others; **sesquiterpenes** including caryophyllene, epoxydihydrocaryophyllene, β-elemem-7α-ol and cadinene; **diterpenes** including geijerone, and the acids isocommunic, isopimaric, and torulosic and others; **flavonoids** such as quercetin, isoquercitrin, apigenin and their glycosides; **tannins**, mainly proanthocyanidins (condensed), gallocatechin and epigallocatechin and the **lignan**, desoxypodophyllotoxin.

Use and indications

Traditionally, juniper is used as a diuretic, and for dyspepsia, cystitis, arteriosclerosis and inflammatory or rheumatic conditions, where the essential oil is applied topically to the joints or muscles. Juniper berries are used as a flavouring in foods and drinks.

Pharmacokinetics

No relevant pharmacokinetic data found. For information on the pharmacokinetics of individual flavonoids present in juniper, see under flavonoids, page 213.

Interactions overview

An isolated case of lithium toxicity has been reported in a patient who took a herbal diuretic containing juniper among other ingredients, see under Parsley + Lithium, page 364. For information on the interactions of individual flavonoids present in juniper, see under flavonoids, page 213.

Interactions monographs

- Food, page 312
- Herbal medicines, page 312

J

Juniper + Food

No interactions found. Juniper berries are used as a flavouring in foods and drinks.

Juniper + Herbal medicines

No interactions found.

Juniper + Lithium

For mention of a case of lithium toxicity in a woman who had been taking a non-prescription herbal diuretic containing corn silk, *Equisetum hyemale,* juniper, buchu, parsley and bearberry, all of which are believed to have diuretic actions, see under Parsley + Lithium, page 364.

J

Karela

Momordica charantia L. (Cucurbitaceae)

Synonym(s) and related species

Balsam pear, Bitter cucumber, Bitter gourd, Bitter melon, Cundeamor, Ku gua.

Constituents

The active constituents of the fruits are **triterpenes** including momordicin and momordicinin, and a series of cucurbitanes, momordicosides, goyaglycosides and kuguacins; **proteins** including α, β and γ-momorcharins, and momordins a and b and **polypeptide P**, also known as vegetable or plant insulin (v- or p-insulin). **Pyrimidines** such as such as vicine and charine are found particularly in the seed, and many sterols (including charantin), fatty acids and volatile compounds have also been identified in the fruit. The chemical composition of the leaf is less well-known, but it does contain goyasaponins.

Use and indications

The fruits of karela are eaten all over the world, as a food as well as for their medicinal properties. The leaves are occasionally consumed as 'bush tea'. Most commonly karela has been used for the treatment of type 2 diabetes. Despite well-documented hypoglycaemic effects, a Cochrane review has concluded that the evidence is conflicting and issues of standardisation must be addressed before it can be recommended for clinical use.[1] Other traditional uses include the treatment of gastrointestinal cramps, cancer, viral infections, and immune disorders. Karela is contraindicated in pregnant women as it can induce abortion in animals. Hepatotoxicity has been reported in animal studies and ingestion of vicine (from the seed) may cause favism (an acute haemolytic crisis in patients with glucose-6-phosphate dehydrogenase (G6PD) deficiency often seen in response to broad beans).

Pharmacokinetics

In an *in vitro* study, an aqueous extract of karela leaves inhibited the 4-hydroxylation of diclofenac by CYP2C9.[2] In another *in vitro* study, an alcoholic extract of karela was found to inhibit P-glycoprotein activity.[3] Whether these effects are clinically relevant is unclear.

Interactions overview

Karela appears to have blood glucose-lowering effects and can potentiate the effects of chlorpropamide and other antidiabetics.

Interactions monographs

- Antidiabetics, page 314
- Food, page 314
- Herbal medicines, page 314

1. Ooi CP, Yassin Z, Hamid TA. *Momordica charantia* for type 2 diabetes mellitus (), .
2. Appiah-Opong R, Commandeur JNM, Axson C, Vermeulen NPE. Interactions between cytochromes P450, glutathione S-transferases and Ghanaian medicinal plants. *Food Chem Toxicol* (2008) 46, 3598–3603.
3. Konishi T, Satsu H, Hatsugai Y, Aizwa K, Inakuma T, Nagata S, Sakuda S, Nagasawa H, Shimizu M. Inhibitory effect of a bitter melon extract on the P-glycoprotein activity in intestinal Caco-2 cells. *Br J Pharmacol* (2004) 143, 379–87.

K

Karela + Antidiabetics

The blood glucose-lowering effects of chlorpropamide and other antidiabetics can be increased by karela.

Clinical evidence

A report of a patient whose diabetes was poorly controlled on diet and **chlorpropamide**, but much better controlled when she ate curry containing karela, provides some evidence that the blood glucose-lowering effects of karela and conventional oral antidiabetics can be additive.[1] Small, non-controlled studies have subsequently shown that karela produces a significant improvement in glucose tolerance in patients with type 2 diabetes, both when they are taking **chlorpropamide**,[2] **tolbutamide**,[2] **glibenclamide**,[2,3] **glymidine**[2] or **metformin**,[3] and when they are not taking antidiabetics.[4–6] In these studies, karela was given orally as a juice from the fruit,[2,4] dried powdered fruit,[5,6] fried fruits,[2] aqueous extract,[6] or solvent extract from the fruit.[3]

However, in a small, randomised, placebo-controlled study in 40 patients with type 2 diabetes given karela capsules (*Charantia*) three times daily after meals for 3 months, both karela and placebo had no statistically significant effect on HbA1c (there was a very slight *increase* of 0.28% and 0.5%, respectively) and there was no change in fasting blood glucose (slight decrease with karela and an increase with placebo). In this study, karela was taken in addition to standard **oral antidiabetics** (types not stated) and patients included both those newly diagnosed and those with established diabetes, with HbA1c levels of 7 to 9%.[7]

A case report describes hypoglycaemic coma and seizures in two young non-diabetic children after they were given karela tea.[8]

Experimental evidence

In a study in *rats,* the combination of an alcoholic extract of karela with rosiglitazone 2 mg/kg or 5 mg/kg caused a greater reduction in serum glucose levels than either dose of rosiglitazone alone, in both an oral glucose tolerance test and streptozotocin-induced diabetes. In addition, the combination of karela extract with low-dose rosiglitazone had an effect on serum glucose concentrations similar to that seen with high-dose of rosiglitazone alone.[9]

Mechanism

The blood glucose-lowering effects of karela may be due to the constituent polypeptide P[10] (see under constituents, page 313) This substance is effective when given subcutaneously,[11] but its oral activity is uncertain.[12] Other constituents with blood glucose-lowering effects include charantin and vicine. Karela may have both insulin-like effects and stimulate insulin secretion.[12]

Importance and management

The blood glucose-lowering activity of karela appears to be established, although the best controlled clinical study so far found its effects to be minimal. Health professionals should therefore be aware that patients may possibly be using karela as well as more conventional drugs to control their diabetes. Irregular consumption of karela as part of the diet could possibly contribute to unexplained fluctuations in diabetic control.

1. Aslam M, Stockley IH. Interaction between curry ingredient (karela) and drug (chlorpropamide) *Lancet* (1979) i, 607.
2. Leatherdale BA, Panesar KR, Singh G, Atkins TW, Bailey CJ, Bignell AHC. Improvement in glucose tolerance due to Momordica charantia (karela). *BMJ* (1981) 282, 1823–4.
3. Tongia A, Tongia SK, Dave M. Phytochemical determination and extraction of Momordica charantia fruit and its hypoglycemic potentiation of oral hypoglycemic drugs in diabetes mellitus (NIDDM). *Indian J Physiol Pharmacol* (2004) 48, 241–4.
4. Welihinda J, Karunanayake EH, Sheriff MHR, Jaysinghe KSA. Effect of *Momordica charantia* on the glucose tolerance in maturity onset diabetes. *J Ethnopharmacol* (1986) 17, 277–82.
5. Akhtar MS. Trial of Momordica Charantia Linn (Karela) powder in patients with maturity-onset diabetes. *J Pakistan Med Assoc* (1982) 32, 106–7.
6. Srivastava Y, Venkatakrishna-Bhatt H, Verma Y, Venkaiah K, Raval BH. Antidiabetic and adaptogenic properties of *Momordica charantia* extract: an experimental and clinical evaluation. *Phytother Res* (1993) 7, 285–9.
7. Dans AML, Villarruz MVC, Jimeno CA, Javelosa MAU, Chua J, Bautista R, Velez CGB. The effect of *Momordica charantia* capsule preparation on glycemic control in type 2 diabetes mellitus needs further studies. *J Clin Epidemiol* (2007) 60, 554–9.
8. Hulin A, Wavelet M, Desbordes JM. Intoxication aiguë par *Momordica charantia* (sorrossi). A propos de deux cas. *Sem Hop Paris* (1988) 64, 2847–8.
9. Nivitabishekam SN, Asad M, Prasad VS. Pharmacodynamic interaction of *Momordica charantia* with rosiglitazone in rats. *Chem Biol Interact* (2009) 177, 247–53.
10. Khanna P, Jain SC, Panagariya A, Dixit VP. Hypoglycemic activity of polypeptide-p from a plant source. *J Nat Prod* (1981) 44, 648–55.
11. Baldwa VS, Bhandari CM, Pangaria A, Goyal RK. Clinical trial in patients with diabetes mellitus of an insulin-like compound obtained from plant source. *Ups J Med Sci* (1977) 82, 39–41.
12. Raman A, Lau C. Anti-diabetic properties and phytochemistry of *Momordica charantia* (Cucurbitaceae). *Phytomedicine* (1996) 2, 349–62.

Karela + Food

No interactions found.

Karela + Herbal medicines

No interactions found.

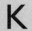

Kava

Piper methysticum G.Forst. (Piperaceae)

Synonym(s) and related species

Intoxicating pepper, Kava kava, Kawa, *Methysticum methysticum*.

Constituents

The main active constituents of the root are pyrone derivatives, the **kavalactones**, which include kawain (kavain), dihydrokawain, methysticin, dihydromethysticin, yangonin, 11-methoxy-nor-yangonin, desmethoxyyangonin and the dimeric trux-yangonins I, II. Other constituents include flavonoids known as flavokavins.

Pyridone alkaloids such as pipermethystine, 3-alpha,4-alpha-epoxy-5-beta-pipermethystine and awaine are also found, but mainly concentrated in the stem and leaf.

Use and indications

Kava root is used to make a ceremonial and mildly psychoactive drink in the South Pacific islands, for its relaxing and stimulant properties. It was also traditionally used in herbal medicine to treat bronchitis, as well as inflammatory diseases such as rheumatism and gout. More recently it gained popularity for treatment of anxiety disorders.

Kava products are banned in some countries, due to reports of liver toxicity. The mechanism for this toxicity has not been established and could include the plant part used (aerial stem peelings have been used to make commercial extracts rather than the root, and contain higher levels of the alkaloid pipermethystine, which may be more hepatotoxic than the kavalactones). Alternative explanations that are being debated include the presence of mould hepatotoxins in poor quality raw material, or people with genotypes that are predisposed to the way they metabolise kavalactones. In view of the lack of evidence as to the cause of the reported hepatotoxicity, or its mechanism, kava should not be recommended for use.

Pharmacokinetics

Little is known about the pharmacokinetics of kavalactones in humans. A number of studies have investigated the effect of kava extracts on cytochrome P450 isoenzymes and drug transporters. In some *in vitro* studies, kava or its kavalactone constituents inhibited CYP1A2,[1] CYP2C19,[1,2] CYP2C9,[1,2] CYP2D6[1,2] and CYP3A4[1–3] but not CYP2E1.[1]

Of the kavalactones studied, methysticin, dihydromethysticin and desmethoxyyangonin appear to be the most potent inhibitors, with all three inhibiting CYP2C9 and CYP3A4.[1]

In contrast, *in vivo* studies have shown no effect on CYP1A2 (see Kava + Caffeine, page 317), CYP3A4 (see Kava + Benzodiazepines, page 316) or CYP2D6[3,4] activity, but have shown inhibition of CYP2E1 (see Kava + Chlorzoxazone, page 317).

In vitro studies have suggested that kava may inhibit P-glycoprotein, however there is no evidence from human pharmacokinetic studies that kava has a clinically important effect on P-glycoprotein substrates, see Kava + Digitalis glycosides, page 317.

Interactions overview

Kava may increase the CNS depression caused by alcohol and benzodiazepines, potentiate the effects of anaesthetics, and might antagonise the effects of levodopa. Kava does not affect the pharmacokinetics of caffeine, chlorzoxazone or digoxin to a clinically relevant extent.

Interactions monographs

- Alcohol, page 316
- Anaesthetics, general, page 316
- Benzodiazepines, page 316
- Caffeine, page 317
- Chlorzoxazone, page 317
- Digitalis glycosides, page 317
- Food, page 317
- Herbal Medicines, page 317
- Levodopa, page 318
- Paracetamol (Acetaminophen), page 318

1. Matthews JM, Etheridge AS, Black SR. Inhibition of human cytochrome P450 activities by kava extract and kavalactones. *Drug Metab Dispos* (2002) 30, 1153–7.
2. Matthews JM, Etheridge AS, Valentine JL, Black SR, Coleman DP, Patel P, So J, Burka LT. Pharmacokinetics and disposition of the kavalactone kawain: interaction with kava extract and kavalactones in vivo and in vitro. *Drug Metab Dispos* (2005) 33, 1555–63.
3. Gurley BJ, Gardner SF, Hubbard MA, Williams DK, Gentry WB, Khan IA, Shah A. In vivo effects of goldenseal, kava kava, black cohosh, and valerian on human cytochrome P450 1A2, 2D6, 2E1, and 3A4/5 phenotypes. *Clin Pharmacol Ther* (2005) 77, 415–26.
4. Gurley BJ, Swain A, Hubbard MA, Williams DK, Barone G, Hartsfield F, Tong Y, Carrier DJ, Cheboyina S, Battu SK. Clinical assessment of CYP2D6-mediated herb-drug interactions in humans: effects of milk thistle, black cohosh, goldenseal, kava kava, St. John's wort and Echinacea. *Mol Nutr Food Res* (2008) 52, 755–63.

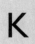

K

Kava + Alcohol

There is some evidence that kava may worsen the CNS depressant effects of alcohol.

Clinical evidence

Forty healthy subjects underwent a number of cognitive and visuo-motor tests after taking alcohol alone, kava alone, or both together. The subjects took 0.75 g/kg of alcohol (enough to give blood-alcohol levels above 50 mg%) and the kava dose was 1 g/kg. The kava drink was made by mixing middle grade Fijian kava with water and straining it to produce about 350 mL of kava liquid. It was found that kava alone had no effect on the tests, but when the kava was given with alcohol it potentiated both the perceived and measured impairment that occurred with alcohol alone.[1] However, another study found that a kava extract (WS 1490) did not enhance the negative effects of alcohol on performance tests.[2]

Experimental evidence

A study in *mice* found that when a lipid-soluble extract of kava (kava resin) was given with alcohol, sleeping times and toxicity were increased compared with kava resin or alcohol alone.[3]

Mechanism

Not established. *In vitro*, **kavalactones**, the main active constituents of kava, did not inhibit the activity of alcohol dehydrogenase suggesting no pharmacokinetic interaction via this route.[4] However there may be a pharmacodynamic interaction since kava may cause drowsiness and thus have an additive effect when taken with alcohol.

Importance and management

No very strong conclusions can be drawn from the results of these studies, but it is possible that car driving and handling other machinery may be more hazardous if kava and alcohol are taken together. Note that it has been hypothesised that concurrent use of alcohol and kava might increase the risk of hepatotoxicity.[5] Kava products are banned in some countries, due to reports of liver toxicity, see Useand indications, page 315.

1. Foo H, Lemon J. Acute effects of kava, alone or in combination with alcohol, on subjective measures of impairment and intoxication and on cognitive performance. *Drug Alcohol Rev* (1997) 16, 147–55.
2. Herberg K-W. Zum Einfluß von Kava-Spezialextrakt WS 1490 in Kombination mit Ethylalkohol auf sicherheitsrelevante Leistungsparameter. The influence of kava-special extract WS 1490 on safety-relevant performance alone and in combination with ethyl alcohol. *Blutalkohol* (1993) 30, 96–105.
3. Jamieson DD, Duffield PH. Positive interaction of ethanol and kava resin in mice. *Clin Exp Pharmacol Physiol* (1990) 17, 509–14.
4. Anke J, Fu S, Ramzan I. Kavalactones fail to inhibit alcohol dehydrogenase in vitro. *Phytomedicine* (2006) 13, 192–5.
5. Li XZ, Ramzan I. Role of ethanol in kava hepatotoxicity. *Phytother Res* (2010) 24, 475–80.

Kava + Anaesthetics, general

It has been predicted that kava may prolong or potentiate the effects of anaesthetics. The American Society of Anesthesiologists recommends that all herbal medicines should be stopped two weeks before elective surgery.

Clinical evidence

A review of the anaesthetic implications of patients taking kava suggests that it may potentiate the effects of anaesthetics and prolong sedation.[1] There is a case report of kava potentiating the effect of benzodiazepines (see Kava + Benzodiazepines, below) and some authors suggest that it could also potentiate other CNS depressants including **barbiturates**[2,3] (e.g **thiopental**), which may be used for induction anaesthesia.

Experimental evidence

No relevant data found.

Mechanism

Kava may potentiate the sedative effects of anaesthetics, possibly via GABA receptors.[2,3,1] In addition, kava might cause hypotension[1] and **kavalactones**, the main active constituents of kava, also have skeletal muscle relaxant and local anaesthetic properties.[2,3] Toxic doses can produce muscle weakness and paralysis.[3]

Importance and management

Not established. The evidence presented suggests that some caution may be warranted in patients using kava if they are given general anaesthetics. Because of the limited information, the American Society of Anesthesiologists have recommended discontinuation of all herbal medicines 2 weeks before an elective anaesthetic, and this should be applied to kava.[1]

1. Raduege KM, Kleshinski JF, Ryckman JV, Tetzlaff JE. Anesthetic considerations of the herbal, Kava. *J Clin Anesthesia* (2004) 16, 305–11.
2. Ang-Lee MK, Moss J, Yuan C-S. Herbal medicines and perioperative care. *JAMA* (2009) 286, 208–16.
3. Pepping J. Kava: *Piper methysticum*. *Am J Health-Syst Pharm* (1999) 56, 957–8.

Kava + Benzodiazepines

A man taking alprazolam became semicomatose a few days after starting to take kava, which was suggested to be due to additive sedation. The pharmacokinetics of midazolam are not affected by kava.

Clinical evidence

(a) Alprazolam

A 54-year-old man taking alprazolam, cimetidine and terazosin was hospitalised in a lethargic and disorientated state 3 days after starting to take kava, which he had bought from a local health food store. He denied having overdosed with any of these drugs. The patient became alert again after several hours.[1]

(b) Midazolam

In a study in 6 subjects, who regularly took 7 to 27 g of kavalactones, the main active constituents of kava, weekly as an aqueous kava extract, there was no change in the metabolism of a single 8-mg oral dose of midazolam before or after they stopped kava for 30 days.[2] Similar results were found in two further pharmacokinetic studies. In a study in 16 healthy subjects given kava root extract 1.227 g three times daily (standardised to contain 75 mg kavalactones per capsule) for 14 days before receiving a single 8-mg dose of oral midazolam, the pharmacokinetics of midazolam were unaffected.[3] Likewise, in another study in 12 healthy subjects given kava root extract 1 g twice daily (with no standardisation claim) for 28 days before receiving a single 8-mg dose of oral midazolam, the pharmacokinetics of midazolam were similarly unaffected.[4]

Experimental evidence

In vitro studies using human liver microsomes suggest that kava and some of its kavalactone constituents might inhibit CYP3A4, one study used midazolam 1-hydroxylation as the probe CYP3A4 substrate, see Pharmacokinetics, page 315.

Mechanism

The reason for what happened in the alprazolam case is not known, but the suggested explanation is that kavalactones, the main active constituents of kava, might have had additive sedative effects with those of alprazolam.[1,5] The studies with midazolam confirm that kava does not inhibit CYP3A4 clinically, by which a number of the benzodiazepines, including alprazolam, are metabolised.

Importance and management

The alprazolam case is an isolated report and its general importance is not known, although it fits with the theoretical pharmacological interaction anticipated. Bear the possibility of increased sedation in mind if kava and benzodiazepines are used together. No pharmacokinetic interaction occurs between midazolam and kava, and would not be expected with other similarly metabolised benzodiazepines such as alprazolam and **triazolam**.

1. Almeida JC, Grimsley EW. Coma from the health food store: interaction between kava and alprazolam. *Ann Intern Med* (1996) 125, 940–941.
2. Russmann S, Lauterburg BH, Barguil Y, Choblet E, Cabalion P, Rentsch K, Wenk M. Traditional aqueous kava extracts inhibit cytochrome P450 1A2 in humans: protective effect against environmental carcinogens? *Clin Pharmacol Ther* (2005) 77, 453–4.
3. Gurley BJ, Swain A, Hubbard MA, Hartsfield F, Thaden J, Williams DK, Gentry QWB, Tong Y. Supplementation with Goldenseal (*Hydratis Canadensis*), but not Kava Kava (*Piper methysticum*), inhibits human CYP3A activity in vivo. *Clin Pharmacol Ther* (2008) 83, 61–9.
4. Gurley BJ, Gardner SF, Hubbard MA, Williams DK, Gentry WB, Khan IA, Shah A. In vivo effects of goldenseal, kava kava, black cohosh, and valerian on human cytochrome P450 1A2, 2D6, 2E1, and 3A4/5 phenotypes. *Clin Pharmacol Ther* (2005) 77, 415–26.
5. Jussofie A, Schmiz A, Hiemke C. Kavapyrone enriched extract from *Piper methysticum* as modulator of the GABA binding site in different regions of rat brain. *Psychopharmacology (Berl)* (1994) 116, 469–74.

Kava + Caffeine

An aqueous kava extract appeared to inhibit the metabolism of caffeine in one study, whereas another controlled study using kava root extract found no interaction.

Clinical evidence

In a study in 6 subjects (3 of whom smoked tobacco) who regularly took 7 to 27 g of **kavalactones**, the main active constituents of kava, weekly as an aqueous kava extract, the metabolic ratio of caffeine was increased twofold when kava was withheld for 30 days.[1]

However, in a study in 12 non-smoking healthy subjects given kava root extract 1 g twice daily for 28 days before receiving a single 100-mg dose of oral caffeine, no significant change in the metabolic ratio of caffeine was noted.[2]

Experimental evidence

See *Mechanism* below.

Mechanism

Note that *in vitro* studies using human liver microsomes suggest that kava and some of its kavalactone constituents might inhibit the cytochrome P450 isoenzyme CYP1A2, which is responsible for the metabolism of caffeine, see Pharmacokinetics, page 315. The clinical evidence is contradictory.

Importance and management

From the controlled study, it seems unlikely that kava root extract affects the metabolism of caffeine. It is possible that, in the first study, the lack of standardisation of kava intake might have influenced the results. Further study is needed to confirm this.

1. Russman S, Lauterburg BH, Barguil Y, Choblet E, Cabalion P, Rentsch K, Wenk M. Traditional aqueous kava extracts inhibit cytochrome P450 1A2 in humans: protective effect against environmental carcinogens? *Clin Pharmacol Ther* (2005) 77, 451–4.
2. Gurley BJ, Gardner SF, Hubbard MA, Williams DK, Gentry WB, Khan IA, Shah A. In vivo effects of goldenseal, kava kava, black cohosh, and valerian on human cytochrome P450 1A2, 2D6, 2E1, and 3A4/5 phenotypes. *Clin Pharmacol Ther* (2005) 77, 415–26.

Kava + Chlorzoxazone

The metabolism of chlorzoxazone is weakly inhibited by kava.

Clinical evidence

In a study in 12 healthy subjects, kava extract 1 g (no standardisation claim) given twice daily for 28 days reduced the conversion of a single 250-mg dose of chlorzoxazone to 6-hydroxychlorzoxazone by about 40%.[1]

Experimental evidence

See *Mechanism* below.

Mechanism

Chlorzoxazone is a probe substrate for the cytochrome P450 isoenzyme CYP2E1. This clinical study suggests that kava is an inhibitor of this isoenzyme. However, *in vitro* studies suggest that kava is not an inhibitor of CYP2E1, see Pharmacokinetics, page 315.

Importance and management

Evidence is limited to this one study, which suggests that the metabolism of chlorzoxazone is weakly inhibited by kava, but this effect is probably not clinically relevant.

1. Gurley BJ, Gardner SF, Hubbard MA, Williams DK, Gentry WB, Khan IA, Shah A. In vivo effects of goldenseal, kava kava, black cohosh, and valerian on human cytochrome P450 1A2, 2D6, 2E1, and 3A4/5 phenotypes. *Clin Pharmacol Ther* (2005) 77, 415–26.

Kava + Digitalis glycosides

A standardised kava extract did not alter the pharmacokinetics of digoxin.

Clinical evidence

A study in 20 healthy subjects given a single 500-microgram dose of digoxin before and on the last day of treatment with a standardised kava extract 1227 mg three times daily for 14 days, found no changes in the pharmacokinetics of digoxin. The product used was standardised for kavalactone content.[1]

Experimental evidence

See *Mechanism* below.

Mechanism

Digoxin is a P-glycoprotein substrate. It has been suggested that kava may alter digoxin pharmacokinetics by affecting P-glycoprotein, since kava and kavalactones, the main active constituents of kava, are modulators of P-glycoprotein *in vitro*.[2,3]

Importance and management

Direct evidence is limited to one clinical study, which showed that kava does not cause clinically relevant changes in digoxin pharmacokinetics. Therefore no changes in digoxin levels would be anticipated on concurrent use, the caveat being that, as with all herbal medicines, these results may not be applicable to all kava products.[1]

1. Gurley BJ, Swain A, Barone GW, Williams DK, Breen P, Yates CR, Stuart LB, Hubbard MA, Tong Y, Cheboyina S. Effect of goldenseal (*Hydrastis canadensis*) and kava kava (*Piper methysticum*) supplementation on digoxin pharmacokinetics in humans. *Drug Metab Dispos* (2007) 35, 240–245.
2. Weiss J, Sauer A, Frank A, Unger M. Extracts and kavalactones of Piper methysticum G. Forst (kava-kava) inhibit P-glycoprotein in vitro. *Drug Metab Dispos* (2005) 33, 1580–1583.
3. Burka LT. Pharmacokinetics and disposition of the kavalactone kawain: interaction with kava extract and kavalactones in vivo and in vitro. *Drug Metab Dispos* (2005) 33, 1555–63.

Kava + Food

No interactions found.

Kava + Herbal medicines

For mention of a case of myoglobinuria in a patient taking guarana and kava, see Guarana + Herbal medicines, page 280. For mention

K

of the synergistic sedative effects of passiflora and kava in *animals,* see Passiflora + Amfetamines, page 367, and Passiflora + Anxiolytics and Hypnotics, page 367.

Kava + Levodopa

An isolated case report suggests that kava may antagonise the effects of levodopa.

Clinical evidence

A case report describes a 76-year-old woman with Parkinson's disease taking levodopa 500 mg (plus benserazide 125 mg) daily who noted an increase in the duration and number of "off-periods" within 10 days of starting a kava preparation containing 150 mg kava extract. The patient's normal baseline pattern of "off-periods" was restored within 2 days of stopping the kava preparation.[1]

Acute dystonic reactions have been described with kava alone in 4 non-Parkinson's disease patients after taking one dose or multiple doses of various kava preparations over four to ten days.[1] One case resolved spontaneously within about 40 minutes and two cases immediately resolved on administration of biperiden.[1] In the remaining case, symptoms were more severe and persistent and the authors note that this may have been influenced by a genetic predisposition.[2]

Experimental evidence

An *animal* study showed that kava extract and some individual **kavalactones**, the main active constituents of kava, both increased and decreased dopamine concentrations in the brains of *rats*.[3]

Mechanism

No mechanism established. It is possible that kava antagonises the effects of levodopa via its effects on the dopaminergic system.

Importance and management

Evidence of a direct interaction between kava and levodopa is limited to an isolated case report and its clinical importance is unclear. However, this report and the small number of cases of Parkinson-like effects occurring after kava intake, suggest that this should be borne in mind if a patient with Parkinson's disease stabilised on levodopa experiences a relapse in symptom control from their normal baseline after starting kava.

1. Schelosky L, Raffauf C, Jendroska K, Poewe W. Kava and dopamine antagonism. *J Neurol Neurosurg Psychiatry* (1995) 58, 639–40.
2. Meseguer E, Taboada T, Sánchez B, Mena MA, Campos V, Garcia De Yébenes J. Life-threatening parkinsonism induced by kava-kava. *Mov Disord* (2002) 17, 195–6.
3. Baum SS, Hill R, Rommelspacher H. Effect of kava extract and individual kavapyrones on neurotransmitter levels in the nucleus accumbens of rats. *Prog Neuropsychopharmacol Biol Psychiatry* (1998) 22, 1105–20.

Kava + Paracetamol (Acetaminophen)

The information regarding the use of kava with paracetamol is based on experimental evidence only.

Clinical evidence

No interactions found.

Experimental evidence

A study in *rat* hepatocytes found that kava (at a concentration of 200 micrograms/mL) did not affect cell viability compared with control. However, when tested with paracetamol, kava potentiated paracetamol-induced glutathione depletion and increased mitochondrial damage, which resulted in 100% cell death compared with about 40 to 60% for paracetamol alone.[1]

Mechanism

Paracetamol-induced liver injury is related to glutathione depletion and the disruption of mitochondrial function, and, since these effects are potentiated by kava, there might be an increased risk of liver injury on concurrent use.

Importance and management

Evidence appears to be limited to the experimental study cited, which suggests that paracetamol-induced liver cell injury might be potentiated by kava. This evidence, coupled with the fact that kava is known to cause hepatotoxicity (the mechanism for which is not understood), suggests that it might be prudent to avoid using kava supplements with paracetamol. Note that kava products are banned in some countries, due to reports of liver toxicity, see Use and indications, page 315.

1. Yang X, Salminen WF. Kava extract, an herbal alternative for anxiety relief, potentiates acetaminophen-induced cytotoxicity in rat hepatic cells. *Phytomedicine* (2011) 18, 592–600.

Kelp

Fucus vesiculosus L. and other species (Fucaceae)

Synonym(s) and related species

Black tang, Bladder fucus, Bladderwrack, Cutweed, Kelpware, Rockweed, Seawrack.

Fucus serratus L., (known as Toothed wrack). *Ascophyllum nodosum* (L.) Le Jolis (known as Knotted wrack) is also used in a similar way to *Fucus* species.

Technically, kelps are species of *Laminaria* and *Macrocystis*.

Pharmacopoeias

Kelp (*BP 2012, PhEur 7.5*).

Constituents

The thallus of kelp contains polysaccharides including **alginic acid** (the major component), fucoidan and laminarin (sulfated polysaccharide esters), free phloroglucinol and its high molecular weight polymers the phlorotannins and fucols and galactolipids. The **iodine** content can be high, and kelp may be standardised to the total iodine content. Kelp also contains vitamins and minerals, particularly ascorbic acid (vitamin C), and it is a moderate source of vitamin K_1 (phytomenadione). Kelp may be contaminated with various heavy metals such as arsenic, and it may be standardised to a maximum limit of these.

Use and indications

Traditionally kelp has been used as a source of minerals such as iodine for thyroid deficiency. It has also been used as a slimming supplement. Note that the iodine content in kelp may precipitate hyperthyroidism, and prolonged or excessive intake is inadvisable.

Pharmacokinetics

No relevant pharmacokinetic data found.

Interactions overview

Kelp is probably unlikely to interact with warfarin, because, although it is a moderate source of vitamin K_1, and therefore has the potential to reduce the effect of warfarin and related anticoagulants, sufficient vitamin K is very unlikely to be attained with usual doses of kelp supplements. Note also that anticoagulant fucoidans in kelp are unlikely to be orally active.

Interactions monographs

- Anticoagulants, page 320
- Food, page 320
- Herbal medicines, page 320

K

Kelp + Anticoagulants

Unintentional and unwanted antagonism of warfarin occurred in one patient when she ate seaweed sushi. It has been suggested that kelp contains substances with anticoagulant activity, but the evidence for this is theoretical.

Clinical evidence

An isolated report describes a patient taking **warfarin** who had, on two occasions, reduced INRs of 1.6 and 1.8 (usual range 2 to 3) within 24 hours of eating sushi with **seaweed** (*asakusa-nori*). It was estimated that she had consumed only about 45 micrograms of vitamin K_1, which would not usually be sufficient to interact. However, if her vitamin K stores were low, this amount could have accounted for a large percentage of her vitamin K intake or stores, and might therefore have interacted.[1] Note that kelp is a moderate source of vitamin K, having about 66 micrograms per 100 g.[2] However, this means that supplements containing 1 g of kelp will contain very little vitamin K (0.66 micrograms). Also, when the kelp is used to prepare an infusion, it would be unlikely to contain much vitamin K_1, because the vitamin is not water soluble.

Experimental evidence

In experimental studies, fucoidans from brown seaweeds including kelp have demonstrated anticoagulant activity. For example, in one *in vitro* study, the fucoidan from *Fucus serratus* had anticoagulant activity, as measured by activated partial thromboplastin time; this was roughly equivalent to 19 units of heparin per mg. The fucoidin inhibited thrombin-induced human platelet activation. The fucoidans from *Fucus vesiculosus* and *Ascophyllum nodosum* had a smaller effect (roughly equivalent to 9 and 13 units of heparin per mg, respectively).[3]

Mechanism

Kelp is a moderate source of vitamin K, and therefore, if eaten in sufficient quantities, would antagonise the effects of coumarins and indanediones, because these anticoagulants act as vitamin K antagonists. Fucoidans from kelp may act like heparin and inhibit thrombin activity, and therefore have some anticoagulant effects. However, they are large polysaccharides, and are therefore unlikely to be orally active.

Importance and management

The interaction of warfarin with vitamin K from foods is a very well established, well documented and clinically important drug-food interaction, expected to occur with every coumarin or indanedione anticoagulant because they have a common mode of action. However, the evidence suggests that, in patients with normal vitamin K_1 status, in general, clinically relevant changes in coagulation status require large continued changes in intake of vitamin K_1 from foods, which would be highly unlikely to be attained from usual doses of kelp supplements. This interaction would therefore be more applicable to kelp eaten as a food.

Fucoids in kelp are very unlikely to be orally active, so kelp supplements would be unlikely to have any anticoagulant activity.

Taking the evidence together, there appears to be no reason why patients taking warfarin should particularly avoid taking kelp supplements.

1. Bartle WR, Madorin P, Ferland G. Seaweed, vitamin K, and warfarin. *Am J Health-Syst Pharm* (2001) 58, 2300.
2. USDA National Nutrient Database for Standard Reference, Release 17. Vitamin K (phylloquinone) (μg) Content of selected foods per common measure. http://www.nal.usda.gov/fnic/foodcomp/Data/SR17/wtrank/sr17a430.pdf (accessed 20/11/2008).
3. Cumashi A, Ushakova NA, Preobrazhenskaya ME, D'Incecco A, Piccoli A, Totani L, Tinari N, Morozevich GE, Berman AE, Bilan MI, Usov AI, Ustyuzhanina NE, Grachev AA, Sanderson CJ, Kelly M, Rabinovich GA, Iacobelli S, Nifantiev NE. Consorzio Interuniversitario Nazionale per la Bio-Oncologia, Italy. A comparative study of the anti-inflammatory, anticoagulant, antiangiogenic, and antiadhesive activities of nine different fucoidans from brown seaweeds. *Glycobiology* (2007) 17, 541–52.

Kelp + Food

No interactions found.

Kelp + Herbal medicines

No interactions found.

Kudzu

Pueraria montana (Lour.) Merr. (Fabaceae)

Synonym(s) and related species

Ge Gen.

Pueraria hirsuta (Thunb.) C. Schneider, *Pueraria lobata* (Willd.) Ohwi, *Pueraria lobata* (Willd.) Ohwi var. *thomsonii* (Benth.) Maesen, *Pueraria thunbergiana* (Sieb. & Zucc.) Benth., *Dolichos lobatus* Willd.

Other species used include *Pueraria mirifica* Airy Shaw & Suvatabandhu (Thai kudzu, Kwao Kreu Kao) and *Pueraria phaseoloides* (Roxb.) Benth. (Puero, Tropical kudzu).

Constituents

The major **isoflavone** constituent of the root of *Pueraria lobata* is **puerarin**, which is the 8-C-glucoside of daidzein, but there are many others, such as puerarin hydroxy- and methoxy- derivatives and their glycosides; daidzein and its O-glycoside daidzin; biochanin A, genistein, and formononetin derivatives. Pterocarpans are also present, including medicarpin glycinol and tuberosin. The flowers contain the phytoestrogens kakkalide and tectoridin.

Pueraria mirifica root contains similar constituents to *Pueraria lobata,* the major difference being lower amounts of daidzein.

Much of the research carried out on kudzu has been on the effects of isolated **puerarin**.

Use and indications

Kudzu contains isoflavones and is used as a phytoestrogen for menopausal symptoms, with a particular emphasis on bone metabolism for use in postmenopausal osteoporosis. It also has a popular reputation for being able to lower alcohol consumption and to treat symptoms of alcohol intoxication. This effect has not been reported for other isoflavone-containing herbs and the possible mechanism of action is unknown. Kudzu has also been used for migraine and hypertension, pain and stiffness, and angina. The phytoestrogenic properties are well known, and puerarin is thought to be the major component with this effect, which has been well documented in *animals*. For further details about the general and specific effects of isoflavones, see isoflavones, page 300.

Pharmacokinetics

No relevant pharmacokinetic data for kudzu found. For information on the pharmacokinetics of its main isoflavone constituent puerarin, see isoflavones, page 300.

Interactions overview

Studies in *rats* suggest that kudzu can increase the effects of methotrexate. Kudzu contains oestrogenic compounds and therefore it may interact with oestrogens and oestrogen antagonists. Potential interactions of isoflavone constituents of kudzu are covered under isoflavones; see antibacterials, page 302, antidiabetics, page 302, benzodiazepines, page 302, miscellaneous cardiovascular drugs, page 302, digoxin, page 302, fexofenadine, page 303, nicotine, page 303, paclitaxel, page 303, and theophylline, page 305.

Interactions monographs

- Food, page 322
- Herbal medicines, page 322
- Methotrexate, page 322
- Oestrogens or Oestrogen antagonists, page 322

K

Kudzu + Antibacterials

No data for kudzu found. For the theoretical possibility that broad-spectrum antibacterials might reduce the metabolism of the isoflavone constituents of kudzu, such as puerarin and daidzin, by colonic bacteria, and so alter their efficacy, see Isoflavones + Antibacterials, page 302.

Kudzu + Antidiabetics

No data for kudzu found. For comment on the blood-glucose lowering effects of puerarin, a major isoflavone constituent of kudzu, see Isoflavones + Antidiabetics, page 302.

Kudzu + Benzodiazepines

No data for kudzu found. Puerarin, a major isoflavone constituent of kudzu, has been reported to be a weak benzodiazepine antagonist, see Isoflavones + Benzodiazepines, page 302.

Kudzu + Cardiovascular drugs; Miscellaneous

No data for kudzu found. For a discussion of the evidence that puerarin, an isoflavone present in kudzu, might inhibit platelet aggregation, see Isoflavones + Cardiovascular drugs; Miscellaneous, page 302.

Kudzu + Digoxin

No data for kudzu found. For the possibility that high-dose biochanin A, an isoflavone present in kudzu, might increase digoxin levels, see Isoflavones + Digoxin, page 302.

Kudzu + Fexofenadine

For the possibility that high-dose biochanin A, an isoflavone in kudzu, may slightly decrease fexofenadine levels in *rats*, see Isoflavones + Fexofenadine, page 303.

Kudzu + Food

No interactions found.

Kudzu + Herbal medicines

No interactions found.

Kudzu + Methotrexate

The interaction between kudzu and methotrexate is based on experimental evidence only.

Clinical evidence
No interactions found.

Experimental evidence
In a pharmacokinetic study in *rats,* the use of a kudzu root decoction significantly decreased the elimination and resulted in markedly increased exposure of methotrexate.[1] *Animals* were given methotrexate, orally or intravenously, alone or with the decoction. Giving the decoction at a dose of 4 g/kg and 2 g/kg significantly increased the AUC of oral methotrexate by about 3-fold and 2.3-fold, respectively. This resulted in high mortalities (57.1% and 14.3%). With intravenous methotrexate, the concurrent use of the kudzu decoction at 4 g/kg increased the half-life by 54% and decreased the clearance by 48%.

Mechanism
Kudzu markedly reduces the elimination of methotrexate. This might occur because of competition for renal of biliary excretion, possibly via organic anion transporter (OAT).[1]

Importance and management
Evidence is limited to data in *rats,* and the doses of kudzu used in this study are very high. Nevertheless, the findings suggest that kudzu might markedly increase the effects of methotrexate. Until more is known, caution might be appropriate on concurrent use. The risks are likely to be greatest with high-dose methotrexate (for neoplastic diseases) and in patients with impaired renal function, but less in those given low doses (5 to 25 mg weekly) for psoriasis or rheumatoid arthritis and with normal kidney function. Note that the use of methotrexate requires routine monitoring (e.g. of LFTs), and patients should be advised to report any sign or symptom suggestive of infection, particularly sore throat (which might possibly indicate that white cell counts have fallen) or dyspnoea or cough (suggestive of pulmonary toxicity).

1. Chiang H-M, Fang S-H, Wen K-C, Hsiu S-L, Tsai S-Y, Hou Y-C, Chi Y-C, Chao P-DL. Life-threatening interaction between the root extract of *Pueraria lobata* and methotrexate in rats. *Toxicol Appl Pharmacol* (2005) 209, 263–8.

Kudzu + Nicotine

For discussion of a study showing that daidzein and genistein present in kudzu caused a minor decrease in the metabolism of nicotine, see Isoflavones + Nicotine, page 303.

Kudzu + Oestrogens or Oestrogen antagonists

Kudzu contains oestrogenic compounds. This may result in additive effects with oestrogens or it may oppose the effects of oestrogens. Similarly, kudzu may have additive effects with oestrogen antagonists or oppose the effects of oestrogen antagonists (e.g. tamoxifen).

Evidence, mechanism, importance and management
Kudzu has a long history of use for menopausal symptoms, and is known to contain isoflavones (plant oestrogens). Numerous *in vitro* and *animal* studies have demonstrated oestrogenic effects for the herb (too many to cite here). However, few clinical studies

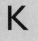

have been conducted. In one study,[1] *Pueraria mirifica* alleviated menopausal symptoms in perimenopausal women, but in another study in postmenopausal women,[2] *Pueraria lobata* did not alter menopausal symptoms or lipids or hormone levels, and was less effective than conventional HRT.

Theoretically, the isoflavones from kudzu might have oestrogen antagonistic effects when they are given with potent oestrogenic drugs, as their oestrogenic effects are weaker and they might competitively inhibit the conventional oestrogenic drugs. Conversely, because of their oestrogenic effects it is possible that they might reduce the efficacy of potent oestrogen antagonists.

Although many studies have been carried out, clinical information on the potential interaction of kudzu with oestrogens or oestrogen antagonists is sparse. On the basis of the postulated oestrogenic effects of kudzu and the theoretical mechanisms of antagonism, some have recommended caution if kudzu is given with other oestrogens including hormonal contraceptives, or with oestrogen antagonists such as tamoxifen. However, isoflavones from plants are widely consumed as part of the traditional diet in many parts of the world, and there is no clear evidence that this affects response to hormonal contraceptives or oestrogen antagonists such as tamox-

ifen. For further information on the oestrogenic effects of isoflavone supplements, see Isoflavones + Tamoxifen, page 304.

1. Lamlertkittikul S, Chandeying V. Efficacy and safety of *Pueraria mirifica* (Kwao Kruea Khao) for the treatment of vasomotor symptoms in perimenopausal women: phase II study. *J Med Assoc Thai* (2004) 87, 33–40.
2. Woo J, Lau E, Ho SC, Cheng F, Chan C, Chan ASY, Haines CJ, Chan TYK, Li M, Sham A. Comparison of *Pueraria lobata* with hormone replacement therapy in treating the adverse health consequences of menopause. *Menopause* (2003) 10, 352–61.

Kudzu + Paclitaxel

No data for kudzu found. For the possibility that the isoflavones biochanin A and genistein present in kudzu might increase paclitaxel levels, see Isoflavones + Paclitaxel, page 303. Note that paclitaxel is used intravenously, and the effect of biochanin A on intravenous paclitaxel does not appear to have been evaluated.

Kudzu + Theophylline

No data for kudzu found. For the possibility that high doses of daidzein present in kudzu might modestly increase theophylline levels, see Isoflavones + Theophylline, page 305.

Lapacho

Tabebuia avellanedae Lorentz ex Griseb. (Bignoniaceae)

Synonym(s) and related species

Pau D'arco, Taheebo.

Tabebuia impetiginosa, *Tabebuia pentaphylla*, *Tabebuia rosea* Bertol., *Tabebuia serratifolia* (Vahl) Nicholson.

Constituents

Naphthoquinones are the major active constituents of the inner bark, the most important of which is **lapachol**, with deoxylapachol and α- and β-lapachone and others. **Flavonoids** and natural coumarins are also present.

Other constituents that may contribute to the pharmacological activity of lapacho include iridoid glycosides such as ajugol; lignans based on secoisolariciresinol and cycloolivil; isocoumarin glycosides based on 6-hydroxymellein; phenolic glycosides of methoxyphenol derivatives and vanillyl 4-hydroxybenzoate; various aldehydes; and volatile constituents such as 4-methoxybenzaldehyde, elemicin, trans-anethole, and 4-methoxybenzyl alcohol.

Use and indications

Lapacho is used traditionally for infectious diseases of bacterial, protozoal, fungal and viral origin, to enhance the immune system, and as an anti-inflammatory agent. It is also used as an anticancer therapy, especially in South America, and although there is experimental evidence to support some of these uses, good clinical evidence is not available. Lapachol is toxic in high doses.

Pharmacokinetics

No relevant pharmacokinetic data found.

Interactions overview

Lapachol is reported to have anticoagulant properties, which may be additive with those of conventional anticoagulants.

Interactions monographs

- Anticoagulants, page 325
- Food, page 325
- Herbal medicines, page 325

L

Lapacho + Anticoagulants

Lapacho may have anticoagulant effects and therefore, theoretically, concurrent use of conventional anticoagulants may be additive.

Clinical evidence

No interactions data found. However, it has been stated that lapachol (the main active constituent of lapacho) was originally withdrawn from clinical study because of its anticoagulant adverse effects,[1] but the original data does not appear to be available.

Experimental evidence

An *in vitro* study in *rat* liver microsomes found that lapachol is a potent inhibitor of vitamin K epoxide reductase. These effects were said to be similar to those of warfarin.[1]

Mechanism

Anticoagulants such as warfarin exert their effects by antagonising the effects of vitamin K, which is necessary to produce some clotting factors. They do this by inhibiting vitamin K epoxide reductase, which reduces the synthesis of vitamin K. This action appears to be shared by lapachol, and therefore the concurrent use of lapacho and anticoagulants may be additive.

Importance and management

Evidence is extremely limited, but the fact that lapachol was withdrawn from clinical studies due to its anticoagulant effects adds weight to the theoretical mechanism. Until more is known it would seem prudent to discuss the possible increase in anticoagulant effects with any patient taking an anticoagulant, who also wishes to take lapacho. If concurrent use is considered desirable it may be prudent to refer the patient to have their INR, or other suitable clotting parameters, checked.

1. Preusch PC, Suttie JW. Lapachol inhibition of vitamin K epoxide reductase and vitamin K quinine reductase. *Arch Biochem Biophys* (1984) 234, 405–12.

Lapacho + Food

No interactions found.

Lapacho + Herbal medicines

No interactions found.

L

Lemon balm

Melissa officinalis L. (Lamiaceae)

Synonym(s) and related species

Balm, Cure-all, Honeyplant, Melissa, Sweet balm.

Faucibarba officinalis (L.) Dulac, *Melissa bicornis* Klokov, *Mutelia officinalis* (L.) Gren. ex Mutel, *Thymus melissa* (L.) Krause.

Bee balm has been used for both lemon balm and some unrelated Monarda species, and care should be taken to avoid any confusion.

Pharmacopoeias

Lemon Balm (*BP 2012*); Lemon Balm Dry Extract (*BP 2012*); Melissa Leaf (*PhEur 7.5*); Melissa Leaf Dry Extract (*PhEur 7.5*).

Constituents

Lemon balm contains an essential oil composed mainly of aldehydes of mono- and sesquiterpenes, including citronellal, geranial, neral, citronellol, geraniol, nerol, β-ocimene, β-caryophyllene and germacrene D. **Flavonoids** including glycosides of luteolin, quercetin, apigenin and kaempferol, and polyphenolic acids including caffeic, hydroxycinnamic, protocatechuic, chlorogenic and rosmarinic acids are also present.

Use and indications

Lemon balm has been used traditionally for its sedative, carminative and spasmolytic properties. It has most commonly been used for nervousness, to aid sleep and for the symptomatic relief of gastrointestinal disorders. Lemon balm has also been used topically to treat herpes simplex labialis.

Pharmacokinetics

No relevant pharmacokinetic data found. For information on the pharmacokinetics of individual flavonoids present in lemon balm, see under flavonoids, page 213.

Interactions overview

No interactions with lemon balm found. For information on the interactions of individual flavonoids present in lemon balm, see under flavonoids, page 213.

L

Lime flower

Synonym(s) and related species

Lime tree, Lindenflowers, Linden tree,

Tilia cordata Mill, (also known as Small-leaved Lime), *T. officinarum* Crantz, *T. officinarum* Crantz subsp. *officinarum* pro parte.

Tilia × *vulgaris* Hayne, hybrid of the above (also known as Lime), *T.* × *europaea* auct. non L.

Other species are also used in various parts of the world.

Constituents

The flowers contain the **flavonoids** astragalin, tiliroside, myricetin, quercetin and kaempferol and their glycosides. A mucilage is also present, which is composed of **polysaccharides** including arabinose, galactose, rhamnose, glucose, mannose, xylose, galacturonic and glucuronic acids. The **volatile oil** contains citral, citronellal, citronellol, eugenol, limonene, nerol, α-pinene, terpineol, farnesol and many other components. The coumarin scopoletin, condensed tannins, tocopherol, and amino acids including GABA (gamma amino benzoic acid) have also been identified.

Use and indications

Traditionally the flowers are used as a sedative, antispasmodic, diaphoretic, diuretic and mild astringent. They have also been used in the treatment of migraine, hysteria, and arterial hypertension.

Pharmacokinetics

No relevant pharmacokinetic data found. For information on the pharmacokinetics of individual flavonoids present in lime flower, see under flavonoids, page 213.

Interactions overview

Lime flower tea may reduce the absorption of iron compounds. For information on the interactions of individual flavonoids present in lime flower, see under flavonoids, page 213.

Interactions monographs

- Food, page 328
- Herbal medicines, page 328
- Iron compounds, page 328

L

Lime flower + Food

No interactions found.

Lime flower + Herbal medicines

No interactions found.

Lime flower + Iron compounds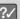

Lime flower tea caused a modest reduction in iron absorption in one study.

Clinical evidence

In a study in 10 healthy subjects, a 275 mL serving of lime flower tea reduced the absorption of iron in a 50 g bread roll by about 52%. The tea was prepared by adding 300 mL of boiling water to 3 g of the herbal tea, then infusing for 10 minutes before straining and serving. In this study, the inhibitory effect of lime flower tea on iron absorption was less than that of black tea (Assam tea, *Camellia sinensis* L.), which is known to inhibit iron absorption.[1] Consider also, Tea + Iron compounds, page 467.

Experimental evidence

No relevant data found.

Mechanism

The polyphenols in lime flower may bind to iron in the intestine and reduce its absorption.

Importance and management

The clinical relevance of the interaction between lime flower tea and iron compounds is unclear, as the effect on absorption was smaller than that of black tea (Assam tea, *Camellia sinensis* L.), which is known to inhibit iron absorption to a clinically relevant extent (see Tea + Iron compounds, page 467.) Until more is known it may be prudent to consider lime flower tea intake in patients requiring iron supplementation and in patients that are particularly unresponsive to iron replacement therapy.

1. Hurrell RF, Reddy M, Cook JD. Inhibition of non-haem iron absorption in man by polyphenolic-containing beverages. *Br J Nutr* (1999) 81, 289–95.

L

Liquorice

Glycyrrhiza glabra L. (Fabaceae)

Synonym(s) and related species

Licorice.

Spanish and Italian liquorice is *Glycyrrhiza glabra* var *typica* Reg. et Herd.

Persian or Turkish liquorice is *Glycyrrhiza glabra* L var *violacea* Boiss.

Russian liquorice is *Glycyrrhiza glabra* L var *glandulifera*.

Chinese liquorice is the closely related *Glycyrrhiza uralensis* Fisch., also known as Gancao.

Pharmacopoeias

Licorice (*USP35–NF30 S1*); Liquorice (*BP 2012*); Liquorice Dry Extract for Flavouring Purposes (*BP 2012, PhEur 7.5*); Liquorice Liquid Extract (*BP 2012*); Liquorice Root (*PhEur 7.5*); Liquorice Root for use in THM (*BP 2012*); Powdered Licorice (*USP35–NF30 S1*); Powdered Licorice Extract (*USP35–NF30 S1*); Processed Liquorice Root for use in THMP (*BP 2012*); Standardised Liquorice Ethanolic Liquid Extract (*BP 2012, PhEur 7.5*).

Constituents

Liquorice has a great number of active compounds of different classes that act in different ways. The most important constituents are usually considered to be the oleanane-type triterpenes, mainly **glycyrrhizin** (glycyrrhizic or **glycyrrhizinic acid**), to which it is usually standardised, and its aglycone glycyrrhetinic acid. There are also numerous phenolics and **flavonoids** of the chalcone and isoflavone type, and many natural coumarins such as liqcoumarin, umbelliferone, glabrocoumarones A and B, herniarin, and glycyrin. It also contains polysaccharides such as glycyrrhizan GA, and a small amount of volatile oil.

Use and indications

The dried root and stolons of liquorice are used as an expectorant, antispasmodic, anti-inflammatory and to treat peptic and duodenal ulcers. Liquorice is widely used in traditional oriental systems of medicine, and as a flavouring ingredient in food. It has mineralocorticoid and oestrogenic activity in large doses, as a result of glycyrrhetinic acid, and has many other reputed pharmacological effects.

Pharmacokinetics

Prolonged intake of high doses of liquorice extract, or its constituent glycyrrhizin, on probe cytochrome P450 isoenzyme substrates was investigated in *mice*.[1] With repeated treatment, both liquorice extract and glycyrrhizin significantly induced hepatic CYP3A and to a lesser extent, CYP1A2.

In a single-dose study in 2 healthy subjects, plasma levels of glycyrrhetic acid were much lower after administration of aqueous liquorice root extract 21 g (containing 1600 mg glycyrrhizin) than after the same 1600-mg dose of pure glycyrrhizin. This suggests that the biological activity of a given dose of glycyrrhizin might be greater if taken as the pure form than as liquorice. This confirmed data from a study in *rats*.[2] Note that much of the evidence relating to possible interactions is for pure constituents. These findings therefore suggest that the effect of liquorice might be less than that of pure glycyrrhizin at the same dose.

Interactions overview

Liquorice appears to diminish the effects of antihypertensives and may have additive effects on potassium depletion if given in large quantities with laxatives and corticosteroids. A case report describes persistent diarrhoea and raised lopinavir levels when evening primrose oil and a product containing aloes, rhubarb and liquorice were started, see under Evening primrose oil + Lopinavir, page 207. Iron absorption may be decreased by liquorice, whereas antibacterials may diminish the effects of liquorice. One case report describes raised digoxin levels and toxicity in a patient taking liquorice and another case report attributes pseudoaldosteronism to the use of cilostazol and glycyrrhizin, a major constituent of liquorice. Although it has been suggested that liquorice may enhance the effects of warfarin, there appears to be no evidence to support this. Note that liquorice is a constituent of a number of Chinese herbal medicines. See under bupleurum, page 98, for possible interactions of liquorice given as part of these preparations.

Interactions monographs

- Antihypertensives, page 330
- Cilostazol, page 330
- Corticosteroids, page 330
- Digitalis glycosides, page 331
- Food, page 331
- Herbal medicines, page 332
- Iron compounds, page 332
- Laxatives, page 332
- Midazolam, page 332
- Ulcer-healing drugs, page 333
- Warfarin, page 333

1. Paolini M, Pozzetti L, Sapone A, Cantelli-Forti G. Effect of licorice and glycyrrhizin on murine liver CYP-dependent monooxygenases. *Life Sci* (1998) 62, 571–82.
2. Cantelli-Forti G, Maffei F, Hrelia P, Bugamelli F, Bernardi M, D'Intino P, Maranesi M, Raggi MA. Interaction of licorice on glycyrrhizin pharmacokinetics. *Environ Health Perspect* (1994) 102 (Suppl 9), 65–8.

L

Liquorice + Antihypertensives

Liquorice may cause fluid retention and therefore reduce the effects of antihypertensives. Additive hypokalaemia may also occur with loop and thiazide diuretics.

Clinical evidence

In 11 patients with treated hypertension, liquorice 100 g daily for 4 weeks (equivalent to glycyrrhetinic acid 150 mg daily) increased mean blood pressure by 15.3/9.3 mmHg. Smaller rises (3.5/3.6 mmHg) were seen in 25 normotensive subjects taking the same dose of liquorice.[1] In another study in healthy subjects liquorice 50 to 200 mg daily for 2 to 4 weeks (equivalent to glycyrrhetinic acid 75 to 540 mg daily) increased systolic blood pressure by 3.1 to 14.4 mmHg. The group taking the largest quantity of liquorice experienced the greatest rise in systolic blood pressure, and was the only group to have a statistically significant rise in diastolic blood pressure.[2]

There are many published case reports of serious hypertension occurring in people consuming, often, but not always, excessive doses of liquorice from various sources (confectionery, alcoholic drinks, flavoured chewing tobacco, herbal teas, herbal medicines).

Experimental evidence

Because of the quality of the clinical evidence, experimental data have not been cited. There is extensive literature, which has been the subject of a review.[3]

Mechanism

Ingestion of liquorice inhibits 11 β-hydroxysteroid dehydrogenase type 2, thereby preventing the inactivation of cortisol to cortisone.[3,4] This results in mineralocorticoid effects including sodium and water retention (leading to hypertension) and hypokalaemia.[3] This effect would oppose the effects of drugs used to lower blood pressure. In addition, the potassium-depleting effect of liquorice would be expected to be additive with loop and thiazide diuretics. The mineralocorticoid effect of liquorice is due to the content of glycyrrhetinic acid (a metabolite of glycyrrhizic acid), and therefore deglycyrrhizinated liquorice would not have this effect.

Importance and management

The ability of liquorice to increase blood pressure is well established. The dose required to produce this effect might vary between individuals, and the evidence from the study cited suggests that patients with hypertension might be more sensitive to its effect. It is probably not appropriate for patients taking antihypertensive drugs to be treated with liquorice, especially if their hypertension is not well controlled. Although liquorice-containing confectionery and other foodstuffs have also been implicated in this interaction it is usually when it has been consumed to excess. It seems unlikely that the occasional consumption of small amounts of these products will cause a notable effect. Nevertheless, in patients with poorly controlled blood pressure it may be prudent to ask about liquorice consumption to establish whether this could be a factor.

Note also that the potassium-depleting effect of liquorice would be additive with that of potassium-depleting diuretics such as loop diuretics and thiazides. Deglycyrrhizinated liquorice would not be expected to have these effects.

1. Sigurjonsdottir HA, Manhem K, Axelson M, Wallerstedt S. Subjects with essential hypertension are more sensitive to the inhibition of 11 β -HSD by liquorice. *J Hum Hypertens* (2003) 17, 125–31.
2. Sigurjónsdóttir HÁ, Franzson L, Manhem K, Ragnarsson J, Sigurdsson G, Wallerstedt S. Liquorice-induced rise in blood pressure: a linear dose-response relationship. *J Hum Hypertens* (2001) 15, 549–52.
3. Walker BR, Edwards CRW. Licorice-induced hypertension and syndromes of apparent mineralocorticoid excess. *Endocrinol Metab Clin North Am* (1994) 23, 359–77.
4. Hammer F, Stewart PM. Cortisol metabolism in hypertension. *Best Pract Res Clin Endocrinol Metab* (2006) 20, 337–53.

Liquorice + Caffeine

For mention that sho-saiko-to (of which liquorice is one of 7 constituents) only slightly reduced the metabolism of caffeine in one study, see Bupleurum + Caffeine, page 99.

Liquorice + Carbamazepine

For mention that sho-saiko-to (of which liquorice is one of 7 constituents) did not affect the metabolism of carbamazepine in an *animal* study, see Bupleurum + Carbamazepine, page 99.

Liquorice + Cilostazol

A case report describes a case of pseudoaldosteronism which was attributed to an interaction between glycyrrhizin and cilostazol.

Clinical evidence

A case report describes a 65-year-old man who was admitted to hospital with palpitations. Investigations revealed an elevated blood pressure (158/98 mmHg) and low potassium concentrations (2.5 mmol/L), with aldosterone concentrations within the normal range, and he was diagnosed with pseudoaldosteronism. His drug regimen, which included glycyrrhizin, a major constituent of liquorice, for alcoholic liver injury, had remained unchanged for a year, apart from the addition of cilostazol about 7 months earlier. The authors therefore attributed the pseudoaldosteronism to an interaction between cilostazol and glycyrrhizin.[1]

Experimental evidence

No relevant data found.

Mechanism

Liquorice alone can cause pseudoaldosteronism. The authors of the case suggested that competition for protein binding between cilostazol and glycyrrhizin caused an increase in free glycyrrhizin resulting in the effects seen. However, note that protein binding alone has largely been discredited as a mechanism of drug interactions.

Importance and management

Evidence for an interaction between liquorice and cilostazol appears limited to this case report involving glycyrrhizin, a major constituent of liquorice, and an interaction is not established. As such, no general recommendations can be made on the basis of this case report.

1. Maeda Y, Inaba N, Aoyagi M, Tanase T, Shiigai T. Pseudoaldosteronism caused by combined administration of cilostazol and glycyrrhizin. *Intern Med* (2008) 47, 1345–8.

Liquorice + Corticosteroids

Liquorice, if given in large quantities with corticosteroids, may cause additive hypokalaemia.

Clinical evidence

(a) Dexamethasone

In a parallel group study, 6 patients were given **glycyrrhizin** 225 mg daily for 7 days, and 6 patients were given the same dose of glycyrrhizin and dexamethasone 1.5 mg daily for 7 days. The mineralocorticoid effects of glycyrrhizin were significantly reduced by dexamethasone; cortisol plasma concentrations and urinary excretions were reduced by up to 70%.[1]

(b) Hydrocortisone

Glycyrrhizin slightly increased the AUC of cortisol by 13.6% in 4 patients with adrenocorticol insufficiency taking oral hydrocortisone 20 to 40 mg daily. Note that glycyrrhizin had no effect on endogenous cortisol levels in 7 control subjects without adrenal insufficiency.[2]

In a study in 23 healthy subjects, topical **glycyrrhetinic acid** markedly potentiated the activity of topical hydrocortisone, as assessed by cutaneous vasoconstrictor effect.[3]

(c) Prednisolone

A study in 6 healthy subjects found that after taking four 50-mg oral doses of **glycyrrhizin** at 8 hourly intervals, followed by a bolus injection of prednisolone hemisuccinate 96 micrograms/kg, the AUC of total prednisolone was increased by 50% and the AUC of free prednisolone was increased by 55%.[4] This confirms previous findings in which the glycyrrhizin 200 mg was given by intravenous infusion.[5]

Glycyrrhizin slightly increased the AUC of prednisolone by about 16 to 20% in 12 patients who had been taking oral prednisolone 10 to 30 mg daily for at least 3 months.[2]

Experimental evidence

Several experimental studies have found that glycyrrhizin and glycyrrhetinic acid, (from liquorice), inhibit the conversion of cortisol to the inactive steroid cortisone by 11 β-hydroxysteroid dehydrogenase, thereby having mineralocorticoid effects.[1-3,6]

In vitro, glycyrrhetinic acid (the aglycone of glycyrrhizin), inhibited 20-hydroxysteroid dehydrogenase, which reduced the conversion of prednisolone to its metabolite 20-dihydroprednisolone.[2]

Mechanism

Inhibition of 11 β-hydroxysteroid dehydrogenase by glycyrrhetinic acid may slightly delay the clearance of hydrocortisone and prednisolone and thereby enhance their effects. However, note that whether a mineralocorticoid or glucocorticoid is a substrate for this enzyme system depends on its chemical structure. Therefore, it cannot be assumed that liquorice will inhibit the inactivation of all corticosteroids.

Dexamethasone appears to attenuate the mineralocorticoid effects of glycyrrhizin because it suppresses endogenous cortisol secretion (causes adrenal suppression). Other corticosteroids would be expected to interact similarly if given in adrenal-suppressant doses.

Deglycyrrhizinated liquorice would not have these effects.

Importance and management

The clinical importance of these observations is uncertain. Doses of corticosteroids sufficient to cause adrenal suppression would be expected to reduce the mineralocorticoid activity of liquorice, but mineralocorticoid activity might still occur. Glycyrrhizin (an active constituent of liquorice) and its metabolite glycyrrhetinic acid slightly increased the plasma levels of hydrocortisone and prednisolone and markedly potentiated the cutaneous effects of hydrocortisone. This suggests that liquorice will slightly potentiate the effects of these steroids. However, this might not apply to other corticosteroids (see *Mechanism*, above). Nevertheless, it might be prudent to monitor the concurrent use of liquorice and corticosteroids, especially if liquorice ingestion is prolonged or if large doses are taken, as additive effects on water and sodium retention, and potassium depletion may occur.

1. Kageyama Y, Suzuki H, Saruta T. Glycyrrhizin induces mineralocorticoid activity through alterations in cortisol metabolism in the human kidney. *J Endocrinol* (1992) 135, 147–52.
2. Ojima M, Satoh K, Gomibuchi T, Itoh N, Kin S, Fukuchi S, Miyachi Y. The inhibitory effects of glycyrrhizin and glycyrrhetinic acid on the metabolism of cortisol and prednisolone - in vivo and in vitro studies. *Nippon Naibunpi Gakkai Zasshi* (1990) 66, 584–96.

3. Teelucksingh S, Mackie ADR, Burt D, McIntyre MA, Brett L, Edwards CRW. Potentiation of hydrocortisone activity in skin by glycyrrhetinic acid. *Lancet* (1990) 335, 1060–1063.
4. Chen M-F, Shimada F, Kato H, Yano S, Kanaoka M. Effect of oral administration of glycyrrhizin on the pharmacokinetics of prednisolone. *Endocrinol Jpn* (1991) 38, 167–74.
5. Chen M-F, Shimada F, Kato H, Yano S, Kanaoka M. Effect of glycyrrhizin on the pharmacokinetics of prednisolone following low dosage of prednisolone hemisuccinate. *Endocrinol Jpn* (1990) 37, 331–41.
6. Whorwood CB, Sheppard MC, Stewart PM. Licorice inhibits 11β-hydroxysteroid dehydrogenase messenger ribonucleic acid levels and potentiates glucocorticoid hormone action. *Endocrinology* (1993) 132, 2287–92.

Liquorice + Digitalis glycosides

An isolated case of digoxin toxicity reported in an elderly patient was attributed to the use of a herbal laxative containing kanzo (liquorice).

Clinical evidence

An 84-year-old man taking digoxin 125 micrograms daily and furosemide complained of loss of appetite, fatigue and oedema of the lower extremities 5 days after starting to take a Chinese herbal laxative containing liquorice (kanzo) 400 mg and **rhubarb** (daio) 1.6 g three times daily. He was found to have a raised digoxin level of 2.9 nanograms/mL (previous level 1 nanogram/mL) with a pulse rate of 30 bpm, and a slightly low potassium level (2.9 mmol/L).[1]

Experimental evidence

No relevant data found.

Mechanism

The reason for the increase in digoxin levels is unclear. Digoxin inhibits the sodium-potassium ATP-ase pump, which is concerned with the transport of sodium and potassium ions across the membranes of the myocardial cells. Potassium loss caused by a combination of the liquorice, rhubarb and diuretics exacerbated the potassium loss from the myocardial cells, thereby enhancing the bradycardia already caused by an elevated digoxin level. Hypokalaemia also promotes the binding of digoxin to myocardial cells. Pre-existing cardiovascular disease might have predisposed the patient to enhanced digoxin effects.

Importance and management

Evidence for an interaction between digoxin and liquorice appears to be limited to one case. It is likely that the effects of the elevated digoxin levels were exacerbated by the hypokalaemia, which might have been caused by the herbal laxative. The theoretical basis for an interaction between liquorice and digoxin is well established, but there are few actual cases. Any herbal preparation that can reduce potassium levels would be expected to increase the risk of digoxin toxicity. This is likely to be additive with other concurrent medications a patient may also be taking that can cause hypokalaemia, such as loop diuretics. It would be prudent to exercise caution in patients who are taking digitalis glycosides and who regularly use/abuse laxatives including liquorice and/or anthraquinone-containing substances such as rhubarb. However, note that if these laxatives are used as recommended (at a dose producing a comfortable soft-formed motion), then this interaction is probably unlikely to be important.

1. Harada T, Ohtaki E, Misu K, Sumiyoshi T, Hosoda S. Congestive heart failure caused by digitalis toxicity in an elderly man taking a licorice-containing chinese herbal laxative. *Cardiology* (2002) 98, 218.

Liquorice + Food

No interactions found. Note that liquorice is consumed as part of the diet.

L

Liquorice + Herbal medicines

See under Liquorice + Laxatives, below.

Liquorice + Iron compounds

The interaction between liquorice and iron compounds is based on experimental evidence only.

Clinical evidence
No interactions found.

Experimental evidence
Liquorice extract 5 g/100 mL slightly enhanced the absorption index of iron by about 44% in *rats*.[1]

Mechanism
Unknown, it may be related to the content of iron and vitamin C (which promotes iron absorption) in the liquorice extract.

Importance and management
The experimental evidence suggests that liquorice might slightly enhance the bioavailability of medicinal iron, but further study is needed to assess the clinical relevance of this. At present, no action is considered necessary.

1. El-Shobaki FA, Saleh ZA, Saleh N. The effect of some beverage extracts on intestinal iron absorption. *Z Ernahrungswiss* (1990) 29, 264–9.

Liquorice + Laxatives

Liquorice may cause additive hypokalaemia if given in large quantities with laxatives.

Evidence and mechanism

(a) Additive potassium depletion
Liquorice root may cause water retention and potassium depletion. Chronic diarrhoea caused by the long-term use or abuse of stimulant laxatives such as aloes and senna may lead to excessive loss of water and potassium, and can also lead to potassium deficiency. Theoretically, concurrent use of these herbs might have additive effects on potassium loss. Although the increased potential for potassium deficiency on combined use is mentioned in some reviews,[1] there appear to be few clinical reports of this having occurred. Moreover, laxatives containing both senna and liquorice are available in some countries. One report describes four cases of pseudohyperaldosteronism (hypertension, hypokalaemia, and suppression of the renin-aldosterone axis) in patients taking liquorice-containing laxatives for chronic constipation. In three of the patients, the preparation had been prepared by a herbalist and the fourth patient was taking a proprietary preparation containing senna and liquorice (*Midro*). The liquorice doses were high, varying from 0.5 to 8 g daily. Patients had the liquorice laxative withdrawn and replaced by glycerine suppositories or lactulose, and received spironolactone 200 mg daily for 2 weeks to correct blood pressure and potassium. Two months later, the patients had no signs or symptoms of hyperaldosteronism.[2] It is not possible to say what contribution senna had to these cases, as the effects seen could be attributed to liquorice alone. Note that a similar combination laxative of liquorice with **rhubarb** caused mild hypokalaemia and digoxin toxicity, see Liquorice + Digitalis glycosides, page 331.

(b) Reduced absorption of liquorice
The introduction to an *animal* study briefly reported that, in a study in healthy subjects, the AUC and maximum levels of glycyrrhetic

acid were much lower after oral administration of Onpito, a Kampo medicine composed of five herbs including liquorice and **rhubarb**, than after other Kampo medicines containing liquorice and not containing **rhubarb**.[3] In a series of experiments in *rats,* the AUC of glycyrrhetic acid, a major component of liquorice, was reduced by up to about 70% by sennoside A, an anthraquinone derivative found in **rhubarb**.[3] The authors propose that competitive inhibition of the anthraquinones on glycyrrhetic acid transportation by monocarboxylic acid transporter (MCT1) and induction of P-glycoprotein in the intestinal tract may be possible mechanisms for reducing the absorption of glycyrrhetic acid.[3]

In a study in *rats,* the AUC and maximum level of glycyrrhetic acid were reduced by 80% and 85% respectively, when a single dose of shaoyao-gancao-tang was given 5 hours after a single dose of **sodium picosulfate**.[4] However, it was found that the reduction in glycyrrhetic acid levels seen with the laxative could be markedly attenuated by the repeated administration of shaoyao-gancao-tang.[4]

It was suggested that **sodium picosulfate** could reduce the metabolism of the glycoside glycyrrhizin to its active metabolite glycyrrhetic acid.[4] Note that shaoyao-gancao-tang is a traditional Chinese medicine containing liquorice (gancao), of which glycyrrhizin is a major constituent.

Importance and management
The possible additive potassium depletion in patients given liquorice and anthraquinone-containing laxatives (such as senna and rhubarb) is a theoretical interaction, but bear it in mind in patients who are taking liquorice and who are regular users or abusers of anthraquinone-containing substances. If anthraquinone laxatives are used as recommended (at a dose producing a comfortable soft-formed motion), this interaction is unlikely to be important.

It is unclear if sodium picosulfate affects the efficacy of liquorice as a laxative, and combination products are common.

Consider also, Evening primrose oil + Lopinavir, page 207 for a case report describing persistent diarrhoea and raised lopinavir levels when evening primrose oil and a product containing aloes, rhubarb and liquorice were started.

1. Hadley SK, Petry JJ. Medicinal herbs: A primer for primary care. *Hosp Pract* (1999) 34, 105–23.
2. Scali M, Pratesi C, Zennaro MC, Zampollo V, Armanini D. Pseudohyperaldosteronism from liquorice-containing laxatives. *J Endocrinol Invest* (1990) 10, 847–8.
3. Mizuhara Y, Takizawa Y, Ishihara K, Asano T, Kushida H, Morota T, Kase Y, Takeda S, Aburada M, Nomura M, Yokogawa K. The influence of the sennosides on absorption of glycyrrhetic acid in rats. *Biol Pharm Bull* (2005) 28, 1897–1902.
4. Goto E, He J-X, Akao T, Tani T. Bioavailability of glycyrrhizin from Shaoyao-Gancao-Tang in laxative-treated rats. *J Pharm Pharmacol* (2005) 57, 1359–63.

Liquorice + Lopinavir

For mention of a case of persistent diarrhoea and raised lopinavir levels in an HIV-positive man after starting evening primrose oil and a product containing aloes, rhubarb and liquorice, see Evening primrose oil + Lopinavir, page 207.

Liquorice + Midazolam

Glycyrrhizin, a constituent of liquorice, very slightly reduces midazolam exposure.

Clinical evidence
In a study, 16 healthy subjects were given a single 7.5-mg dose of midazolam after taking glycyrrhizin 150 mg twice daily for 14 days. Glycyrrhizin decreased the AUC of midazolam by 24% and increased its maximum plasma concentration by 19%.[1]

Experimental evidence

In vitro study, and a study in *rats,* found that glycyrrhetinic acid inhibited the formation of 1-hydroxymidazolam and decreased the exposure to midazolam.[2]

Mechanism

Midazolam is a substrate of the cytochrome P450 isoenzyme CYP3A4. It seems likely that glycyrrhizin, and its metabolite, glycyrrhetinic acid, induce CYP3A4, resulting in an increase in the metabolism of midazolam, and a decrease in its bioavailability.

Importance and management

Direct evidence about an interaction between midazolam and liquorice appears to be limited to one clinical study with the constituent, glycyrrhizin, and experimental data with the glycyrrhizin metabolite, glycyrrhetinic acid. However, the effects of glycyrrhizin on midazolam exposure were slight and unlikely to be of clinical relevance. Midazolam is used as a probe drug for CYP3A4 activity, and therefore these results also suggest that a pharmacokinetic interaction between glycyrrhizin or liquorice and other substrates of CYP3A4 is unlikely.

1. Tu J-H, He Y-J, Chen Y, Fan L, Zhang W, Tan Z-R, Huang Y-F, Guo D, Hu D-L, Wang D, Zhou H-H. Effect of glycyrrhizin on the activity of CYP3A enzyme in humans *Eur J Clin Pharmacol* (2010) 66, 805–10.
2. Li HY, Xu W, Su J, Zhang X, Hu LW, Zhang WD. In vitro and in vivo inhibitory effects of glycyrrhetinic acid on cytochrome P450 3A activity *Pharmacology* (2010) 86, 287–92.

Liquorice + Ofloxacin

For mention that sho-saiko-to and sairei-to (of which liquorice is one of the constituents) did not affect the metabolism of ofloxacin, see Bupleurum + Ofloxacin, page 99.

Liquorice + Tolbutamide

For conflicting evidence from *animal* studies that sho-saiko-to (of which liquorice is one of 7 constituents) might increase or decrease the rate of absorption of tolbutamide, see Bupleurum + Tolbutamide, page 99.

Liquorice + Ulcer-healing drugs

The interaction between liquorice and ulcer-healing drugs is based on experimental evidence only.

Clinical evidence

No interactions found.

Experimental evidence

In a study in *rats,* a single oral dose of shaoyao-gancao-tang was given alone and on the last day of a number of different drugs given twice daily for 7 doses. Pretreatment with **amoxicillin** with **metronidazole** or **clarithromycin** with **metronidazole** markedly reduced the AUC of glycyrrhetic acid by about 90%. **Hyoscine** or **omeprazole** had no effect on the AUC of glycyrrhetic acid. **Cimetidine** decreased the AUC of glycyrrhetic acid by 42%, but this was not statistically significant.[1] However, in a further study, it was found that the reduction in glycyrrhetic acid levels seen with

the antibacterials could be markedly attenuated by the repetitive administration of shaoyao-gancao-tang.[2]

Mechanism

It was suggested that amoxicillin, clarithromycin and metronidazole decimate intestinal bacteria and so reduce the hydrolysis of the glycoside glycyrrhizin to glycyrrhetic acid, which is the form absorbed.[1] Note that shaoyao-gancao-tang is a traditional Chinese medicine containing liquorice (gancao), of which glycyrrhizin is a major constituent.

Importance and management

There appears to be no clinical data regarding an interaction between liquorice and ulcer-healing drugs. The findings of the single-dose experimental study suggested that the clinical efficacy of shaoyao-gancao-tang in peptic ulcer disease might be reduced by the concurrent use of antibacterials used to eliminate *Helicobacter pylori* infection. However, the multiple-dose study suggests that with repeated doses of the herbal medicine, the interaction might not be clinically relevant.

1. He J-X, Akao T, Nishino T, Tani T. The influence of commonly prescribed synthetic drugs for peptic ulcer on the pharmacokinetic fate of glycyrrhizin from Shaoyao-Gancao-tang. *Biol Pharm Bull* (2001) 24, 1395–9.
2. He J-X, Akao T, Tani T. Repetitive administration of Shaoyao-Gancao-tang to rats restores the bioavailability of glycyrrhizin reduced by antibiotic treatment. *J Pharm Pharmacol* (2003) 55, 1569–75.

Liquorice + Warfarin

The interaction between liquorice and warfarin is based on experimental evidence only.

Clinical evidence

No interactions found.

Experimental evidence

In a study in *rats,* pretreatment with gancao aqueous extract 900 mg/kg daily by gastric lavage for 6 days, reduced the AUC of a single 2-mg/kg dose of intravenous warfarin by about 38% and increased its clearance by 57%.[1]

Mechanism

The authors of the study in *rats* suggest that gancao increases the metabolism of warfarin by the activation of the pregnane X receptor (PXR), which increases the expression of cytochrome P450 subfamily CYP3A, and isoenzyme CYP2C9.[1]

Importance and management

Evidence appears to be limited to one experimental study in *rats*. It has been hypothesised that liquorice (gancao) might increase the effect of warfarin because of its natural coumarin content,[2] but the coumarin constituents of liquorice are not known to be anticoagulants, and there is no evidence of liquorice acting as an anticoagulant. Furthermore, liquorice is not known as a food substance that reduces the activity of warfarin anticoagulation, neither is it know to induce the metabolism of other drugs; however, the experimental study introduces the possibility that it might. The evidence presented is too slim to make any specific recommendations regarding concurrent use.

1. Mu Y, Zhang J, Zhang S, Zhou H-H, Toma D, Ren S, Huang L, Yaramus M, Baum A, Venkataramanan R, Xie W. Traditional Chinese medicines Wu Wei Zi (*Schisandra chinensis Baill*) and Gan Cao (*Glycyrrhiza uralensis Fisch*) activate pregnane X receptor and increase warfarin clearance in rats. *J Pharmacol Exp Ther* (2006) 316, 1369–77.
2. Heck AM, DeWitt BA, Lukes AL. Potential interactions between alternative therapies and warfarin. *Am J Health-Syst Pharm* (2000) 57, 1221–7.

L

Lycium

Lycium barbarum L. (Solanaceae)

Synonym(s) and related species

Chinese wolfberry, Goji berries, Matrimony vine, Wolfberry.

Lycium chinense.

Constituents

Lycium fruit contains carotenoids such as betacarotene and **zeaxanthin**, beta-sitosterol, linoleic acid, betaine and various polysaccharides, vitamins and amino acids. The root bark contains beta-sitosterol and betaine among other constituents.

Use and indications

Lycium (dried berries or root bark) has been used to treat diabetes, ophthalmic disorders, hypertension and erectile dysfunction, and is thought to possess anti-inflammatory, antioxidant and anticancer properties. The dried berries are also used as a foodstuff.

Pharmacokinetics

In vitro studies suggest that lycium may be a weak inhibitor of the cytochrome P450 isoenzyme CYP2C9, although this is considered insufficient to cause a drug interaction,[1] see warfarin, page 335.

Interactions overview

Lycium has antidiabetic effects, which may be additive with conventional antidiabetics, although evidence for this is largely experimental. A case report suggests that lycium may enhance the effects of warfarin, but this does not appear to be as a result of inhibiting CYP2C9, as has been suggested by some sources.

Interactions monographs

- Antidiabetics, page 335
- Food, page 335
- Herbal medicines, page 335
- Warfarin, page 335

1. Lam AY, Elmer GW, Mohutsky M. Possible interaction between warfarin and *Lycium barbarum* L. *Ann Pharmacother* (2001) 35, 1199–1201.

L

Lycium + Antidiabetics

The interaction between lycium and antidiabetics is based on experimental evidence only.

Clinical evidence

No interactions found.

Experimental evidence

In an experimental study in *rats* with streptozotocin-induced type 2 diabetes,[1] *Lycium barbarum* polysaccharide (extracted from the fruit of lycium) decreased insulin resistance, and reduced fasting insulin and postprandial glucose levels. In another study, a fruit extract of *Lycium barbarum* 10 mg/kg twice daily for 10 days significantly reduced blood-glucose levels in diabetic *rabbits* but did not reduce blood-glucose levels in healthy *mice*.[2]

Mechanism

Lycium appears to improve glucose transport and increase insulin signalling thereby reducing blood-glucose levels. In theory, these effects may be additive with conventional antidiabetics.

Importance and management

The evidence is limited and purely experimental but what there is suggests that lycium may have antidiabetic properties. This is supported by the traditional use of lycium, in diabetes. Therefore, there is a theoretical possibility that lycium may enhance the blood-glucose-lowering effects of conventional antidiabetics. However, until more is known, it would be unwise to advise anything other than general caution.

1. Zhao R, Li Q, Xiao B. Effect of *Lycium barbarum* polysaccharide on the improvement of insulin resistance in NIDDM rats. *Yakugaku Zasshi* (2005) 125, 981–8.
2. Luo Q, Cai Y, Yan J, Sun M, Corke H. Hypoglycemic and hypolipidemic effects and antioxidant activity of fruit extracts from *Lycium barbarum*. *Life Sci* (2004) 76, 137–49.

Lycium + Food

No interactions found. Note that lycium berries are used as a foodstuff.

Lycium + Herbal medicines

No interactions found.

Lycium + Warfarin

A case report suggests that lycium may enhance the effects of warfarin.

Clinical evidence

A 61-year-old Chinese woman stabilised on warfarin (INRs normally 2 to 3) had an unexpected rise in her INR to 4.1, which was identified during a routine monthly check. No bleeding was seen. She was also taking atenolol, benazepril, digoxin and fluvastatin. It was found that 4 days before visiting the clinic she had started to take one glass (about 170 mL) 3 or 4 times daily of a Chinese herbal tea made from the fruits of lycium to treat blurred vision caused by a sore eye. When the herbal treatment was stopped, her INRs rapidly returned to normal.[1] In another case report, goji juice (said to contain *Lycium barbarum*) was considered to have been responsible for an increase in the INR of a 71-year-old woman who had been taking warfarin for about 3 months. Four days before her admission, with nose bleeds, bruising and rectal bleeding, she had starting drinking goji juice: her prothrombin time was more than 120 seconds.[2]

Experimental evidence

See under *Mechanism*, below.

Mechanism

Warfarin is metabolised by a number of isoenzymes, the most important being CYP2C9. Inhibition of this isoenzyme may therefore lead to increased warfarin levels and effects. The authors also carried out an *in vitro* study and concluded that although lycium is a weak inhibitor of the cytochrome P450 isoenzyme CYP2C9, this is insufficient to cause an interaction. However, they note that other mechanisms cannot be ruled out.[1]

Importance and management

Although the authors suggest avoiding the concurrent use of lycium and warfarin,[1,2] because of the many other factors influencing anticoagulant control, it is not possible to reliably ascribe a change in INR specifically to a drug interaction in a single case report without other supporting evidence. It may be better to advise patients to discuss the use of any herbal products they wish to try, and to increase monitoring if this is thought advisable. Cases of uneventful use should be reported, as they are as useful as possible cases of adverse effects. It should be noted that lycium berries are also used as an ingredient in Chinese foods.

1. Lam AY, Elmer GW, Mohutsky M. Possible interaction between warfarin and *Lycium barbarum* L. *Ann Pharmacother* (2001) 35, 1199–1201.
2. Rivera CA, Ferro CL, Bursua AJ, Gerber BS. Probable interaction between Lycium barbarum (Goji) and warfarin. *Pharmacotherapy* (2012) 32, 298.

L

Lycopene

Lycium barbarum L. (Solanaceae)

Types, sources and related compounds

E160(d).

Pharmacopoeias

Lycopene (*USP35–NF30 S1*); Lycopene preparation (*USP35–NF30 S1*); Tomato extract containing lycopene (*USP35–NF30 S1*).

Use and indications

Lycopene is a **carotenoid**; a natural red pigment found in plants including some fruit and vegetables (such as tomatoes), and is therefore eaten as part of a healthy diet, and is also used as a food-colouring. It has been used for age-related macular degeneration and its antioxidant properties have been investigated for possible use in cardiovascular disease and cancer prevention, especially prostate cancer.

Pharmacokinetics

Lycopene is similar to betacarotene, the most widely studied carotenoid, but unlike betacarotene, it is not a precursor to vitamin A. A study in 25 healthy men found that the amount of lycopene absorbed from a single dose of up to 120 mg was less than 6 mg in 80% of subjects, regardless of dose.[1]

Interactions overview

There is very little information on the interactions of lycopene supplements, but there is some information on dietary lycopene. Combined use with sucrose polyesters, colestyramine, probucol or betacarotene modestly reduces dietary lycopene absorption. Lycopene does not appear to affect the absorption of betacarotene. A low-fat diet does not alter dietary lycopene absorption when dietary intake is high. Colchicine and orlistat modestly reduce the absorption of the related carotenoid, betacarotene, probably because of their effects on fat absorption. If the mechanism is correct, lycopene levels could also be affected, see Betacarotene + Colchicine, page 70 and Betacarotene + Orlistat, page 71.

Interactions monographs

- Food, page 337
- Herbal medicines; Betacarotene, page 337
- Lipid regulating drugs, page 337
- Sucrose polyesters, page 338

1. Diwadkar-Navsariwala V, Novotny JA, Gustin DM, Sosman JA, Rodvold KA, Crowell JA, Stacewicz-Sapuntzakis M, Bowen PE. A physiological pharmacokinetic model describing the disposition of lycopene in healthy men. *J Lipid Res* (2003) 44, 1927–39.

L

Lycopene + Colchicine

Colchicine modestly reduces the absorption of the related carotenoid, betacarotene, potentially because of its effects on fat absorption. Because lycopene levels tended to be lower in those taking low-fat diets (see food, page 337), if the mechanism is correct, lycopene levels may also be affected by colchicine, see Betacarotene + Colchicine, page 70.

Lycopene + Food

A low-fat diet is unlikely to alter the absorption of lycopene when the dietary intake of lycopene is high.

Clinical evidence

There do not appear to be any studies on the effect of food on the absorption of lycopene from supplements; however, there are studies on the effect of foods on absorption of *dietary* lycopene. In one crossover study in 13 healthy men eating a diet with a controlled carotenoid content and high in lycopene, there was no significant difference in the serum levels of lycopene between a high-fat monounsaturated-fat-enriched diet, or a high-carbohydrate low-fat diet. Lycopene was consumed as 300 g tomato soup and 60 g of tomato paste every day for 14 days.[1] Similarly, no change in serum lycopene levels or betacarotene levels were found in a 12-month study in women randomised to a control diet or a low-fat diet, although plasma lycopene levels tended to be lower in those on the low-fat diet.[2]

Experimental evidence

In an experimental study in *rats* fed a diet including lycopene 250 mg/kg for 3 weeks, food restriction of 20% significantly increased the accumulation of lycopene in the liver by about 70% and reduced the serum lycopene levels by about 90%.[3]

Mechanism

Carotenoids are transported in plasma in lipoprotein cholesterol. The study in humans indicates that in situations of abundant lycopene intake, the fat content of the diet does not affect absorption. In a situation of food restriction, the distribution of carotenoids is also restricted because the circulating total lipid concentrations are reduced, thus resulting in a reduction in the serum levels, and accumulation in the liver.

Importance and management

The available data suggest that diet, especially dietary fat, is unlikely to alter the absorption of lycopene when the dietary intake of lycopene is high. This might therefore apply to lycopene supplements, but further study is needed to confirm the absence of an effect of food on their absorption.

1. Ahuja KDK, Ashton EL, Ball MJ. Effects of a high monounsaturated fat, tomato-rich diet on serum levels of lycopene. *Eur J Clin Nutr* (2003) 57, 832–41.
2. Djuric Z, Ren J, Mekjovich O, Venkatramanamoorthy R, Heilbrun L. Effects of high fruit-vegetable and/or low-fat intervention on plasma micronutrient levels. *J Am Coll Nutr* (2006) 25, 178–87.
3. Boileau TW-M, Clinton SK, Zaripheh S, Monaco MH, Donovan SM, Erdman JW. Testosterone and food restriction modulate hepatic lycopene isomer concentrations in male F344 rats. *J Nutr* (2001) 131, 1746–52.

Lycopene + Herbal medicines; Betacarotene

The absorption of endogenous lycopene and lycopene given as a supplement may be altered by betacarotene supplementation. The absorption of betacarotene appears to be unaffected.

Clinical evidence

In a study in 10 healthy subjects, a single 60-mg dose of betacarotene given with a single 60-mg dose of lycopene appeared to significantly increase the AUC of lycopene by about fourfold when compared with lycopene given alone. Betacarotene levels remained the same when given alone and when given with lycopene. However, it was unclear whether absorption was complete by the 24-hour time point, and there was large variation in the absorption of the carotenoids between subjects in this study.[1]

In contrast, in a study in 5 healthy subjects (not taking any lycopene supplements), very high-dose betacarotene 300 mg daily for 21 days decreased the levels of endogenous lycopene by about 30%.[2]

Experimental evidence

In a study in *ferrets,* although the serum levels of betacarotene following a single 10-mg/kg dose were reduced by a single 10-mg/kg dose of lycopene, the average reduction was not significant.[3]

Mechanism

Unclear. There is some debate as to whether these two carotenoids share the same biochemical pathways and compete for absorption, or whether the chemical nature of the preparations in which the supplements are taken affect absorption kinetics.

Importance and management

The evidence is limited, but it suggests that absorption of betacarotene from supplements is affected only modestly, if at all, by lycopene supplements, whereas betacarotene supplements might increase absorption of lycopene supplements taken at the same time. However, the clinical relevance of this, if any, is uncertain. Note that the doses of betacarotene used in the studies are much higher than the maximum daily dose of supplements of 7 mg recommended by the Food Standards Agency in the UK.[4]

1. Johnson EJ, Qin J, Krinsky NI, Russell RM. Ingestion by men of a combined dose of β-carotene and lycopene does not affect the absorption of β-carotene but improves that of lycopene. *J Nutr* (1997) 127, 1833–7.
2. Prince MR, Frisoli JK, Goetschkes MM, Stringham JM, LaMuraglia GM. Rapid serum carotene loading with high-dose β-carotene: clinical implications. *J Cardiovasc Pharmacol* (1991) 17, 343–7.
3. White WS, Peck KM, Bierer TL, Gugger ET, Erdman JW. Interactions of oral β-carotene and canthaxanthin in ferrets. *J Nutr* (1993) 123, 1405–13.
4. Food Standards Agency Betacarotene http://www.eatwell.gov.uk/healthydiet/nutrition essentials/vitaminsandminerals/betacarotene/ (accessed 14/10/2008).

Lycopene + Lipid regulating drugs

Colestyramine and probucol reduce the serum levels of lycopene eaten as part of a normal diet.

Clinical evidence

There do not appear to be any studies on the effect of lipid regulating drugs on the absorption of lycopene from supplements; however, one 3-year study of 303 hypercholesterolaemic subjects given **colestyramine** in doses of 8 g to 16 g daily, according to tolerance, found that the serum levels of *dietary*-derived lycopene were reduced by about 30% after 2 months. When **probucol** 500 mg twice daily was then added, the serum levels of lycopene were reduced by another 30% after a further 2 months. After the initial 6-month period, patients were randomised to receive **probucol** or placebo, and all continued to take **colestyramine**. In those patients randomised to the placebo group, it took about 1 year for the lycopene levels to return to the pre-**probucol** level, and in those randomised to **probucol**, lycopene levels remained at the same low level and did not drop further.[1]

Experimental evidence

No relevant data found.

L

Mechanism

Colestyramine and probucol are lipid regulating drugs that reduce the levels of low-density lipoprotein-cholesterol and high-density lipoprotein-cholesterol respectively. Colestyramine also reduces the intestinal absorption of lipids and the authors suggest that probucol may also displace lycopene from very-low-density lipoprotein-cholesterol in the liver. All these factors may contribute to the reduction of lycopene serum levels because lycopene is fat soluble and therefore its absorption and distribution is dependent on the presence of lipoproteins.

Importance and management

This long-term study suggests that colestyramine and probucol reduce the serum levels of lycopene eaten as part of a normal diet. Supplemental lycopene does not appear to have been studied, but be aware that its desired effect may be reduced by colestyramine and probucol.

1. Elinder LS, Hådell K, Johansson J, Mølgaard J, Holme I, Olsson AG, Walldius G. Probucol treatment decreases serum concentrations of diet-derived antioxidants. *Arterioscler Thromb Vasc Biol* (1995) 15, 1057–63.

Lycopene + Orlistat

Orlistat modestly reduces the absorption of the related carotenoid, betacarotene, probably because of its effects on fat absorption. Because lycopene levels tended to be lower in those taking low-fat diets (see food, page 337) they may also be affected by orlistat, see Betacarotene + Orlistat, page 71.

Lycopene + Sucrose polyesters

Olestra **reduces the serum levels of lycopene eaten as part of a normal diet.**

Clinical evidence

There do not appear to be any studies on the effect of sucrose polyesters on the absorption of lycopene from supplements; however, in one study in 194 healthy subjects, the serum levels of *dietary* lycopene were reduced by up to about 30% by *Olestra* 18 g daily. *Olestra* is a sucrose polyester that is a non-absorbable, non-calorific fat ingredient in snack foods.[1]

Experimental evidence

No relevant data found.

Mechanism

Olestra is thought to reduce the absorption of fat soluble vitamins when present at the same time in the gastrointestinal tract.

Importance and management

Evidence is limited to data on dietary lycopene and it is not known whether *Olestra* or other sucrose polyesters will reduce the absorption of supplemental lycopene; however, it has been found that the base line levels of **vitamin A** have been maintained when subjects take **vitamin A** supplements with *Olestra*, and theoretically at least, this may also be the case with lycopene.[1] The manufacturers of *Olestra* state that because snacking is just a part of the normal balanced diet and because there is a lack of scientific agreement on the health benefits of carotenoids, it is not necessary to take carotenoid supplements with *Olestra*.[2] It should also be pointed out that the intake of *Olestra* in this study is far higher than the average daily intake from snack foods. Nevertheless, separating the intake of lycopene and sucrose polyesters should be enough to avoid any possible interaction.

1. Koonsvitsky BP, Berry DA, Jones MB, Lin PYT, Cooper DA, Jones DY, Jackson JE. Olestra affects serum concentrations of α-Tocopherol and carotenoids but not vitamin D or vitamin K status in free-living subjects. *J Nutr* (1997) 127, 1636S–1645S.
2. Procter and Gamble. Olean® (Olestra) Frequently asked questions. http://www.olean.com/default.asp?p=faq#11 (accessed 04/04/2008).

L

Maté

Ilex paraguariensis A.St.-Hil. (Aquifoliaceae)

Synonym(s) and related species

Ilex, Jesuit's Brazil tea, Paraguay tea, St Bartholomew's tea, Yerba maté.

Constituents

Maté leaves contain xanthine derivatives, mainly **caffeine** (0.2 to 2%) and theobromine, with minor amounts of theophylline. They also contain various **flavonoids** of the flavonol subclass (quercetin, kaempferol and rutin) and polyphenolics, tannins and caffeic acid derivatives. Others include triterpenoid saponins and volatile oil.

Use and indications

Maté leaves are used as a stimulant, diuretic and analgesic, effects which can be attributed to the caffeine content. Maté is used to make a tea-like beverage in South America. High consumption of this tea appears to be associated with a high incidence of cancers of the oropharynx and oesophagus.

Pharmacokinetics

For the pharmacokinetics of caffeine, see caffeine, page 106. For information on the pharmacokinetics of individual flavonoids present in maté, see under flavonoids, page 213.

Interactions overview

The interactions of maté are mainly due to its caffeine content, see caffeine, page 106. For information on the interactions of individual flavonoids found in maté, see under flavonoids, page 213.

M

Meadowsweet

Filipendula ulmaria (L.) Maxim. (Rosaceae)

Synonym(s) and related species

Bridewort, Queen of the meadow.

Spiraea ulmaria L.

Pharmacopoeias

Meadowsweet (*BP 2012, PhEur 7.5*).

Constituents

Meadowsweet contains the phenolic glycosides spiraein, monotropin, and gaultherin, and the essential oil is composed of up to 75% salicylaldehyde, with methylsalicylate and other salicylates. It also contains **flavonoids**, tannins, traces of natural coumarin and ascorbic acid. It may be standardised to a minimum content of steam volatile substances.

Use and indications

Meadowsweet is used as an anti-inflammatory and antacid. Surprisingly for a herb containing salicylates, meadowsweet is used traditionally to treat stomach complaints, and anti-ulcer activity has been demonstrated in some *animal* studies. Extracts from the flowers have been reported to have bacteriostatic activity *in vitro*.

Pharmacokinetics

No relevant pharmacokinetic data found.

Interactions overview

No interactions with meadowsweet have been found. Note however, that it contains salicylates, although it is unknown whether the salicylates are at sufficient levels to have antiplatelet effects and thereby interact with warfarin. For more information about salicylate-containing herbs, see willow, page 485.

Interactions monographs

- Anticoagulants and Antiplatelet drugs, page 341
- Food, page 341
- Herbal medicines, page 341

Meadowsweet + Anticoagulant or Antiplatelet drugs ☑

The information regarding the use of meadowsweet with anticoagulants and antiplatelet drugs is based on a prediction only.

Evidence, mechanism, importance and management

No evidence found. However, note that meadowsweet contains salicylates, and conventional salicylate drugs increase the risk of bleeding with anticoagulants such as **warfarin**, and may have additive effects with antiplatelet drugs, because of their antiplatelet effects.

Whether there are sufficient salicylates in meadowsweet to have an equivalent antiplatelet effect to low-dose aspirin, is unknown. Further study of the *in vitro* antiplatelet potential of meadowsweet is required, using aspirin as a control. See also, *Interactions overview*, under willow, page 485.

Meadowsweet + Food

No interactions found.

Meadowsweet + Herbal medicines

No interactions found.

M

Melatonin

N-[2-(5-Methoxyindol-3-yl)ethyl]acetamide

Types, sources and related compounds

N-Acetyl-5-methoxytryptamine.

Pharmacopoeias

Melatonin (*BP 2012*); Melatonin Capsules (*BP 2012*).

Use and indications

Melatonin is a hormone that is produced in the pineal gland of the brain and influences the circadian rhythm. Supplements are therefore principally used for treating sleep disturbances and disorders such as jet lag, insomnia, sleep walking, and shift-work sleep disorder. It is also believed to have anticancer and antihypertensive properties, and has been used to treat cluster headaches. Melatonin has also been detected in a large number of plant species, including those used as foods. Concentrations detected have been very variable, the reasons for which are currently uncertain. In addition, the importance of dietary melatonin is unclear.

Pharmacokinetics

When an oral melatonin supplement 3 mg was given to 17 healthy subjects the AUC and maximum serum levels of melatonin were about 18-fold and 100-fold greater, respectively, than overnight endogenous melatonin secretion, although there was a wide variation between individuals.[1] The oral bioavailability was approximately 15% after oral doses of 2 or 4 mg, possibly due to significant first-pass metabolism. The half-life has been found to be about 1 hour.[2]

Melatonin has been found to be extensively metabolised by the cytochrome P450 isoenzymes CYP1A1 and CYP1A2 *in vitro*.[3,4] This has been supported by *in vivo* studies, see fluvoxamine, page 345 and caffeine, page 343. *In vitro,* melatonin had no inhibitory effect on CYP3A4, CYP2D6, CYP2C9 and CYP2C19 and a modest inhibitory effect on CYP1A2 in one study,[3] and was reported to *induce* CYP3A (but at supra-therapeutic doses) in another.[4]

Interactions overview

Fluvoxamine markedly increases melatonin levels and increases its effects (drowsiness). Similarly, combined oral contraceptives modestly increase melatonin levels, and other estrogens are predicted to interact similarly. Other drugs that inhibit CYP1A2 are predicted to similarly interact with melatonin. These include some quinolone antibacterials such as ciprofloxacin, the oral psoralens, and, to a lesser extent, cimetidine. Caffeine also modestly increases melatonin levels. Increased cognitive impairment or similar has been seen when melatonin was used with zolpidem, imipramine and thioridazine, and might be expected with any CNS depressant drug. Alcohol is expected to decrease the efficacy of melatonin on sleep. Tobacco smoking reduces melatonin levels, and carbamazepine might be expected to have the same effect, but melatonin had no effect on carbamazepine levels. A few cases of increased or decreased effects of warfarin have been noted, but the relevance of this is uncertain. Melatonin slightly increased mean 24-hour blood pressure when given to patients taking nifedipine.

Interactions monographs

- Alcohol, page 343
- Antipsychotics, page 343
- Benzodiazepines and related drugs, page 343
- Buspirone, page 343
- Caffeine, page 343
- Carbamazepine, page 344
- Cimetidine, page 344
- Food, page 344
- Herbal medicines, page 344
- Imipramine, page 344
- Nifedipine, page 344
- Oestrogens, page 345
- Propofol, page 345
- Psoralens, page 345
- SSRIs, page 345
- Tobacco, page 346
- Warfarin, page 346

1. Kovács J, Brodner W, Kirchlechner V, Arif T, Waldhauser F. Measurement of urinary melatonin: a useful tool for monitoring serum melatonin after its oral administration. *J Clin Endocrinol Metab* (2000) 85, 666–70.
2. DeMuro RL, Nafziger AN, Blask DE, Menhinick AM, Bertino JS. The absolute bioavailability of oral melatonin. *J Clin Pharmacol* (2000) 40, 781–4.
3. Yeleswaram K, Vachharajani N, Santone K. Involvement of cytochrome P-450 isozymes in melatonin metabolism and clinical implications. *J Pineal Res* (1999) 26, 190–191.
4. Circadin Melatonin. Lundbeck Ltd. UK Summary of product characteristics, June 2010.

M

Melatonin + Alcohol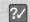

Alcohol may reduce the effects of melatonin on sleep.

Evidence, mechanism, importance and management

The manufacturer briefly notes that alcohol reduces the effectiveness of melatonin on sleep, and that it should not be taken with melatonin.[1] Given the known effects of alcohol on sleep, if melatonin is being taken to improve quality of sleep then this is sensible advice.

1. Circadin (Melatonin). Lundbeck Ltd. UK Summary of product characteristics, July 2008.

Melatonin + Antipsychotics

The concurrent use of thioridazine and melatonin led to increased CNS effects in a pharmacodynamic study.

Evidence, mechanism, importance and management

In a single-dose controlled study, there was no pharmacokinetic interaction between **thioridazine** 50 mg and melatonin 2 mg. However, there was a possible pharmacodynamic interaction, with increased feelings of 'muzzy-headedness' when compared with **thioridazine** alone.[1,2] However, in a placebo-controlled, clinical efficacy study in 22 patients with antipsychotic-induced tardive dyskinesia taking various antipsychotics (13 taking **haloperidol**, 4 taking **chlorpromazine**, 3 taking **perphenazine**, and 2 taking **zuclopenthixol**), the addition of controlled-release melatonin 10 mg in the evening for 6 weeks did not cause any apparent adverse effects.[3] It is possible that the sedative effects of melatonin and antipsychotics might be additive. Bear this possibility in mind.

1. Circadin (Melatonin). Lundbeck Ltd. UK Summary of product characteristics, August 2011.
2. EMEA Assessment report for Circadin. Procedure No. EMEA/H/C/695. 2007 http://www.ema.europa.eu/ema/index.jsp?curl=pages/medicines/human/medicines/000695/human_med_000701.jsp|=WC0b01ac058001d124 (accessed 14/06/2012).
3. Shamir E, Barak Y, Shalman I , Laudon M, Zisapel N, Tarrasch R, Elizur A, Weizman R. Melatonin treatment for tardive dyskinesia: a double-blind, placebo-controlled, crossover study. *Arch Gen Psychiatry* (2001) 58, 1049–52.

Melatonin + Benzodiazepines and related drugs

The CNS effects of benzodiazepines and related hypnotics, such as zolpidem, might be additive with those of melatonin.

Clinical evidence

In a well-controlled single-dose study in 16 healthy subjects aged 55 years and older, giving prolonged-release melatonin 2 mg with **zolpidem** 10 mg at bedtime enhanced the impairment of cognitive function seen with **zolpidem** alone at 1 hour and 4 hours post-dose, but not the next morning. Melatonin alone had no effect on cognitive function. No pharmacokinetic interaction was found.[1]

Experimental evidence

In three experiments in *hamsters* and *mice,* melatonin at doses of 300 micrograms/kg, 20 mg/kg and 50 mg/kg given intraperitoneally was found to significantly reduce locomotor activity, increase pain thresholds when placed on hot plates and prolong the onset of seizures when convulsions were induced, respectively. The benzodiazepine antagonist, flumazenil 5 mg/kg, 10 mg/kg and 50 mg/kg given intraperitoneally, respectively, reduced the activity of melatonin back to approximate normal levels.[2]

Mechanism

The activity of melatonin is thought to involve similar interactions at the GABA (gamma-aminobutyric acid) receptors in the brain to benzodiazepines. Melatoinin might therefore enhance the activity of benzodiazepines and related drugs. Flumazenil is a benzodiazepine antagonist and may have blocked the direct effect of the melatonin, thus causing the GABA activity to fall below the level required to have the effects seen in the experimental study.

Importance and management

The evidence available suggests that melatonin might enhance the sedative properties of benzodiazepines and related hypnotics such as zolpidem. Although in the study of zolpidem, the enhanced effect was not apparent the morning after dosing, it would be wise to be aware that increased drowsiness is a possibility if melatonin is also given, especially with longer-acting hypnotics.

1. Otmani S, Demazières A, Staner C, Jacob N, Nir T, Zisapel N, Staner L. Effects of prolonged-release melatonin, zolpidem, and their combination on psychomotor functions, memory recall, and driving skills in healthy middle aged and elderly volunteers. *Hum Psychopharmacol* (2008) 23, 693–705.
2. Golombek DA, Escolar E, Burin LJ, De Brito Sánchez MG, Fernández Duque D, Cardinali DP. Chronopharmacology of melatonin: inhibition by benzodiazepine antagonism. *Chronobiol Int* (1992) 9, 124–31.

Melatonin + Buspirone

For a case report describing anxiety, with episodes of over-sleeping and memory deficits in a woman taking fluoxetine and buspirone with St John's wort, ginkgo and melatonin, see St John's wort + Buspirone, page 443.

Melatonin + Caffeine

Caffeine may moderately raise melatonin levels.

Clinical evidence

A crossover study in 12 healthy subjects found that a single 200-mg dose of caffeine (equivalent to one large or two small cups of coffee), taken 1 hour before and 1 and 3 hours after a single 6-mg oral dose of melatonin, increased the average AUC and maximum levels of melatonin by 120% and 137%, respectively, although the half-life of melatonin was not significantly affected. The interaction was less pronounced in smokers (6 subjects) than in non-smokers (6 subjects).[1] In a similar study, taking caffeine 12 or 24 hours before melatonin did not affect the melatonin levels, although 2 subjects had raised melatonin levels when caffeine was taken 12 hours, but not 24 hours, before melatonin.[2]

In 12 healthy subjects given a single 200-mg dose of caffeine, taken in the evening, *endogenous,* nocturnal melatonin levels were found to be increased, and the AUC of melatonin was increased by 32%.[3]

Experimental evidence

No relevant data found.

Mechanism

Caffeine is thought to reduce the metabolism of melatonin by competing for metabolism by the cytochrome P450 isoenzyme CYP1A2.

Importance and management

It appears that caffeine significantly increases the levels of single doses of supplementary melatonin; however, the long-term effects of caffeine and concurrent multiple dosing of melatonin do not appear to have been studied. Melatonin can cause drowsiness when taken on its own, so patients who take melatonin should be advised that this effect may be increased (because of increased melatonin levels) if they also take caffeine, including that from beverages. This increased drowsiness may oppose the stimulating effect of caffeine, or alternatively caffeine may diminish the sedating effects of melatonin; the outcome of concurrent use does not appear to have been studied.

1. Härtter S, Nordmark A, Rose D-M, Bertilsson L, Tybring G, Laine K. Effects of caffeine intake on the pharmacokinetics of melatonin, a probe drug for CYP1A2 activity. *Br J Clin Pharmacol* (2003) 56, 679–82.
2. Härtter S, Korhonen T, Lundgren S, Rane A, Tolonen A, Turpeinen M, Laine K. Effect of caffeine intake 12 or 24 hours prior to melatonin intake and *CYP1A2*1F* polymorphism on CYP1A2 phenotyping by melatonin. *Basic Clin Pharmacol Toxicol* (2006) 99, 300–304.
3. Ursing C, Wikner J, Brismar K, Röjdmark S. Caffeine raises the serum melatonin level in healthy subjects: an indication of melatonin metabolism by cytochrome P450 (CYP)1A2. *J Endocrinol Invest* (2003) 26, 403–6.

Melatonin + Carbamazepine

Carbamazepine levels are not affected by melatonin. Melatonin levels are predicted to be reduced by carbamazepine.

Evidence, mechanism, importance and management

In a placebo-controlled study on the effects of melatonin on antioxidant enzymes, melatonin 6 to 9 mg/kg daily for 14 days was given to children with epilepsy taking carbamazepine monotherapy. Serum levels of carbamazepine and its metabolite carbamazepine-10,11-epoxide were not affected by melatonin. Melatonin appeared to antagonise the accumulation of reactive oxygen species caused by carbamazepine.[1]

One manufacturer predicts that carbamazepine may increase the metabolism of melatonin (by induction of the cytochrome P450 isoenzyme CYP1A2), decreasing its levels (magnitude unknown).[2] However, note that carbamazepine is not a particularly potent inducer of this isoenzyme.

It appears that carbamazepine dose adjustments are unlikely to be needed when melatonin is taken. Nevertheless, be aware that melatonin may be less effective.

1. Gupta M, Gupta YK, Agarwal S, Aneja S, Kalaivani M, Kohli K. Effects of add-on melatonin administration on antioxidant enzymes in children with epilepsy taking carbamazepine monotherapy: a randomized, double-blind, placebo-controlled trial. *Epilepsia* (2004) 45, 1636–9.
2. Circadin (Melatonin). Lundbeck Ltd. UK Summary of product characteristics, July 2008.

Melatonin + Cimetidine

Cimetidine slightly increases melatonin levels.

Evidence, mechanism, importance and management

In a single-dose controlled study, cimetidine 800 mg increased the plasma concentration of melatonin after a 2 mg oral dose (magnitude not stated), whereas the plasma levels of cimetidine were unaffected. The pharmacodynamics of melatonin were not affected.[1,2] Cimetidine is a weak inhibitor of the cytochrome P450 isoenzyme CYP1A2 by which melatonin is principally metabolised. The pharmacokinetic interaction would be unlikely to be clinically relevant. Nevertheless, the manufacturer recommends caution.[1] Be aware of a possible interaction if there is an increase in adverse effects of melatonin (e.g. irritability, dry mouth, dizziness) on concurrent use. Other H$_2$-receptor antagonists are unlikely to interact as they are not known to have enzyme-inhibiting effects.

1. Circadin (Melatonin). Lundbeck Ltd. UK Summary of product characteristics, July 2008.
2. EMEA Assessment report for Circadin. Procedure No. EMEA/H/C/695. 2007 http://www.emea.europa.eu/humandocs/PDFs/EPAR/circadin/H-695-en6.pdf (accessed 21/11/2008).

Melatonin + Food

No interactions found, but caffeine-containing beverages might increase melatonin levels, see Melatonin + Caffeine, page 343.

Melatonin + Herbal medicines

No interactions found, but note that caffeine from caffeine-containing herbs might increase melatonin levels, see Melatonin + Caffeine, page 343.

Melatonin + Imipramine

The concurrent use of imipramine and melatonin may lead to increased CNS effects.

Evidence, mechanism, importance and management

In a single-dose controlled study, there was no pharmacokinetic interaction between melatonin 2 mg and imipramine 75 mg. However, there was a possible pharmacodynamic interaction, with increased feelings of tranquillity and difficulty in performing tasks (undefined) when compared with imipramine alone.[1,2] Patients should be warned of a possible additive effect.

1. Circadin (Melatonin). Lundbeck Ltd. UK Summary of product characteristics, July 2008.
2. EMEA Assessment report for Circadin. Procedure No. EMEA/H/C/695. 2007 http://www.emea.europa.eu/humandocs/PDFs/EPAR/circadin/H-695-en6.pdf (accessed 21/11/2008).

Melatonin + Nifedipine

Melatonin may have some modest effects on blood pressure in patients taking nifedipine.

Clinical evidence

Forty-seven subjects with mild to moderate hypertension well-controlled on nifedipine GITS 30 mg or 60 mg daily for the past 3 months were given melatonin immediate-release capsules 5 mg each evening for 4 weeks. At the end of the 4 weeks, there was a modest increase in mean 24-hour systolic and diastolic blood pressure of 6.5 mmHg and 4.9 mmHg, respectively, and an increase in heart rate of 3.9 bpm. However, there was no difference in single-time point 'clinic' blood pressure (136/85 mmHg versus 138/87 mmHg) and heart rate. While taking melatonin, there was a greater incidence of drowsiness, during the morning, and weakness. One subject dropped out of the study complaining of marked weakness.[1]

Experimental evidence

No relevant data found.

Mechanism

Unknown. Melatonin has been reported to possess blood pressure-lowering properties when used alone and was expected to have additive effects with nifedipine.[1]

Importance and management

Chronic use of melatonin appears to modestly impair the hypotensive effects of nifedipine and *increase* the blood pressure and heart rates of patients. However, this was only detected on 24-hour blood pressure monitoring, and was not apparent with single-measures of blood pressure at the clinic. Therefore, the clinical relevance of the effect is probably minor. The mechanism is not clear, and until more is known, bear in mind the possibility of an interaction if patients taking calcium-channel blockers have increased blood pressure while also taking melatonin supplements.

1. Lusardi P, Piazza E, Fogari R. Cardiovascular effects of melatonin in hypertensive patients well controlled by nifedipine: a 24-hour study. *Br J Clin Pharmacol* (2000) 49, 423–7.

Melatonin + Oestrogens

Oestrogens, from combined hormonal contraceptives, appear to increase melatonin levels.

Clinical evidence

In a clinical study, the AUC and maximum level of a single 6-mg dose of melatonin was about 4 times higher in subjects taking a combined oral contraceptive than those not. Melatonin alone did not significantly affect alertness in this study, and no reduced alertness was noted in those taking oral contraceptives. Oral contraceptives being used by the women included **ethinylestradiol** with either cyproterone acetate, desogestrel, drospirenone or gestodene. There did not appear to be any obvious differences between these contraceptives, but the numbers of women taking each were too small for this to be conclusive.[1]

Experimental evidence

No relevant data found.

Mechanism

Ethinylestradiol is a moderate inhibitor of the cytochrome P450 isoenzyme CYP1A2, by which melatonin is principally metabolised.

Importance and management

Women taking combined oral contraceptives may have higher levels of melatonin after using supplements. Although in the study cited, this did not decrease alertness, it would be prudent to bear in mind the possibility of increased drowsiness. One UK manufacturer extends this caution to hormone replacement therapy,[2] although it is unclear whether the oestrogens used for HRT will have the same effect as ethinylestradiol.

1. Hilli J, Korhonen T, Turpeinen M, Hokkanen J, Mattila S, Laine K. The effect of oral contraceptives on the pharmacokinetics of melatonin in healthy subjects with CYP1A2 g.-163C>A polymorphism. *J Clin Pharmacol* (2008) 48, 986–94.
2. Circadin (Melatonin). Lundbeck Ltd. UK Summary of product characteristics, July 2008.

Melatonin + Propofol

Melatonin slightly reduces the dose of propofol needed for the induction of anaesthesia.

Clinical evidence

A study in 45 adult patients found that the induction dose of intravenous propofol, as measured by bispectral index and loss of eyelash reflex, was 15% lower in patients who had received a single 3 or 5-mg oral dose of melatonin 100 minutes preoperatively, compared with patients who had received placebo. The time to recover from the anaesthetic was not affected by premedication with melatonin. Propofol was given in an incremental dose fashion in this study so that any difference could be assessed, but is usually given as a bolus dose.[1]

Experimental evidence

No relevant data found.

Mechanism

Melatonin appears to have anxiolytic and sedative effects, which might reduce the required induction dose of propofol.

Importance and management

This study was conducted to assess the clinical value of using melatonin premedication, which is not an established use. The reduction in required dose of propofol was small, and on the basis of these data, it is unlikely that any untoward effects would be seen in the situation where a patient who had recently taken a melatonin supplement was anaesthetised with propofol.

1. Turkistani A, Abdullah KM, Al-Shaer AA, Mazen KF, Alkatheri K. Melatonin premedication and the induction dose of propofol. *Eur J Anaesthesiol* (2007) 24, 399–402.

Melatonin + Psoralens

Psoralens are predicted to increase melatonin levels.

Evidence, mechanism, importance and management

The manufacturer briefly notes that **methoxsalen** and **5-methoxypsoralen** inhibit the metabolism of melatonin and increases its levels (magnitude not stated).[1] Note that 5-methoxypsoralen has been shown to increase *endogenous* melatonin levels (one study is cited as an example[2]).

Psoralens are potent inhibitors of the cytochrome P450 isoenzyme CYP1A2 by which melatonin is principally metabolised, and the manufacturer recommends caution on concurrent use,[1] which seems prudent as the adverse effects of melatonin may be increased. Any interaction would only apply to these psoralens used orally, and not when they are used topically. Be aware of a possible interaction if there is an increase in adverse effects of melatonin (e.g. irritability, dry mouth, dizziness) in patients also taking psoralens.

1. Circadin (Melatonin). Lundbeck Ltd. UK Summary of product characteristics, July 2008.
2. Souetre E, Salvati E, Belugou JL, Krebs B, Darcourt G. 5-Methoxypsoralen as a specific stimulating agent of melatonin secretion in humans. *J Clin Endocrinol Metab* (1990) 71, 670–674.

Melatonin + SSRIs

Fluvoxamine raises melatonin levels. Limited evidence suggests that citalopram does not affect melatonin levels, and no effect would be expected with other SSRIs.

Clinical evidence

(a) Citalopram

In a study in 7 healthy subjects, citalopram 40 mg had no effect on the levels of *endogenous* melatonin or its excretion from the body. Extrapolating these findings to an instance where melatonin is given exogenously as a supplement is difficult, but they suggest that citalopram does not inhibit melatonin metabolism.[1]

(b) Fluvoxamine

In a study in 5 healthy subjects, a single 50-mg dose of fluvoxamine taken 3 hours before a single 5-mg oral dose of melatonin markedly increased the AUC and maximum levels of melatonin by 17-fold and 12-fold, respectively, although the half-life of melatonin was not significantly affected. The interaction was more pronounced in the one subject who was of a CYP2D6-poor metaboliser phenotype (meaning that this patient was lacking or deficient in this isoenzyme). All subjects reported marked drowsiness after melatonin intake, and this was even more pronounced after fluvoxamine was also given.[2]

Similarly, fluvoxamine 75 mg raised the levels of oral melatonin 5 mg by about 20-fold and significantly improved the sleep behaviour of a 51-year-old insomniac.[3]

In another study in 7 healthy subjects, fluvoxamine 50 mg doubled the maximum serum levels and excretion of *endogenous* melatonin and increased the AUC by about threefold.[1]

Experimental evidence

No relevant data found.

Mechanism

Fluvoxamine is a potent inhibitor of the cytochrome P450 isoenzyme CYP1A2, which is the principal isoenzyme involved in the metabolism of melatonin.

Importance and management

Fluvoxamine markedly increases the bioavailability of endogenous melatonin and melatonin given as a supplement. However the long-term effects of fluvoxamine and concurrent multiple dosing of melatonin do not appear to have been studied. Be aware that excessive drowsiness and related adverse effects may occur on concurrent use. Note that one UK manufacturer advises that the combination should be avoided.[4] Other inhibitors of CYP1A2 may interact similarly (although to a lesser extent as fluvoxamine is currently the most potent CYP1A2 inhibitor in clinical use). The UK manufacturer specifically mentions the quinolones.[4] Of the quinolones in common usage, **ciprofloxacin** is an example of a clinically important CYP1A2 inhibitor.

Note that this effect would not be expected with other SSRIs, as these are not CYP1A2 inhibitors, and the study looking at the effects of citalopram on endogenous melatonin somewhat supports this suggestion.

For a case report describing anxiety, with episodes of oversleeping and memory deficits in a woman taking **fluoxetine** and buspirone with St John's wort, ginkgo and melatonin, see St John's wort + Buspirone, page 443.

1. von Bahr C, Ursing C, Yasui N, Tybring G, Bertilsson L, Röjdmark S. Fluvoxamine but not citalopram increases serum melatonin in healthy subjects - an indication that cytochrome P_{450} CYP1A2 and CYP2C19 hydroxylate melatonin. *Eur J Clin Pharmacol* (2000) 56, 123–7.
2. Härtter S, Grözinger M, Weigmann H, Röschke J, Hiemke C. Increased bioavailability of oral melatonin after fluvoxamine coadministration. *Clin Pharmacol Ther* (2000) 67, 1–6.
3. Grözinger M, Härtter S, Wang X, Röschke J, Hiemke C. Fluvoxamine strongly inhibits melatonin metabolism in a patient with low-amplitude melatonin profile. *Arch Gen Psychiatry* (2000) 57, 812.
4. Circadin (Melatonin). Lundbeck Ltd. UK Summary of product characteristics, July 2008.

Melatonin + Tobacco

Tobacco smoking reduces melatonin levels.

Evidence, mechanism, importance and management

In a study in 8 tobacco smokers, the AUC of a single 25-mg dose of melatonin was almost threefold higher when the melatonin was taken after 7 days of smoking abstinence than when taken while smoking.[1]

Constituents of tobacco smoke are minor to moderate inducers of the cytochrome P450 isoenzyme CYP1A2, by which melatonin is principally metabolised.

The finding of this study suggests that melatonin might not be as effective in smokers. Be aware of this possibility, and consider trying an increased melatonin dose if it is not effective in a smoker.

1. Ursing C, von Bahr C, Brismar K, Röjdmark S. Influence of cigarette smoking on melatonin levels in man. *Eur J Clin Pharmacol* (2005) 61, 197–201.

Melatonin + Warfarin

Case reports suggest that melatonin may raise or lower the INR in response to warfarin.

Clinical evidence

Six case reports of a suspected interaction between melatonin and **warfarin** have been documented by the WHO Uppsala Monitoring Centre, and have been briefly summarised in a review of melatonin.[1] In three cases, the prothrombin time was increased, with bleeding events in two (nosebleed, eye haemorrhage, bruising) occurring up to 8 days after starting to take melatonin. The other three cases reports describe a prothrombin time decrease.[1]

Experimental evidence

See *Mechanism*, below.

Mechanism

Unknown. Melatonin did not inhibit the cytochrome P450 isoenzyme CYP2C9 *in vitro*,[2] and would not therefore be expected to alter warfarin metabolism via this mechanism.

Importance and management

These appear to be the only reports in the literature of a possible interaction between melatonin and warfarin. They are difficult to interpret, since they include both increased and decreased warfarin effects, and it is possible that they are just idiosyncratic cases. Because of these cases, a study designed to exclude a pharmacokinetic/pharmacodynamic interaction would be useful. Until more is known, bear these cases in mind in the event of an unexpected change in coagulation status in patients also taking melatonin supplements.

1. Herxheimer A, Petrie KKJ. Melatonin for the prevention and treatment of jet lag. Available in the Cochrane Database of Systematic Reviews; Issue 1. Chichester: John Wiley; 2009..
2. Yeleswaram K, Vachharajani N, Santone K. Involvement of cytochrome P-450 isozymes in melatonin metabolism and clinical implications. *J Pineal Res* (1999) 26, 190–191.

M

Melilot

Melilotus officinalis (L.) Pall. (Fabaceae)

Synonym(s) and related species

King's clover, Sweet clover, Ribbed melilot, Yellow melilot, Yellow sweet clover.

Melilotus arvensis Wallr.

Not to be confused with Red clover, page 398 (*Trifolium pratense*), which is known as Cow clover, Meadow clover or Purple clover.

Pharmacopoeias

Melilot (*BP 2012, PhEur 7.5*).

Constituents

The main active constituents of melilot are natural coumarin and its derivatives, melilotin (3,4-dihydrocoumarin), melilotol, umbelliferone and scopoletin, which are formed on drying from the glycoside melilotoside. If spoilage and subsequent fermentation occurs, some coumarin derivatives can be transformed into the potent anticoagulant dicoumarol (bishydroxycoumarin). Other constituents present are **flavonoids** (including quercetin), and a number of saponins.

Use and indications

Melilot is used mainly to treat inflammation, oedema and capillary fragility.

Pharmacokinetics

No relevant pharmacokinetic data for melilot found. For information on the pharmacokinetics of individual flavonoids present in melilot, see under flavonoids, page 213.

Interactions overview

A case report describes bleeding and a raised INR in a woman taking acenocoumarol while using a topical cream containing melilot and butcher's broom, but an interaction has not been established. For information on the interactions of individual flavonoids present in melilot, see under flavonoids, page 213.

Interactions monographs

- Food, page 348
- Herbal medicines, page 348
- Warfarin and related drugs, page 348

M

Melilot + Food

No interactions found.

Melilot + Herbal medicines

No interactions found.

Melilot + Warfarin and related drugs

The INR of a patient taking acenocoumarol was increased after she used a melilot-containing topical cream, and a woman who had been drinking large quantities of a herbal tea containing melilot developed a prolonged prothrombin time.

Clinical evidence

A 66-year-old taking **acenocoumarol**, levothyroxine and prazepam had an increase in her INR after massaging a proprietary topical cream (*Cyclo 3*) containing melilot and butcher's broom on her legs three times daily. On the first occasion her INR rose from about 2 to 5.8 after 7 days of use, and on a later occasion it rose to 4.6 after 10 days of use.[1] In another report, a woman with unexplained abnormal menstrual bleeding was found to have a prothrombin time of 53 seconds, and laboratory tests showed that her blood clotting factors were abnormally low. When given parenteral vitamin K her prothrombin time rapidly returned to normal (suggesting that she was taking a vitamin K antagonist of some kind). She strongly denied taking any anticoagulant drugs, but it was eventually dis-covered that she had been drinking large quantities of a herbal tea containing among other ingredients tonka beans, melilot and sweet woodruff, all of which might contain natural coumarins.[2]

Experimental evidence

No relevant data found.

Mechanism

Unknown. Melilot is known to contain natural coumarins, although these do not possess the minimum structural requirements required for anticoagulant activity (see Natural coumarins + Warfarin and related drugs, page 360), and coumarin does not inhibit CYP2C9, by which acenocoumarol and the other coumarin anticoagulants are metabolised. It seems that fermentation and spoilage of the melilot by mould is necessary for anticoagulant effects to occur.

Importance and management

Evidence appears to be limited to these isolated cases, which are not established. Many factors influence anticoagulant control, and therefore it is not possible to reliably ascribe a change in INR specifically to a drug interaction in a single case report without other supporting evidence. It may be better to advise patients to discuss the use of any herbal products they wish to try, and to increase monitoring if this is thought advisable. Cases of uneventful use should be reported, as they are as useful as possible cases of adverse effects. However, while recognising that there is no mechanistic basis for an interaction, the EMEA Committee on Herbal Medicinal Products (HMPC) does nevertheless say that self-medication with melilot should be contraindicated in patients taking anticoagulant therapy.

1. Chiffoleau A, Huguenin H, Veyrac G, Argaiz V, Dupe D, Kayser M, Bourin M, Jolliet P. Interaction entre mélilot et acénocoumarol ? (mélilot-*ruscus aculeatus*). *Therapie* (2001) 56, 321–7.
2. Hogan RP. Hemorrhagic diathesis caused by drinking an herbal tea. *JAMA* (1983) 249, 2679–80.

M

Milk thistle

Silybum marianum (L.) Gaertn. (Asteraceae)

Synonym(s) and related species

Lady's thistle, Marian thistle, Mediterranean milk thistle, St Mary's thistle.

Carduus marianus, *Mariana lactea* Hill.

Not to be confused with Blessed thistle, page 83, which is *Cnicus benedictus*.

Pharmacopoeias

Milk Thistle (*USP35–NF30 S1*); Milk Thistle Capsules (*USP35–NF30 S1*); Milk Thistle Fruit (*BP 2012, PhEur 7.5*); Milk Thistle Tablets (*USP35–NF30 S1*); Powdered Milk Thistle (*USP35–NF30 S1*); Powdered Milk Thistle Extract (*USP35–NF30 S1*); Refined and Standardised Milk Thistle Dry Extract (*BP 2012, PhEur 7.5*).

Constituents

The mature fruit (seed) of milk thistle contains **silymarin**, which is a mixture of the flavonolignans silibinin (silybin), silicristin (silychristin), silidianin (silydianin), isosilibinin and others. It may be standardised to contain not less than 1.5% (*PhEur 7.5*), or not less than 2% (*USP35–NF30 S1*) of **silymarin**, expressed as silibinin (dried drug). Standardised extracts, containing high levels of **silymarin**, are often used. Milk thistle fruit also contains various other flavonoids, page 213, such as quercetin, and various sterols.

Note that milk thistle leaves do not contain **silymarin**, and contain the flavonoids, page 213, apigenin and luteolin, and the triterpene, beta-sitosterol.

Use and indications

Milk thistle is reported to have hepatoprotective properties and is mainly used for liver diseases and jaundice. Traditionally milk thistle was used by nursing mothers for stimulating milk production, as a bitter tonic, demulcent, as an antidepressant, and for dyspeptic complaints. Both the fruit and leaves are used as a herbal medicine, but currently the fruit is the main target of investigation because it contains the pharmacologically active silymarin component. Standardised extracts of silymarin are also commonly used. A water-soluble salt of the individual flavonolignan silibinin is used intravenously for preventing hepatotoxicity after poisoning with the death cap mushroom *Amanita phalloides*.

Pharmacokinetics

Several studies have investigated the effect of milk thistle extracts on cytochrome P450 isoenzymes and drug transporters. In some *in vitro* studies[1-7] milk thistle or its flavonolignan constituents inhibited CYP3A4. Although some clinical pharmacokinetic studies suggest that milk thistle may raise the levels of some CYP3A4 substrates, several other studies have found no effect on CYP3A4 substrates, see midazolam, page 351, and HIV-protease inhibitors, page 352. These conflicting findings may be due, in part, to the dose of milk thistle used. Indeed, some *in vitro* studies found that the effect of milk thistle on CYP3A4 was sometimes minor or seen only at higher concentrations.[2,4-7]

Other *in vitro* studies have found that milk thistle or its flavonolignan constituents were minor or moderate inhibitors of CYP2C19[4] and CYP2C8[5] but the clinical relevance of this seems likely to be limited. Milk thistle might also affect CYP2C9[3,4,7] but it is unclear if this is clinically relevant or not, see angiotensin II receptor antagonists, page 351. It has been suggested that, while *in vitro* levels of silymarin may cause moderate inhibition of several cytochrome P450 isoenzymes, *in vivo* levels do not reach inhibitory concentrations and so milk thistle would not be expected to exhibit inhibition at pharmacologically effective concentrations.[5,6,8]

Other *in vivo* and *in vitro* studies, have found that milk thistle is unlikely to affect the metabolism of drugs that are substrates of CYP1A2[4,5,9] (see caffeine, page 351), CYP2E1[5,9] (see chlorzoxazone, page 351), or CYP2D6.[4,5,9]

In vitro studies have suggested that silymarin may affect P-glycoprotein substrate binding. However, there is no evidence from human pharmacokinetic studies that milk thistle has a clinically important effect on the levels of drugs that are P-glycoprotein substrates, see digoxin, page 351.

Silymarin has also been found to inhibit several UDP-glucuronosyltransferases *in vitro*.[1,3] These enzymes are involved in phase II glucuronidation, a process that affects the metabolism of several drugs (such as irinotecan, paracetamol, and zidovudine), and reduced activity could theoretically lead to raised drug levels, although the clinical implications of this are, as yet, unclear.

Silibinin dihemisuccinate has also been found to inhibit several of the organic anion-transporting polypeptide (OATP) family *in vitro,* which could theoretically lead to reduced cellular uptake, and therefore raised levels, of drugs that are OATP substrates.[10] For information on the pharmacokinetics of individual flavonoids present in milk thistle, see under flavonoids, page 213.

Interactions overview

In vitro studies have suggested that milk thistle may interact with a number of drugs by inhibiting their metabolism by various cytochrome P450 isoenzymes or affecting their transport by P-glycoprotein. However, *in vivo* studies suggest that any such inhibition is unlikely to be clinically relevant, although the outcome of the concurrent use of milk thistle and losartan remains to be established. Milk thistle may raise the levels of a hepatotoxic metabolite of pyrazinamide. For information on the interactions of individual flavonoids present in milk thistle, see under flavonoids, page 213.

Interactions monographs

1. Venkataramanan R, Ramachandran V, Komoroski BJ, Zhang S, Schiff PL, Strom SC. Milk thistle, a herbal supplement, decreases the activity of CYP3A4 and uridine diphosphoglucuronosyl transferase activity in human hepatocyte cultures. *Drug Metab Dispos* (2000) 28, 1270–1273.
2. Budzinski JW, Foster BC, Vandenhoek S, Arnason JT. An in vitro evaluation of human cytochrome P450 3A4 inhibition by selected commercial herbal extracts and tinctures. *Phytomedicine* (2000) 7, 273–82.
3. Sridar C, Goosen TC, Kent UM, Williams JA, Hollenberg PF. Silybin inactivates cytochromes P450 3A4 and 2C9 and inhibits major hepatic glucuronosyltransferases. *Drug Metab Dispos* (2004) 32, 587–94.
4. Zou L, Harkey MR, Henderson GL. Effects of herbal components on cDNA-expressed cytochrome P450 enzyme catalytic activity. *Life Sci* (2002) 71, 1579–89.
5. Etheridge AS, Black SR, Patel PR, So J, Mathews JM. An *in vitro* evaluation of cytochrome P450 inhibition and P-glycoprotein interaction with Goldenseal, *Ginkgo biloba*, grape seed, milk thistle, and ginseng extracts and their constituents. *Planta Med* (2007) 73, 731–41.
6. Zuber R, Modrianský M, Dvořák Z, Rohovský P, Ulrichová J, Simánek V, Anzenbacher P. Effect of silybin and its congeners on human liver microsomal cytochrome P450 activities. *Phytother Res* (2002) 16, 632–8.
7. Beckmann-Knopp S, Rietbrock S, Weyhenmeyer R, Bocker RH, Beckerts KT, Lang W, Hunz M, Fuhr U. Inhibitory effects of silibinin on cytochrome P-450 enzymes in human liver microsomes. *Pharmacol Toxicol* (2000) 86, 250–256.
8. Fuhr U, Beckmann-Knopp S, Jetter A, Lück H, Mengs U. The effect of silymarin on oral nifedipine pharmacokinetics. *Planta Med* (2007) 73, 1429–35.
9. Gurley BJ, Gardner SF, Hubbard MA, Williams DK, Gentry WB, Carrier J, Khan IA, Edwards DJ, Shah A. In vivo assessment of botanical supplementation on human cytochrome P450 phenotypes: *Citrus aurantium, Echinacea purpurea,* milk thistle, and saw palmetto. *Clin Pharmacol Ther* (2004) 76, 428–40.
10. Letschert K, Faulstich H, Keller D, Keppler D. Molecular characterization and inhibition of amanitin uptake into human hepatocytes. *Toxicol Sci* (2006) 91, 140–149.

M

Milk thistle + Angiotensin II receptor antagonists

Milk thistle appears to decrease the metabolism of losartan to its active metabolite, E-3174.

Clinical evidence

In a randomised, placebo-controlled study, 12 healthy Chinese subjects were given a single 50-mg dose of losartan after a 14-day course of a standardised extract of milk thistle three times daily. The subjects were divided into two groups: heterozygous CYP2C9 extensive metabolisers (6) and CYP2C9 poor metabolisers (6). The AUC of losartan and its metabolite, E-3174 were increased by 108% and decreased by 17%, respectively, in the extensive metabolisers, whereas in the poor metabolisers the AUC of losartan was not affected, whereas that of E-3174 was decreased by 13%. The plasma levels of losartan and its metabolite, E-3174 were increased by 89% and decreased by 17%, respectively, in the extensive metabolisers, whereas in the poor metabolisers there was no effect on plasma concentrations. In this study the milk thistle extract was standardised to contain 140 mg of silymarin.[1]

Experimental evidence

No relevant data found.

Mechanism

Milk thistle appears to decrease the metabolism of losartan to its active metabolite, E-3174, by the cytochrome P450 isoenzyme CYP2C19. In poor metabolisers, the metabolism of losartan is less affected as they are deficient in active CYP2C19.

Importance and management

This appears to be the only study examining the effects of milk thistle on angiotensin II receptor antagonists, and it did not determine the effect of the pharmacokinetic changes on losartan efficacy. The increase in losartan exposure might be expected to increase its blood pressure lowering effects, but this might be attenuated by the reduction in the exposure to the active metabolite, E-3174, which is much more potent than the parent, losartan. **Irbesartan** is also metabolised by CYP2C9 and might therefore also interact with gingko, but the outcome of any such interaction is also unclear. There is insufficient evidence to generally recommend that milk thistle should be avoided in patients taking losartan or irbesartan; however, the potential for changes in the blood pressure-lowering effects of these drugs should be born in mind if they are taken with milk thistle.

1. Han Y, Guo D, Chen Y, Chen Y, Tan Z-R, Zhou H-H. Effect of silymarin on the pharmacokinetics of losartan and its active metabolite E-3174 in healthy Chinese volunteers *Eur J Clin Pharmacol* (2009) 65, 585–91.

Milk thistle + Benzodiazepines

Milk thistle does not appear to affect the pharmacokinetics of midazolam.

Evidence, mechanism, importance and management

In a study 19 healthy subjects were given milk thistle 300 mg three times daily for 14 days (standardised to silymarin 80%) with a single 8-mg oral dose of **midazolam** on the last day. There was no change in the pharmacokinetics of **midazolam**, and milk thistle had no effect on the duration of midazolam-induced sleep.[1] Similarly, in another study in 12 healthy subjects, milk thistle 175 mg (standardised to silymarins 80%) given twice daily for 28 days had no significant effects on the metabolism of a single 8-mg dose of **midazolam**.[2]

These studies show that the pharmacokinetics of **midazolam** are not affected by the concurrent use of milk thistle. As midazolam is used as a probe substrate for the cytochrome P450 isoenzyme CYP3A4 this study also suggests that milk thistle is unlikely to affect the metabolism of other drugs that are substrates of this isoenzyme. This suggestion is supported by the finding that the metabolism of other known CYP3A4 substrates is not affected by milk thistle.

See also Milk thistle + HIV-protease inhibitors, page 352.

1. Gurley B, Hubbard MA, Williams DK, Thaden J, Tong Y, Gentry WB, Breen P, Carrier DJ, Cheboyina S. Assessing the clinical significance of botanical supplementation on human cytochrome P450 3A activity: comparison of a milk thistle and black cohosh product to rifampin and clarithromycin. *J Clin Pharmacol* (2006) 46, 201–13.
2. Gurley BJ, Gardner SF, Hubbard MA, Williams DK, Gentry WB, Carrier J, Khan IA, Edwards DJ, Shah A. In vivo assessment of botanical supplementation on human cytochrome P450 phenotypes: *Citrus aurantium, Echinacea purpurea,* milk thistle, and saw palmetto. *Clin Pharmacol Ther* (2004) 76, 428–40.

Milk thistle + Caffeine

Milk thistle does not appear to affect the pharmacokinetics of caffeine.

Evidence, mechanism, importance and management

In a study in 12 healthy subjects, milk thistle 175 mg (standardised to silymarins 80%) given twice daily for 28 days had no significant effects on the metabolism of a single 100-mg dose of caffeine.[1]

This study suggests that the pharmacokinetics of caffeine are not affected by the concurrent use of milk thistle. As caffeine is used as a probe substrate for the cytochrome P450 isoenzyme CYP1A2 this study also suggests that milk thistle is unlikely to affect the metabolism of other drugs that are substrates of this isoenzyme.

1. Gurley BJ, Gardner SF, Hubbard MA, Williams DK, Gentry WB, Carrier J, Khan IA, Edwards DJ, Shah A. In vivo assessment of botanical supplementation on human cytochrome P450 phenotypes: *Citrus aurantium, Echinacea purpurea,* milk thistle, and saw palmetto. *Clin Pharmacol Ther* (2004) 76, 428–40.

Milk thistle + Chlorzoxazone

Milk thistle does not appear to affect the pharmacokinetics of chlorzoxazone.

Evidence, mechanism, importance and management

In a study in 12 healthy subjects, milk thistle 175 mg (standardised to silymarins 80%) given twice daily for 28 days had no significant effects on the metabolism of a single 250-mg dose of chlorzoxazone.[1]

This study suggests that the pharmacokinetics of chlorzoxazone are not affected by the concurrent use of milk thistle. As chlorzoxazone is used as a probe substrate for the cytochrome P450 isoenzyme CYP2E1 this study also suggests that milk thistle is unlikely to affect the metabolism of other drugs that are substrates of this isoenzyme.

1. Gurley BJ, Gardner SF, Hubbard MA, Williams DK, Gentry WB, Carrier J, Khan IA, Edwards DJ, Shah A. In vivo assessment of botanical supplementation on human cytochrome P450 phenotypes: *Citrus aurantium, Echinacea purpurea,* milk thistle, and saw palmetto. *Clin Pharmacol Ther* (2004) 76, 428–40.

Milk thistle + Digoxin

Milk thistle does not appear to affect the pharmacokinetics of digoxin.

Clinical evidence

In a study, 16 healthy subjects were given a single 400-microgram dose of digoxin before and on the last day of a 14-day course of a milk thistle extract (standardised to 80% silymarin) 300 mg three times daily. No statistically significant changes in the pharmacokinetics of digoxin were found, although there was a trend towards a minor 10% reduction in the AUC of digoxin.[1]

Experimental evidence

See *Mechanism*, below.

Mechanism

In vitro,[2] P-glycoprotein ATPase activity, which is the energy source for the active transport of drugs across cell membranes by P-glycoprotein, was inhibited by silymarin, suggesting a direct interaction with P-glycoprotein substrate binding. Digoxin is a P-glycoprotein substrate, and it had been suggested that milk thistle would therefore affect digoxin pharmacokinetics.

Importance and management

Direct evidence appears to be limited to one clinical study, which showed that milk thistle does not cause clinically relevant changes in digoxin pharmacokinetics. It would therefore appear that the dose of digoxin would not need to be adjusted in patients also given milk thistle. As digoxin is used as a probe substrate for P-glycoprotein this study also suggests that milk thistle is unlikely to affect the metabolism of other drugs that are substrates of this transporter protein.

1. Gurley BJ, Barone GW, Williams DK, Carrier J, Breen P, Yates CR, Song P-f, Hubbard MA, Tong Y, Cheboyina S. Effect of milk thistle (*Silybum marianum*) and black cohosh (*Cimicifuga racemosa*) supplementation on digoxin pharmacokinetics in humans. *Drug Metab Dispos* (2006) 34, 69–74.
2. Zhang S, Morris ME. Effects of the flavonoids biochanin A, morin, phloretin, and silymarin on P-glycoprotein-mediated transport. *J Pharmacol Exp Ther* (2003) 304, 1258–67.

Milk thistle + Food

No interactions found.

Milk thistle + Herbal medicines

No interactions found.

Milk thistle + HIV-protease inhibitors

Milk thistle does not appear to have an important effect on the pharmacokinetics of indinavir. *In vitro* studies suggests that silibinin does not affect the pharmacokinetics of ritonavir.

Clinical evidence

Milk thistle 175 mg three times daily (*Thisilyn*; *Nature's Way,* standardised for 80% silymarin content) for 3 weeks caused a 9% reduction in the AUC of **indinavir** and a 25% reduction in its trough plasma level after four doses of **indinavir** 800 mg every 8 hours, but only the value for the trough level reached statistical significance.[1] The authors suggested that the effect on the trough level could represent a time-dependent effect of **indinavir** pharmacokinetics, as the plasma levels without milk thistle were found to be similarly lowered after a washout phase.[1] In another similar study, in 10 healthy subjects, milk thistle standardised for silymarin 160 mg (*General Nutrition Corp.*) three times daily for 13 days and then with **indinavir** 800 mg every 8 hours for 4 doses did not cause any statistically significant changes in the **indinavir** pharmacokinetics (6% reduction in AUC and 32% reduction in minimum level).[2] In

yet another similar study, in 8 healthy subjects, milk thistle capsules (standardised for silymarins 456 mg; *Kare and Hope Ltd.*), three times daily for 28 days had no effect on the pharmacokinetics of **indinavir** 800 mg every 8 hours for four doses when compared with 6 subjects in a control group not receiving milk thistle extract. Both the control and **indinavir** group had a lower **indinavir** AUC after the second and third time of administration compared with the first, and this decline was greater in the control group.[3] A meta-analysis of these 3 studies showed no effect of milk thistle on **indinavir** levels.[3]

Experimental evidence

In a series of experiments on human cell lines and *rat* hepatocytes, silibinin, the major active constituent of the silymarin flavonolignan mixture found in milk thistle, was found not to affect the pharmacokinetics of **ritonavir**.[4]

Mechanism

Based on *animal* data, milk thistle might be expected to increase indinavir levels by inhibiting its metabolism,[1] or transport by P-glycoprotein.[2] However, silibinin was found not to have a significant effect on P-glycoprotein or cytochrome P450 isoenzyme CYP3A4 activity when given with ritonavir.[4]

Importance and management

The available data suggest that milk thistle extract does not have an effect on the pharmacokinetics of indinavir (and possibly ritonavir), although this is not totally conclusive. The reduction in indinavir levels appears to be just a time-dependent effect rather than an effect of the milk thistle, but further study is needed with longer exposure to indinavir than just four doses. Evidence appears to be too slim to prohibit concurrent use, but until more is known it may be prudent to give milk thistle cautiously to patients taking indinavir.

1. Piscitelli SC, Formentini E, Burstein AH, Alfaro R, Jagannatha S, Falloon J. Effect of milk thistle on the pharmacokinetics of indinavir in healthy volunteers. *Pharmacotherapy* (2002) 22, 551–6.
2. DiCenzo R, Shelton M, Jordan K, Koval C, Forrest A, Reichman R, Morse G. Coadministration of milk thistle and indinavir in healthy subjects. *Pharmacotherapy* (2003) 23, 866–70.
3. Mills E, Wilson K, Clarke M, Foster B, Walker S, Rachlis B, DeGroot N, Montori VM, Gold W, Phillips E, Myers S, Gallicano K. Milk thistle and indinavir: a randomized controlled pharmacokinetics study and meta-analysis. *Eur J Clin Pharmacol* (2005) 61, 1–7.
4. Patel J, Buddha B, Dey S, Pal D, Mitra AK. In vitro interaction of the HIV protease inhibitor ritonavir with herbal constituents: changes in P-gp and CYP3A4 activity. *Am J Ther* (2004) 11, 262–77.

Milk thistle + Irinotecan

Milk thistle does not appear to affect the pharmacokinetics of irinotecan.

Evidence, mechanism, importance and management

A pharmacokinetic study was undertaken in 6 patients who were receiving intravenous irinotecan 125 mg/m² weekly for 4 weeks, followed by a 2 week rest period. Four days before the second dose of irinotecan, a 14-day course of milk thistle seed extract 200 mg (containing silymarin 80%) three times daily was started. The pharmacokinetics of irinotecan and its metabolites did not differ between week one (no milk thistle), week two (4 days of milk thistle) or week three (12 days of milk thistle).[1] No dose alterations would therefore be expected to be needed if milk thistle (standardised with silymarin 80%) is given with irinotecan.

1. van Erp NPH, Baker SD, Zhao M, Rudek MA, Guchelaar H-J, Nortier JWR, Sparreboom A, Gelderblom H. Effect of milk thistle (*Silybum marianum*) on the pharmacokinetics of irinotecan. *Clin Cancer Res* (2005) 11, 7800–7806.

Milk thistle + Metronidazole

Silymarin (the active constituent of milk thistle) modestly reduces metronidazole levels.

Evidence, mechanism, importance and management

Silymarin (*Silybon*) 140 mg daily was given to 12 healthy subjects for 9 days, with metronidazole 400 mg three times daily on days 7 to 10. Silymarin reduced the AUC of metronidazole and hydroxymetronidazole (a major active metabolite) by 28% and the maximum serum levels by 29% and 20%, respectively.

The authors suggest that silymarin causes these pharmacokinetic changes by inducing P-glycoprotein and the cytochrome P450 isoenzyme CYP3A4, which are involved in the transport and metabolism of metronidazole.[1] But evidence from other interactions suggests that a clinically relevant effect on P-glycoprotein and CYP3A4 is unlikely. See Milk thistle + Benzodiazepines, page 351, and Milk thistle + HIV-protease inhibitors, page 352. The general importance of this interaction is unclear, but a 28% reduction in the AUC of metronidazole would not be expected to be of much clinical significance.

1. Rajnarayana K, Reddy MS, Vidyasagar J, Krishna DR. Study on the influence of silymarin pretreatment on metabolism and disposition of metronidazole. *Arzneimittelforschung* (2004) 54, 109–13.

Milk thistle + Nifedipine

Milk thistle does not appear to alter the haemodynamic effects of nifedipine.

Clinical evidence

In a study in 16 healthy subjects, silymarin 280 mg was given 10 hours, and 90 minutes, before a 10-mg dose of nifedipine. Silymarin increased the AUC of nifedipine by about 10% and reduced its maximum serum levels by about 30%, but these effects varied greatly between subjects. Silymarin did not alter the haemodynamic effects of nifedipine.[1] One capsule of the product used in this study (*Legalon*) contains 173 to 186 mg dry extract from milk thistle fruits, equivalent to silymarin 140 mg calculated as silibinin.

Experimental evidence

Two *in vitro* studies found that silymarin flavonolignans moderately inhibited the oxidation of nifedipine[2] and denitronifedipine,[3] a closely related nifedipine derivative, as marker substrates for CYP3A4 activity.

Mechanism

The maximum serum levels of nifedipine were reduced slightly but the AUC was not, suggesting a delay in nifedipine absorption. This could be due to irregular gastric emptying in the presence of silymarin, or an interaction with drug transporters such as OATP. While the experimental evidence suggests an inhibitory effect on CYP3A4, this has not been found to be clinically significant (see under benzodiazepines, page 351).

Importance and management

Evidence appears to be limited to these three studies. The clinical study found that milk thistle may modestly delay the absorption of nifedipine with an apparent high intra-individual variability. However, as there was no considerable change in the pharmacokinetics or pharmacodynamic effects of nifedipine (blood pressure and heart rate), this is probably not clinically relevant. It would appear that the modest effects found *in vitro* do not translate in to a clinically relevant effect.

1. Fuhr U, Beckmann-Knopp S, Jetter A, Lück H, Mengs U. The effect of silymarin on oral nifedipine pharmacokinetics. *Planta Med* (2007) 73, 1429–35.

2. Zuber R, Modrianský M, Dvořák Z, Rohovský P, Ulrichová J, Simánek V, Anzenbacher P. Effect of silybin and its congeners on human liver microsomal cytochrome P450 activities. *Phytother Res* (2002) 16, 632–8.
3. Beckmann-Knopp S, Rietbrock S, Weyhenmeyer R, Bocker RH, Beckerts KT, Lang W, Hunz M, Fuhr U. Inhibitory effects of silibinin on cytochrome P-450 enzymes in human liver microsomes. *Pharmacol Toxicol* (2000) 86, 250–256.

Milk thistle + Pyrazinamide

The interaction between milk thistle and pyrazinamide is based on experimental evidence only.

Clinical evidence

No interactions found.

Experimental evidence

In a study in *rats*,[1] pyrazinamide and its active metabolite, pyrazinoic acid, were given after either long-term, or short-term exposure to silibinin, the major active constituent of the silymarin flavonolignan mixture found in milk thistle. The first group of *rats* received intravenous silibinin 100 mg/kg for 3 days before an intravenous dose of pyrazinamide 50 mg/kg or pyrazinoic acid 30 mg/kg concurrently on the fourth day. The second group received intravenous silibinin 30 mg/kg 10 minutes before an intravenous dose of pyrazinamide 50 mg/kg or pyrazinoic acid 30 mg/kg.

Silibinin had no effect on the pharmacokinetics of pyrazinamide, but increased the AUC of pyrazinoic acid by 3.5-fold in the long-term exposure group and 4-fold in the short-term exposure group. The maximum serum levels of pyrazinoic acid were increased by about 60% and 70% respectively.

Mechanism

It is thought that silibinin may inhibit xanthine oxidase, which is involved in pyrazinamide and pyrazinoic acid hydroxylation. Silibinin may also decrease the hepatobiliary excretion of pyrazinoic acid.

Importance and management

Evidence appears to be limited to experimental data. While no pharmacokinetic changes were seen when milk thistle was given with pyrazinamide, milk thistle appears to increase the levels of the active metabolite, pyrazinoic acid. So far, this has only been shown in *rats* so determining the clinical relevance of this interaction is difficult. Nevertheless, because of the dose-related hepatotoxic adverse effects associated with pyrazinamide, it would be prudent to bear this possible interaction in mind in case of an unexpected response to treatment.

1. Wu J-W, Tsai T-H. Effect of silibinin on the pharmacokinetics of pyrazinamide and pyrazinoic acid in rats. *Drug Metab Dispos* (2007) 35, 1603–10.

Milk thistle + Ranitidine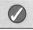

Silymarin, a major constituent of milk thistle, does not appear to affect the pharmacokinetics of single-dose ranitidine.

Evidence, mechanism, importance and management

In a study in 12 healthy subjects, silymarin capsules (*Sivylar*) 140 mg three times daily for 7 days did not significantly affect the pharmacokinetics of a single 150-mg dose of ranitidine.[1] No particular precautions would appear to be necessary if patients take milk thistle and ranitidine together.

1. Rao BN, Srinivas M, Kumar YS, Rao YM. Effect of silymarin on the oral bioavailability of ranitidine in healthy human volunteers. *Drug Metab Drug Interact* (2007) 22, 175–85.

Milk thistle + Rosuvastatin

Silymarin, a major constituent of milk thistle, does not appear to affect the pharmacokinetics of single-dose rosuvastatin.

Clinical evidence

In a randomised study, 8 healthy subjects were given silymarin (*Legalon*) 140 mg three times daily for 5 days. On day 4 they were given a single 10-mg oral dose of rosuvastatin. Silymarin did not significantly affect the pharmacokinetics of rosuvastatin.[1]

Experimental evidence

An *in vitro* study found that silymarin inhibited the uptake of rosuvastatin mediated by the drug transporter proteins OATP1B1 and BCRP.[1]

Mechanism

In vitro study suggests that silymarin may inhibit drug transporter proteins, but this was not shown by any changes in the pharmacokinetics of rosuvastatin in a small clinical study.

Importance and management

No particular precautions would appear to be necessary if patients decide to take milk thistle and rosuvastatin together.

1. Deng JW, Shon J-H, Shin H-J, Park S-J, Yeo C-W, Zhou H-H, Song I-S, Shin J-G. Effect of silymarin supplement on the pharmacokinetics of rosuvastatin. *Pharm Res* (2008) 25, 1807–14.

Milk thistle + Talinolol

Milk thistle slightly increases the exposure to talinolol.

Clinical evidence

In a crossover study, 18 healthy subjects took a placebo or milk thistle extract (standardised to contain silymarin 140 mg) three times daily for 15 days with a single 100-mg dose of talinolol on day 15. The AUC and maximum plasma levels of talinolol were increased by 30% and 27%, respectively, in the presence of silymarin, but the elimination half life, and time to reach maximum plasma levels were not affected.[1]

Experimental evidence

See *Mechanism* below.

Mechanism

In vitro study suggests that silymarin is an inhibitor of P-glycoprotein (for more information see *Mechanism* under Milk thistle + Digoxin, page 351. Talinolol is a substrate of this transporter protein and therefore it might be expected that milk thistle will affect talinolol pharmacokinetics, increasing its bioavailability. However, note that milk thistle did not alter the pharmacokinetics of digoxin, another P-glycoprotein substrate, see Milk thistle + Digoxin, page 351.

Importance and management

Evidence for an interaction between milk thistle and talinolol appears to be limited to this one study, which was designed to establish the pharmacokinetics of any interaction. However, the evidence suggests that milk thistle causes only a small increase in exposure to talinolol, which is unlikely to be clinically relevant.

1. Han Y, Guo D, Chen Y, Tan Z-R, Zhou H-H. Effect of continuous silymarin administration on oral talinolol pharmacokinetics in healthy volunteers. *Xenobiotica* (2009) 39, 694–9.

M

Motherwort

Leonurus cardiaca L. (Lamiaceae)

Synonym(s) and related species

Leonurus, Lion's tail.

Leonurus heterophyllus Sweet, *Leonurus sibiricus* L., and *Leonurus japonicus* Houtt. f. *albiflorus* (Migo) Y.C.Zhu (sometimes known as Chinese motherwort), have been referred to by the name Siberian motherwort and are used similarly.

Pharmacopoeias

Motherwort (*BP 2012, PhEur 7.5*).

Constituents

Motherwort contains **iridoids** such as leonuride, ajugol, ajugoside and galiridoside; labdane-type **diterpenes** including leocardin; and **triterpenoids** such as ursolic acid. **Flavonoids** based on apigenin, kaempferol, quercetin and their glycosides, hyperoside (to which it may be standardised), and many others; caffeic acid derivatives, and the **alkaloid** stachydrine are also present.

Leonurus heterophyllus, Leonurus sibiricus and *Leonurus japonicus* contain similar compounds, with the alkaloid leonurine (which may or may not be present in *Leonurus cardiaca*) also documented.

Use and indications

Motherwort is used as a cardiac tonic, antispasmodic and sedative although few clinical or pharmacological studies are available to support its use. There is limited *in vitro* evidence for cardioactivity of motherwort, and for uterotonic activity of leonurine.

Pharmacokinetics

No relevant pharmacokinetic data found. For information on the pharmacokinetics of individual flavonoids present in motherwort, see under flavonoids, page 213.

Interactions overview

No interactions with motherwort found. For information on the interactions of individual flavonoids present in motherwort, see under flavonoids, page 213.

M

Natural coumarins

Natural coumarins are widespread in herbal medicines and vegetables. There is a misconception that if a plant contains natural coumarins it will have anticoagulant properties, but very specific structural requirements are necessary for this; namely there must be a non-polar carbon substituent at the 3-position of 4-hydroxycoumarin. Moreover, at present, there are no established interactions between warfarin and herbal medicines that have been attributed to the natural coumarin content of the herb. Even in the classic case of haemorrhagic death of livestock that led to the discovery of dicoumarol, it was the action of the mould on the natural coumarin in the sweet clover (melilot, page 347) that led to the production of the anticoagulant, so consumption of a spoiled product would seem to be necessary for this specific interaction to occur. This suggests that the occurrence of natural coumarins in dietary supplements or herbal medicines should not trigger immediate concern as regards interactions with anticoagulants.

The information in this family monograph relates to the individual natural coumarins, and the reader is referred back to the herb (and vice versa) where appropriate. Note that, to avoid confusion with the synthetic anticoagulant coumarins, such as warfarin, the term natural coumarins has been used to describe those that are of plant origin.

Types, sources and related compounds

Natural coumarins are aromatic lactones and phenyl-propanoids based on 1,2-benzopyrone (coumarin). They usually occur naturally bound to one or more sugar molecules as glycosides rather than as the free aglycone. There are three major classes of natural coumarins based on the structure of the aglycone:

- **Hydroxycoumarins:** such as umbelliferone, aesculetin (esculetin), herniarin, scopoletin and osthol, occur in many plants. Some are further derivatised or prenylated, and coumarins in this class are generally harmless. However, some of the substituted 4-hydroxyderivatives have potent anticoagulant properties. The classic example that occurs naturally is dicoumarol (bishydroxycoumarin), which can occur in mouldy forage crops when coumarin itself is transformed into dicoumarol by microbial action. This compound has been used therapeutically as an anticoagulant, and is also the causative agent of haemorrhagic sweet clover disease (caused by ingestion of mouldy *Melilotus officinalis*) in cattle. See melilot, page 347. Note that the coumarin anticoagulants used clinically (acenocoumarol, phenprocoumon, warfarin) are all synthetic 4-hydroxycoumarins.
- **Furanocoumarins (furocoumarins):** have an additional furan ring attached, and this group can be further divided into linear compounds including psoralen, 5-methoxypsoralen (bergapten) and methoxsalen (xanthotoxin or 8-methoxypsoralen), and angular compounds such as angelicin (isopsoralen) and pimpinellin (5,6-dimethoxyangelicin). Some furanocoumarins may have additional prenyl substitution (e.g. bergamottin, alloimperatorin) and some occur as dimers, for example the paradisins, which are found in grapefruit juice. Others are more complex, such as the highly toxic aflatoxin B1, which is produced by microbial contamination of food crops with *Aspergillus niger*. Furanocoumarins are commonly found in food items. They are mainly present in the two large plant families Rutaceae and Apiaceae, but occur in others. The Rutaceae family includes grapefruit, page 270, and prickly ash, page 390. The Apiaceae family includes aniseed, page 37, asafoetida, page 43, celery, page 138, Chinese angelica, page 145, carrot, parsnip, and many other herbs and spices. Note that the furanocoumarins are thought to be principally responsible for the main drug interactions of grapefruit juice, page 270 and possibly bitter orange, page 75.
- **Pyranocoumarins:** have a fused pyran ring attached, and can be divided into linear or angular.[1]

There is also a minor class of coumarins, the **4-phenylcoumarins** such as mammeisin, which can also be classified as neoflavonoids.

Isocoumarins (1,4-benzopyrones) are more commonly known as **chromones**; the most important of these is khellin, a compound found in *Ammi visnaga* which was the basis for the development of the anti-allergic drug cromoglicate and the class III antiarrhythmic amiodarone. Apart from khellin, which is a smooth muscle relaxant with bronchodilatory and vasodilatory effects, little is known of their activities or toxicities.

Coumarin (1,2-benzopyrone) was initially isolated from the tonka bean, and is found in other herbs such as melilot, page 347, and in many vegetables, fruits, and spices. It has a sweet scent, recognisable as the odour of new-mown hay.

Use and indications

Natural coumarins have a wide spectrum of activity ranging from the beneficial to the highly toxic. Generally, the furanocoumarins are more biologically active than the other types. Unlike the flavonoids, page 213, and isoflavones, page 300, it is not possible to generalise about their group actions, and this also applies to their toxic and drug interaction effects. In addition, coumarin supplements are not marketed or taken in the way that isoflavone or flavonoid (bioflavonoid) products are. Therefore only the most notable actions of the natural coumarin derivatives will be outlined here.

(a) Anticoagulant activity

The anticoagulant activity possessed by some natural coumarins is not universal and should not be attributed to all of them. In order to have anticoagulant activity, there must be a nonpolar carbon substituent at the 3-position of 4-hydroxycoumarin.[2,3] The best known natural example is dicoumarol (bishydroxycoumarin), which is formed by the action of moulds on coumarin in sweet clover, see melilot, page 347. It functions as a vitamin K antagonist and has been used therapeutically as an anticoagulant, but the anticoagulant coumarins commonly used clinically are all fully synthetic compounds (e.g. acenocoumarol, phenprocoumon, warfarin).

(b) Photosensitization and PUVA

Many furanocoumarins cause phototoxicity by sensitizing the skin to UV light. This can cause hyperpigmentation of the skin, and extracts of plants containing these compounds have been used in traditional medicine to treat vitiligo. This property is also responsible for the allergenicity that is characteristic of some plants in the Apiaceae and Rutaceae families, particularly giant hogweed (*Heracleum mantegazzianum*) and rue (*Ruta graveolens*).

Photochemotherapy or PUVA (Psoralen plus UVA) is a recognised conventional treatment for certain skin disorders such as cutaneous T-cell lymphoma, chronic graft-versus-host disease, and psoriasis. UVA irradiation can help these conditions and the effect is enhanced by oral treatment with psoralen and other furanocoumarin derivatives (including methoxsalen), which cause photosensitization. The doses of psoralens used for these treatments (up to 1.2 mg/kg) are very unlikely to be achieved with herbs containing methoxsalen, and therefore interactions involving the oral psoralens are probably unlikely to occur with herbs containing these substances.

(c) Antioxidant effects

The phenolic structure of the natural coumarins means that most will have free radical scavenging and therefore antioxidant effects.[4,5] Many natural coumarins are potent metal chelating agents, and powerful chain-breaking antioxidants.[4] However, these properties have, as yet, only been studied experimentally.

(d) Anti-inflammatory activity

There is experimental evidence from *in vitro* and *animal* studies to suggest that various natural coumarins have anti-inflammatory activity. Esculetin, herniarin, scopoletin and scopolin have been used in Spanish traditional medicine against inflammation,[5] and scopoletin has been shown to be pharmacologically active,[6] as has esculin, extracted from the stem bark of *Fraxinus ornus*.[7]

Coumarin itself is an anti-inflammatory agent. This has been demonstrated in *animal* studies where a coumarin-containing extract of *Melilotus officinalis* was found to have similar anti-inflammatory action to that of hydrocortisone.[8] Coumarin has also been used in the treatment of lymphoedema.[9]

(e) Chemopreventive and cytotoxic effects

Experimental work has suggested that natural coumarins may prevent carcinogenesis, or have cytotoxic effects. Further work is required to confirm whether this is a potential therapeutic use of these substances.[10,11]

(f) Miscellaneous effects

Insecticidal, anti-diabetic, antifungal and larvicidal, activities have all been described for natural coumarin derivatives. It has also been suggested that some of the natural coumarins may be reverse transcriptase, protease or integrase inhibitors, and may warrant further investigation for possible use in the management of HIV infection.[12]

Coumarin has also been used in perfumery, and as a flavour. However, it has been banned as a food additive in numerous countries, or limits have been set on its use, because it is moderately toxic to the liver and kidneys.

Pharmacokinetics

(a) Coumarin

Coumarin is completely absorbed after oral administration, and in humans subject to extensive first pass hepatic metabolism, by the cytochrome P450 isoenzyme CYP2A6, to 7-hydroxycoumarin (umbelliferone), which is less toxic and also occurs widely in plants. However, in some people, coumarin is much more hepatotoxic than in others, and this is thought to be due to reduced metabolism of coumarin by CYP2A6, and greater dependence on metabolism by CYP3A4 to form the more toxic 3-hydroxycoumarin and intermediates.[9,13]

(b) Bergamottin and related products

Bergamottin is metabolised *in vivo* to 6',7'-dihydroxybergamottin. In a study in 12 healthy subjects given single 6-mg or 12-mg doses of bergamottin, 8 subjects had measurable levels of bergamottin, and 3 had detectable levels of 6',7'-dihydroxybergamottin.[14]

(c) Effect on cytochrome P450 isoenzymes

Furanocoumarins are now recognised as major cytochrome P450 enzyme inhibitors. They are mainly responsible for the complex drug interaction profile of grapefruit products, as shown by a study using furanocoumarin-free grapefruit juice (see Natural coumarins + Felodipine, page 359), although other constituents contribute to the effect (see *pharmacokinetics*, under grapefruit, page 270). The furanocoumarins, bergamottin, bergaptol, dihydroxybergamottin, geranylcoumarin and paradisin A have been shown to have inhibitory effects on CYP3A4, CYP2D6, and CYP2C9 *in vitro*,[15] and paradisin B has also been found to be a potent inhibitor of human CYP3A4.[16] Methoxsalen and 5-methoxypsoralen (bergapten) are inhibitors of CYP1A2. In clinical pharmacokinetic drug interaction studies oral methoxsalen 1.2 mg/kg has been shown to markedly inhibit CYP1A2 using caffeine and theophylline as probe substrates.[17,18] In another study, oral methoxsalen slightly increased ciclosporin levels.[19] It is very unlikely that these doses of methoxsalen would be achieved using herbs containing psoralens including methoxsalen. However, the findings are presented for information.

(d) Effect on P-glycoprotein

In vitro data[20] suggests that some of the furanocoumarins present in grapefruit juice, such as 6',7'-dihydroxybergamottin and 6',7'-epoxybergamottin, are able to inhibit

N

P-glycoprotein activity, raising the possibility of interactions between drugs that are substrates of this transporter protein and furanocoumarins, see Talinolol, page 360. However, another *in vitro* study has suggested that 6′7′-dihydroxybergamottin does *not* affect the function of P-glycoprotein.[21]

Interactions overview

None of the individual natural coumarins are used as dietary supplements or herbal medicines on their own, but rather as the herbs that contain them. Any interactions of the herbal medicines containing natural coumarins are covered under the specific herb.

Coumarin itself and the psoralens such as methoxsalen are used in conventional medicine. The doses used for these treatments are very unlikely to be achieved by taking herbal medicines containing these substances, and therefore the interactions of drugs such as methoxsalen are not covered here.

The drug interaction potential of some of the furanocoumarins is well established, and has been identified by investigating the mechanism of the interactions involving grapefruit juice, page 270.

This monograph does not contain any of the interactions of the synthetic 4-hydroxycoumarin derivatives that are used as anticoagulants, such as warfarin, because these are not natural coumarins.

Interactions monographs

1. Curini M, Cravotto G, Epifano F, Giannone G. Chemistry and biological activity of natural and synthetic prenyloxycoumarins. *Curr Med Chem* (2006) 13, 199–222.
2. Overman RS, Stahmann MA, Huebner CF, Sullivan WR, Spero L, Doherty DG, Ikawa M, Graf L, Roseman S, Link KP. Studies on the hemorrhagic sweet clover disease. XIII. Anticoagulant activity and structure in the 4-hydroxycoumarin group. *J Biol Chem* (1944) 153, 5–24.
3. Majerus PW, Tollefsen DM. Blood coagulation and anticoagulant, thrombolytic, and antiplatelet drugs. In: Brunton LL, Lazo JS, Parker KL, eds. Goodman & Gilman's The Pharmacological Basis of Therapeutics 11th ed. New York: McGraw-Hill; 2005. p. 1467–88.
4. Kostova I. Synthetic and Natural Coumarins as Antioxidants. *Mini Rev Med Chem* (2006) 6, 365–74.
5. Fylaktakidou KC, Hadjipavlou-Litina DJ, Litinas KE, Nicolaides DN. Natural and synthetic coumarin derivatives with anti-inflammatory/antioxidant activities. *Curr Pharm Des* (2004) 10, 3813–33.
6. Moon P-D, Lee B-H, Jeong H-J, An H-J, Park S-J, Kim H-R, Ko S-G, Um J-Y, Hong S-H, Kim H-M. Use of scopoletin to inhibit the production of inflammatory cytokines through inhibition of the I κ B/NF- κ B signal cascade in the human mast cell line HMC-1. *Eur J Pharmacol* (2007) 555, 218–25.
7. Stefanova Z, Neychev H, Ivanovska N, Kostova I. Effect of a total extract from *Fraxinus ornus* stem bark and esculin on zymosan- and carrageenan-induced paw oedema in mice. *J Ethnopharmacol* (1995) 46, 101–6.
8. Pleşca-Manea L, Pârvu AE, Pârvu M, Taămaş M, Buia R, Puia M. Effects of *Melilotus officinalis* on acute inflammation. *Phytother Res* (2002) 16, 316–19.
9. Farinola N, Piller NB. *CYP2A6* polymorphisms: is there a role for pharmacogenomics in preventing coumarin-induced hepatotoxicity in lymphedema patients? *Pharmacogenomics* (2007) 8, 151–8.
10. Kaneko T, Tahara S, Takabayashi F. Inhibitory effect of natural coumarin compounds, esculetin and esculin, on oxidative DNA damage and formation of aberrant crypt foci and tumors induced by 1,2-dimethylhydrazine in rat colons. *Biol Pharm Bull* (2007) 30, 2052–7.
11. Kostova I. Synthetic and natural coumarins as cytotoxic agents. *Curr Med Chem Anti-Canc Agents* (2005) 5, 29–46.
12. Kostova I, Mojzis J. Biologically active coumarins as inhibitors of HIV-1. *Future HIV Ther* (2007) 1, 315–29.
13. Lake BG. Coumarin metabolism, toxicity and carcinogenicity: relevance for human risk assessment. *Food Chem Toxicol* (1999) 37, 423–53.
14. Goosen TC, Cillié D, Bailey DG, Yu C, He K, Hollenberg PF, Woster PM, Cohen L, Williams JA, Rheeders M, Dijkstra HP. Bergamottin contribution to the grapefruit juice-felodipine interaction and disposition in humans. *Clin Pharmacol Ther* (2004) 76, 607–17.
15. Girennavar B, Jayaprakasha GK, Patil BS. Potent inhibition of human cytochrome P450 3A4, 2D6, and 2C9 isoenzymes by grapefruit juice and its furocoumarins. *J Food Sci* (2007) 72, C417–C421.
16. Oda K, Yamaguchi Y, Yoshimura T, Wada K, Nishizono N. Synthetic models related to furanocoumarin-CYP 3A4 interactions. Comparison of furanocoumarin, coumarin, and benzofuran dimers as potent inhibitors of CYP3A4 activity. *Chem Pharm Bull (Tokyo)* (2007) 55, 1419–21.
17. Mays DC, Camisa C, Cheney P, Pacula CM, Nawoot S, Gerber N. Methoxsalen is a potent inhibitor of the metabolism of caffeine in humans. *Clin Pharmacol Ther* (1987) 42, 621–6.
18. Apseloff G, Shepard DR, Chambers MA, Nawoot S, Mays DC, Gerber N. Inhibition and induction of theophylline metabolism by 8-methoxypsoralen. In vitro study in rats and humans. *Drug Metab Dispos* (1990) 18, 298–303.
19. Rheeders M, Bouwer M, Goosen TC. Drug-drug interaction after single oral doses of the furanocoumarin methoxsalen and cyclosporine. *J Clin Pharmacol* (2006) 46, 768–75.
20. de Castro WV, Mertens-Talcott S, Derendorf H, Butterweck V. Grapefruit juice-drug interactions: Grapefruit juice and its components inhibit P-glycoprotein (ABCB1) mediated transport of talinolol in Caco-2 cells. *J Pharm Sci* (2007) 96, 2808–17.
21. Edwards DJ, Fitzsimmons ME, Scguetz EG, Yasuda K, Ducharme MP, Warbasse LH, Woster PM, Scuetz JD, Watkins P. 6′7′-dihydroxybergamottin in grapefruit juice and Seville orange juice: effects on cyclosporine disposition, enterocyte CYP3A4, and P-glycoprotein. *Clin Pharmacol Ther* (1999) 65, 237–44.

Natural coumarins + Ciclosporin

A citrus soft drink containing furanocoumarins increased the bioavailability of ciclosporin in an isolated case.

Clinical evidence

A lung transplant patient taking ciclosporin had large variations in his ciclosporin levels, which ranged between 319 and 761 nanograms/mL, on discharge from hospital, which were unexplained by changes in his current medication or ciclosporin dose changes. It was found that on the days when the ciclosporin levels were increased, the patient had drunk a citrus soft drink (*Sun Drop*) at breakfast. These fluctuations resolved when he stopped drinking the soft drink.[1] However, a subsequent pharmacokinetic study in 12 healthy subjects found that neither *Sun Drop* nor another citrus soft drink, *Fresca,* had any significant effects on the pharmacokinetics of a single 2.5-mg/kg dose of ciclosporin. Both *Sun Drop* and *Fresca* were tested, and found to contain the furanocoumarin **bergamottin** 0.078 and 6.5 mg/L, respectively (note that grapefruit, which is known to interact with ciclosporin, contains about 5.6 mg/L). The authors note that factors such as genetic and disease-related variability in ciclosporin metabolism, as well as changes in the **bergamottin** content between batches of the drinks, may account for the contrasting results.[2]

Experimental evidence

No relevant data found.

Mechanism

The authors of the report of an interaction with a citrus soda drink confirmed with the manufacturers that it contained furanocoumarins, such as bergamottin, which are thought to inhibit the cytochrome P450 isoenzyme CYP3A4,[1,2] which is the major isoenzyme involved in the metabolism of ciclosporin.

Importance and management

The isolated report of an interaction between a citrus soft drink (containing furanocoumarins) and ciclosporin was not confirmed by a subsequent single-dose pharmacokinetic study in healthy subjects[2] and therefore its significance is unclear. The case does highlight the influence diet can have on ciclosporin levels and it should be borne in mind should any unexpected changes in ciclosporin levels occur.

1. Johnston PE, Milstone A. Probable interaction of bergamottin and cyclosporine in a lung transplant recipient. *Transplantation* (2005) 79, 746.
2. Schwarz UI, Johnston PE, Bailey DG, Kim RB, Mayo G, Milstone A. Impact of citrus soft drinks relative to grapefruit juice on ciclosporin disposition. *Br J Clin Pharmacol* (2005) 62, 485–91.

Natural coumarins + Felodipine

Clinical studies demonstrate that bergamottin and other furanocoumarins may cause a clinically relevant increase in the levels of felodipine, but note that other active constituents also present in grapefruit juice, may interact by additive or synergistic mechanisms.

Clinical evidence

In a single-dose study in healthy subjects, the maximum plasma level of felodipine was increased by 33%, 35% and 40% by **bergamottin** 2, 6 and 12 mg, respectively, and by 86% by grapefruit juice 250 mL containing about 1.7 mg of bergamottin. The AUC_{0-12} of felodipine was increased by 37% by **bergamottin** 12 mg, and by 48% by the grapefruit juice. There was however a wide variation between individuals.[1] In another study, one-quarter strength lime juice, which contained the same concentration of **bergamottin** as grapefruit juice, had much less effect on the AUC

of felodipine than grapefruit juice (20% increase versus 80% increase).[2]

A further study in 18 healthy subjects found that furanocoumarin-free grapefruit juice had no consistent effect on the pharmacokinetics of felodipine relative to orange juice, with AUC changes ranging between a decrease of 46% to an increase of 44%. The median increase in the AUC of felodipine was 104% (range 6% to 230%) in those subjects given grapefruit juice with furanocoumarins present. Furanocoumarins identified in the grapefruit juice included **6',7'-dihydroxybergamottin**, **bergamottin**, **bergamottin**-like substances, and **spiro-esters**.[3]

A study in 12 healthy subjects, which investigated the effects of grapefruit juice and fractions of grapefruit juice on the pharmacokinetics of felodipine, found that **6',7'-dihydroxybergamottin** was not one of the main active ingredients. The fraction with the greatest **6',7'-dihydroxybergamottin** concentration caused a smaller increase in the AUC of felodipine than the fraction with one-third the amount of **6',7'-dihydroxybergamottin**.[4]

Experimental evidence

No relevant data found.

Mechanism

The furanocoumarins inhibit the activity of the cytochrome P450 isoenzyme CYP3A subfamily in the intestinal wall so that the first-pass metabolism of felodipine is reduced, thereby increasing its bioavailability and its effects. However, individually, bergamottin does not cause as great effect as grapefruit juice. Similarly, 6',7'-dihydroxybergamottin is not as active as grapefruit juice.

Importance and management

These studies demonstrate that bergamottin and other furanocoumarins may cause a clinically relevant increase in the levels of felodipine, but that other active constituents are also present in grapefruit juice, which may interact by additive or synergistic mechanisms.

Note that the interaction of grapefruit juice and felodipine, page 272 is established and the manufacturers of felodipine[5,6] say that it should not be taken with grapefruit juice.

Because any interaction between furanocoumarins and felodipine appears to depend upon interactions between the individual furanocoumarin constituents present, it is difficult to predict what the effects of individual herbs may be. The effects of the individual furanocoumarins appear to be modest.

1. Goosen TC, Cillié D, Bailey DG, Yu C, He K, Hollenberg PF, Woster PM, Cohen L, Williams JA, Rheeders M, Dijkstra HP. Bergamottin contribution to the grapefruit juice-felodipine interaction and disposition in humans. *Clin Pharmacol Ther* (2004) 76, 607–17.
2. Bailey DG, Dresser GK, Bend JR. Bergamottin, lime juice, and red wine as inhibitors of cytochrome P450 3A4 activity: comparison with grapefruit juice. *Clin Pharmacol Ther* (2003) 73, 529–37.
3. Paine MF, Widmer WW, Hart HL, Pusek SN, Beavers KL, Criss AB, Brown SS, Thomas BF, Watkins PB. A furanocoumarin-free grapefruit juice establishes furanocoumarins as the mediators of the grapefruit juice-felodipine interaction. *Am J Clin Nutr* (2006) 83, 1097–1105.
4. Bailey DG, Kreeft JH, Munoz C, Freeman DJ, Bend JR. Grapefruit juice-felodipine interaction: effect of naringin and 6'7'-dihydroxybergamottin in humans. *Clin Pharmacol Ther* (1998) 64, 248–56.
5. Plendil (Felodipine). AstraZeneca UK Ltd. UK Summary of product characteristics, September 2007.
6. Vascalpha (Felodipine). Actavis UK Ltd. UK Summary of product characteristics, June 2007.

Natural coumarins + Food

No interactions found.

Natural coumarins + Herbal medicines

No interactions found.

N

Natural coumarins + Saquinavir

The interaction between natural coumarins and saquinavir is based on experimental evidence only.

Evidence, mechanism, importance and management

In an *in vitro* study in which human liver microsomes were incubated with **bergamottin** and with **6',7'-dihydroxybergamottin** (furanocoumarins), the metabolism of saquinavir by the cytochrome P450 isoenzyme CYP3A4 was inhibited by both compounds to a similar extent to ketoconazole, a known CYP3A4 inhibitor. The transport of saquinavir by P-glycoprotein was also, to an extent, inhibited by **6',7'-dihydroxybergamottin**.[1]

Note that grapefruit juice, of which these furanocoumarins are a principal constituent, is known to modestly increase saquinavir levels.

It is difficult to extrapolate these findings to the clinical situation, but if the effect of these furanocoumarins is similar to that of grapefruit juice, any interaction with herbal medicines containing these constituents would be expected to be mild, and of limited clinical relevance.

1. Eagling VA, Profit L, Back DJ. Inhibition of the CYP3A4-mediated metabolism and P-glycoprotein-mediated transport of the HIV-1 protease inhibitor saquinavir by grapefruit juice components. *Br J Clin Pharmacol* (1999) 48, 543–52.

Natural coumarins + Statins

The interaction between natural coumarins and statins is based on experimental evidence only.

Evidence, mechanism, importance and management

An *in vitro* study demonstrated that **bergamottin** (a furanocoumarin) inhibited the metabolism of **simvastatin** in human and *rat* liver microsomes.[1] Note that grapefruit juice, of which furanocoumarins such as **bergamottin** are a principal constituent, is known to markedly increase **simvastatin** levels, which may lead to myopathy and rhabdomyolysis, and avoidance of concurrent use is therefore advised. These experimental studies suggest that **bergamottin** plays a part in this interaction, and therefore, until more is known, a cautious approach would be to advise patients taking **simvastatin** (or **lovastatin**, which is similarly metabolised) to avoid taking supplements containing **bergamottin**, particularly in large quantities. If concurrent use is considered desirable, patients should be advised of the symptoms of myopathy (muscle pain, cramps, brown urine), and advised to promptly seek medical attention if they occur.

1. Le Goff Klein N, Koffel J-C, Jung L, Ubeaud G. In vitro inhibition of simvastatin metabolism, a HMG-CoA reductase inhibitor in human and rat liver by bergamottin, a component of grapefruit juice. *Eur J Pharm Sci* (2003) 18, 31–5.

Natural coumarins + Talinolol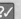

The interaction between natural coumarins and talinolol is based on experimental evidence only.

Evidence, mechanism, importance and management

In an *in vitro* study the effects of several furanocoumarins on P-glycoprotein were assessed using talinolol, a probe substrate for P-glycoprotein. **Bergamottin** did not affect the transport of talinolol, but **6',7'-dihydroxybergamottin** and **6',7'-epoxybergamottin** inhibited the P-glycoprotein transport of talinolol 5-fold and 2.5-fold, respectively, when used in similar concentrations to those found in grapefruit juice.[1] Note that grapefruit juice, of which furanocoumarins are a principal constituent, has been shown to modestly decrease talinolol levels without altering its haemodynamic effects.

It is difficult to extrapolate these findings to the clinical situation, but if the effect of these furanocoumarins is similar to that of grapefruit juice, any interaction with herbal medicines containing these constituents would be expected to be mild, and of limited clinical relevance.

1. de Castro WV, Mertens-Talcott S, Derendorf H, Butterweck V. Grapefruit juice-drug interactions: Grapefruit juice and its components inhibit P-glycoprotein (ABCB1) mediated transport of talinolol in Caco-2 cells. *J Pharm Sci* (2007) 96, 2808–17.

Natural coumarins + Warfarin and related drugs

The interaction between natural coumarins and warfarin and related drugs is based on a prediction only.

Evidence, mechanism, importance and management

It has been suggested that herbal medicines containing naturally occurring coumarins might interact with warfarin and other anticoagulants by causing additive anticoagulant effects. On this basis, some authors have produced lists of plants that might increase the effect of warfarin solely because they contain natural coumarins.[1]

It is known that, to have anticoagulant activity, a coumarin needs to be a 4-hydroxycoumarin with a nonpolar carbon substituent at the 3-position.[2,3] Natural coumarins differ widely in their structures, as discussed under Types, sources and related compounds, page 356, and many do not meet this structural requirement. Moreover, even if anticoagulant activity for a natural coumarin was likely based on its structure, it would need to be determined whether it could occur in sufficiently high enough levels in a plant to be expected to be active.[4] Also, it would need to be demonstrated that it is absorbed when given orally.[4]

There are no established interactions between warfarin and herbal medicines that have been shown to be due to the natural coumarin content of the herb. Even in the classic case of haemorrhagic death of livestock after eating mouldy hay that led to the discovery of dicoumarol, it was the action of the mould on the natural coumarin in the sweet clover (melilot, page 347) that led to the production of the anticoagulant, so consumption of a spoiled product would seem to be necessary for this interaction to occur.

On this basis, the occurrence of natural coumarins in herbal medicines should not cause immediate concern.[4]

1. Heck AM, DeWitt BA, Lukes AL. Potential interactions between alternative therapies and warfarin. *Am J Health-Syst Pharm* (2000) 57, 1221–7.
2. Overman RS, Stahmann MA, Huebner CF, Sullivan WR, Spero L, Doherty DG, Ikawa M, Graf L, Roseman S, Link KP. Studies on the hemorrhagic sweet clover disease. XIII. Anticoagulant activity and structure in the 4-hydroxycoumarin group. *J Biol Chem* (1944) 153, 5–24.
3. Majerus PW, Tollefsen DM. Blood coagulation and anticoagulant, thrombolytic, and antiplatelet drugs. In: Brunton LL, Lazo JS, Parker KL, eds. Goodman & Gilman's The Pharmacological Basis of Therapeutics 11th ed. New York: McGraw-Hill; 2005. p. 1467–88.
4. Booth NL, Nikolic D, van Breemen RB, Geller SE, Banuvar S, Shulman LP, Farnsworth NR. Confusion regarding anticoagulant coumarins in dietary supplements. *Clin Pharmacol Ther* (2004) 76, 511–16.

Nettle

Urtica dioica L. (Urticaceae)

Synonym(s) and related species

Stinging nettle, Urtica.

Note that *Urtica urens* L. has been referred to as Dwarf nettle.

Pharmacopoeias

Common Stinging Nettle for Homeopathic Preparations (BP 2012, PhEur 7.5); Nettle Leaf (*BP 2012, PhEur 7.5*); Powdered Stinging Nettle (*USP35–NF30 S1*); Powdered Stinging Nettle Extract (*USP35–NF30 S1*); Stinging Nettle (*USP35–NF30 S1*).

Constituents

Nettle root contains sterols including **beta-sitosterol**, and lignans, such as pinoresinol, secoisolariciresinol, dehydro-coniferyl alcohol, and neo-olivil. The triterpenes, oleanolic acid and ursolic acid, and their derivatives, and a lectin mixture known as *Urtica dioica* agglutinin (UDA) are also present. Root extracts may be standardised to its content of **beta-sitosterol**, **scopoletin** and amino acids (*USP 32*).

The leaves contain **flavonoids**, mainly kaempferol, isorhamnetin and quercetin glycosides, and caffeic acid derivatives. Extracts may be standardised to caffeoylmalic acid and chlorogenic acid expressed as **chlorogenic acid** (*BP 2009, Ph Eur 6.4*). Note that histamine, formic acid, acetylcholine, acetic acid and 5-hydroxytryptamine, which form the 'sting' when the fresh leaf is touched, are denatured during drying and processing.

Use and indications

The root is used mainly to treat benign prostatic hyperplasia in men, and difficulties in passing urine. There is some pharmacological evidence to support this use, but clinical evidence is equivocal and further trials are required. Leaf extracts have been used for treating allergies. Whole nettle extracts have been shown to have anti-inflammatory activity and may improve symptoms of osteoarthritis.

Pharmacokinetics

No relevant pharmacokinetic data found. For information on the pharmacokinetics of individual flavonoids present in nettle, see under flavonoids, page 213.

Interactions overview

No interactions with nettle found. For information on the interactions of individual flavonoids present in nettle, see under flavonoids, page 213.

Oregon grape

Mahonia aquifolium Nutt. (Berberidaceae)

Synonym(s) and related species

Holly-leaved berberis, Mountain grape.

Berberis aquifolium (Pursh), *Mahonia aquifolium* Nutt.

Constituents

The root, rhizome and stem bark contain the isoquinoline alkaloids **berberine**, berbamine, columbamine, jatrorrhizine, oxyacanthine, oxyberberine, and others.

Use and indications

Used for many conditions, particularly diarrhoea, gastritis and skin diseases such as psoriasis.

Pharmacokinetics

No relevant pharmacokinetic data found for Oregon grape, but see berberine, page 63, for details on this constituent of Oregon grape.

Interactions overview

No interactions with Oregon grape found. However, for the interactions of one of its constituents, berberine, see under berberine, page 63.

Parsley

Petroselinum crispum (Mill.) Fuss (Apiaceae)

Synonym(s) and related species

Apium petroselinum L., *Carum petroselinum* (L.) Benth., *Petroselinum peregrinum* (L.) Lag., *Petroselinum sativum* Hoffm., *Petroselinum vulgare* Lag.

Constituents

All parts of the parsley plant contain similar compounds but possibly in different proportions. The most important constituents are the **natural coumarins (furanocoumarins** including bergapten, psoralen, 8- and 5-methoxypsoralen), and the phthalides Z-ligustilide, cnidilide, neocnidilide and senkyunolide. **Flavonoids** present include apigenin, luteolin and others. There is also a small amount of volatile oil present, in all parts but especially the seed, containing apiole, myristicin, eugenol, osthole, carotol and others.

Use and indications

Parsley root and seed are traditionally used as a diuretic, carminative and for arthritis, rheumatism and other inflammatory disorders. The leaves are used as a culinary herb in foods.

Pharmacokinetics

A small study in *mice* reported that a parsley root extract reduced the liver content of cytochrome P450 when compared with control animals. The general significance of this is unclear and further study is needed.[1] For information on the pharmacokinetics of individual flavonoids present in parsley, see under flavonoids, page 213.

Interactions overview

A single case reports lithium toxicity in a patient who took a herbal diuretic containing parsley, among many other ingredients. A patient taking warfarin had an increase in his INR when he stopped taking a regular supplement containing various vitamin K-containing plants, including parsley. For information on the interactions of individual flavonoids present in parsley, see under flavonoids, page 213.

Interactions monographs

- Aminophenazone, page 364
- Food, page 364
- Herbal medicines, page 364
- Lithium, page 364
- Paracetamol, page 364
- Pentobarbital, page 364
- Warfarin and related drugs, page 364

1. Jakovljevic V, Raskovic A, Popovic M, Sabo J. The effect of celery and parsley on pharmacodynamic activity of drugs involving cytochrome P450 in their metabolism. *Eur J Drug Metab Pharmacokinet* (2002) 27, 153–6.

P

Parsley + Aminophenazone

The interaction between parsley and aminophenazone is based on experimental evidence only.

Evidence, mechanism, importance and management

A study in *mice* found that parsley (extracted from the rhizome and mixed with water and olive oil in a ratio of 4:3:3), given 2 hours before a single 60-mg/kg dose of aminophenazone, potentiated and prolonged, the analgesic action of aminophenazone.[1]

The authors of this study suggest that it is possible that the parsley extract reduced the metabolism of aminophenazone by cytochrome P450, as the overall content of cytochrome P450 in the livers of the *mice* given parsley was significantly reduced, when compared with the control group.

The clinical relevance of this small preliminary study is unclear and further study is needed, particularly as parsley is commonly used in food.

1. Jakovljevic V, Raskovic A, Popovic M, Sabo J. The effect of celery and parsley juices on pharmacodynamic activity of drugs involving cytochrome P450 in their metabolism. *Eur J Drug Metab Pharmacokinet* (2002) 27, 153–6.

Parsley + Food

No interactions found. Parsley is commonly used in food.

Parsley + Herbal medicines

No interactions found.

Parsley + Lithium

A woman developed lithium toxicity after taking a herbal diuretic remedy.

Evidence, mechanism, importance and management

A 26-year-old woman who had been taking lithium 900 mg twice daily for 5 months, with hydroxyzine, lorazepam, propranolol, risperidone and sertraline, came to an emergency clinic complaining of nausea, diarrhoea, unsteady gait, tremor, nystagmus and drowsiness, (all symptoms of lithium toxicity). Her lithium level, which had previously been stable at 1.1 mmol/L, was found to be 4.5 mmol/L. For the past 2 to 3 weeks she had been taking a non-prescription herbal diuretic containing **corn silk**, *Equisetum hyemale*, **juniper**, **ovate buchu**, **parsley** and **bearberry**, all of which are believed to have diuretic actions. The other ingredients were bromelain, paprika, potassium and vitamin B_6.[1]

The most likely explanation for what happened is that the herbal diuretic caused the lithium toxicity. It is impossible to know which herb or combination of herbs actually caused the toxicity, or how, but this case once again emphasises that herbal remedies are not risk-free just because they are natural. It also underscores the need for patients to avoid self-medication without first seeking informed advice and supervision if they are taking potentially hazardous drugs like lithium.

1. Pyevich D, Bogenschutz MP. Herbal diuretics and lithium toxicity. *Am J Psychiatry* (2001) 158, 1329.

Parsley + Paracetamol (Acetaminophen)

The interaction between parsley and paracetamol (acetaminophen) is based on experimental evidence only.

Evidence, mechanism, importance and management

A study in *mice* found that parsley (extracted from the rhizome and mixed with water and olive oil in a ratio of 4:3:3), given 2 hours before a single 80-mg/kg dose of paracetamol, potentiated and prolonged, the analgesic action of paracetamol to an extent that was statistically significant.

The authors suggest that it is possible that the parsley extract reduced the metabolism of paracetamol by cytochrome P450, as the overall content of cytochrome P450 in the livers of the *mice* given parsley was significantly reduced, when compared with the control group.[1]

The clinical relevance of this small preliminary study is unclear and further study is needed, particularly as parsley is commonly used in food.

1. Jakovljevic V, Raskovic A, Popovic M, Sabo J. The effect of celery and parsley juices on pharmacodynamic activity of drugs involving cytochrome P450 in their metabolism. *Eur J Drug Metab Pharmacokinet* (2002) 27, 153–6.

Parsley + Pentobarbital

The interaction between parsley and pentobarbital is based on experimental evidence only.

Evidence, mechanism, importance and management

A study in *mice* found that parsley (extracted from the rhizome and mixed with water and olive oil in a ratio of 4:3:3), given 2 hours before a single 40-mg/kg dose of pentobarbital significantly extended the sleeping time, when compared with a control group of *animals* who received pentobarbital alone. This effect was not seen when the same parsley extract was given 30 minutes before pentobarbital.[1]

The authors suggest that it is possible that the parsley extract reduced the metabolism of pentobarbital by cytochrome P450, as the overall content of cytochrome P450 in the livers of the *mice* given parsley was significantly reduced compared with the control group.

The clinical relevance of this small preliminary study is unclear and further study is needed, particularly as parsley is commonly used in food.

1. Jakovljevic V, Raskovic A, Popovic M, Sabo J. The effect of celery and parsley juices on pharmacodynamic activity of drugs involving cytochrome P450 in their metabolism. *Eur J Drug Metab Pharmacokinet* (2002) 27, 153–6.

Parsley + Warfarin and related drugs

A man had a rise in his INR after stopping taking a herbal nutritional supplement *(Nature's Life Greens)*, which contained a number of plants including parsley.

Clinical evidence

A 72-year-old man stabilised on warfarin was found to have an INR of 4.43 at a routine clinic visit, which was increased from 3.07 six weeks previously. The patient had stopped taking a herbal product *Nature's Life Greens* that month because he did not have enough money to buy it. He had been taking it for the past 7 years as a vitamin supplement because he had previously been instructed to limit his intake of green leafy vegetables. He was eventually restabilised on warfarin and the same nutritional product.

Experimental evidence

No relevant data found.

Mechanism

The product label listed 25 vegetables without stating the amounts or concentrations,[1] but at least 5 of the listed ingredients are known to contain high levels of vitamin K_1 including parsley, green tea leaves, spinach, broccoli, and cabbage. It is therefore likely the supplement contained sufficient vitamin to antagonise the effect of the warfarin so that when it was stopped warfarin requirements fell, and without an appropriate adjustment in dose, this resulted in an increased INR.

Importance and management

The interaction of vitamin K_1 from vegetables with warfarin is well-established. However, the evidence suggests that, in patients with normal vitamin K_1 status, in general, clinically relevant changes in coagulation status require large continued changes in intake of vitamin K_1 from foods. It is unlikely that the parsley alone caused this effect, and there appear to be no other published cases of parsley reducing the efficacy of warfarin and related anticoagulants. Because of the many other factors influencing anticoagulant control, it is not possible to reliably ascribe a change in INR specifically to a drug interaction in a single case report without other supporting evidence. It may be better to advise patients to discuss the use of any herbal products they wish to try, and to increase monitoring if this is thought advisable. Cases of uneventful use should be reported, as they are as useful as possible cases of adverse effects.

Nevertheless, some consider that increased INR monitoring is required in any patient wanting to stop or start any herbal medicine or nutritional supplement.

P

1. Bransgrove LL. Interaction between warfarin and a vitamin K-containing nutritional supplement: a case report. *J Herb Pharmacother* (2001) 1, 85–9.

Passiflora

Passiflora incarnata L. (Passifloraceae)

Synonym(s) and related species

Apricot vine, Maypop, Passion flower, Passion vine.

Note that *Passiflora edulis* Sims is the source of the edible passion fruit.

Pharmacopoeias

Passion Flower (*BP 2012, PhEur 7.5*); Passion Flower Dry Extract (*BP 2012, PhEur 7.5*).

Constituents

The major constituents of passiflora leaf and flower are C-glycosides of **flavonoids** based on apigenin and luteolin, to which it may be standardised. Other **flavonoids** present include chrysin (5,7-hydroxyflavone), quercetin and kaempferol. The indole alkaloids of the β-carboline type (e.g. harman, harmol, and others) are minor constituents or may not even be detectable. Other minor constituents include a cyanogenic glycoside gynocardin, γ-benzopyrones maltol and ethylmaltol, a polyacetylene passicol, and an essential oil.

Use and indications

Passiflora is used as a sedative, hypnotic and anxiolytic and has been reported to have antiepileptic and anti-inflammatory effects. Some clinical studies in patients appear to support the anxiolytic and sedative effects of passiflora, and *animal* data suggest that some of the flavonoid constituents, chrysin and apigenin, may be responsible for these effects.

Pharmacokinetics

No relevant pharmacokinetic data found. For information on the pharmacokinetics of individual flavonoids present in passiflora, see under flavonoids, page 213.

Interactions overview

Passiflora is used for its sedative effects; additive sedation is therefore a theoretical possibility with other drugs with sedative properties, whereas the effects of stimulant drugs may be reduced. For information on the interactions of individual flavonoids present in passiflora, see under flavonoids, page 213.

Interactions monographs

- Amfetamines, page 367
- Anxiolytics and Hypnotics, page 367
- Food, page 367
- Herbal medicines; Kava, page 367

Passiflora + Amfetamines

The interaction between passiflora and amfetamines is based on experimental evidence only.

Evidence, mechanism, importance and management

A study in *rats* reported that a passiflora extract 250 mg/kg reduced the hyperactivity induced by subcutaneous **amfetamine** by 39%, when compared with a control group who received **amfetamine** alone. This effect was reduced by 83% when a *Piper methysticum* (kava) extract 100 mg/kg was also given.[1]

Although this was a high-dose study in *animals,* these results appear to be in line with the known sedative effects of passiflora. Bear in mind the possibility of antagonistic effects when passiflora is given with stimulants.

1. Capasso A, Sorrentino L. Pharmacological studies on the sedative and hypnotic effect of *Kava kava* and *Passiflora* extracts combination. *Phytomedicine* (2005) 12, 39–45.

Passiflora + Anxiolytics and Hypnotics

The interaction between passiflora and phenobarbital is based on experimental evidence only.

Evidence, mechanism, importance and management

A study in *rats* found an additive sedative effect when a passiflora extract 250 mg/kg was given with **phenobarbital**. This was reported as a 53% increase in sleep duration. This effect was greater (92%) when *Piper methysticum* (kava) extract 100 mg/kg was also given.[1]

Although this was a high-dose study in *animals,* these results appear to be in line with the known sedative effects of passiflora. Bear in mind the possibility of additive sedative effects when passiflora is taken with other known sedative drugs.

1. Capasso A, Sorrentino L. Pharmacological studies on the sedative and hypnotic effect of *Kava kava* and *Passiflora* extracts combination. *Phytomedicine* (2005) 12, 39–45.

Passiflora + Food

No interactions found.

Passiflora + Herbal medicines; Kava

The effects of passiflora extract and *Piper methysticum* (kava) extract were synergistic in one *animal* study, see Passiflora + Amfetamines, above, and Passiflora + Anxiolytics and Hypnotics, above.

P

Pelargonium

Pelargonium sidoides DC. and *Pelargonium reniforme* Curtis (Geraniaceae)

Synonym(s) and related species

Geranium, South African geranium.

Pharmacopoeias

Pelargonium Root (*BP 2012, PhEur 7.5*).

Constituents

The active constituents of pelargonium root are not conclusively known, although they are thought to be proanthocyanidin oligomers based on epigallo- and gallo-catechin. A unique series of O-galloyl-C-glucosylflavones, and novel ellagitannins with a (1)C(4) glucopyranose core (trivially named pelargoniins), have been found in *Pelargonium reniforme*. There are also oxygenated benzopyranones such as 6,7,8-trihydroxycoumarin and 8-hydroxy-5,6,7-trimethoxycoumarin, predominantly as sulphated derivatives. The **natural coumarins** found in *Pelargonium sidoides* do not possess the structure required for anticoagulant activity.

Use and indications

Pelargonium is used in the treatment of acute bronchitis, tonsillitis and upper respiratory tract infections.

Pharmacokinetics

No relevant pharmacokinetic data found.

Interactions overview

Pelargonium does not appear to affect either the pharmacokinetics or the anticoagulant response to warfarin.

Interactions monographs

- Food, page 369
- Herbal medicines, page 369
- Warfarin and related drugs, page 369

Pelargonium + Food

No interactions found.

Pelargonium + Herbal medicines

No interactions found.

Pelargonium + Warfarin and related drugs

The interaction between pelargonium and warfarin is based on experimental evidence only.

Clinical evidence

No interactions found.

Experimental evidence

In a study in *rats*,[1] pelargonium 500 mg/kg (alcoholic extract of *Pelargonium sidoides* root, *Umckaloabo*) given for 14 days had no significant effect on the pharmacokinetics of a single 0.2-mg/kg dose of warfarin given on day 15. In a separate study, the coagulation parameters (thromboplastin time, partial thromboplastin time and thrombin time) of *rats* remained unchanged when they were given pelargonium up to 500 mg/kg daily for 2 weeks. Furthermore, coagulation parameters in response to warfarin 0.05 mg/kg did not differ when pelargonium 500 mg/kg was also given.[1]

Mechanism

It has been suggested that the natural coumarins present in pelargonium may affect the anticoagulant response to warfarin.

Importance and management

Evidence is limited to this one study in *rats,* but the coumarin constituents of pelargonium have not been found to possess anticoagulant activity (consider also coumarins, page 356). The manufacturers of a UK product containing *Pelargonium sidoides* (*Kaloba*) state that it may theoretically have an effect on coagulation and therefore interact with anticoagulants.[2] However, the natural coumarins found in *Pelargonium sidoides* do not possess the structure required for anticoagulant activity,[1,3] and the evidence above supports the conclusion that an interaction is unlikely. Therefore, the dose of warfarin does not need adjusting if *Pelargonium sidoides* extracts are also given.

1. Koch E, Biber A. Treatment of rats with the pelargonium sidoides extract EPs 7630 has no effect on blood coagulation parameters or on the pharmacokinetics of warfarin. *Phytomedicine* (2007) 14, 40–45.
2. Kaloba Oral Drops (*Pelargonium sidoides* DC). Schwabe Pharma UK Ltd. UK Summary of product characteristics, May 2008.
3. Schwabe Pharma UK Ltd. August 2008.

P

Pennyroyal

Mentha pulegium L. or *Hedeoma pulegioides* Pers. (Lamiaceae)

Synonym(s) and related species

Mentha pulegium L.: European pennyroyal. *Mentha pulegioides* Dumort.Fl.Belg., *Pulegium erectum* Mill., *Pulegium parviflorum* (Req.) Samp., *Pulegium vulgare* Mill.

Hedeoma pulegioides Pers.: American pennyroyal, Squaw mint.

Melissa pulegioides L.

Constituents

The main constituent of pennyroyal is the toxic volatile oil **pulegone**. Other components include menthone, isomenthone, piperitone, neomenthol, 2-octanol, camphene, and limonene. Pennyroyal also contains polyphenolic acids and **flavonoids**.

Use and indications

Traditionally, pennyroyal has been used for dyspepsia, colds, skin eruptions, delayed menstruation, and it is reported to be an effective antibacterial and antifungal. It is also believed to be carminative, abortifacient and diaphoretic and it has been used as an insect repellent. The oil from pennyroyal (pulegium oil) is toxic to the liver, kidneys and nerves, and its use is generally considered unsafe.

Pharmacokinetics

The toxic effects of pennyroyal are thought to be principally due to metabolites of pulegone such as menthofuran. The metabolism to toxic metabolites and then inactivation has been shown to be subject to cytochrome P450 isoenzyme-mediated metabolism.[1-5] Preclinical experiments are inconclusive as to which isoenzyme is principally involved. One study using human isoenzymes found that CYP2E1 is the main metaboliser of pulegone and its metabolite menthofuran, with CYP1A2, CYP2C19 and CYP2A6 also contributing to some extent.[2] In contrast, a study in *mice* found that CYP1A2 is the major metabolising enzyme with CYP2E1 playing a lesser role.[3]

Note that peppermint, page 379, contains only small amounts of pulegone.

Interactions overview

Pennyroyal may reduce the absorption of iron compounds.

Interactions monographs

- Food, page 371
- Herbal medicines, page 371
- Iron compounds, page 371

1. Mizutani T, Nomura H, Nakanishi K, Fujita S. Effects of drug metabolism modifiers on pulegone-induced hepatotoxicity in mice. *Res Commun Chem Pathol Pharmacol* (1987) 58, 75–83.
2. Khojasteh-Bakht SC, Chen W, Koenigs LL, Peter RM, Nelson SD. Metabolism of (*R*)-(+)-pulegone and (*R*)-(+)-menthofuran by human liver cytochrome P-450s: Evidence for formation of a furan epoxide. *Drug Metab Dispos* (1999) 27, 574–80.
3. Sztajnkrycer MD, Otten EJ, Bond GR, Lindsell CJ, Goetz RJ. Mitigation of pennyroyal oil hepatotoxicity in the mouse. *Acad Emerg Med* (2003) 10, 1024–8.
4. Gordon WP, Huitric AC, Seth CL, McClanahan RH, Nelson SD. The metabolism of the abortifacient terpene, (*R*)-(+)-pulegone, to a proximate toxin, menthofuran. *Drug Metab Dispos* (1987) 15, 589–94.
5. Thomassen D, Slattery JT, Nelson SD. Menthofuran-dependent and independent aspects of pulegone hepatotoxicity: roles of glutathione. *J Pharmacol Exp Ther* (1990) 253, 567–72.

Pennyroyal + Food

No interactions found.

Pennyroyal + Herbal medicines

No interactions found.

Pennyroyal + Iron compounds

Pennyroyal tea reduces iron absorption similarly to conventional tea.

Clinical evidence

In a study in 9 healthy subjects, a 275 mL serving of pennyroyal tea reduced the absorption of iron in a 50 g bread roll by about 70%. The tea was prepared by adding 300 mL of boiling water to 3 g of the herbal tea, then infusing for 10 minutes before straining and serving. In this study, the inhibitory effect of pennyroyal tea on iron absorption was only slightly less than that of black tea (Assam tea, *Camellia sinensis* L.), which is known to inhibit iron absorption.[1] Consider also, Tea + Iron compounds, page 467.

Experimental evidence

No relevant data found.

Mechanism

The polyphenols in pennyroyal may bind to iron in the intestine and influence its absorption.

Importance and management

The clinical impact of this interaction is not fully known, but be aware that some herbal teas such as pennyroyal reduce iron absorption similarly to conventional tea, which is not generally considered to be a suitable drink for babies and children, because of its effects on iron absorption. Furthermore, the safety of pennyroyal tea is not established, and there are concerns about the toxicity of its major volatile oil, pulegone.

1. Hurrell RF, Reddy M, Cook JD. Inhibition of non-haem iron absorption in man by polyphenolic-containing beverages. *Br J Nutr* (1999) 81, 289–95.

P

Pepper

Piper nigrum L. (Piperaceae)

Synonym(s) and related species

Black and white pepper are derived from the fruits of the same species, *Piper nigrum* L. Black pepper is the unripe fruit which has been immersed in hot water and dried in the sun, during which the outer pericarp shrinks and darkens into a thin, wrinkled black layer. White pepper consists of the seed only, prepared by soaking the fully ripe berries, removing the pericarp and drying the naked seed.

Long pepper, *Piper longum* L., is a closely related species where the fruits are smaller and occur embedded in flower 'spikes', which form the seed heads.

Constituents

Alkaloids and alkylamides, the most important being **piperine**, with piperanine, piperettine, piperlongumine, pipernonaline, lignans, and minor constituents such as the piperoleins, have been isolated from the fruits of both species of pepper. Black pepper and long pepper also contain a volatile oil which may differ in constitution, but is composed of bisabolene, sabinene and many others; white pepper contains very little. The pungent taste of pepper is principally due to **piperine**, which acts at the vanilloid receptor.

Use and indications

Pepper is one of the most popular spices in the world, and it is also used as a folk medicine in many countries. It is used as a stimulant and carminative, and is reputed to have anti-asthmatic, anti-oxidant, antimicrobial, hepatoprotective, and hypocholesterolaemic effects. Most of the pharmacological effects reported to date are attributed to piperine. A black pepper extract containing 95% piperine is used in a number of herbal supplements.

Both long pepper and black pepper are important ingredients of many Ayurvedic herbal medicines where they are intended to enhance absorption of other medicines, for example in the traditional formula known as **Trikatu**, which contains *Piper nigrum, Piper longum* and *Zingiber officinale* (ginger, page 235) in a ratio of 1:1:1. There is increasing evidence to support this rationale as well as some of the other traditional uses, but it should be noted that the actions of **Trikatu** are not always the same as for pepper extracts or pure piperine, and **Trikatu** has been implicated in reducing rather than enhancing bioavailability of some drugs. **Trikatu** is also used as a digestive aid.

Pharmacokinetics

Piperine, given to *mice* has been shown to delay gastrointestinal transit time in a dose-dependent manner.[1,2] A non-significant trend towards a delay in gastrointestinal transit has also been seen in a study in 14 healthy fasting subjects given 1.5 g black pepper.[3] This has been suggested as one way that piperine might increase the absorption of drugs, but its clinical significance is unclear, as pepper is normally ingested as part of a meal.

It has been known for some time that pepper, and piperine in particular, inhibit cytochrome P450,[4,5] but it is only more recently that activity against specific human isoenzymes has been tested. Piperine has been found to inhibit the cytochrome P450 isoenzyme CYP3A4, see verapamil, page 378, *in vitro*. The bisalkaloids, dipiperamides D and E have also been shown *in vitro* to inhibit this isoenzyme using nifedipine as a probe substrate.[6] Similarly, methanolic and ethanolic extracts of *Piper nigrum* fruit inhibited CYP3A4 and CYP2D6 *in vitro* using erythromycin and dextromethorphan as probe substrates, although only the activity of the methanolic extract against CYP3A4 had a low IC_{50} value.[7] These findings have also been published elsewhere.[8] Piperine did not alter CYP2C, see verapamil, page 378.

In vitro studies suggest that piperine may inhibit P-glycoprotein, see digoxin, page 375, and ciclosporin, page 374.

It has also been suggested, using data from *in vitro* studies using *guinea pig* cell cultures,[9] and *in vivo* studies in *rats*[5] that piperine may inhibit glucuronidation via the UDP-glucuronyltransferase enzyme system, which is involved in the metabolism of a number of drugs.

Interactions overview

Piperine, the active alkaloidal constituent of pepper, increased the AUC of a single dose of nevirapine and of theophylline when given at a dose that might easily be achieved with piperine-containing supplements. Some caution might be appropriate with these combinations. The AUC of a single-dose of propranolol and of steady-state carbamazepine have also been increased by piperine, but these changes are of little or no clinical importance. Increases in phenytoin levels have also been demonstrated, and high-dose piperine also increased the AUC of rifampicin.

Various *animal* studies have shown increased levels of amoxicillin, barbiturates, NSAIDs and oxytetracycline with piperine, but little effect on cefadroxil. Piperine also had an antithyroid effect in *animals*. In other *animal* studies, Trikatu decreased diclofenac and isoniazid levels.

Interactions monographs

- Barbiturates, page 374
- Beta-lactam antibacterials, page 374
- Carbamazepine, page 374
- Ciclosporin, page 374
- Digoxin, page 375
- Food, page 375
- Herbal medicines; Coenzyme Q_{10}, page 375
- Herbal medicines; Rhodiola, page 375

1. Izzo AA, Capasso R, Pinto L, Di Carlo G, Mascolo N, Capasso F. Effect of vanilloid drugs on gastrointestinal transit in mice. *Br J Pharmacol* (2001) 132, 1411–16.
2. Bajad S, Bedi KL, Singla AK, Johri RK. Piperine inhibits gastric emptying and gastrointestinal transit in rats and mice. *Planta Med* (2001) 67, 176–9.
3. Vazquez-Olivencia W, Shah P, Pitchumoni CS. The effect of red and black pepper on orocecal transit time. *J Am Coll Nutr* (1992) 11, 228–31.
4. Srinivasan K. Black pepper and its pungent principle piperine: a review of diverse physiological effects. *Crit Rev Food Sci Nutr* (2007) 47, 735–48.
5. Atal CK, Dubey RK, Singh J. Biochemical basis of enhanced drug bioavailability of piperine: Evidence that piperine is a potent inhibitor of drug metabolism. *J Pharmacol Exp Ther* (1985) 232, 258–62.
6. Tsukamoto S, Tomise K, Miyakawa K, Cha B-C, Abe T, Hamada T, Hirota H, Ohta T. CYP3A4 inhibitory activity of new bisalkaloids, dipiperamides D and E, and cognates from white pepper. *Bioorg Med Chem* (2002) 10, 2981–5.
7. Usia T, Iwata H, Hiratsuka A, Watabe T, Kadota S, Tezuka Y. CYP3A4 and CYP2D6 inhibitory activities of Indonesian medicinal plants. *Phytomedicine* (2006) 13, 67–73.
8. Subehan , Usia T, Kadota S, Tezuka Y. Mechanism-based inhibition of CYP3A4 and CYP2D6 by Indonesian medicinal plants. *J Ethnopharmacol* (2006) 105, 449–55.
9. Singh J, Dubey RK, Atal CK. Piperine-mediated inhibition of glucuronidation activity in isolated epithelial cells of the guinea-pig small intestine: evidence that piperine lowers the endogeneous [sic] UDP-glucuronic acid content. *J Pharmacol Exp Ther* (1986) 236, 488–93.

P

Pepper + Barbiturates

The interaction between piperine and pentobarbital or pheno-barbital is based on experimental evidence only.

Clinical evidence

No interactions found.

Experimental evidence

In a single-dose study in *rats,* pre-treatment with increasing doses of oral **piperine** from 10 to 50 mg/kg increased the **pentobarbital** sleeping time (up to twofold). Blood levels of **pentobarbital** were raised (by 38% at 45 minutes). **Piperine** at a lower dose of 5 mg/kg had no significant effect on the **pentobarbital** sleeping time. When the study was repeated after pre-treatment with **pheno-barbital** 100 mg/kg for 7 days, the **pentobarbital** sleeping time was still prolonged after administration of **piperine**, but the length of sleeping time was much less than without barbiturate pretreatment.[1]

Mechanism

It was suggested that the increase in sleeping time induced by pentobarbital and phenobarbital was a result of inhibition of drug metabolising enzymes by piperine.[1]

Importance and management

This preclinical study provides some limited evidence that piperine, the main active constituent of pepper, might increase the effects of pentobarbital and possibly also phenobarbital. While it is not possible to directly apply these data to the clinical situation, it should be noted that the doses used are probably unlikely to be ingested from pepper itself, or from piperine-containing supplements.

1. Mujumdar AM, Dhuley JN, Deshmukh VK, Raman PH, Thorat SL, Naik SR. Effect of piperine on pentobarbitone induced hypnosis in rats. *Indian J Exp Biol* (1990) 28, 483–7.

Pepper + Beta-lactam antibacterials

The interaction or lack of interaction between piperine and amoxicillin, cefadroxil or cefotaxime is based on experimental evidence only.

Clinical evidence

No interactions found.

Experimental evidence

(a) Amoxicillin

In a single-dose study in *rats,* giving **piperine** 10 mg/kg or 20 mg/kg followed 30 minutes later by oral amoxicillin 100 mg/kg significantly increased the maximum amoxicillin plasma concentration by 90% and 124%, respectively, and the AUC by 66% and 107%, respectively. The time to reach maximum levels was reduced, and the half-life increased.[1]

(b) Cefadroxil

In a single-dose study in *rats,* giving piperine 10 mg/kg or 20 mg/kg followed 30 minutes later by oral cefadroxil 100 mg/kg had no effect on the pharmacokinetics of cefadroxil.[1]

(c) Cefotaxime

In a single-dose study in *rats,* giving piperine 10 mg/kg or 20 mg/kg followed 30 minutes later by intraperitoneal cefotaxime 10 mg/kg significantly increased the maximum cefotaxime plasma concentration by 51% and 71%, respectively, the AUC by 71% and 118%, respectively, and the half-life by 44% and 65%, respectively.[1]

Mechanism

Unknown. The increase in elimination half-life of amoxicillin and cefotaxime suggests a mechanism affecting drug clearance, and not a mechanism of increased gastrointestinal absorption. Although the authors suggest that an effect on drug metabolising enzymes cannot be ruled out, this is unlikely as none of these antibacterials undergoes significant metabolism by this route.

Importance and management

This preclinical study provides some evidence that piperine, the main active constituent of pepper, might increase exposure to some antibacterials. While it is not possible to directly apply these data to the clinical situation, the level of increases seen would not be expected to be clinically important. It should be noted that the doses used are probably unlikely to be ingested from pepper itself, or from piperine-containing supplements

1. Hiwale AR, Dhuley JN, Naik SR. Effect of co-administration of piperine on pharma-cokinetics of beta-lactam antibiotics in rats. *Indian J Exp Biol* (2002) 40, 277–81.

Pepper + Carbamazepine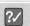

Piperine causes a negligible increase in the exposure to carba-mazepine.

Clinical evidence

In a study, 10 patients with epilepsy taking carbamazepine 300 or 500 mg twice daily for at least 2 months were given a single 20-mg dose of piperine. The AUC of carbamazepine was increased by 10% and 13% for the 300 mg and 500 mg doses, respectively, whereas the maximum concentration was only increased in the 500 mg group, and then only by 11%.[1]

Experimental evidence

No relevant data found.

Mechanism

It was proposed that piperine might have inhibited the metabolism of carbamazepine by the cytochrome P450 isoenzyme CYP3A4.

Importance and management

Evidence for an interaction between pepper and carbamazepine comes from one study using the constituent piperine. Although piperine increases carbamazepine exposure the effect is almost certainly not of clinical relevance.

1. Pattanaik S, Hota D, Prabhakar S, Kharbanda P, Pandhi P. Pharmacokinetic interaction of single dose of piperine with steady-state carbamazepine in epilepsy patients. *Phytother Res* (2009) 23, 1281–6.

Pepper + Ciclosporin

The interaction between piperine and ciclosporin is based on experimental evidence only.

Evidence, mechanism, importance and management

In an *in vitro* study, the transport of ciclosporin by P-glycoprotein was modestly inhibited in the presence of **piperine**, in a concentration-dependent manner.[1] It is difficult to apply the findings of one experimental study to human intake of pepper and a clinical study is needed to assess whether ingestion of pepper or piperine-containing supplements actually alters ciclosporin levels. Until more is known, bear this finding in mind in the event of unexpected outcomes in patients taking ciclosporin and piperine-containing supplements.

1. Bhardwaj RK, Glaeser H, Becquemont L, Klotz U, Gupta SK, Fromm MF. Piperine, a major constituent of black pepper, inhibits human P-glycoprotein and CYP3A4. *J Pharmacol Exp Ther* (2002) 302, 645–50.

Pepper + Digoxin

The interaction between piperine and digoxin is based on experimental evidence only.

Clinical evidence

No interactions found.

Experimental evidence and mechanism

In two *in vitro* studies, **piperine** inhibited the transport of digoxin by P-glycoprotein in a concentration-dependent manner.[1,2] In one of these studies, **piperine** 50 micromol had an effect comparable to verapamil 100 micromol, a known P-glycoprotein inhibitor.[2]

Importance and management

Unclear. It is difficult to apply this finding to human intake of pepper. The authors of one of the studies suggest that an inhibitory concentration of piperine could potentially be achieved *in vivo* after ingestion of soup containing 1 g black pepper.[1] This amount could have the effect of increasing plasma digoxin levels. However, a clinical study is needed to assess whether ingestion of pepper or piperine-containing supplements actually alters digoxin levels. Until more is known, bear this finding in mind in the event of unexpected outcomes in patients taking digoxin and piperine-containing supplements.

1. Bhardwaj RK, Glaeser H, Becquemont L, Klotz U, Gupta SK, Fromm MF. Piperine, a major constituent of black pepper, inhibits human P-glycoprotein and CYP3A4. *J Pharmacol Exp Ther* (2002) 302, 645–50.
2. Han Y, Tan TMC, Lim L-Y. *In vitro* and *in vivo* evaluation of the effects of piperine on P-gp function and expression. *Toxicol Appl Pharmacol* (2008) 230, 283–9.

Pepper + Food

No interactions found between pepper and food. Note that pepper is an ingredient in many foods. For mention that piperine increased the absorption of one green tea catechin, see Tea + Herbal medicines; Pepper, page 467.

Pepper + Herbal medicines; Coenzyme Q$_{10}$

For a study showing that piperine modestly increased the AUC of one dose of coenzyme Q$_{10}$, see Coenzyme Q$_{10}$ + Herbal medicines; Pepper, page 160.

Pepper + Herbal medicines; Rhodiola

For mention that piperine might reduce the antidepressant activity of rhodiola, see Rhodiola + Herbal medicines; Pepper, page 405

Pepper + Herbal medicines; Turmeric

For mention that piperine increased the bioavailability of curcumin, see Turmeric + Herbal medicines; Pepper, page 474.

Pepper + Isoniazid

The interaction between piperine and isoniazid is based on experimental evidence only.

Clinical evidence

No interactions found.

Experimental evidence

In a single-dose study,[1] *rabbits* were given isoniazid 14 mg/kg alone or with **Trikatu** 500 mg, which contained 10 mg of the active principle **piperine**. **Trikatu** was found to significantly reduce the maximum plasma levels and AUC of isoniazid by 35% and 39%, respectively. **Trikatu** is an Ayurvedic medicine which contains ginger, black pepper and long pepper in a 1:1:1 ratio.

Mechanism

It has been suggested that Trikatu delays gastric motility, causing retention of the isoniazid in the stomach. Since isoniazid is largely absorbed from the intestine, this might explain the decrease in plasma isoniazid concentrations.

Importance and management

If the findings of the study in *animals* were also replicated in humans, it would seem possible that ingestion of Trikatu with isoniazid may reduce isoniazid levels to below the required minimum inhibitory concentration. However, the widespread use of pepper in cooking and lack of reports of treatment failure with isoniazid provide some reassurance that an interaction is unlikely. Nevertheless, bear in mind the possibility of an interaction if there is any indication of a lack of isoniazid efficacy in a patient taking Trikatu.

1. Karan RS, Bhargava VK, Garg SK. Effect of Trikatu (piperine) on the pharmacokinetic profile of isoniazid in rabbits. *Indian J Pharmacol* (1998) 30, 254–6.

Pepper + Nevirapine

Piperine markedly increases the AUC of a single dose of nevirapine in healthy subjects.

Clinical evidence

In a well-controlled study in 8 healthy subjects who received **piperine** 20 mg daily for 7 days, with a single 200-mg dose of nevirapine at the same time as the **piperine** on day 7, the maximum plasma concentration and AUC of nevirapine were markedly increased by about twofold and 2.6-fold, respectively. The estimated elimination half-life of nevirapine was not significantly altered. In this single-dose study there was no difference in the incidence of adverse events.[1]

Experimental evidence

No relevant data found.

Mechanism

Uncertain. It was suggested that piperine inhibited the cytochrome P450 isoenzyme CYP3A4, which is involved in the metabolism of nevirapine.[1] However, since the elimination half-life of nevirapine was unaltered, it is unlikely that hepatic CYP3A4 was affected. Also, inhibition of gastrointestinal CYP3A4 would not explain the marked increase in nevirapine levels seen, because nevirapine is already over 90% bioavailable. On repeated dosing nevirapine induces its own metabolism (hence the need to increase the dose after 2 weeks), but in this study nevirapine was given as a single dose, so autoinduction would not have played any part. Subjects in this study were fasting, but food does not affect nevirapine pharmacokinetics.

Importance and management

This study appears to show that piperine markedly increases the exposure to single-dose nevirapine that might easily be achieved with piperine-containing supplements or even from consuming black pepper. However, at present there is no clear explanation for the finding, and further investigation is clearly warranted. Furthermore, how the findings relate to the use of multiple-dose nevirapine is unknown, especially as nevirapine induces its own metabolism. Although no adverse effects were seen in this small single-dose study in healthy subjects, nevirapine is known to cause a dose-related rash, and to be hepatotoxic. Until more it known, it would be prudent to be cautious with the use of piperine-containing supplements in patients taking nevirapine.

1. Kasibhatta R, Naidu MUR. Influence of piperine on the pharmacokinetics of nevirapine under fasting conditions: a randomised, crossover, placebo-controlled study. *Drugs R D* (2007) 8, 383–91.

Pepper + NSAIDs

The interaction between piperine and diclofenac, indometacin and oxyphenbutazone is based on experimental evidence only.

Clinical evidence

No interactions found.

Experimental evidence

(a) Diclofenac

In a single-dose study in *rabbits,* the AUC of diclofenac 25 mg/kg was markedly reduced by about 80% when given with **Trikatu** 500 mg/kg. In this study, a suspension of a combination of diclofenac and **Trikatu** was used. The anti-inflammatory effects of diclofenac 25 mg/kg were also reduced by **Trikatu** 500 mg/kg when the combination was given to *rats*.[1] **Trikatu** is an Ayurvedic medicine that contains ginger, black pepper and long pepper in a 1:1:1 ratio.

(b) Indometacin

In a single-dose study in *rabbits,* **Trikatu** 500 mg/kg modestly increased the maximum plasma levels of indometacin 7 mg/kg by 29%, without affecting the AUC or other pharmacokinetic parameters.[2] **Trikatu** is an Ayurvedic medicine that contains ginger, black pepper and long pepper in a 1:1:1 ratio.

(c) Oxyphenbutazone

A single-dose study in *rats* and *mice* found that giving **piperine** 10 mg/kg at the same time as oxyphenbutazone 50 mg/kg modestly increased the AUC and maximum plasma levels of oxyphenbutazone by 28% and 36%, respectively. The anti-inflammatory activity of oxyphenbutazone in an *animal* model was increased.[3]

Mechanism

Unknown. It was expected that Trikatu might increase the bioavailability of diclofenac and indometacin. It is possible that there was an incompatibility between diclofenac and a constituent of Trikatu in the single suspension that resulted in the decreased absorption. The increased bioavailability of oxyphenbutazone with piperine was attributed to increased gastric absorption and inhibition of hepatic metabolism of oxyphenbutazone.[3]

Importance and management

The relevance of these disparate findings in *animal* studies to humans is unclear. Both ginger and pepper, which make up the Trikatu herbal formulation, are used extensively as food ingredients, and as there appear to be no reports of an interaction in humans, the clinical impact of the diclofenac and indometacin findings is probably minor. Similarly, while the modestly increased exposure to oxyphenbutazone with piperine cannot be directly extrapolated

to humans, increased levels of oxyphenbutazone of this magnitude are unlikely to be of much clinical relevance.

1. Lala LG, D'Mello PM, Naik SR. Pharmacokinetic and pharmacodynamic studies on interaction of "Trikatu" with diclofenac sodium. *J Ethnopharmacol* (2004) 91, 277–80.
2. Karan RS, Bhargava VK, Garg SK. Effect of Trikatu on the pharmacokinetic profile of indomethacin in rabbits. *Indian J Pharmacol* (1999) 31, 160–161.
3. Mujumdar AM, Dhukey JN, Deshmukh VK, Naik SR. Effect of piperine on bioavailability of oxyphenylbutazone in rats. *Indian Drugs* (1999) 36, 123–6.

Pepper + Oxytetracycline

The interaction between long pepper and oxytetracycline is based on experimental evidence only.

Clinical evidence

No interactions found.

Experimental evidence

In a study in *hens,* giving long pepper, equivalent to piperine 15 mg/kg, for 7 days, increased the AUC of a single 10-mg/kg oral dose of oxytetracycline given on day 8 by 27%. The elimination half life was also increased by 29%. The rate of absorption of oxytetracycline was not affected by the pepper. Note that oxytetracycline levels were determined by microbial assay.[1]

Mechanism

The authors of the study attributed the increased bioavailability to inhibition of microsomal metabolising enzymes by piperine in the long pepper.[1]

Importance and management

This *animal* study provides some evidence that pepper might increase exposure to oxytetracycline. While it is not possible to directly apply these data to the clinical situation, the level of increases seen would not be expected to be clinically important.

1. Singh M, Varshneya C, Telang RS, Srivastava AK. Alteration of pharmacokinetics of oxytetracycline following oral administration of *Piper longum* in hens. *J Vet Sci* (2005) 6, 197–200.

Pepper + Phenytoin

Piperine appears to increase the maximum levels and AUC of phenytoin, although the effect may be less in patients receiving long-term phenytoin.

Clinical evidence

Pepper or its active alkaloid **piperine** have been reported to enhance the oral bioavailability of phenytoin in three clinical studies. In one crossover study, 6 healthy subjects received a single 300-mg dose of phenytoin 30 minutes after a soup with or without **black pepper**, 1 g per 200 mL. The presence of pepper increased the AUC_{0-48}, $AUC_{0-\infty}$ and maximum plasma concentration of phenytoin by 49%, 133% and 13%, respectively, and the elimination half-life was increased from 22.48 to 49.71 hours. The pepper was added to the soup after preparation, and the piperine content of the soup was analysed and found to be 44 mg per 200 mL.[1]

In another crossover study, 5 healthy subjects received a single 300-mg dose of phenytoin orally alone, or after pretreatment with **piperine** 20 mg daily for 7 days. **Piperine** increased the AUC and maximum plasma level of phenytoin by 50% and 27%, respectively. The rate of absorption of phenytoin was higher when given after **piperine**.[2]

In a study in patients with epilepsy taking phenytoin 150 mg twice daily (10 patients) or 200 mg twice daily (10 patients), there was a minor increase in the AUC and maximum plasma concentrations of phenytoin when they were given a single 20-mg dose of **piperine** with their morning dose of phenytoin. The increase in AUC and maximum plasma concentrations of phenytoin were about 9% in the 150-mg phenytoin group, and 17% and 22%, respectively, in the 200-mg phenytoin group, and the elimination half-life was unchanged.[3]

Experimental evidence

A study in *mice* found that the rate and extent of absorption of a single 10-mg oral dose of phenytoin were increased by the concurrent administration of oral **piperine** 0.6 mg, and the rate of elimination was reduced. Similarly oral **piperine** reduced the rate of elimination of phenytoin after an intravenous dose. [1]

Mechanism

The increase in bioavailability of phenytoin caused by piperine may be the result of increased gastrointestinal absorption and decreased elimination. The effects of piperine in patients already taking phenytoin were far less marked than those in the healthy subjects given single doses of phenytoin. This might be because a single dose of piperine was given simultaneously with the phenytoin in the study in patients, rather than prior to the phenytoin. Alternatively, it could be that after long-term use of phenytoin, piperine has little effect on the elimination of phenytoin.

Importance and management

The increases in AUC of single-dose phenytoin in the studies in healthy subjects with pretreatment with pepper or piperine would be considered clinically relevant. However, more minor, clinically irrelevant increases were seen when a single dose of piperine was given simultaneously with a dose of phenytoin in patients on established phenytoin therapy. It is unclear if, had the administration schedules in the healthy subject studies been used in the patient study, a greater effect might have been seen. However, the widespread use of pepper in cooking and Ayurvedic medicine, and the lack of any reports of phenytoin toxicity, provide some reassurance that an interaction is unlikely. Nevertheless, bear the possibility of an interaction in mind if a patient who starts taking piperine-containing supplements presents with unexpectedly high phenytoin levels.

1. Velpandian T, Jasuja R, Bhardwaj RK, Jaiswal J, Gupta SK. Piperine in food: interference in the pharmacokinetics of phenytoin. *Eur J Drug Metab Pharmacokinet* (2001) 26, 241–8.
2. Bano G, Amla V, Raina RK, Zutschi U, Chopra CL. The effect of piperine on pharmacokinetics of phenytoin in healthy volunteers. *Planta Med* (1987) 53, 568–9.
3. Pattanaik S, Hota D, Prabhakar S, Kharbanda P, Pandhi P. Effect of piperine on the steady-state pharmacokinetics of phenytoin in patients with epilepsy. *Phytother Res* (2006) 20, 683–6.

Pepper + Propranolol

Piperine pretreatment increased the AUC of a single dose of propranolol by twofold in a study in healthy subjects.

Clinical evidence

In a study in 6 healthy subjects who received a single 40-mg dose of propranolol alone, and after taking **piperine** 20 mg daily for 7 days, the bioavailability of propranolol was significantly increased, with a twofold increase in both the AUC and maximum plasma concentration. However, the rate of elimination of propranolol was unaffected by **piperine**.[1]

Experimental evidence

No relevant data found.

Mechanism

Piperine is known to increase the absorption of some substances from the gastrointestinal tract, but the exact mechanism is unclear.

Importance and management

The effect of piperine on propranolol in this study was fairly large, but increases of this level are not usually considered clinically relevant with drugs such as propranolol that have marked variation in levels between individuals, and are titrated to effect. Also, this dose of piperine is easily achievable by the consumption of black pepper in the diet, and there do not appear to any reports of interactions. Moreover, because it involved only a single dose of propranolol, its findings might not be replicated in the clinical situation. Nevertheless, bear the possibility of an interaction in mind if a patient who starts taking piperine-containing supplements presents with an unexpected increase in adverse effects of propranolol, such as hypotension or bradycardia.

1. Bano G, Raina RK, Zutshi U, Bedi KL, Johri RK, Sharma SC. Effect of piperine on bioavailability and pharmacokinetics of propranolol and theophylline in healthy volunteers. *Eur J Clin Pharmacol* (1991) 41, 615–17.

Pepper + Rifampicin (Rifampin)

Piperine increased the AUC of rifampicin, but a small dose of Trikatu had no effect.

Clinical evidence

In a study, 14 patients with pulmonary tuberculosis were given a single 450-mg dose of rifampicin alone, repeated 5 days later with a 50-mg dose of **piperine**, extracted from *Piper nigrum*. The maximum plasma level and AUC of rifampicin were significantly increased by **piperine**, by 29% and 70%, respectively.[1]

In contrast, in a single-dose study in 6 healthy subjects, when rifampicin 450 mg was given with a small dose of **Trikatu** extract 50 mg the maximum level was slightly reduced by 18% and the time to maximum level was slightly delayed, but these changes were not statistically significant. **Trikatu** is an Ayurvedic medicine which contains ginger, black pepper and long pepper in a 1:1:1 ratio.[2] Although the preparation used was not analysed for **piperine** content, it is estimated that this could have been about 1 mg in the 50 mg of **Trikatu**, based on findings of other studies.

Experimental evidence

In a placebo-controlled study in *rabbits,* a single dose of **Trikatu** 500 mg/kg was given with rifampicin 24 mg/kg. The *rabbits* were then given the same dose of **Trikatu** once daily for 7 days, with a single 24-mg/kg dose of rifampicin on day 7. In the single-dose study, the maximum plasma concentration of rifampicin was reduced by just 15%. The AUC was also reduced to a similar extent, but this was not statistically significant. In the multiple-dose study, **Trikatu** did not significantly alter the pharmacokinetics of rifampicin. The quantity of **piperine** in the **Trikatu** was estimated to be 1 mg per 50 mg.[3]

Mechanism
Unknown.

Importance and management

These are conflicting results, which may be caused, in part, by the use of markedly different doses of piperine, as well as the use of the plant extract and pure piperine. The findings are difficult to interpret, but the widespread use of pepper in cooking and lack of reports of interactions with rifampicin give some reassurance that any interaction is unlikely to be clinically important.

1. Zutshi RK, Singh R, Zutshi U, Johri RK, Atal CK. Influence of piperine on rifampicin blood levels in patients of pulmonary tuberculosis. *J Assoc Physicians India* (1984) 33, 223–4.
2. Dahanukar SA, Kapadia AB, Karandikar SM. Influence of Trikatu on rifampicin bioavailability. *Indian Drugs* (1982) 12, 271–3.
3. Karan RS, Bhargava VK, Garg SK. Effect of trikatu, an Ayurvedic prescription, on the pharmacokinetic profile of rifampicin in rabbits. *J Ethnopharmacol* (1999) 64, 259–64.

P

P

Pepper + Theophylline

Piperine almost doubled the AUC of a single dose of theophylline.

Clinical evidence

In a study in 6 healthy subjects who received a single 150-mg dose of theophylline alone, and after taking **piperine** 20 mg daily for 7 days, the bioavailability of theophylline was significantly increased, with an increase in the AUC and maximum plasma concentration of 96% and 61%, respectively. The elimination half-life of theophylline was extended from about 6.6 to 10.8 hours.[1] Although not specifically stated, it is assumed that this study used a standard-release theophylline preparation.

Experimental evidence

No relevant data found.

Mechanism

Piperine is known to increase the absorption of some substances from the gastrointestinal tract, but the exact mechanism is unclear. However, theophylline already has high oral bioavailability. The finding of an increased elimination half-life suggests a mechanism of reduced metabolism or clearance. Piperine is known to inhibit some of the cytochrome P450 isoenzymes, although there do not appear to be any data specifically on CYP1A2, which is mainly involved in the metabolism of theophylline.

Importance and management

This study appears to show a marked increase in exposure to single-dose theophylline when given with a dose of piperine that might easily be achieved with piperine-containing supplements or even from consuming black pepper. How the findings relate to the use of multiple-dose theophylline or sustained-release formulations is also unknown. The widespread use of pepper in cooking and lack of reports of interactions with theophylline gives some reassurance that any interaction is unlikely to be clinically important. Nevertheless, until more it known, it would be prudent to be cautious with the use of piperine-containing supplements in patients taking theophylline.

1. Bano G, Raina RK, Zutshi U, Bedi KL, Johri RK, Sharma SC. Effect of piperine on bioavailability and pharmacokinetics of propranolol and theophylline in healthy volunteers. *Eur J Clin Pharmacol* (1991) 41, 615–17.

Pepper + Thyroid and Antithyroid drugs

The interaction between piperine and thyroid drugs, such as levothyroxine, or antithyroid drugs, such as carbimazole, is based on experimental evidence only.

Clinical evidence

No interactions found.

Experimental evidence

Piperine was evaluated for its thyroid-hormone and glucose-regulatory effects in a study in *mice*. Oral **piperine** 2.5 mg/kg daily for 15 days lowered the serum levels of the thyroid hormones thyroxine (T4) and triiodothyronine (T3) as well as glucose concentrations. The decreases were comparable to that of the antithyroid drug, **propylthiouracil**. A 10-fold lower dose of **piperine** (0.25 mg/kg) had little effect.[1]

Mechanism

Not known. Piperine appears to have antithyroid activity.

Importance and management

This preclinical study provides some evidence that piperine, the main active constituent of pepper, might have antithyroid effects. Theoretically this may have additive effects with other antithyroid drugs, such as propylthiouracil or **carbimazole**, and could antagonise the effects of **levothyroxine**. It is not possible to directly apply these data to the clinical situation, and how the doses used relate to usual human consumption of pepper or the dose of piperine in supplements is unclear. Note that there appears to be no evidence of pepper or piperine being a problem in patients with thyroid disorders. This study does not provide sufficient evidence to recommend caution in patients requiring thyroid supplementation. Bear in mind the possibility of an interaction in a patient requiring an increase in levothyroxine dose after starting piperine-containing supplements.

1. Panda S, Kar A. Piperine lowers the serum concentrations of thyroid hormones, glucose and hepatic 5'D activity in adult male mice. *Horm Metab Res* (2003) 35, 523–6.

Pepper + Verapamil

The interaction between piperine and verapamil is based on experimental evidence only.

Evidence, mechanism, importance and management

In an *in vitro* study, the CYP3A4-mediated metabolism of verapamil to norverapamil was inhibited by the presence of **piperine**, but that the CYP2C-mediated metabolism of verapamil was not significantly altered by **piperine**.[1] It is difficult to apply this finding to human intake of pepper. However, a clinical study is needed to assess whether ingestion of pepper or **piperine**-containing supplements actually alters verapamil levels. Until more is known, bear this finding in mind in the event of unexpected outcomes in patients taking verapamil and **piperine**-containing supplements.

1. Bhardwaj RK, Glaeser H, Becquemont L, Klotz U, Gupta SK, Fromm MF. Piperine, a major constituent of black pepper, inhibits human P-glycoprotein and CYP3A4. *J Pharmacol Exp Ther* (2002) 302, 645–50.

Peppermint

Mentha × piperita L. (Lamiaceae)

Synonym(s) and related species

Black mint (*Mentha piperita* Sole), White mint (*Mentha piperita* Sole).

Note that *Mentha × piperita* L. is a hybrid between *Mentha spicata* L. and *Mentha viridis* L.

Pharmacopoeias

Concentrated Peppermint Emulsion (*BP 2012*); Gastro-resistant Peppermint Oil Capsules (*BP 2012*); Peppermint (*USP35–NF30 S1*); Peppermint Leaf (*BP 2012, PhEur 7.5*); Peppermint Leaf Dry Extract (*BP 2012, PhEur 7.5*); Peppermint Oil (*BP 2012, PhEur 7.5, USP35–NF30 S1*); Peppermint Spirit (*BP 2012, USP35–NF30 S1*); Peppermint Water (*USP35–NF30 S1*).

Constituents

Essential oils, including **menthol**, menthone, menthyl acetate as the main components, and cineole, isomenthone, neomenthol, piperitone, pulegone and limonene. A maximum level of pulegone is permitted, since this is toxic, see pennyroyal, page 370. Peppermint also contains **flavonoids** such as rutin, menthoside, luteolin and phenolic acids and lactones.

Use and indications

Peppermint leaf and distilled oil have carminative, antispasmodic, diaphoretic and antiseptic properties and are mainly used to relieve symptoms of indigestion. Peppermint is commonly used as a flavouring ingredient in food, cosmetics and medicines.

Pharmacokinetics

Peppermint tea was found to inhibit the activity of the cytochrome P450 subfamily CYP2E by up to 40% in a study in *rats* pretreated for 4 weeks with the tea.[1] In an *in vitro* study, peppermint oil 20 to 500 micrograms/mL was found to moderately inhibit the activity of the cytochrome P450 isoenzymes CYP2C8, CYP2C9, CYP2C19, and CYP2D6.[2]

Both these studies found that there was no significant inhibition of CYP3A4 by peppermint,[1,2] but see also calcium-channel blockers, page 380 and ciclosporin, page 381. Peppermint oil does not appear to have any clinically relevant effects on the cytochrome P450 isoenzyme CYP1A2, see caffeine, page 380. For information on the pharmacokinetics of individual flavonoids present in peppermint, see under flavonoids, page 213.

Interactions overview

Food and antacids may compromise the enteric coating of some commercially available peppermint oil capsules. Peppermint oil appears to increase ciclosporin and felodipine levels and topically, in high doses, it may also enhance the skin penetration of some topical medicines. Peppermint tea contains digoxin-like constituents, which could, in theory, have additive effects with digoxin or digitoxin, or interfere with their assays, but the clinical relevance of this is unclear. It may also impair iron absorption, and is unlikely to have a significant effect on the pharmacokinetics of caffeine.

For information on the interactions of individual flavonoids present in peppermint, see under flavonoids, page 213.

Interactions monographs

- Antacids, page 380
- Caffeine, page 380
- Calcium-channel blockers, page 380
- Ciclosporin, page 381
- Digitalis glycosides, page 381
- Food, page 381
- Herbal medicines, page 381
- Iron compounds, page 381
- Miscellaneous, page 382

1. Maliakal PP, Wanwimolruk S. Effect of herbal teas on hepatic drug metabolizing enzymes in rats. *J Pharm Pharmacol* (2001) 53, 1323–9.
2. Unger M, Frank A. Simultaneous determination of the inhibitory potency of herbal extracts on the activity of six major cytochrome P450 enzymes using liquid chromatography/mass spectrometry and automated online extraction. *Rapid Commun Mass Spectrom* (2004) 18, 2273–81.

Peppermint + Antacids

Antacids may compromise the enteric coating of some commercially available peppermint oil capsules. H_2-receptor antagonists and proton pump inhibitors may interact similarly.

Evidence, mechanism, importance and management

The manufacturers of some enteric-coated peppermint oil preparations advise that indigestion remedies (antacids) should not be taken at the same time as peppermint oil.[1] This is presumably because a marked rise in pH caused by antacids might cause premature dissolution of the enteric coating and release of the peppermint oil in the stomach, which increases the risk of heartburn with the preparation. Separation of administration by a couple of hours usually avoids this type of interaction with antacids. Some monographs extend this advice to H_2-receptor antagonists and proton pump inhibitors and suggest that these drugs should be avoided.

1. Colpermin (Peppermint oil). McNeil Ltd. UK Summary of product characteristics, May 2008.

Peppermint + Caffeine

Peppermint oil does not appear to affect the metabolism of caffeine but might slightly delay its absorption.

Clinical evidence

In a crossover study in 11 healthy women, a single 100-mg capsule of menthol (a major constituent of peppermint oil) taken with decaffeinated coffee, to which 200 mg of caffeine had been added, had no effect on caffeine pharmacokinetics except for an increase in time to maximum caffeine concentration of about 30 minutes. The maximum decrease in heart rate seen with caffeine was less in the presence of menthol (about 4 bpm difference), but menthol had no effect on the small changes in blood pressure seen with caffeine.[1]

Experimental evidence

One in vitro[2] study and one *animal* study[3] found that peppermint oil or tea inhibited the cytochrome P450 isoenzyme CYP1A2.

Mechanism

Experimental evidence[2,3] suggests that peppermint might inhibit cytochrome P450 isoenzyme CYP1A2, for which caffeine is a probe substrate the clinical evidence with menthol (a major constituent of peppermint oil) found that caffeine metabolism was not altered. Menthol slightly delayed the absorption of caffeine.

Importance and management

The clinical evidence suggests that peppermint oil might not have clinically relevant effects on the metabolism of substrates of CYP1A2, which would be in keeping with the fact that no such interactions appear to have been reported. Peppermint oil might slightly delay the absorption of caffeine, and presumably other drugs, but the delay of 30 minutes suggests that this is usually unlikely to be clinically relevant.

1. Gelal A, Guven H, Balkan D, Artok L, Benowitz NL. Influence of menthol on caffeine disposition and pharmacodynamics in healthy female volunteers. *Eur J Clin Pharmacol* (2003) 59, 417–22.
2. Unger M, Frank A. Simultaneous determination of the inhibitory potency of herbal extracts on the activity of six major cytochrome P450 enzymes using liquid chromatography/mass spectrometry and automated online extraction. *Rapid Commun Mass Spectrom* (2004) 18, 2273–81.
3. Maliakal PP, Wanwimolruk S. Effect of herbal teas on hepatic drug metabolizing enzymes in rats. *J Pharm Pharmacol* (2001) 53, 1323–9.

Peppermint + Calcium-channel blockers

Peppermint oil capsules appear to increase the bioavailability of felodipine, and therefore may increase the incidence of adverse effects such as headache, light-headedness and flushing. *In vitro* experiments suggests peppermint oil is a moderate inhibitor of nifedipine metabolism.

Clinical evidence

In a randomised, single-dose study in 12 healthy subjects[1] peppermint oil capsules 600 mg increased the AUC and maximum serum levels of extended-release **felodipine** 10 mg by about 55% and 40%, respectively, without affecting the half-life. The AUC and maximum serum levels of dehydrofelodipine, the metabolite of **felodipine**, were increased by 37% and 25%, respectively.[1] In a randomised study, 10 healthy subjects were given a single 10-mg dose of extended-release felodipine with either menthol 100 mg or placebo. Menthol did not affect the pharmacokinetics of felodipine, and, in the 8 subjects assessed, there were no differences in heart rate or blood pressure between menthol and placebo.[2]

Experimental evidence

Peppermint oil and two of its components, menthol and menthyl acetate, were found to be moderate reversible inhibitors of **nifedipine** metabolism in *in vitro* investigations in human liver microsomes.[1]

Mechanism

Unknown. Although it has been suggested that menthol may account for a substantial portion of the interactions reported for peppermint oil, the study using menthol found no interaction with felodipine. Felodipine undergoes at least two sequential metabolic steps mediated by CYP3A4 and the authors of one study suggested that peppermint may selectively inhibit the secondary step as opposed to the primary step but further study is needed.[1] In contrast, two other *in vitro* studies found that peppermint did not affect CYP3A4, see Pharmacokinetics, page 379.

Importance and management

The clinical study suggests that peppermint oil may modestly increase the bioavailability of felodipine, which might therefore increase the incidence of adverse effects such as headache, light-headedness and flushing. Further study is needed, but until then, it would be prudent to be aware of this possibility in any patient taking felodipine if they are given oral peppermint oil. It is possible that not all calcium-channel blockers will be affected, since some, unlike felodipine, are highly bioavailable. This interaction is similar to that of grapefruit juice, which affects felodipine and nisoldipine (low oral bioavailability), but only minimally affects amlodipine and diltiazem (high oral bioavailability).

The data would only be expected to have relevance to therapeutic doses of oils, and not to herbal teas, or small amounts in foods, where no clinically relevant interaction is anticipated. Similarly, menthol does not appear to interact with felodipine and therefore seems unlikely to interact with other calcium-channel blockers.

1. Dresser GK, Wacher V, Wong S, Wong HT, Bailey DG. Evaluation of peppermint oil and ascorbyl palmitate as inhibitors of cytochrome P4503A4 activity in vitro and in vivo. *Clin Pharmacol Ther* (2002) 72, 247–55.
2. Gelal A, Balkan D, Ozzeybek D, Kaplan YC, Gurler S, Guven H, Benowitz NL. Effect of menthol on the pharmacokinetics and pharmacodynamics of felodipine in healthy subjects. *Eur J Clin Pharmacol* (2005) 60, 785–90.

Peppermint + Ciclosporin

The interaction between peppermint oil and ciclosporin is based on experimental evidence only.

Clinical evidence

No interactions found.

Experimental evidence

In a single-dose study in *rats,* peppermint oil 100 mg/kg mixed with ciclosporin (*Sandimmune* formulation) almost tripled the AUC and maximum serum levels of ciclosporin 25 mg/kg.[1]

In vitro studies also found that peppermint oil 50 micrograms/mL inhibits ciclosporin metabolism in *rat* liver microsomes by up to 85%.[1]

Mechanism

Unclear. The authors rule out P-glycoprotein inhibition as a potential mode of action. They say that inhibition of the cytochrome P450 subfamily CYP3A may have a role, and enhanced gastrointestinal permeability may also be a factor.

Importance and management

Although clinical data is lacking, the experimental study demonstrates that peppermint oil significantly enhances the oral bioavailability of ciclosporin in *rats*. Further study is needed to see if a similar effect occurs in humans. Until then, it may be prudent to be aware of the possibility that peppermint oil might increase ciclosporin levels. If patients taking ciclosporin are given peppermint oil it may be prudent to monitor ciclosporin levels within a few weeks of starting concurrent use, if this is not already planned.

The data would only have relevance to therapeutic doses of oils, and not to herbal teas, or small amounts in foods, which would not be expected to interact to a clinically relevant extent.

1. Wacher VJ, Wong S, Wong HT. Peppermint oil enhances cyclosporine oral bioavailability in rats: Comparison with d-α-tocopheryl poly(ethylene glycol 1000) succinate (TPGS) and ketoconazole. *J Pharm Sci* (2002) 91, 77–90.

Peppermint + Digitalis glycosides

Many herbal medicines contain cardiac glycosides, which could in theory have additive effects with digoxin or digitoxin, or interfere with their assays. However, there appear to be few such interactions reported.

Evidence, mechanism, importance and management

In an *in vitro* study, 46 commercially packaged herb teas and 78 teas prepared from herbs were assayed for digoxin-like factors by their cross-reactivity with digoxin antibody, and these values were used to give approximate equivalent daily doses of digoxin. Peppermint was found to contain greater than 30 micrograms of digoxin equivalents per cup and was suggested that this would provide a therapeutic daily dose of digoxin if 5 cups of peppermint tea a day were drunk.[1] However, note that some common teas sampled in this study (e.g. English Breakfast, Earl Grey) contained over 20 micrograms of digoxin equivalents per cup. Given that these teas are commonly consumed in the UK and an interaction with digoxin has not been reported the interpretation of the findings of this study is unclear.

Theoretical interactions with herbal medicines are not always translated into practice. On the basis of this one study, no special precautions would be expected to be necessary in patients taking digoxin who drink peppermint tea.

1. Longerich L, Johnson E, Gault MH. Digoxin-like factors in herbal teas. *Clin Invest Med* (1993) 16, 210–218.

Peppermint + Food

Food may compromise the enteric coating of some commercially available peppermint oil capsules.

Evidence, mechanism, importance and management

The manufacturers of some enteric-coated peppermint oil preparations advise that they should not be taken immediately after food.[1,2] This is presumably because presence of food in the stomach will delay gastric emptying and might cause premature dissolution of the enteric coating and release of the peppermint oil before it reaches the intestine. This may result in adverse effects, such as indigestion.

1. Colpermin (Peppermint oil). McNeil Ltd. UK Summary of product characteristics, May 2008.
2. Mintec (Peppermint oil). Shire Pharmaceuticals Ltd. UK Summary of product characteristics, March 2001.

Peppermint + Herbal medicines

No interactions found.

Peppermint + Iron compounds

Peppermint tea appears to reduce iron absorption similarly to conventional tea.

Clinical evidence

In a study in 9 healthy subjects a 275 mL serving of peppermint tea reduced the absorption of iron from a 50 g bread roll by about 85%. The tea was prepared by adding 300 mL of boiling water to 3 g of the herb tea, then infusing for 10 minutes before straining and serving. In this study, the inhibitory effect of peppermint tea on iron absorption was equivalent to that of black tea (Assam tea, *Camellia sinensis* L.), which is known to inhibit iron absorption, see Tea + Iron compounds, page 467.[1]

Experimental evidence

Peppermint leaf tea 2.2 g/kg daily was found to inhibit iron absorption in *rats*.[2] Serum iron and ferritin levels were reduced by about 20%. Conversely, a tea prepared from *Mentha spicata* did not inhibit iron absorption to a significant extent and so the authors suggested that menthol, a major constituent of peppermint, but not *Mentha spicata*, is involved.

Mechanism

The polyphenols in peppermint tea may bind to iron in the gastrointestinal tract and reduce its absorption.

Importance and management

The clinical impact of this interaction between peppermint tea and iron is not fully known, but be aware that some herbal teas such as peppermint reduce iron absorption similarly to conventional tea. See Tea + Iron compounds, page 467. Note that tea and coffee are not generally considered to be suitable drinks for babies and children, because of their effects on iron absorption.

1. Hurrell RF, Reddy M, Cook JD. Inhibition of non-haem iron absorption in man by polyphenolic-containing beverages. *Br J Nutr* (1999) 81, 289–95.
2. Akdogan M, Gultekin F, Yontem M. Effect of *Mentha piperita* (Labiatae) and *Mentha spicata* (Labiatae) on iron absorption in rats. *Toxicol Ind Health* (2004) 20, 119–22.

P

Peppermint + Miscellaneous

The information regarding the use of topical peppermint oil preparations is based on experimental evidence only.

Evidence, mechanism, importance and management

Preliminary *in vitro* experiments using human skin samples[1] have found that low dose peppermint oil (0.1% and 1%) on the skin surface can significantly reduce the amount of topical **benzoic acid** penetrating the dermal barrier. Conversely, at higher concentrations (5%), peppermint oil decreased the integrity of the dermal barrier.[1] In another study, peppermint oil enhanced the **fluorouracil** permeation across *rat* skin.[2]

These experimental studies suggest that topical peppermint oil might increase the absorption of other topical drugs; however, there is currently insufficient evidence to make any clinical recommendations.

1. Nielsen JB. Natural oils affect the human skin integrity and the percutaneous penetration of benzoic acid dose-dependently. *Basic Clin Pharmacol Toxicol* (2006) 98, 575–81.
2. Abdullah D, Ping QN, Liu GJ. Enhancing effect of essential oils on the penetration of 5-fluorouracil through rat skin. *Yao Xue Xue Bao* (1996) 31, 214–21.

Plantain

Plantago major L. (Plantaginaceae)

Synonym(s) and related species

Broad-leaf plantain, Common plantain, Greater plantain, Not to be confused with Ribwort plantain, page 408 (*Plantago lanceolata*), Psyllium (*Plantago afra* (*P. psyllium*) or *P. indica* (*P. arenaria*), or Ispaghula, page 306 (*Plantain ovata*).

Constituents

Plantain leaves contain **flavonoids** including baicalein, scutellarein, plantagoside, hispidulin, luteolin and apigenin glycosides, and others; **iridoids** including catalpol, aucubin, plantarenaloside and others; **caffeic acid derivatives** and other organic acids; **triterpenes** such as ursolic and oleanolic acids; fatty acids; traces of the alkaloid boschniakine and its derivatives; **tannins** and **mucilage**.

Use and indications

Plantain is traditionally used for its diuretic, antihaemorrhagic and anti-inflammatory properties for the treatment of a wide range of complaints including haemorrhage, haemorrhoids and cystitis.

Pharmacokinetics

No relevant pharmacokinetic data found. For general information on the pharmacokinetics of flavonoids, see under flavonoids, page 213.

Interactions overview

No interactions with plantain found. An *in vitro* study found that plantain had no effect on digoxin assays. For information on the interactions of individual flavonoids present in plantain, see under flavonoids, page 213.

Interactions monographs

- Food, page 384
- Herbal medicines, page 384
- Laboratory tests, page 384

P

Plantain + Food

No interactions found.

Plantain + Herbal medicines

No interactions found.

Plantain + Laboratory tests

The information regarding the use of plantain and digoxin assays is based on experimental evidence only.

Clinical evidence, mechanism, importance and management

In an *in vitro* study, plantain extract from capsules, liquid extract, or dry leaf did not affect the results of digoxin assays when using fluorescence polarization immunoassay or microparticle enzyme immunoassay.[1] It would therefore seem unlikely that the therapeutic drug monitoring of digoxin would be affected by patients taking plantain. Note that contamination of plantain with *Digitalis lanata* has been reported.[2]

1. Dasgupta A, Davis B, Wells A. Effect of plantain on therapeutic drug monitoring of digoxin and thirteen other common drugs. *Ann Clin Biochem* (2006) 43, 223–5.
2. Slifman NR, Obermeyer WR, Aloi BK, Musser SM, Correll WA, Cichowicz SM, Betz JM, Love LA. Contamination of botanical dietary supplements by Digitalis lanata. *N Engl J Med* (1998) 339, 806–11.

Pleurisy root

Asclepias tuberosa L. (Asclepiadaceae)

Synonym(s) and related species

Butterfly milkweed, Butterfly weed, Chieger flower, Chigger flower, Indian paintbrush, Orange milkweed.

Constituents

Little is known about the chemistry of pleurisy root, but the major constituents are steroidal glycosides of the cardenolide type, based on the aglycones ikemagenin, lineolon, pleurogenin, uzarigenin, coroglaucigenin and corotoxigenin. Other glycosides present include ascandroside, thiazolidinone derivatives, Δ^5-calotropin and its derivatives, and many others.

Use and indications

Pleurisy root has traditionally been used for respiratory tract disorders including bronchitis, pneumonitis, influenza, and pleurisy. It is a constituent of many herbal cough preparations due to its expectorant effects.

Pharmacokinetics

No relevant pharmacokinetic data found.

Interactions overview

Pleurisy root contains digoxin-like constituents, which could, in theory, have additive effects with digoxin or digitoxin, or interfere with their assays, but the clinical relevance of this is unclear.

Interactions monographs

- Digitalis glycosides, page 386
- Food, page 386
- Herbal medicines, page 386

Pleurisy root + Digitalis glycosides

Many herbal medicines contain cardiac glycosides, which could, in theory, have additive effects with digoxin or digitoxin, or interfere with their assays. However, there appear to be few such interactions reported.

Evidence, mechanism, importance and management

In an *in vitro* study, 46 commercially packaged herb teas and 78 teas prepared from herbs were assayed for digoxin-like factors by their cross-reactivity with digoxin antibody, and these values were used to give approximate equivalent daily doses of digoxin. Pleurisy root was found to contain greater than 30 micrograms of digoxin equivalents per cup and it was suggested that this would provide a therapeutic daily dose of digoxin if 5 cups of pleurisy root tea a day were drunk.[1] However, note that some common teas sampled in this study (e.g. English Breakfast, Earl Grey) contained over 20 micrograms of digoxin equivalents per cup. Given that these teas are commonly consumed in the UK, and an interaction with digoxin has not been reported, the interpretation of the findings of this study is unclear.

Theoretical interactions with herbal medicines are not always translated into practice. On the basis of this one study, no special precautions would be expected to be necessary in patients taking digoxin who drink pleurisy root tea.

1. Longerich L, Johnson E, Gault MH. Digoxin-like factors in herbal teas. *Clin Invest Med* (1993) 16, 210–218.

Pleurisy root + Food

No interactions found.

Pleurisy root + Herbal medicines

No interactions found.

Policicosanol

Asclepias tuberosa L. (Asclepiadaceae)

Types, sources and related compounds

Octacosanol.

Constituents

Policicosanol consists of a mixture of alcohols with octacosanol being the major component. Triacontanol and hexacosanol are also present but in lesser amounts.

Use and indications

Policicosanol is isolated from sugar cane wax and because of its lipid lowering and antiplatelet properties, is mainly used for cardiovascular disorders. It is also being investigated for possible use in the treatment of Parkinson's disease, and for enhancing athletic performance.

Pharmacokinetics

Policicosanol did not alter the metabolism of phenazone (antipyrine) in *dogs*.[1] Phenazone is used as a probe drug to assess the effects of other drugs on hepatic enzyme induction and inhibition. This finding therefore suggests that policicosanol is unlikely to induce or inhibit the metabolism of other drugs that are substrates of hepatic enzymes.

Interactions overview

Policicosanol has antiplatelet effects, which may be additive with other antiplatelet drugs. Policicosanol does not affect the pharmacokinetics of warfarin; however its antiplatelet effects could theoretically increase the risk of bleeding in patients taking anticoagulants. Policicosanol may also enhance the blood pressure-lowering effects of some antihypertensives.

Interactions monographs

- Antiplatelet drugs, page 388
- Beta blockers, page 388
- Food, page 388
- Herbal medicines, page 388
- Nifedipine, page 388
- Phenazone (Antipyrine), page 388
- Sodium nitroprusside, page 389
- Warfarin and related drugs, page 389

1. Pérez-Souto N, Acosta PC, Mederos CM, Reyes JL, Martınez O. Efecto del ateromixol (PPG) sobre la farmacocinetica de la antipirina. *Rev Cenic Cien Biol* (1991) 22, 77–8.

P

Policosanol + Antiplatelet drugs

Policosanol has antiplatelet effects, which may be additive with those of other antiplatelet drugs.

Clinical evidence

In a randomised study, four groups, each containing 10 or 11 subjects, were given placebo, policosanol 20 mg daily, **aspirin** 100 mg daily, or both drugs together, for 7 days. Adrenaline-induced platelet aggregation was reduced in the group given **aspirin** and policosanol by about 35% more than in the group given **aspirin** alone: the effects of aspirin and policosanol were approximately additive. Furthermore, collagen-induced platelet aggregation was reduced in the group given **aspirin** and policosanol by about 10% more than in the group given **aspirin** alone. One patient taking both drugs suffered from bleeding gums. There was no significant effect on coagulation time.[1] A 3-year study, primarily designed to assess the safety and efficacy of policosanol in patients taking beta blockers, included 32 patients taking antiplatelet drugs (mainly **aspirin**). No adverse effects related to bleeding were reported.[2]

Experimental evidence

No relevant data found.

Mechanism

Additive antiplatelet effects.

Importance and management

The concurrent use of two conventional antiplatelet drugs is not uncommon, and so concurrent use of policosanol and aspirin need not be avoided. However, because platelet aggregation was reduced significantly, and a bleeding event was experienced, caution is perhaps warranted when taking policosanol supplements with aspirin or any other antiplatelet drug.

1. Arruzazabala ML, Valdés S, Más R, Carbajal D, Fernández L. Comparative study of policosanol, aspirin and the combination therapy policosanol-aspirin on platelet aggregation in healthy volunteers. *Pharmacol Res* (1997) 36, 293–7.
2. Castaño G, Mas R, Gámez R, Fernández J, Illnait J, Fernández L, Mendoza S, Mesa M, Gutiérrez JA, López E. Concomitant use of policosanol and β-blockers in older patients. *Int J Clin Pharmacol Res* (2004) 24, 65–77.

Policosanol + Beta blockers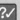

Policosanol appears to increase the blood pressure-lowering effects of beta blockers.

Clinical evidence

In a randomised study in patients aged 60 to 80 years taking beta blockers, the addition of policosanol 5 mg tablets daily (titrated to a dose of 2 to 4 tablets) reduced the average blood pressure from 141/83 mmHg to 131/81 mmHg after one year, and to 126/79 mmHg after 3 years. The efficacy of policosanol was not reduced and adverse effects were actually slightly lower in the policosanol group.[1]

Experimental evidence

In a study in hypertensive *rats,* a single 200-mg/kg oral dose of policosanol enhanced the blood pressure-lowering effects of intravenous and oral **propranolol** without increasing the reduction in heart rate induced by **propranolol**.[2]

Mechanism

Policosanol is thought to reduce vascular resistance.

Importance and management

Policosanol increased the blood pressure-lowering effects of beta blockers and the clinical study suggests that the effect is gradual and

beneficial. Furthermore, adverse effects related to hypotension were not reported. It therefore appears that, as with other conventional antihypertensives policosanol may increase the effects of the beta blockers and so some caution is warranted, but no adverse effects such as first-dose hypotension would be expected.

1. Castaño G, Mas R, Gámez R, Fernández J, Illnait J, Fernández L, Mendoza S, Mesa M, Gutiérrez JA, López E. Concomitant use of policosanol and β-blockers in older patients. *Int J Clin Pharmacol Res* (2004) 24, 65–77.
2. Molina Cuevas V, Arruzazabala ML, Carbajal Quintana D, Mas Ferreiro R, Valdes Garcia S. Effect of policosanol on arterial blood pressure in rats. Study of the pharmacological interaction with nifedipine and propranolol. *Arch Med Res* (1998) 29, 21–4.

Policosanol + Food

No interactions found.

Policosanol + Herbal medicines

No interactions found.

Policosanol + Nifedipine

Policosanol does not appear to affect the blood pressure-lowering effects of nifedipine.

Clinical evidence

A 3-year study, primarily designed to assess the safety and efficacy of policosanol in patients taking beta blockers, included 28 patients taking calcium-channel blockers (unnamed). No adverse effects related to hypotension were reported.[1]

Experimental evidence

In a study in hypertensive *rats,* a single 200-mg/kg oral dose of policosanol did not affect the blood pressure-lowering effects of intravenous nifedipine 300 micrograms/kg given 2 hours later.[2]

Mechanism

Policosanol is thought to reduce vascular resistance.

Importance and management

There appears to be no reason to avoid taking policosanol supplements with nifedipine. However, additive blood pressure-lowering effects seem possible, see, beta blockers, above.

1. Castaño G, Mas R, Gámez R, Fernández J, Illnait J, Fernández L, Mendoza S, Mesa M, Gutiérrez JA, López E. Concomitant use of policosanol and β-blockers in older patients. *Int J Clin Pharmacol Res* (2004) 24, 65–77.
2. Molina Cuevas V, Arruzazabala ML, Carbajal Quintana D, Mas Ferreiro R, Valdes Garcia S. Effect of policosanol on arterial blood pressure in rats. Study of the pharmacological interaction with nifedipine and propranolol. *Arch Med Res* (1998) 29, 21–4.

Policosanol + Phenazone (Antipyrine)

The information regarding the use of policosanol with phenazone (antipyrine) is based on experimental evidence only.

Clinical evidence

No interactions found.

Experimental evidence

A study in *dogs* found that the pharmacokinetics of an intravenous dose of phenazone 10 mg/kg were not affected by oral treatment with policosanol, 25 mg/kg daily for 21 days.[1]

Mechanism

No mechanism expected.

Importance and management

On the basis of the results from this *animal* study, there appears to be no reason to avoid taking policosanol supplements with phenazone.

1. Pérez-Souto N, Acosta PC, Mederos CM, Reyes JL, Martrnez O. Efecto del ateromixol (PPG) sobre la farmacocinetica de la antipirina. *Rev Cenic Cien Biol* (1991) 22, 77–8.

Policosanol + Sodium nitroprusside

The interaction between policosanol and sodium nitroprusside is based on experimental evidence only.

Clinical evidence

No interactions found.

Experimental evidence

A study found that the antiplatelet and hypotensive effect of sodium nitroprusside was greater in *rats* that had been pre-treated with a single 200-mg/kg oral dose of policosanol, than in *animals* that had not received policosanol.[1]

Mechanism

Both policosanol and sodium nitroprusside have antiplatelet effects. These appear to be additive. Policosanol reduces vascular resistance and has been shown to enhance the blood pressure-lowering effects of other antihypertensives.

Importance and management

The clinical significance of this finding is unclear, but bear it in mind in case of an unexpected response to treatment.

1. Arruzazabala ML, Carbajal D, Más R, Valdés S, Molina V. Pharmacological interaction between policosanol and nitroprusside in rats. *J Med Food* (2001) 4, 67–70.

Policosanol + Warfarin and related drugs

Echinacea does not appear to affect the pharmacokinetics or pharmacodynamics of warfarin; however, policosanol has antiplatelet effects which could theoretically increase the risk of bleeding in patients taking anticoagulants.

Clinical evidence

In a randomised study, 12 healthy subjects were given a single 25-mg dose of warfarin before and after taking policosanol 10 mg twice daily for 14 days; policosanol was continued for a further 7 days during the assessment of warfarin pharmacokinetics. Policosanol did not affect the pharmacokinetics of *R*- or *S*-warfarin and, in the 11 subjects assessed, there was no change in the INR in response to warfarin in the presence of policosanol.[1]

Experimental evidence

Policosanol 200 mg/kg did not prolong the bleeding time of **warfarin** 200 micrograms/kg given for 3 days in *rats*.[2]

Mechanism

Policosanol does not appear to affect the metabolism of warfarin.

Importance and management

Evidence for an interaction between policosanol and warfarin appears to be limited to this one well-designed study, which suggests that policosanol does not interact with warfarin. Although other coumarins do not appear to have been studied, they are metabolised similarly to warfarin, and therefore would also seem unlikely to interact with policosanol. Although a dose adjustment seems unlikely to be necessary if policosanol is given with a coumarin, policosanol has antiplatelet properties and increased bleeding has been reported when it was given with aspirin, page 388, so bear this in mind if excessive bleeding is seen in a patient taking any **anticoagulant** with policosanol.

1. Abdul MIM, Jiang X, Williams KM, Day RO, Roufogalis BD, Liauw WS, Xu H, Matthias A, Lehmann RP, McLachlan AJ. Pharmacokinetic and pharmacodynamic interactions of echinacea and policosanol with warfarin in healthy subjects. *Br J Clin Pharmacol* (2010) 69, 508–15.
2. Carbajal D, Arruzazabala ML, Valdés S, Más R. Interaction policosanol-warfarin on bleeding time and thrombosis in rats. *Pharmacol Res* (1998) 38, 89–91.

P

Prickly ash

Zanthoxylum americanum Mill., *Zanthoxylum clava-herculis* L. (Rutaceae)

Synonym(s) and related species

Toothache tree, Xanthoxylum, Yellow wood, Zanthoxylum.

Constituents

The main constituents of prickly ash bark include the isoquinoline alkaloids magnoflorine, laurifoline, nitidine, chelerythrine, tambetarine and candicine. Various natural coumarins, tannins, lignans including sesamin and asarinin, resins, and volatile oil are also present.

Use and indications

Prickly ash is traditionally used for cramps and Raynaud's syndrome. The bark is mainly used as an antirheumatic, analgesic, and carminative, and is believed to possess cardioprotective effects. It is also used to treat toothache and fevers, and is used as a flavouring agent in food and drink. It is also used as a fish poison. Because of doubts about the toxicity of the alkaloids it contains (which are said to have hypotensive, anti-inflammatory and neuromuscular blocking activity), some sources do not recommend its use.

Pharmacokinetics

No relevant pharmacokinetic data found.

Interactions overview

No interactions with prickly ash found.

Pumpkin

Cucurbita pepo L. (Cucurbitaceae)

Synonym(s) and related species

Cucurbita, Gourd, Melon pumpkin seeds, Squash.

Cucurbita maxima Duchesne, and other *Cucurbita* species.

Constituents

Pumpkin seeds contain a fixed oil, the predominant fatty acids of which are linoleic, oleic, palmitic, and stearic. There is a high sterol content with cholestanol and lathostanol derivatives present, and vitamin E, particularly gamma-tocopherol. The seeds also contain a number of cucurbitacins such as cucurbitin, the type and concentration depending on growth and variety.

Use and indications

Pumpkin seeds are widely used as a foodstuff. Traditionally, they were used to treat tapeworm infection (cucurbitin has anthelmintic effects), but more recently they have begun to be more widely used to treat benign prostatic hyperplasia.

Pharmacokinetics

No relevant pharmacokinetic data found.

Interactions overview

For mention of a case of an elderly man stable taking **warfarin** and simvastatin who had a raised INR after starting *Curbicin* (saw palmetto, pumpkin and vitamin E), see under Saw palmetto + Anticoagulants, page 416. Note that pumpkin seeds are widely used as a foodstuff.

Interactions monographs

- Food, page 392
- Herbal medicines, page 392

P

Pumpkin + Anticoagulants

For mention of a case of an elderly man stable taking **warfarin** and simvastatin who had a raised INR after starting *Curbicin* (saw palmetto, pumpkin and vitamin E), see under Saw palmetto + Anticoagulants, page 416.

Pumpkin + Food

No interactions found. Pumpkin seeds are widely used as food.

Pumpkin + Herbal medicines

No interactions found.

Pycnogenol

Pinus pinaster Aiton (Pinaceae)

Synonym(s) and related species

French maritime pine.

Pinus maritima Lam.

Note that Pycnogenol is a trademark for the extract from the bark of the French maritime pine which grows in the southern coastal area of France.

Pharmacopoeias

Maritime Pine (*USP35–NF30 S1*).

Constituents

Pycnogenol is a standardised water extract of the bark of French maritime pine, containing a range of **flavonoid** polyphenols and procyanidins, including catechin, and to a lesser degree, epicatechin. Other constituents are polyphenolic monomers, which include taxifolin, ferulic acid, benzoic acid, and cinnamic acid and their glycosides.

Use and indications

Pycnogenol is used for a wide variety of disease states and is promoted for its antioxidant effects. Clinical studies indicate that it can be effective in the treatment of chronic venous insufficiency, cardiovascular disorders, asthma, vascular retinopathies, and inflammatory conditions such as systemic lupus erythematosus.

Pharmacokinetics

No relevant pharmacokinetic data found. For information on the pharmacokinetics of individual flavonoids present in pycnogenol, see under flavonoids, page 213.

Interactions overview

Pycnogenol only modestly increases the antiplatelet effects of aspirin. For information on the interactions of individual flavonoids present in pycnogenol, see under flavonoids, page 213.

Interactions monographs

- Antiplatelet drugs, page 394
- Food, page 394
- Herbal medicines, page 394

Pycnogenol + Antiplatelet drugs

The interaction between pycnogenol and antiplatelet drugs is based on experimental evidence only.

Clinical evidence

No interactions found.

Experimental evidence

An *in vitro* study using blood samples from 38 healthy subjects found that pycnogenol dissolved in alcohol inhibited ADP-stimulated platelet aggregation, but only slightly enhanced the platelet inhibition caused by **aspirin**. Pycnogenol dissolved in water did not affect platelet inhibition caused by **aspirin**.[1]

Mechanism

Pycnogenol inhibits both COX-1 and COX-2, which it is suggested, may account for its antiplatelet effects.[2]

Importance and management

Evidence is limited to one experimental study, which suggests that pycnogenol may inhibit platelet aggregation; however, it does not appear to particularly enhance the effects of aspirin. Therefore concurrent use seems likely to be safe, although this needs confirmation in clinical studies. The use of pycnogenol with other antiplatelet drugs does not appear to have been studied.

1. Golański J, Muchova J, Golański R, Durackova Z, Markuszewski L, Watała C. Does pycnogenol intensify the efficacy of acetylsalicylic acid in the inhibition of platelet function? *In vitro* experience. *Postepy Hig Med Dosw* (2006) 60, 316–21.
2. Schäfer A, Chovanová Z, Muchová J, Sumegová K, Liptáková A, Ďuračková Z, Högger P. Inhibition of COX-1 and COX-2 activity by plasma of human volunteers after ingestion of French maritime pine bark extract (Pycnogenol). *Biomed Pharmacother* (2005) 60, 5–9.

Pycnogenol + Food

No interactions found.

Pycnogenol + Herbal medicines

No interactions found.

Pygeum

Prunus africana (Hook.f.) Kalkman (Rosaceae)

Synonym(s) and related species

African prune.

Pygeum africanum (Gaert).

Pharmacopoeias

Pygeum (*USP35–NF30 S1*); Pygeum Africanum Bark (*PhEur 7.5*); Pygeum Bark (*BP 2012*), Pygeum Capsules (*USP35–NF30 S1*); Pygeum Extract (*USP35–NF30 S1*).

Constituents

Pygeum bark contains phytosterols including beta-sitosterol and beta-sitostenone, pentacyclic triterpenes based on oleanolic and ursolic acids, and ferulic esters.

Use and indications

Pygeum bark is used to treat benign prostatic hyperplasia. Several clinical and pharmacological studies suggest that it may be effective.

Pharmacokinetics

No relevant pharmacokinetic data found.

Interactions overview

No interactions with pygeum found.

P

No interactions have been included for herbal medicines or dietary supplements beginning with the letter Q

Q

Raspberry leaf

Rubus idaeus L. (Rosaceae)

Synonym(s) and related species

Frambuesa, Rubus.

Constituents

The leaves contain **flavonoids**, mainly derivatives of kaempferol and quercetin, including their glycosides quercetin-3-*O*-β-D-glucoside, quercetin- and kaempferol-3-*O*-β-D-galactosides, kaempferol-3-*O*-β-L-arabinopyranoside and kaempferol-3-*O*-β-D-(6'-*p*-coumaroyl)-glucoside (tiliroside). Other **polyphenols**, such as gallo- and ellagitannins; **volatile components** such as E-2-hexenal, Z-3-hexenol, and glycosides of C_{13}-norisoprenoids; and **vitamin C** are also present.

Use and indications

Raspberry leaf is traditionally used as a tea to help in childbirth and is taken during the later stages of pregnancy, to stimulate and facilitate labour and shorten its duration. It has also been used for its astringent properties as a treatment for diarrhoea, stomatitis, tonsillitis (as a mouthwash), and conjunctivitis (as an eye lotion). The evidence for its use in pregnancy is weak and contradictory, and although it appears to be safe, no studies have been carried out to confirm this.

Pharmacokinetics

No relevant pharmacokinetic data found. For information on the pharmacokinetics of individual flavonoids present in raspberry leaf, see under flavonoids, page 213.

Interactions overview

No interactions with raspberry leaf found. For information on the interactions of individual flavonoids present in raspberry leaf, see under flavonoids, page 213.

R

Red clover

Trifolium pratense L. (Fabaceae)

Synonym(s) and related species

Cow clover, Meadow clover, Purple clover, Trefoil.

Trifolium borysthenicum Gruner, *Trifolium bracteatum* Schousb., *Trifolium lenkoranicum* (Grossh.) Rosk., *Trifolium ukrainicum* Opp.

Not to be confused with Melilot, page 347 (*Melilotus officinalis*), which is known as King's clover, Sweet clover or Yellow sweet clover.

Pharmacopoeias

Powdered Red Clover (*USP35–NF30 S1*); Powdered Red Clover Extract (*USP35–NF30 S1*); Red Clover (*USP35–NF30 S1*); Red Clover tablets (*USP35–NF30 S1*).

Constituents

Red clover flowers contain **isoflavones**, to which they may be standardised. The major isoflavones are **biochanin A** and **formononetin**, with small amounts of genistein and daidzein and others, and their glycoside conjugates. Other constituents include clovamides, coumestrol, and the natural coumarins medicagol and coumarin.

Use and indications

Red clover was traditionally used for skin conditions, such as eczema and psoriasis. However, the isoflavone fraction is now more commonly used as a form of HRT in women to reduce the symptoms of the menopause, although randomised controlled studies show only a slight benefit at best.[1,2] It is also used for mastalgia, premenstrual syndrome and cancer prevention.

Pharmacokinetics

In an *in vitro* study, an extract of red clover reduced the activity of CYP1A2, CYP2C8, CYP2C9, CYP2C19, CYP2D6 and CYP3A4. The effects on CYP2C8 and CYP2C9 were the most significant.[3] Biochanin A, a major component of red clover, can inhibit P-glycoprotein and OATP, see Isoflavones + Digoxin, page 302 and Isoflavones + Paclitaxel, page 303.

For further information on the pharmacokinetics of the specific isoflavones genistein, daidzein and biochanin A, see isoflavones, page 300. Note that biochanin A is metabolised to genistein, and formononetin to daidzein.[4]

Interactions overview

It has been suggested that red clover may interact with anticoagulants, but evidence for this is largely lacking. Potential interactions of isoflavone constituents of red clover are covered under isoflavones; see antibacterials, page 302, digoxin, page 302, fexofenadine, page 303, paclitaxel, page 303, and tamoxifen, page 304.

Interactions monographs

- Anticoagulants, page 399
- Food, page 399
- Herbal medicines, page 399

1. Nelson HD, Vesco KK, Haney E, Fu R, Nedrow A, Miller J, Nicolaidis C, Walker M, Humphrey L. Nonhormonal therapies for menopausal hot flashes: systematic review and meta-analysis. *JAMA* (2006) 295, 2057–71.
2. Coon JT, Pittler MH, Ernst E. *Trifolium pratense* isoflavones in the treatment of menopausal hot flushes: a systematic review and meta-analysis. *Phytomedicine* (2007) 14, 153–9.
3. Unger M, Frank A. Simultaneous determination of the inhibitory potency if herbal extracts on the activity of six major cytochrome P450 enzymes using liquid chromatography/mass spectrometry and automated online extraction. *Rapid Commun Mass Spectrom* (2004) 18, 2273–81.
4. Tolleson WH, Doerge DR, Churchwell MI, Marques MM, Roberts DW. Metabolism of biochanin A and formononetin by human liver microsomes in vitro. *J Agric Food Chem* (2002) 50, 4783–90.

R

Red clover + Antibacterials

No data for red clover found. For the theoretical possibility that broad-spectrum antibacterials might reduce the metabolism of the isoflavone constituents of red clover, such as daidzin, by colonic bacteria, and so alter their efficacy, see Isoflavones + Antibacterials, page 302.

Red clover + Anticoagulants

The interaction between red clover and anticoagulants is based on a prediction only.

Evidence, mechanism, importance and management

Some reviews list red clover as having the potential to increase the risk of bleeding or potentiate the effects of warfarin,[1] based on the fact that red clover contains natural coumarins. Although red clover contains coumarin, it is not itself an active anticoagulant. With melilot, page 347, which has a high content of coumarin, the action of moulds on the herb can result in the formation of an active anticoagulant, dicoumarol, from the coumarin, and bleeding disorders have occurred in animals fed spoiled hay containing melilot. There appears to be no published evidence of haemorrhagic disorders in animals fed red clover silage or hay. It might be that the coumarin content of red clover is too low to be a problem. Note that mouldy red clover hay has caused poisoning in animals, but this is because of mycotoxins such as slaframine. However, there is one case report of spontaneous subarachnoid haemorrhage in a 53-year-old woman, which was attributed to a herbal supplement containing red clover, and also wild yam, black cohosh, Chinese angelica, raspberry leaf, agnus castus, Siberian ginseng, partridge berry and nettle leaf, which she had been taking for 4 months.[2] With case reports, it is not possible to say, conclusively, which, if any, of these constituents might have contributed to the adverse effect. However, of the constituents in this preparation, Chinese angelica has been associated with bleeding events, see Chinese angelica + Warfarin and related drugs, page 147.

Taken together, the evidence suggests that no special precautions are likely to be required when red clover supplements are used with anticoagulants.

1. Heck AM, DeWitt BA, Lukes AL. Potential interactions between alternative therapies and warfarin. *Am J Health-Syst Pharm* (2000) 57, 1221–7.
2. Friedman JA, Taylor SA, McDermott W, Alikhani P. Multifocal and recurrent subarachnoid hemorrhage due to an herbal supplement containing natural coumarins. *Neurocrit Care* (2007) 7, 76–80.

Red clover + Digoxin

No data for red clover found. For the possibility that high-dose biochanin A, an isoflavone present in red clover, might increase digoxin levels, see Isoflavones + Digoxin, page 302.

Red clover + Fexofenadine

No data for red clover found. For the possibility that high-dose biochanin A, a major isoflavone in red clover, has been shown to slightly decrease fexofenadine levels in *rats,* see Isoflavones + Fexofenadine, page 303.

Red clover + Food

No interactions found.

Red clover + Herbal medicines

No interactions found.

Red clover + Paclitaxel

No data for red clover found. For the possibility that biochanin A and genistein present in red clover might markedly increase paclitaxel levels, see Isoflavones + Paclitaxel, page 303. Note that paclitaxel is used intravenously, and the effect of biochanin A on intravenous paclitaxel does not appear to have been evaluated.

Red clover + Tamoxifen

No data for red clover found. Data relating to the use of the isoflavone constituents of red clover, such as biochanin A, daidzein and genistein, with tamoxifen are covered under Isoflavones + Tamoxifen, page 304.

R

Red vine leaf

Vitis vinifera L. (Vitaceae)

Synonym(s) and related species

Vitis vinifera is the Grape vine, of which there are many cultivars. Red vine leaf is a cultivar with red leaves.

Constituents

Red vine leaf contains a range of polyphenolics, mainly **flavonoids**, proanthocyanins and anthocyanins. The major **flavonoids** in the extract are quercetin and isoquercitrin. Catechins present include gallocatechin and epigallocatechin and their polymers. The red colour is due to the anthocyanins, which are mainly glucosides of malvidin, but also of delphinidin, cyanidin and pertunidin. Hydroxycinnamic acids (e.g. caffeic acid) and **resveratrol** are also present.

Use and indications

Red vine leaf extract is used both internally and externally to improve blood circulation, particularly in the legs for varicose veins. There is some clinical evidence to support its use in venous insufficiency.

Pharmacokinetics

No relevant pharmacokinetic data found. See under flavonoids, page 213, for information on the individual flavonoids present in red vine leaf, and see under resveratrol, page 401, for the pharmacokinetics of resveratrol.

Interactions overview

No interactions with red vine leaf found. For information on the interactions of flavonoids, see under flavonoids, page 213, and for the interactions of resveratrol, see under resveratrol, page 401.

R

Resveratrol

Vitis vinifera L. (Vitaceae)

Types, sources and related compounds

Resveratrol is a polyphenol present in most grape and wine products and is the compound largely credited with providing the health benefits of red wine. However the concentration is very variable between foods and supplements, so it is difficult to evaluate the clinical relevance of the available information.

Use and indications

Resveratrol is used for its reputed anti-ageing effects. It is said to have antioxidant properties and antiplatelet effects, and is therefore promoted as having benefits in a variety of cardiovascular diseases, including atherosclerosis. It also has some oestrogenic and anti-inflammatory activity, and is under investigation in the prevention and treatment of cancer, because it appears to reduce cell proliferation.

Pharmacokinetics

An *in vitro* study reported that resveratrol inhibited the cytochrome P450 isoenzyme CYP3A4, but was much less potent than erythromycin,[1] a known, clinically relevant, moderate CYP3A4 inhibitor. Similar results were found in other studies.[2,3] Interestingly, red wine also inhibited CYP3A4, but this effect did not correlate with the resveratrol content.[1,4]

In other studies resveratrol had only very weak inhibitory effects on CYP1A2, which are unlikely to be of any clinical relevance.[3,5,6] Similarly, one study[3] suggests that resveratrol and its primary metabolite do not inhibit CYP2C9 (see Resveratrol + Diclofenac, page 402) and CYP2D6, and resveratrol only weakly inhibits CYP2C19 (see Resveratrol + Mephenytoin, page 402).

Interactions overview

Resveratrol may have clinically significant antiplatelet effects which may be additive with antiplatelets and anticoagulant drugs as well as other drugs that may cause bleeding such as NSAIDs. An *in vitro* study reports that resveratrol had no significant effect on the metabolism of diclofenac and only weakly inhibited the metabolism of (*S*)-mephenytoin. Therefore clinically relevant pharmacokinetic interactions between resveratrol and substrates of CYP2C9 and CYP2C19, respectively, would not be expected. An *in vitro* study also found that resveratrol moderately inhibited the metabolism of paclitaxel, however the clinical relevance of this is unclear.

Interactions monographs

- Anticoagulant or Antiplatelet drugs, page 402
- Diclofenac, page 402
- Food, page 402
- Herbal medicines, page 402
- Mephenytoin, page 402
- Paclitaxel, page 403

1. Chan WK, Delucchi AB. Resveratrol, a red wine constituent, is a mechanism-based inactivator of cytochrome P450 3A4. *Life Sci* (2000) 67, 3103–12.
2. Chang TK, Yeung RK. Effect of trans-resveratrol on 7-benzyloxy-4-trifluoromethylcoumarin O-dealkylation catalyzed by human recombinant CYP3A4 and CYP3A5. *Can J Physiol Pharmacol* (2001) 79, 220–226.
3. Yu C, Shin YG, Kosmeder JW, Pezzuto JM, van Breemen RB. Liquid chromatography/tandem mass spectrometric determination of inhibition of human cytochrome P450 isozymes by resveratrol and resveratrol-3-sulfate. *Rapid Commun Mass Spectrom* (2003) 17, 307–13.
4. Piver B, Berthou F, Dreano Y, Lucas D. Inhibition of CYP3A, CYP1A and CYP2E1 activities by resveratrol and other non volatile red wine components. *Toxicol Lett* (2001) 125, 83–91.
5. Chun YJ, Kim MY, Guengerich FP. Resveratrol is a selective human cytochrome P450 1A1 inhibitor. *Biochem Biophys Res Commun* (1999) 262, 20–24.
6. Chang TK, Chen J, Lee WB. Differential inhibition and inactivation of human CYP1 enzymes by trans-resveratrol: evidence for mechanism-based inactivation of CYP1A2. *J Pharmacol Exp Ther* (2001) 299, 874–82.

R

Resveratrol + Anticoagulant or Antiplatelet drugs

The interaction between resveratrol and anticoagulants or antiplatelet drugs is based on experimental evidence only.

Clinical evidence

No interactions found.

Experimental evidence

An *ex-vivo* study using samples of platelet-rich plasma from 50 high-risk cardiac patients taking aspirin, found that resveratrol significantly reduced platelet aggregation in response to collagen and adrenaline (epinephrine) in the samples taken from aspirin-resistant patients, but only had a minimal effect in those taken from aspirin-sensitive patients. Resveratrol had minimal effects on ADP-induced platelet aggregation in both groups of patients.[1] Another *in vitro* study found that a low concentration of resveratrol (2 or 5 micromoles) increased the inhibitory effect of prostaglandins E_1 and I_2 on platelet aggregation in response to collagen, although it did not itself affect collagen-induced platelet aggregation.[2] This subject has been extensively studied and is the subject of a number of review articles.[3,4]

Mechanism

Resveratrol appears to enhance the inhibitory response to platelet aggregation. This effect may be additive with the effects of other drugs with antiplatelet effects.

Importance and management

Although there appears to be a plethora of *in vitro* studies to support the antiplatelet role of resveratrol, there is a lack of clinical data in humans. Therefore it is difficult to confirm if a clinically significant enhancement of antiplatelet effects would occur in patients taking resveratrol with antiplatelet drugs. Concurrent use need not be avoided (indeed combinations of antiplatelet drugs are often prescribed together) but it may be prudent to be aware of the potential for increased bleeding if resveratrol is given with other antiplatelet drugs such as **aspirin** and **clopidogrel**. Patients should discuss any episode of prolonged bleeding with a healthcare professional.

Drugs that enhance antiplatelet effects may also increase the risk of bleeding in patients receiving anticoagulants such as **warfarin**. Clinically, the use of an antiplatelet drug with an anticoagulant should generally be avoided in the absence of a specific indication. However, if concurrent use is felt desirable it would seem sensible to warn patients to be alert for any signs of bruising or bleeding, and report these immediately, should they occur.

1. Stef G, Csiszar A, Lerea K, Ungvari Z, Veress G. Resveratrol inhibits aggregation of platelets from high-risk cardiac patients with aspirin resistance. *J Cardiovasc Pharmacol* (2006) 48, 1–5.
2. Wu C-C, Wu C-I, Wang W-Y, Wu Y-C. Low concentrations of resveratrol potentiate the antiplatelet effect of prostaglandins. *Planta Med* (2007) 73, 439–43.
3. Bradamante S, Barenghi L, Villa A. Cardiovascular protective effects of resveratrol. *Cardiovasc Drug Rev* (2004) 22, 169–88.
4. Olas B, Wachowicz B. Resveratrol, a phenolic antioxidant with effects on blood platelet functions. *Platelets* (2005) 16, 251–60.

Resveratrol + Diclofenac

The information regarding the use of resveratrol with diclofenac is based on experimental evidence only.

Clinical evidence

No interactions found.

Experimental evidence

An *in vitro* study using human liver microsomes found that resveratrol had no significant effect on the metabolism of diclofenac.[1]

Mechanism

Nothing expected. Diclofenac can be used as a probe substrate for cytochrome P450 isoenzyme CYP2C9 activity.

Importance and management

Evidence is limited to this one *in vitro* study. Although there are no *in vivo* data available, it seems unlikely that resveratrol will affect the metabolism of diclofenac and therefore no dosage adjustments are likely to be needed if they are given together. Note that resveratrol may have some antiplatelet effects, which may be additive with those of NSAIDs such as diclofenac, consider also Resveratrol + Anticoagulant or Antiplatelet drugs, above. Diclofenac can be used as a probe drug for CYP2C9 activity, and therefore these results also suggest that a pharmacokinetic interaction between resveratrol and other CYP2C9 substrates is unlikely.

1. Yu C, Shin YG, Kosmeder JW, Pezzuto JM, van Breemen RB. Liquid chromatography/tandem mass spectrometric determination of inhibition of human cytochrome P450 isozymes by resveratrol and resveratrol-3-sulfate. *Rapid Commun Mass Spectrom* (2003) 17, 307–13.

Resveratrol + Food

No interactions found.

Resveratrol + Herbal medicines

No interactions found.

Resveratrol + Mephenytoin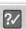

The information regarding the use of resveratrol with mephenytoin is based on experimental evidence only.

Clinical evidence

No interactions found.

Experimental evidence

An *in vitro* study using human liver microsomes found that resveratrol only weakly inhibited the metabolism of (*S*)-mephenytoin.[1]

Mechanism

Nothing expected. Mephenytoin can be used as a probe substrate for cytochrome P450 isoenzyme CYP2C19 activity.

Importance and management

Evidence is limited to this one *in vitro* study. Although there are no *in vivo* data available, it seems unlikely that resveratrol will affect the metabolism of mephenytoin and therefore no dosage adjustments are likely to be needed if they are given together. Mephenytoin can be used as a probe drug for CYP2C19 activity, and therefore these results also suggest that a pharmacokinetic interaction between resveratrol and other CYP2C19 substrates is unlikely.

1. Yu C, Shin YG, Kosmeder JW, Pezzuto JM, van Breemen RB. Liquid chromatography/tandem mass spectrometric determination of inhibition of human cytochrome P450 isozymes by resveratrol and resveratrol-3-sulfate. *Rapid Commun Mass Spectrom* (2003) 17, 307–13.

Resveratrol + Paclitaxel

The interaction between resveratrol and paclitaxel is based on experimental evidence only.

Clinical evidence

No interactions found.

Experimental evidence

An *in vitro* study in human liver microsomes investigated the effects of resveratrol on the metabolism of paclitaxel. In both *rat* and human liver microsomes, resveratrol moderately inhibited paclitaxel metabolism.[1]

Mechanism

Paclitaxel is metabolised by the cytochrome P450 isoenzyme CYP2C8 and, to a lesser extent CYP3A4. In this study resveratrol appeared to moderately inhibit these isoenzymes.

Importance and management

The clinical relevance of this study is unknown. Further study is needed to confirm if this inhibition produces a clinically relevant increase in paclitaxel levels, which could also potentially increase the adverse effects of paclitaxel. However, the authors also suggested that, as the metabolites of paclitaxel are less active than paclitaxel itself, inhibiting its metabolism may be beneficial. There is currently insufficient evidence on which to base any clinical recommendations.

1. Václavříková R, Horský S, Šimek P, Gut I. Paclitaxel metabolism in rat and human liver microsomes is inhibited by phenolic antioxidants. *Naunyn Schmiedebergs Arch Pharmacol* (2003) 368, 200–209.

Rhodiola

Rhodiola rosea L. (Crassulaceae)

Synonym(s) and related species

Arctic root, Golden root, Rodiola, Rose root.

Sedum rosea (L.) Scop., *Sedum roseum* (L.) Scop.

Other *Rhodiola* species may also used, particularly in Chinese medicine.

Constituents

The main active constituents of rhodiola rhizome and root are thought to be the rosavins (a complex series of monoterpene alcohol and phenylpropanoid glycosides such as rosin, rosarin and rosavin), rosiridin, and tyrosol. Rhodiola also contains **flavonoids** such as kaempferol and its glycoside derivatives; sterols (β-sitosterol); tannins; and rhodiolosides or salidrosides (a series of hydroxylated, methoxylated and methylated octadienyl and octenyl glucosides). There is also a small amount of essential oil (about 0.05%).

Use and indications

Rhodiola is widely used throughout the world, and the different species are used for similar purposes. It is considered to be an adaptogen, used for coping with stress, improving mood and alleviating depression. There is a large amount of pharmacological evidence available in support of its use and studies have shown that it can improve both physical and mental performance, reduce fatigue and prevent altitude sickness. However the evidence is of variable quality and the clinical efficacy of rhodiola remains to be conclusively demonstrated.

Pharmacokinetics

An *in vitro* study found that an extract of rhodiola root inhibited the cytochrome P450 isoenzyme CYP3A4; the extent of the inhibition increased with increasing concentrations of rosarin.[1] The manufacturer[2] of a licensed rhodiola product reports that in an *in vitro* study, a rhodiola extract 10 micrograms/mL inhibited CYP2C9 and CYP2C19. However, in another study, an extract of rhodiola did not affect the metabolism of warfarin, page 405, which is a substrate of CYP2C9. Rhodiola did not affect the metabolism of theophylline, page 405, and therefore seems unlikely to affect the metabolism of other drugs that are substrates of CYP1A2. For information on the pharmacokinetics of individual flavonoids present in rhodiola, see under flavonoids, page 213.

Interactions overview

Rhodiola does not appear to affect the pharmacokinetics of theophylline or warfarin. The concurrent use of pepper may diminish the antidepressant effects of rhodiola. For information on the interactions of individual flavonoids present in rhodiola, see under flavonoids, page 213.

Interactions monographs

- Food, page 405
- Herbal medicines; Pepper, page 405
- Theophylline, page 405
- Warfarin, page 405

1. Scott IM, Leduc RI, Burt AJ, Marles RJ, Arnason JT, Foster BC. The inhibition of human cytochrome P450 by ethanol extracts of North American botanicals. *Pharm Biol* (2006) 44, 315–27.
2. Vitano Film-coated Tablets (Dry extract of *Rhodiola rosea* roots and rhizomes). Schwabe Pharma (UK) Ltd. UK Summary of product characteristics, July 2008.

Rhodiola + Food

No interactions found.

Rhodiola + Herbal medicines; Pepper

The interaction between rhodiola and warfarin is based on experimental evidence only.

Clinical evidence

No interactions found.

Experimental evidence

A study in *rats* found that the addition of **piperine**, an alkaloid found in pepper, to an extract of rhodiola (SHR-5, containing rhodioloside 2.7%, rosavin 6% and tyrosol 0.8%), unexpectedly reduced the antidepressant activity of rhodiola. The maximum plasma concentration of rhodioloside was reduced by 22%, and the AUC and maximum plasma concentration of rosavin were increased by 33% and 82%, respectively.[1]

Mechanism

The exact constituents of rhodiola that are responsible for antidepressant activity are not fully established. Rhodioloside alone possesses some antidepressant activity. Although rosavin alone does not appear to be an antidepressant, when given in combination with other rhodiola constituents including rhodioloside the antidepressant effects are enhanced. Changes in the pharmacokinetics of the constituents of rhodiola by piperine may have diminished its antidepressant activity. The authors suggest that this may be due to the inhibition of the cytochrome P450 isoenzyme CYP1A1 by piperine.[1]

Importance and management

Evidence is limited to one experimental study and extrapolating these findings to a clinical setting is difficult. Although the effect of using both of these herbal medicines in humans is unknown, due to the unpredictable effects that may occur when piperine is taken with rhodiola, notably a reduction in antidepressant effects, the authors of this study suggest that concurrent use should be avoided. Given that the outcome of concurrent use is likely to be opposite to the desired effects, this seems a reasonable recommendation.

1. Panossian A, Nikoyan N, Ohanyan N, Hovhannisyan A, Abrahamyan H, Gabrielyan E, Wikman G. Comparative study of Rhodiola preparations on behavioral despair of rats. *Phytomedicine* (2008) 15, 84–91.

Rhodiola + Theophylline

The interaction between rhodiola and theophylline is based on experimental evidence only.

Clinical evidence

No interactions found.

Experimental evidence

In a study, *rats* were given a standardised rhodiola extract (SHR-5, containing rhodioloside 2.7%, rosavin 6%, and tyrosol 0.8%) twice daily for 3 days with a single dose of **aminophylline**, given one hour after the last dose of rhodiola extract. The pharmacokinetics of theophylline were only slightly affected by the rhodiola extract (less than 15% decrease in AUC and maximum levels).[1]

Mechanism

Unknown.

Importance and management

Information appears to be limited to this one study in *rats*, which may not necessarily extrapolate directly to humans. However, what is known suggests that rhodiola extract is unlikely to have a clinically significant effect on the pharmacokinetics of theophylline.

1. Panossian A, Hovhannisyan A, Abrahamyan H, Gabrielyan E, Wikman G. Pharmacokinetic and pharmacodynamic study of interaction of *Rhodiola rosea* SHR-5 extract with warfarin and theophylline in rats. *Phytother Res* (2008) 23, 351–7.

Rhodiola + Warfarin

The interaction between rhodiola and warfarin is based on experimental evidence only.

Clinical evidence

No interactions found.

Experimental evidence

In a study, *rats* were given a standardised rhodiola extract (SHR-5, containing salidroside 2.5%, rosavin 3.9%, and tyrosol 0.8%) twice daily for 3 days with a single dose of warfarin, given one hour after the last dose of rhodiola extract. The maximum levels of warfarin were increased by a modest 34%, but the AUC and half-life were not altered by rhodiola. Furthermore, the anticoagulant effects of warfarin (assessed by monitoring PTT) were unaffected.[1]

Mechanism

Unknown. In other *in vitro* studies, rhodiola inhibited the activity of the cytochrome P450 isoenzyme CYP2C9, which metabolises the *S*-warfarin isomer. See pharmacokinetics, page 404.

Importance and management

Information appears to be limited to this one study in *rats*, which may not necessarily extrapolate directly to humans. However, what is known suggests that rhodiola extract is unlikely to affect the response to treatment with warfarin.

1. Panossian A, Hovhannisyan A, Abrahamyan H, Gabrielyan E, Wikman G. Pharmacokinetic and pharmacodynamic study of interaction of *Rhodiola rosea* SHR-5 extract with warfarin and theophylline in rats. *Phytother Res* (2008) 23, 351–7.

R

Rhubarb

Rheum officinale Baill., *Rheum palmatum* L. (Polygonaceae)

Synonym(s) and related species

Chinese rhubarb.

Rheum tanguticum Maxim.

Note that Indian rhubarb (Himalayan rhubarb) consists of the dried root of *Rheum emodi* Wall. or some other related species of *Rheum*.

Note also that the root of *Rheum rhaponticum* Willd (English rhubarb, Garden rhubarb) sometimes occurs as an adulterant in rhubarb and pharmacopoeias specify a test for its absence.

Pharmacopoeias

Compound Rhubarb Tincture (*BP 2012*); Rhubarb (*BP 2012, PhEur 7.5*).

Constituents

Anthraquinone glycosides are major components of rhubarb. It contains chrysophanol, emodin, rhein, aloe-emodin, physcion and sennosides A to E. Various tannins, stilbene glycosides, resins, starch and trace amounts of volatile oil are also present.

Indian rhubarb contains similar anthraquinones, but English rhubarb contains only chrysophanol and some of its glycosides.

Use and indications

Rhubarb rhizome and root is used as a laxative, but at low doses it is also used to treat diarrhoea, because of the tannin content. It is also used as a flavouring in food.

Pharmacokinetics

For information on the pharmacokinetics of an anthraquinone glycoside present in rhubarb, see under aloes, page 27.

Interactions overview

A case report describes raised digoxin levels and toxicity in a patient taking a Chinese herbal laxative containing rhubarb (daio), see Liquorice + Digitalis glycosides, page 331 for further details. A case report describes persistent diarrhoea and raised lopinavir levels when evening primrose oil and a product containing aloes, rhubarb and liquorice were started, see under Evening primrose oil + Lopinavir, page 207.

No further interactions with rhubarb found; however, rhubarb (by virtue of its anthraquinone content) is expected to share some of the interactions of a number of other anthraquinone-containing laxatives, such as aloes, page 27 and senna, page 423. Of particular relevance are the interactions with corticosteroids and potassium-depleting diuretics.

Interactions monographs

- Food, page 407
- Herbal medicines, page 407

Rhubarb + Food

No interactions found.

Rhubarb + Herbal medicines

No interactions found.

Rhubarb + Lopinavir

For mention of a case of persistent diarrhoea and raised lopinavir levels in an HIV-positive man after starting evening primrose oil and a product containing aloes, rhubarb and liquorice, see Evening primrose oil + Lopinavir, page 207.

R

Ribwort plantain

Plantago lanceolata L. (Plantaginaceae)

Synonym(s) and related species

Buck-horn plantain, Narrow-leaf plantain, English plantain, Not to be confused with Plantain, page 383 (*Plantago major*), Psyllium (*Plantago afra* (*P. psyllium*) or *Plantago indica* (*P. arenaria*), or Ispaghula, page 306 (*Plantain ovata*).

Pharmacopoeias

Ribwort Plantain (*BP 2012, PhEur 7.5*)

Constituents

The leaves of ribwort plantain contain the phenylethanoids acteoside, plantamajoside, isoacteoside and lavandulifolioside; the iridoids aucubin and catalpol; and **flavonoids** including luteolin, and its derivatives.

Use and indications

Ribwort plantain is traditionally used for the treatment of upper respiratory infections and sinusitis and specifically for bronchial catarrh and inflammation of the mucous membrane of the pharynx. The young leaves are sometimes eaten in salads.

Pharmacokinetics

No relevant pharmacokinetic data found. For general information on the pharmacokinetics of flavonoids, see under flavonoids, page 213.

Interactions overview

No interactions for ribwort plantain found. For information on the interactions of flavonoids, see under flavonoids, page 213.

Rooibos

Aspalathus linearis (Burm.f.) R.Dahlgren (Fabaceae)

Synonym(s) and related species

Red bush tea, Green red bush, Kaffree tea.

Constituents

The needle-like leaves and stems of rooibos contain polyphenolic **flavonoids**. The unfermented product remains green in colour and contains aspalathin, a dihydrochalcone, whereas the fermented product is red in colour due to oxidation of the constituent polyphenols. Oxidation of aspalathin produces dihydro-iso-orientin. Other **flavonoids** present in both green and red rooibos include rutin, iso-quercetin, hyperoside, and quercetin. Rooibos also contains volatile oils and minerals, but does not contain caffeine.[1] The tannin content of rooibos tea is less than 5%.

Use and indications

Rooibos teas have been traditionally used in South Africa for a wide range of aliments including asthma, colic, headache, nausea, depression, diabetes, and hypertension.[1] Currently, rooibos is principally used to produce a tea-like beverage. In experimental studies, it has shown some antioxidant, chemopreventive and immunomodulating effects.[1]

Pharmacokinetics

Rooibos appears to induce the cytochrome P450 isoenzyme CYP3A4, see midazolam, page 410. For information on the pharmacokinetics of individual flavonoids present in rooibos, see under flavonoids, page 213.

Interactions overview

Midazolam levels are reduced by rooibos tea *in vitro* and in *rats,* but clinical evidence for an interaction is lacking. Rooibos tea does not appear to affect iron absorption. For information on the interactions of individual flavonoids present in rooibos, see under flavonoids, page 213.

Interactions monographs

- Food, page 410
- Herbal medicines, page 410
- Iron compounds, page 410
- Midazolam, page 410

1. McKay DL, Blumberg JB. A review of the bioactivity of South African Herbal Teas: Rooibos (*Aspalathus Linearis*) and Honeybush (*Cyclopia intermedia*). *Phytother Res* (2007) 21, 1–16.

R

Rooibos + Food

No interactions found.

Rooibos + Herbal medicines

No interactions found.

Rooibos + Iron compounds

Rooibos tea does not appear to significantly reduce the absorption of iron.

Clinical evidence

In a parallel group study in healthy subjects, mean iron absorption after ingestion of radiolabelled iron 16 mg with a beverage was 7.25% with rooibos tea, 1.7% with tea, and 9.34% with water.[1] Note that tea is known to inhibit iron absorption, see Tea + Iron compounds, page 467.

Experimental evidence

No relevant data found.

Mechanism

Rooibos does not appear to reduce the absorption of iron. It contains some polyphenolic flavonoids which might bind iron in the gut; however, these differ from the polyphenols found in tea, such as the catechins, which have reported to affect iron absorption. Tannins found in tea are also thought to reduce iron absorption, but rooibos tea has less than 5% tannins.

Importance and management

The evidence suggests that rooibos does not reduce the absorption of iron. No special precautions are likely to be required.

1. Hesseling PB, Klopper JF, van Heerden PD. The effect of rooibos tea on iron absorption. [In Afrikaans] *S Afr Med J* (1979) 55, 631–2.

Rooibos + Midazolam

The interaction between rooibos tea and midazolam is based on experimental evidence only.

Clinical evidence

No interactions found.

Experimental evidence

An *in vitro* study investigating the effects of rooibos tea on midazolam pharmacokinetics found that a 10% solution of rooibos tea 4 g/L brewed for 5 minutes reduced the levels of the 4-hydroxy metabolite of midazolam to undetectable levels.[1] A subsequent study in *rats* found that an unrestricted amount of rooibos tea given for 2 weeks reduced the AUC and maximum concentration of a single 20-mg/kg oral dose of midazolam by 70% and 64%, respectively. Intestinal metabolism appeared to be more affected than hepatic metabolism.[1]

Mechanism

Midazolam is a substrate of the cytochrome P450 isoenzyme CYP3A4. These studies suggest that rooibos tea induces CYP3A4, mainly in the intestine, thereby increasing midazolam metabolism and decreasing its levels.

Importance and management

Although the data is limited and there appear to be no clinical studies, it would seem that rooibos tea may have the potential to significantly reduce the levels of midazolam, and therefore reduce its efficacy. However, the amount of rooibos tea required to significantly inhibit CYP3A4 in humans, and produce a clinically important reduction in drug levels, is unknown. Nevertheless, until more is known, it would seem prudent to monitor the outcome of concurrent use, being alert for a decrease in the efficacy of midazolam.

Midazolam is used as a probe drug for CYP3A4 activity, and therefore these results also suggest that a pharmacokinetic interaction between rooibos and other CYP3A4 substrates is possible. See the table Drugs and herbs affecting or metabolised by the cytochrome P450 isoenzyme CYP3A4, page 7 for a list of known CYP3A4 substrates.

1. Matsuda K, Nishimura Y, Kurata N, Iwase M, Yasuhara H. Effects of continuous ingestion of herbal teas on intestinal CYP3A in the rat. *J Pharmacol Sci* (2007) 103, 214–21.

Rosemary

Rosmarinus officinalis L. (Lamiaceae)

Synonym(s) and related species

Rosmarini folium.

Rosmarinus laxiflorus Noë ex Lange.

Pharmacopoeias

Rosemary Leaf (*BP 2012, PhEur 7.5*); Rosemary Oil (*BP 2012, PhEur 7.5*).

Constituents

The major constituents of rosemary leaf are **flavonoids** including apigenin and luteolin and its derivatives; **caffeic acid** derivatives such as rosmarinic (to which rosemary leaf may be standardised), labiatic, chlorogenic and neochlorogenic acids; diterpenes including carnosol, carnosolic acid and rosmanol; and **triterpenes** including oleanolic and ursolic acids. The components of the essential oil (to which rosemary leaf may be standardised) vary, but may include camphor, borneol and cineole (usually the major components), and other monoterpene hydrocarbons.

Use and indications

Rosemary is used traditionally as a carminative and spasmolytic for the symptomatic relief of flatulent dyspepsia, and also for headache, cardiovascular and urinary tract disorders. The oil is often applied topically as a rubefacient and mild analgesic for myalgia and sciatica, and may also be used as an adjuvant for the relief of minor muscular and articular pain, and in minor peripheral circulatory conditions. The pure oil should not be taken internally and should not be applied externally in large amounts, or used by pregnant women. Note that rosemary is also commonly used as a flavouring in foods and as a perfume in toiletries.

Pharmacokinetics

A water-soluble extract of rosemary leaves induced the activity of CYP1A1, CYP1A2, CYP2B1/2, CYP2E1 and CYP3A, glutathione S-transferase (GST) and UDP-glucuronosyltransferase (UGT) in *animals*,[1,2] whereas rosmarinic acid alone did not.[1] Rosemary essential oil induced the activity of CYP1A1, CYP1A2, and especially, CYP2B1/2, and a dichloromethane extract induced GST and UGT (especially UGT1A6).[2] In *in vitro* studies using various cancer cells, rosemary extract,[3] and more specifically its components carnosic acid, carnosol and ursolic acid,[4] inhibited the activity of P-glycoprotein. Rosmarinic acid alone had no effect on P-glycoprotein activity.[4] Whether any of these effects are clinically relevant is unclear. For information on the pharmacokinetics of individual flavonoids present in rosemary, see under flavonoids, page 213.

Interactions overview

Rosemary appears to modestly reduce the absorption of iron. For information on the interactions of individual flavonoids present in rosemary, see under flavonoids, page 213.

Interactions monographs

- Food, page 412
- Herbal medicines, page 412
- Iron compounds, page 412

1. Debersac P, Vernevaut M-F, Amiot M-J, Suschetet M, Siess M-H. Effects of a water-soluble extract of rosemary and its purified component rosmarinic acid on xenobiotic-metabolizing enzymes in rat liver. *Food Chem Toxicol* (2001) 39, 109–17.
2. Debersac P, Heydel J-M, Amiot M-J, Goudonnet H, Artur Y, Suschetet M, Siess M-H. Induction of cytochrome P450 and/or detoxication enzymes by various extracts of rosemary: description of specific patterns. *Food Chem Toxicol* (2001) 39, 907–18.
3. Plouzek CA, Ciolino HP, Clarke R, Yeh GC. Inhibition of P-glycoprotein activity and reversal of multidrug resistance *in vitro* by rosemary extract. *Eur J Cancer* (1999) 35, 1541–5.
4. Nabekura T, Yamaki T, Hiroi T, Ueno K, Kitagawa S. Inhibition of anticancer drug efflux transporter P-glycoprotein by rosemary phytochemicals. *Pharmacol Res* (2010) 61, 259–63.

R

Rosemary + Food

No interactions found. Note that rosemary is used widely as a food ingredient.

Rosemary + Herbal medicines

No interactions found.

Rosemary + Iron compounds

Rosemary extract appears to slightly reduce the absorption of iron.

Clinical evidence

A study in 14 healthy women found that a rosemary extract (about 33 mg phenolic substances) modestly reduced the absorption of iron by about 20%.[1]

Experimental evidence

No relevant data found.

Mechanism

Polyphenolic compounds found in rosemary, such as carnosic acid, carnosol, and rosmarinic acid, primarily consist of catechol groups, which are thought to reduce the bioavailability of non-haem iron.[1]

Importance and management

The general importance of the interaction between rosemary and iron is uncertain, but the available data suggest that rosemary extracts rich in polyphenols have much less of an effect on iron absorption than beverages made from black (fermented) teas, which have well-known effects on iron absorption. Furthermore, a reduction in absorption of 20% would not generally be considered to be clinically relevant. No general restrictions are therefore required.

1. Samman S, Sandström B, Bjørndal Toft M, Bukhave K, Jensen M, Sørensen SS, Hansen M. Green tea or rosemary extract added to foods reduces nonheme-iron absorption. *Am J Clin Nutr* (2001) 73, 607–12.

Sage

Salvia officinalis L. (Lamiaceae)

Synonym(s) and related species

Dalmatian sage, Garden sage, Red sage, Salvia, True sage.

There are many related species, which include *Salvia lavandulifolia* Vahl. (Spanish sage), and *Salvia triloba* L. (Greek sage).

Pharmacopoeias

Three-lobed Sage Leaf (*BP 2012, PhEur 7.5*); Sage Leaf (*BP 2012, PhEur 7.5*); Sage Oil (*BP 2012*); Sage Tincture (*BP 2012, PhEur 7.5*); Spanish Sage Oil (*BP 2012, PhEur 7.5*).

Constituents

The major constituents of sage are **flavonoids** including luteolin and derivatives; caffeic acid derivatives; diterpenes and triterpenes.

The essential oil components vary according to species and origin. *Salvia officinalis* contains the monoterpene hydrocarbons α- and β-thujones as the major components, together with 1,8-cineole, camphor and borneol and others. *Salvia lavandulifolia* does not contain thujones, and *Salvia triloba* only small amounts, making these oils less toxic.

Use and indications

Sage is used traditionally to reduce 'hot flushes' and hyperhidrosis associated with the menopause. It has antiseptic and spasmolytic properties, and a tea infusion is used as a gargle for sore throats. Extracts are also strongly antioxidant. Sage (*Salvia lavandulifolia* in particular because of the absence of thujones) has recently generated interest as a cognition enhancer due to its anticholinesterase properties. The oil may be applied topically as an antiseptic and rubefacient but it should not be taken internally, applied externally in large amounts, or used by pregnant women. Note that sage is widely used as a flavouring in foods.

Pharmacokinetics

An *in vitro* study[1] found that sage does not have a clinically significant inductive effect on the cytochrome P450 isoenzymes CYP1A2, CYP2D6 and CYP3A4. Other *in vitro* studies[2,3] have found that sage does not inhibit CYP2D6, hepatic CYP3A4, or P-glycoprotein to a clinically relevant extent, although it may have some potentially clinically relevant effects on intestinal CYP3A4. In contrast, a further *in vitro* study[4] found that sage had inhibitory effects on CYP2C9, CYP2C19, CYP2D6 and CYP3A4, but these findings should be interpreted with caution, as the study also found St John's wort to be a CYP3A4 inhibitor, whereas clinically, it is a CYP3A4 inducer. Therefore sage appears to have a low potential for causing interactions by these mechanisms, although the potential for a clinically relevant effect on intestinal CYP3A4 warrants further study.

For information on the pharmacokinetics of individual flavonoids present in sage, see under flavonoids, page 213.

Interactions overview

No interactions with sage found. Sage is commonly used as a flavouring in foods. For information on the interactions of individual flavonoids present in sage, see under flavonoids, page 213.

1. Hellum BH, Hu Z, Nilsen OG. The induction of CYP1A2, CYP2D6 and CYP3A4 by six trade herbal products in cultured primary human hepatocytes. *Basic Clin Pharmacol Toxicol* (2007) 100, 23–30.
2. Hellum BH, Nilsen OG. The *in vitro* inhibitory potential of trade herbal products on human CYP2D6-mediated metabolism and the influence of ethanol. *Basic Clin Pharmacol Toxicol* (2007) 101, 350–358.
3. Hellum BH, Nilsen OG. *In vitro* inhibition of CYP3A4 metabolism and P-glycoprotein-mediated transport by trade herbal products. *Basic Clin Pharmacol Toxicol* (2008) 102, 466–75.
4. Foster BC, Vandenhoek S, Hana J, Krantis A, Akhtar MH, Bryan M, Budzinski JW, Ramputh A, Arnason JT. *In vitro* inhibition of human cytochrome P450-mediated metabolism of marker substrates by natural products. *Phytomedicine* (2003) 10, 334–42.

S

Sarsaparilla

Smilax L. species. (Smilacaceae)

Synonym(s) and related species

A number of species are used, including:

Smilax aristolochiifolia Mill., (*Smilax medica* or *Smilax ornata*,), also known as Mexican sarsaparilla.

Smilax febrifuga Kunth, also known as Ecuadorian sarsaparilla.

Smilax regelii Killip and C.V. Morton (*Smilax grandifolia* or Smilax ornata,) also known as Jamaican sarsaparilla or Honduras sarsaparilla.

Smilax glabra Roxb., is used in traditional Chinese medicine.

Not to be confused with German sarsaparilla (Carex arenaria L.), Indian sarsaparilla (*Hemidesmus indicus* Brown) or Wild sarsaparilla (*Arali nudicaulis* L.), which are unrelated to *Smilax*.

Constituents

The major constituents of the root and rhizome are **saponins** based on sarsasapogenin (parigenin) and smilagenin, including sarsasaponin (parillin), smilasaponin (smilacin) and sarsaparilloside; **flavonoids** based on kaempferol and quercetin; **phytosterols** such as β-sitosterol, stigmasterol and pollinastanol and other **polyphenolic compounds** such as caffeoylshikimic acid, ferulic acid and shikimic acid.

Use and indications

Sarsaparilla is reputed to have anti-inflammatory, antirheumatic and antipruritic properties. It is used traditionally to treat a wide variety of complaints including rheumatic disorders, psoriasis and other skin disorders, and has been used for leprosy and syphilis. However, there is little pharmacological or clinical evidence to support these uses. Sarsaparilla has also been used as a vehicle and flavouring agent in pharmaceuticals and is used as a flavouring in soft drinks (it is a major ingredient of traditional root beer).

Pharmacokinetics

No relevant pharmacokinetic data found. For information on the pharmacokinetics of individual flavonoids present in sarsaparilla, see under flavonoids, page 213.

Interactions overview

No interactions with sarsaparilla found. For information on the interactions of individual flavonoids present in sarsaparilla, see under flavonoids, page 213. The German Commission E monograph for sarsaparilla root states that it increases the absorption of simultaneously administered substances such as **digitalis glycosides** or bismuth, presumably because of the stated effect of gastric irritation (bismuth compounds are generally nonabsorbable and absorption might be increased when there is damage to the gastrointestinal mucosa). However, the Editors' Note says that gastric irritation is not a problem with ingestion of sarsaparilla in normal quantities. An interaction via altered gastric absorption therefore seems unlikely. The same monograph also states that the elimination of other substances (e.g. **hypnotics**) is accelerated. We could find no evidence to support either of these statements.

S

Saw palmetto

Serenoa repens (W.Bartram) Small (Arecaceae)

Synonym(s) and related species

American dwarf palm, Sabal, Serenoa.

Brahea serrulata H.Wendl., *Sabal serrulata* (Michx.) Schult f., *Sabal serrulatum* Schult f., *Serenoa serrulata* (Michx.) Hook. f. ex B.D. Jacks.

Pharmacopoeias

Powdered Saw Palmetto (*USP35–NF30 S1*); Saw Palmetto (*USP35–NF30 S1*); Saw Palmetto Capsules (*USP35–NF30 S1*); Saw Palmetto Extract (*USP35–NF30 S1*); Saw Palmetto Fruit (*BP 2012, PhEur 7.5*).

Constituents

The fruit of saw palmetto contains about 25% fatty acids (extracts are often standardised to a minimum of 11% total fatty acids) consisting of capric, caprylic, lauric, palmitic, oleic, linoleic and linolenic acids in the form of fixed oils. Sterols including campesterol, stig masterol and β-sitosterol are also present as are long chain alcohols, carotenoids, various polysaccharides and some **flavonoids**, including rutin, isoquercetin and kaempferol.

Use and indications

The main contemporary use of saw palmetto fruit is to treat the urological symptoms of benign prostatic hyperplasia. It has also been used as a diuretic, a sedative, an endocrine agent, an antiseptic and for treating disorders involving the sex hormones.

Pharmacokinetics

Saw palmetto (*ProstaPro* 160 mg berry extract containing 85 to 95% fatty acids and sterols) was found to inhibit the cytochrome P450 isoenzymes CYP2D6, CYP2C9 and CYP3A4 *in vitro*.[1] However, a clinical study[2] in patients given debrisoquine, a probe substrate for CYP2D6, found that saw palmetto had no effect on this isoenzyme, and other clinical studies suggest that the *in vitro* effects reported for CYP3A4 and CYP2D6 may not be clinically relevant, see benzodiazepines, page 416, and dextromethorphan, page 417, for further information. Clinical studies with chlorzoxazone, page 416, and caffeine, page 416, also suggest that saw palmetto has no clinically relevant effect on CYP1E2 or CYP1A2, respectively. For information on the pharmacokinetics of individual flavonoids present in saw palmetto, see under flavonoids, page 213.

Interactions overview

There may be an increased response to anticoagulant treatment in patients who also take saw palmetto. Saw palmetto does not appear to have a clinically relevant effect on the majority of cytochrome P450 isoenzymes and no other interactions with saw palmetto have been found. For information on the interactions of individual flavonoids present in saw palmetto, see under flavonoids, page 213.

Interactions monographs

- Anticoagulants, page 416
- Benzodiazepines, page 416
- Caffeine, page 416
- Chlorzoxazone, page 416
- Dextromethorphan, page 417
- Food, page 417
- Herbal medicines, page 417

1. Yale SH, Glurich I. Analysis of the inhibitory potential of Ginkgo biloba, Echinacea purpurea, and Serenoa repens on the metabolic activity of cytochrome P450 3A4, 2D6, and 2C9. *J Altern Complement Med* (2005) 11, 433–9.
2. Gurley BJ, Gardner SF, Hubbard MA, Williams DK, Gentry WB, Carrier J, Khan IA, Edwards DJ, Shah A. In vivo assessment of botanical supplementation on human cytochrome P450 phenotypes: *Citrus aurantium, Echinacea purpurea*, milk thistle, and saw palmetto. *Clin Pharmacol Ther* (2004) 76, 428–40.

S

Saw palmetto + Anticoagulants

The INR of one patient taking warfarin modestly increased after he took *Curbicin* (saw palmetto, pumpkin, and vitamin E). This product has also been associated with an increased INR in a patient not taking anticoagulants. Excessive bleeding during surgery has been reported in another patient who had been taking saw palmetto.

Clinical evidence

A 61-year-old man taking **warfarin** and simvastatin, with a stable INR of around 2.4, had an increase in his INR to 3.4 within 6 days of starting to take 5 tablets of *Curbicin* daily. Within a week of stopping the *Curbicin,* his INR had fallen to its previous value. Another elderly man who was not taking any anticoagulants and was taking 3 tablets of *Curbicin* daily was found to have an INR of 2.1 (normal 0.9 to 1.2). His INR decreased (to between 1.3 and 1.4) when he was given vitamin K, but did not normalise until a week after the *Curbicin* was stopped. *Curbicin* is a herbal remedy used for micturition problems, and contains extracts from the fruit of saw palmetto and pumpkin seeds.[1]

In addition, saw palmetto has been attributed to excessive bleeding in a 53-year-old man undergoing a surgical procedure to remove a brain tumour. An estimated 2 litres of blood was lost during surgery and bleeding time did not return to normal for 5 days. The patient denied taking NSAIDs pre-operatively but admitted to taking saw palmetto for benign prostate hypertrophy.[2]

Experimental evidence

Saw palmetto may inhibit the cytochrome P450 isoenzyme CYP2C9 *in vitro* (see pharmacokinetics, page 415), but it is not known if this is clinically relevant.

Mechanism

The authors of the first report suggest that what happened was possibly due to the presence of vitamin E in the *Curbicin* preparation (each tablet contains 10 mg), but vitamin E does not normally affect INRs. Experimental evidence suggests that saw palmetto may inhibit the cytochrome P450 isoenzyme CYP2C9, which is an important route of warfarin metabolism.

Importance and management

Evidence appears to be limited to case reports and an experimental study of unknown clinical relevance. Because of the many other factors influencing anticoagulant control, it is not possible to reliably ascribe a change in INR specifically to a drug interaction in a single case report without other supporting evidence. It may be better to advise patients to discuss the use of any herbal products they wish to try, and to increase monitoring if this is thought advisable. Cases of uneventful use should be reported, as they are as useful as possible cases of adverse effects.

1. Yue Q-Y, Jansson K. Herbal drug Curbicin and anticoagulant effect with and without warfarin: possibly related to the vitamin E component. *J Am Geriatr Soc* (2001) 49, 838.
2. Cheema P, El-Mefty O, Jazieh AR. Intraoperative haemorrhage associated with the use of extract of Saw Palmetto herb: a case report and review of literature. *J Intern Med* (2001) 250, 167–9.

Saw palmetto + Benzodiazepines

No pharmacokinetic interaction appears to occur between saw palmetto and alprazolam or midazolam.

Clinical evidence

In a study in 12 healthy subjects, saw palmetto 320 mg daily for 16 days, did not affect the pharmacokinetics of a single 2-mg dose of **alprazolam** given on day 14.[1] In another study in 12 healthy subjects saw palmetto 160 mg twice daily for 28 days did not affect the metabolism of a single 8-mg dose of **midazolam**.[2]

Experimental evidence

Experimental studies have suggested that saw palmetto may inhibit the cytochrome P450 isoenzyme CYP3A4, see pharmacokinetics, page 415.

Mechanism

Midazolam is metabolised by the cytochrome P450 isoenzyme CYP3A4. *In vitro* study suggested that saw palmetto inhibited this route or metabolism, but this does not appear to be clinically relevant.

Importance and management

The findings of these studies suggest that saw palmetto does not alter the metabolism of alprazolam or midazolam, and therefore no dosage adjustments of these benzodiazepines would be expected to be needed on concurrent use.

Midazolam is used as a probe drug for CYP3A4 activity, and therefore these results also suggest that a pharmacokinetic interaction between saw palmetto and other CYP3A4 substrates is unlikely.

1. Markowitz JS, Donovan JL, DeVane L, Taylor RM, Ruan Y, Wang J-S, Chavin KD. Multiple doses of saw palmetto (*Serenoa repens*) did not alter cytochrome P450 2D6 and 3A4 activity in normal volunteers. *Clin Pharmacol Ther* (2003) 74, 536–42.
2. Gurley BJ, Gardner SF, Hubbard MA, Williams DK, Gentry WB, Carrier J, Khan IA, Edwards DJ, Shah A. In vivo assessment of botanical supplementation on human cytochrome P450 phenotypes: *Citrus aurantium, Echinacea purpurea,* milk thistle, and saw palmetto. *Clin Pharmacol Ther* (2004) 76, 428–40.

Saw palmetto + Caffeine

Saw palmetto does not appear to affect the pharmacokinetics of caffeine.

Clinical evidence

In a randomised study, 12 healthy subjects were given saw palmetto 160 mg twice daily for 28 days, with a single 100-mg dose of caffeine at the end of treatment with saw palmetto. The pharmacokinetics of caffeine were unchanged by saw palmetto.[1]

Experimental evidence

No relevant data found.

Mechanism

Caffeine is metabolised by the cytochrome P450 isoenzyme CYP1A2. Saw palmetto does not appear to inhibit this route of metabolism.

Importance and management

Evidence appears to be limited to the study cited, which suggests that in most patients saw palmetto is unlikely to raise caffeine levels.

Caffeine is used as a probe drug for CYP1A2 activity, and therefore these results also suggest that a pharmacokinetic interaction between saw palmetto and other CYP1A2 substrates is unlikely.

1. Gurley BJ, Gardner SF, Hubbard MA, Williams DK, Gentry WB, Carrier J, Khan IA, Edwards DJ, Shah A. In vivo assessment of botanical supplementation on human cytochrome P450 phenotypes: *Citrus aurantium, Echinacea purpurea,* milk thistle, and saw palmetto. *Clin Pharmacol Ther* (2004) 76, 428–40.

Saw palmetto + Chlorzoxazone

Saw palmetto does not appear to affect the pharmacokinetics of chlorzoxazone.

S

Clinical evidence

In a study in 12 healthy subjects the metabolism of a single 250-mg dose of chlorzoxazone was not affected by saw palmetto 160 mg twice daily for 28 days.[1]

Experimental evidence

No relevant data found.

Mechanism

Chlorzoxazone is used as a probe substrate of the cytochrome P450 isoenzyme CYP2E1. Saw palmetto does not appear to inhibit this route of metabolism.

Importance and management

Evidence appears to be limited to the study cited, which suggests that saw palmetto is unlikely to raise chlorzoxazone levels.

Chlorzoxazone is used as a probe drug for CYP2E1 activity, and therefore these results also suggest that a pharmacokinetic interaction between saw palmetto and other CYP2E1 substrates is unlikely.

1. Gurley BJ, Gardner SF, Hubbard MA, Williams DK, Gentry WB, Carrier J, Khan IA, Edwards DJ, Shah A. In vivo assessment of botanical supplementation on human cytochrome P450 phenotypes: *Citrus aurantium, Echinacea purpurea,* milk thistle, and saw palmetto. *Clin Pharmacol Ther* (2004) 76, 428–40.

Saw palmetto + Dextromethorphan

Saw palmetto does not appear to affect the metabolism of dextromethorphan.

Clinical evidence

In a study in 12 healthy subjects, saw palmetto 320 mg daily for 16 days, did not affect the metabolism of a single 30-mg dose of dextromethorphan given on day 14.[1]

Experimental evidence

No relevant data found.

Mechanism

Dextromethorphan is used as a probe substrate of the cytochrome P450 isoenzyme CYP2D6. Saw palmetto does not appear to inhibit this route of metabolism.

Importance and management

Evidence appears to be limited to the study cited, which suggests that saw palmetto is unlikely to raise dextromethorphan levels.

Dextromethorphan is used as a probe drug for CYP2D6 activity, and therefore these results also suggest that a pharmacokinetic interaction between saw palmetto and other CYP2D6 substrates is unlikely.

This finding is confirmed by a study using debrisoquine, see pharmacokinetics, page 415.

1. Markowitz JS, Donovan JL, DeVane L, Taylor RM, Ruan Y, Wang J-S, Chavin KD. Multiple doses of saw palmetto (*Serenoa repens*) did not alter cytochrome P450 2D6 and 3A4 activity in normal volunteers. *Clin Pharmacol Ther* (2003) 74, 536–42.

Saw palmetto + Food

No interactions found.

Saw palmetto + Herbal medicines

No interactions found.

S

Schisandra

Schisandra chinensis (Turcz.) K.Koch (Schisandraceae)

Synonym(s) and related species

Gomishi (Japanese), Magnolia vine, Wu-Wei-Zi (Chinese).

Kadsura chinensis Turcz. *Schisandra sphenanthera* Rehder & EH Wilson is often used with, or substituted for, *Schisandra chinensis*. Other species of *Schisandra* are also used medicinally in China.

Pharmacopoeias

Schisandra Fruit (*BP 2012, PhEur 7.5*).

Constituents

The major active components of the fruits of *Schisandra chinensis* are dibenzocyclooctene lignans. The identity and nomenclature is confusing, because when originally isolated by different researchers, the same compounds were given different names. The main groups of compounds are the **schisandrins** (schizandrins) and the **gomisins** (some of which were originally called wuweizu esters) and their derivatives. Schisandrin is also referred to in the literature as schisandrol A; gomisin A as schisandrol B; deoxyschisandrin as schisandrin A or wuweizu A; and schisantherin B as gomisin B or wuweizu B, for example. An essential oil contains borneol, 1,8-cineole, citral, sesquicarene and other monoterpenes. Extracts of *Schisandra sphenanthera* are reported to have a fairly similar chemical composition.

Use and indications

Schisandra is a very important herb in Chinese medicine. It is used as a tonic and restorative and considered to have liver-protecting, cardiotonic, hypotensive, immunomodulating, expectorant, hypnotic and sedative effects. It is used in the treatment of asthma, hyper-proliferative and inflammatory skin diseases, night sweats, urinary disorders, chronic diarrhoea, insomnia and many other conditions.

Pharmacokinetics

The effects of extracts of schisandra on cytochrome P450 isoenzymes are reasonably well studied. The gomisins B, C, G, and N and γ-schisandrin have all demonstrated inhibition of CYP3A4 *in vitro*. Gomisin C was the most potent and competitive inhibitor and was even stronger than that of ketoconazole. It has also been suggested that gomisin C also irreversibly inactivates CYP3A4.[1] In contrast, schisandrol B [gomisin A], schisandrin A and schisandrin B [gomisin B] induced CYP3A4 in another *in vitro* study.[2] The conflicting effects found with gomisin B are unclear, but it has been suggested that due to confusion over the naming and identification of these compounds, studies may have been carried out with constituents with the same names but different structures.[3,4] Another suggestion for these contrasting effects is that schisandra may exert a biphasic effect on CYP3A, with inhibition occurring with the initial exposure, and induction following long-term use (see midazolam, page 420). Furthermore, the clinical effects of these extracts on CYP3A4 are unclear, as *in vitro* inhibition has not been replicated in *rats* in one study (see nifedipine, page 420), although one clinical study with the CYP3A4 probe substrate midazolam, page 420 did find clinically relevant CYP3A4 inhibition.

Schisandra may also induce the cytochrome P450 isoenzyme CYP2C9, see warfarin and related drugs, page 422.

In vitro studies using schisandrins A and B, schisandrols A and B [gomisin A] and schisantherin A [gomisin C], suggest that these constituents are inhibitors of P-glycoprotein,[3–8] although schisandrols A and B [gomisin A] had only weak effects in one study.[3]

It has also been demonstrated that schisandrins A and B, schisandrols A and B [gomisin A] and schisantherin A [gomisin C] are inhibitors of MDR1, which is a multidrug resistance-associated protein.[8,9]

A study in *rats* given schisandrin, an aqueous extract of *Schisandra chinensis,* or Sheng-Mai-San (a traditional Chinese medicine containing *Radix ginseng, Radix ophiopogonis* and *Fructus schisandrae*) found that schisandrin was detectable in the plasma after each preparation, but after the aqueous extract or Sheng-Mai-San were given, the half-life and AUC of schisandrin were greater than when schisandrin alone was given. It is therefore possible that components of these products could alter the metabolism of schisandrin.[10] This may be important when extrapolating the effects of multi-constituent herbal preparations to the use of schisandra.

Interactions overview

Schisandra may modestly induce the metabolism of warfarin, modestly increase the bioavailability of talinolol and midazolam, and greatly increase the absorption of tacrolimus, but it appears to have little effect on the metabolism of nifedipine. Bifendate, which is derived from schisandra, appears to cause a modest reduction in ciclosporin levels.

Interactions monographs

- Ciclosporin, page 420
- Food, page 420
- Herbal medicines, page 420
- Midazolam, page 420

1. Iwata H, Tezuka Y, Kadota S, Hiratsuka A, Watabe T. Identification and characterization of potent CYP3A4 inhibitors in Schisandra fruit extract. *Drug Metab Dispos* (2004) 32, 1351–8.
2. Mu Y, Zhang J, Zhang S, Zhou H-H, Toma D, Ren S, Huang L, Yaramus M, Baum A, Venkataramanan R, Xie W. Traditional Chinese medicines Wu Wei Zi (*Schisandra chinensis Baill*) and Gan Cao (*Glycyrrhiza uralensis Fisch*) activate pregnane X receptor and increase warfarin clearance in rats. *J Pharmacol Exp Ther* (2006) 316, 1369–77.
3. Pan Q, Lu Q, Zhang K, Hu X. Dibenzocyclooctadiene lignans: a class of novel inhibitors of P-glycoprotein. *Cancer Chemother Pharmacol* (2006) 58, 99–106.
4. Fong W-F, Wan C-K, Zhu G-Y, Chattopadhyay A, Dey S, Zhao Z, Shen X-L. Schisandrol A from *Schisandra chinensis* reverses P-glycoprotein-mediated multidrug resistance by affecting Pgp-substrate complexes. *Planta Med* (2007) 73, 212–20.
5. Qiangrong P, Wang T, Lu Q, Hu X. Schisandrin B - a novel inhibitor of P-glycoprotein. *Biochem Biophys Res Commun* (2005) 335, 406–11.
6. Yoo HH, Lee M, Lee MW, Lim SY, Shin J, Kim D-H. Effects of *Schisandra* lignans on P-glycoprotein-mediated drug efflux in human intestinal Caco-2 cells. *Planta Med* (2007) 73, 444–50.
7. Wan C-K, Zhu G-Y, Shen X-L, Chattopadhyay A, Dey S, Fong W-F. Gomisin A alters substrate interaction and reverses P-glycoprotein-mediated multidrug resistance in HepG2-DR cells. *Biochem Pharmacol* (2006) 72, 824–37.
8. Sun M, Xu X, Lu Q, Pan Q, Hu X. Schisandrin B: a dual inhibitor of P-glycoprotein and multidrug resistance-associated protein 1. *Cancer Lett* (2007) 246, 300–307.
9. Li L, Pan Q, Sun M, Lu Q, Hu X. Dibenzocyclooctadiene lignans - A class of novel inhibitors of multidrug resistance-associated protein 1. *Life Sci* (2007) 80, 741–8.
10. Xu M, Wang G, Xie H, Huang Q, Wang W, Jia Y. Pharmacokinetic comparisons of schizandrin after oral administration of schizandrin monomer, *Fructus Schisandrae* aqueous extract and Sheng-Mai-San to rats. *J Ethnopharmacol* (2008) 115, 483–8.

S

Schisandra + Ciclosporin

Two case reports suggest that bifendate, which is derived from schisandra, can cause a gradual fall in the serum levels of ciclosporin, and a modest reduction in ciclosporin levels was seen in one study in healthy subjects.

Clinical evidence

Two kidney transplant patients were successfully treated with ciclosporin and prednisolone for 30 months and 36 months. When they were given bifendate 75 mg daily for the treatment of chronic hepatitis, both of them had a gradual fall in their trough serum ciclosporin levels. The ciclosporin levels of the first patient fell from 97.7 nanograms/mL to 78 nanograms/mL at 4 weeks, and fell further, to 49 nanograms/mL, at 6 weeks. The other patient had a fall from 127.5 nanograms/mL to 70.5 nanograms/mL at 8 weeks and to 45 nanograms/mL at 16 weeks. The ciclosporin doses remained unchanged throughout, and despite the low serum levels that occurred, no graft rejection was seen. When the bifendate was stopped, ciclosporin levels gradually climbed again, at about the same rate as their decline, to about their former levels.[1] In a subsequent placebo-controlled study in 18 healthy subjects, bifendate 15 mg three times daily for 14 days decreased the AUC of ciclosporin by 10 to 38% after a single oral dose of ciclosporin, and increased the oral clearance by 10 to 32%.[2]

Experimental evidence

No relevant data found.

Mechanism

The reasons for this interaction are not understood. It is possible that bifendate, which is derived from schisandra, is acting as an inducer of the cytochrome P450 isoenzyme CYP3A4,[2] which is the major isoenzyme involved in ciclosporin metabolism.

Importance and management

The available information suggests that a modest interaction might occur between bifendate and ciclosporin, therefore it would be prudent to monitor the outcome, being alert for the need to increase the ciclosporin dose if bifendate is used. Bifendate is derived from schisandra therefore, until more is known, it might be wise to extend this caution to all herbal preparations containing *Schisandra* species. However, in contrast to the above data, studies suggest that extracts from *Schisandra sphenanthera* increase the levels of midazolam and tacrolimus, which are also substrates of CYP3A4, see Schisandra + Midazolam, below and Schisandra + Tacrolimus, page 421.

1. Kim YS, Kim DH, Kim DO, Lee BK, Kim KW, Park JN, Lee JC, Choi YS, Rim H. The effect of diphenyl-dimethyl-dicarboxylate on cyclosporine-A blood level in kidney transplants with chronic hepatitis. *Korean J Intern Med* (1997) 12, 67–9.
2. Zeng Y, He YJ, He FY, Fan L, Zhou HH. Effect of bifendate on the pharmacokinetics of cyclosporine in relation to the CYP3A4*18B genotype in healthy subjects. *Acta Pharmacol Sin* (2009) 30, 478–84.

Schisandra + Food

No interactions found.

Schisandra + Herbal medicines

No interactions found.

Schisandra + Midazolam

Schisandra appears to increase the bioavailability of oral midazolam. Experimental evidence suggests that the long-term use of schisandra may *reduce* the bioavailability of oral midazolam.

Clinical evidence

In a pharmacokinetic study, 12 healthy subjects were given a single 15-mg dose of oral midazolam before and after taking an extract of *Schisandra sphenanthera* (containing 33.75 mg of deoxyschisandrin) twice daily for 7 days. The extract of *Schisandra sphenanthera* increased the AUC and maximum plasma concentrations of midazolam by 105% and 65%, but did not alter its half-life.[1]

Experimental evidence

A study in *rats* reports that a single dose of schisandra lignan extract 150 mg/kg inhibited the metabolism of oral midazolam (AUC increased, clearance decreased), but did not affect the metabolism of intravenous midazolam.[2] In contrast, when schisandra lignan extract 150 mg/kg was given daily for 15 days to *rats,* the metabolism of oral midazolam was induced (AUC reduced, clearance increased).[2]

Mechanism

The authors of the clinical study suggest that the hepatic and/or intestinal metabolism of midazolam, which is a substrate of the cytochrome P450 isoenzyme CYP3A4, may have been inhibited by schisandra.[1] The study in *rats* suggests that schisandra exerts more of an effect on intestinal CYP3A, and may have a biphasic effect, with inhibition occurring after a single dose, and induction occurring after long-term use.[2]

Importance and management

Clinical evidence for an interaction between schisandra and midazolam comes from one study, which suggests that schisandra may inhibit the metabolism of midazolam. Concurrent use would be expected to result in increased exposure to midazolam, possibly leading to increased and prolonged sedation, although this effect was not studied. If schisandra is given to a patient taking midazolam, it may be prudent to be alert for increased sedative effects, and decrease the dose of midazolam if these become troublesome.

The study in *rats* suggests that schisandra may *induce* CYP3A when given long-term. Although the doses used were much larger than those used clinically, until more is known, if concurrent use is continued it would seem prudent to be alert for a subsequent reduction in the effects of midazolam.

Midazolam is used as a probe drug for CYP3A4 activity, and therefore these results also suggest that a pharmacokinetic interaction between schisandra and other CYP3A4 substrates is possible. See Drugs and herbs affecting or metabolised by the cytochrome P450 isoenzyme CYP3A4, page 7, for a list of known CYP3A4 substrates.

1. Xin H-W, Wu X-C, Li Q, Yu A-R, Xiong L. Effects of *Schisandra sphenanthera* extract on the pharmacokinetics of midazolam in healthy volunteers. *Br J Clin Pharmacol* (2009) 67, 541–6.
2. Lai L, Hao H, Wang Q, Zheng C, Zhou F, Liu Y, Wang Y, Yu G, Kang A, Peng Y, Wang G, Chen X. Effects of short-term and long-term pretreatment of *Schisandra* lignans on regulating hepatic and intestinal CYP3A in rats. *Drug Metab Dispos* (2009) 37, 2399–2407.

Schisandra + Nifedipine

The interaction between schisandra and nifedipine is based on experimental evidence only.

Clinical evidence

No interactions found.

Experimental evidence

In a single-dose study, *rats* were given nifedipine 2-mg/kg 30 minutes after a 50-mg/kg dose of Shoseiryuto. The effects of Shoseiryuto were also studied *in vitro* in *rats*. Although the *in vitro* study found that Shoseiryuto inhibited CYP3A4, the study in *rats* found that the pharmacokinetics of nifedipine were not affected by the preparation. Shoseiryuto contains schisandra fruit, ephedra herb, cinnamon bark, peony root, processed ginger, asiasarum root, pinellia tuber, and glycyrrhiza.[1]

Mechanism

Schisandra has been shown *in vitro* to have an inhibitory effect on the cytochrome P450 isoenzyme CYP3A4, which is involved in the metabolism of nifedipine. This *animal* study does not support the *in vitro* findings.

Importance and management

Evidence appears to be restricted to experimental studies involving *rats,* and the findings, which cannot be directly extrapolated to humans, suggest that the *in vitro* effects do not seem to be clinically relevant *in vivo*. Because of the nature of the evidence, it is difficult to make recommendations on the concurrent use of nifedipine and Shoseiryuto until human studies are conducted; however, a clinically relevant interaction appears unlikely.

1. Makino T, Mizuno F, Mizukami H. Does a Kampo medicine containing schisandra fruit affect pharmacokinetics of nifedipine like grapefruit juice? *Biol Pharm Bull* (2006) 29, 2065–9.

Schisandra + Tacrolimus

Schisandra greatly increases tacrolimus levels.

Clinical evidence

In a pharmacokinetic study, 12 healthy subjects were given an extract of *Schisandra sphenanthera* (containing 33.75 mg deoxyschisandrin) twice daily for 14 days, with a single 2-mg oral dose of tacrolimus on day 14. The extract of *Schisandra sphenanthera* increased the AUC and maximum plasma concentrations of tacrolimus by 164% and 227%, but did not alter its half-life. Six of the 12 subjects experienced indigestion, and burning hands and feet, one hour after both medicines were given. These symptoms resolved over 10 hours.[1] In a further study, when 46 liver transplant patients were given an oral dose of tacrolimus with an extract of *Schisandra sphenanthera* (deoxyschisandrin 23 mg) the tacrolimus blood concentrations were increased approximately 4-fold. Further pharmacokinetic analysis in 14 of the patients established that the oral bioavailability of tacrolimus was increased just over 3-fold. Despite these findings, the adverse effects of tacrolimus (liver function (ALT and AST), diarrhoea, agitation) were said to be improved.[2]

A case study describes a 42-year-old man taking tacrolimus 8 mg daily (recently increased from 6 mg daily) after a liver transplant. Because of a low tacrolimus concentration (2.3 nanograms/mL), accompanied by diarrhoea and a raised ALT level he was admitted to hospital, and was started on deoxyschisandrin 22.5 mg after meals, in an attempt to improve his liver function. After 3 days his ALT had decreased and the diarrhoea had resolved; however, his tacrolimus level was found to be 17.7 nanograms/mL. After successive tacrolimus dose decreases he was stabilised on a dose of 4 mg daily, with a tacrolimus level of 10.7 nanograms/mL.[3]

Experimental evidence

Because of the quality of the clinical evidence (controlled pharmacokinetic studies), experimental data have not been sought.

Mechanism

Not established. P-glycoprotein is involved in the intestinal absorption of tacrolimus. It is therefore possible that the inhibition of P-glycoprotein by schisandrin, and possibly other related compounds, may have resulted in increased absorption of tacrolimus.[4] In addition, it has been suggested that the metabolism of tacrolimus, which is a substrate of the cytochrome P450 isoenzyme CYP3A4, may have been inhibited by schisandrin.[1]

Importance and management

An interaction between schisandra and tacrolimus seems established, although the mechanism is not fully elucidated. Concurrent use appears to result in a large rise in tacrolimus levels, which would be expected to be accompanied by an increase in tacrolimus adverse effects, although not all studies have found this. If the use of both medicines is considered desirable it would seem prudent to monitor the outcome of concurrent use closely, adjusting the tacrolimus dose as necessary. It is important to note that, although the schisandra products used in the studies were standardised for schisandrin content, this constituent has not been established as the cause of the interaction. Therefore the extent of the interaction may vary between different schisandra products, and different batches of the same schisandra product. This may make this interaction difficult to standardise for, and therefore it may be prudent to avoid concurrent use where tacrolimus blood levels are critical, such as in organ transplantation.

1. Xin H-W, Wu X-C, Li Q, Yu A-R, Zhu M, Shen Y, Su D, Xiong L. Effects of *Schisandra sphenanthera* extract on the pharmacokinetics of tacrolimus in healthy volunteers. *Br J Clin Pharmacol* (2007) 64, 469–75.
2. Jiang W, Wang X, Xu X, Kong L. Effect of *Schisandra sphenanthera* extract on the concentration of tacrolimus in the blood of liver transplant patients *Int J Clin Pharmacol Ther* (2010) 48, 224–9.
3. Jiang W, Wang X, Kong L. The effect of deoxyschisandrin on blood tacrolimus levels: a case report. *Immunopharmacol Immunotoxicol* (2010) 32, 177–8.
4. Qin XL, Bi HC, Wang XD, Li JL, Wang Y, Xue XP, Chen X, Wang CX, Xu LJ, Wang YT, Huang M. Mechanistic understanding of the different effects of Wuzhi tablet (*Schisandra sphenanthera* extract) on the absorption and first-pass intestinal and hepatic metabolism of tacrolimus (FK506) *Int J Pharmaceutics* (2010) 389, 114–21.

Schisandra + Talinolol

Bifendate, which is derived from schisandra, causes a minor reduction in the bioavailability of talinolol, whereas schisandra modestly increases the bioavailability of talinolol.

Clinical evidence

(a) Bifendate

In a crossover study, 16 healthy subjects took bifendate 15 mg or a placebo three times daily for 14 days, and a single 100-mg dose of talinolol on day 15. Bifendate slightly reduced the AUC and maximum plasma levels of talinolol by 11% and 10%, respectively, with no effect on the elimination half-life.[1]

(b) Schisandra

In a study, 12 healthy subjects took a single 100-mg dose of talinolol alone, or after taking a standardised schisandra extract 300 mg (containing 16.85 mg deoxyschisandrin) twice daily for 14 days. The AUC and maximum plasma level of talinolol were modestly increased by 52% and 51%, respectively, with little effect on the elimination half-life.[2]

Experimental evidence

Deoxyschisandrin (schisandrin A) has been found to inhibit P-glycoprotein *in vitro*, see *pharmacokinetics,* page 418.

Mechanism

Uncertain. Talinolol is a known substrate of the efflux transporter P-glycoprotein, and possibly also multidrug resistance-protein 2 (MRP2) and the uptake transporter, organic anion transporting protein (OATP).[1,2] Bifendate is derived from schisandra, but they appear to have different effects on talinolol exposure, with bifendate causing a small decrease and schisandra causing a modest increase. Schisandra may have greater inhibitory effects on the efflux transporters, which results in a net increase in talinolol absorption.[2]

Importance and management

The studies of the effects of bifendate and schisandra on talinolol disposition were conducted to assess drug interaction mechanisms. Nevertheless, the study with bifendate shows that it causes only a minor reduction in the AUC and maximum plasma levels of talinolol, which is not considered to be clinically relevant. The effects of schisandra on the bioavailability of talinolol are greater than those of bifendate. Nevertheless the effects are only modest and although the clinical relevance of the effects of schisandra is less certain, it also seems likely to be small.

1. Zeng Y, He F-Y, He Y-J, Dai L-L, Fan L, Zhou H-H. Effect of bifendate on the pharmacokinetics of talinolol in healthy subjects. *Xenobiotica* (2009) 39, 844–9.
2. Fan L, Mao X-Q, Tao G-Y, Wang G, Jiang F, Chen Y, Li Q, Zhang W, Lei H-P, Hu D-L, Huang Y-F, Wang D, Zhou H-H. Effect of *Schisandra chinensis* extract and *Ginkgo biloba* extract on the pharmacokinetics of talinolol in healthy volunteers. *Xenobiotica* (2009) 39, 249–54.

Schisandra + Warfarin and related drugs

The interaction between schisandra and warfarin is based on experimental evidence only.

Clinical evidence

No interactions found.

Experimental evidence

In a study in *rats,* pretreatment with schisandra aqueous extract 500 mg/kg daily by gastric lavage for 6 days, reduced the AUC of a single 2-mg/kg dose of intravenous **warfarin** by 29%, and increased warfarin clearance by 37%. The half-life of **warfarin** was also reduced from 13.1 hours to 11.6 hours.[1]

Mechanism

The authors of the study suggest that schisandra increases the metabolism of warfarin by inducing the cytochrome P450 isoenzyme CYP2C9, the most important isoenzyme involved in the metabolism of warfarin.[1]

Importance and management

Evidence is limited to this one experimental study in *rats,* which suggests that schisandra extracts may modestly increase the metabolism of warfarin. If similar effects occur in humans there may be a slight decrease in the anticoagulant effects of warfarin, although note that a decrease in the AUC of 29% is fairly modest and only small effects would be expected. If schisandra extracts are given to any patient taking warfarin, it may be prudent to consider monitoring the INR within the first week of treatment, if this is not already planned. All coumarin anticoagulants are metabolised by CYP2C9 to a greater or lesser extent, and therefore they may interact similarly. It would seem prudent to use similar precautions if these drugs are given with schisandra.

1. Mu Y, Zhang J, Zhang S, Zhou H-H, Toma D, Ren S, Huang L, Yaramus M, Baum A, Venkataramanan R, Xie W. Traditional Chinese medicines Wu Wei Zi (*Schisandra chinensis Baill*) and Gan Cao (*Glycyrrhiza uralensis Fisch*) activate pregnane X receptor and increase warfarin clearance in rats. *J Pharmacol Exp Ther* (2006) 316, 1369–77.

S

Senna

Cassia senna L., *Cassia angustifolia* Vahl (Fabaceae)

Synonym(s) and related species

Indian senna.

Cassia acutifolia Delile, *Senna alexandrina* Mill.

Senna obtained from *Cassia senna* is also known as Alexandrian senna or Khartoum senna, and senna obtained from *Cassia angustifolia* is also known as Tinnevelly senna.

Pharmacopoeias

Alexandrian Senna Fruit (*BP 2012*); Senna Fluidextract (*USP35–NF30 S1*); Senna Leaf (*BP 2012, PhEur 7.5, USP35–NF30 S1*); Senna Liquid Extract (*BP 2012*); Senna Oral Solution (*USP35–NF30 S1*); Senna Pods (*USP35–NF30 S1*); Senna Pods, Alexandrian (*PhEur 7.5*); Senna Pods, Tinnevelly (*PhEur 7.5*); Senna Tablets (*BP 2012*); Sennosides (*USP35–NF30 S1*); Standardised Senna Granules (*BP 2012*); Standardised Senna Leaf Dry Extract (*BP 2012, PhEur 7.5*); Tinnevelly Senna Fruit (*BP 2012*).

Constituents

Anthraquinone glycosides are major components of senna. In the leaf the anthraquinones include sennosides A, B, C and D and palmidin A, rhein anthrone and aloe-emodin glycosides. The fruit contains sennosides A and B and a closely related glycoside, sennoside A1. Senna is usually standardised to the content of sennosides, generally calculated as sennoside B.

Senna also contains naphthalene glycosides in the leaves and pods, mucilage (arabinose, galactose, galacturonic acid) and various other constituents such as **flavonoids**, volatile oil and resins.

Use and indications

Senna leaf or fruit is used as a laxative.

Pharmacokinetics

For information on the pharmacokinetics of an anthraquinone glycoside present in senna, see under aloes, page 27.

Interactions overview

Although senna has been predicted to interact with a number of drugs that lower potassium (such as the corticosteroids and potassium-depleting diuretics), or drugs where the effects become potentially harmful when potassium is lowered (such as digoxin) there appears to be little or no direct evidence that this occurs in practice. Senna may slightly reduce quinidine levels.

Interactions monographs

- Corticosteroids, page 424
- Digitalis glycosides, page 424
- Diuretics; Potassium-depleting, page 424
- Estradiol, page 424
- Food, page 425
- Herbal medicines; Liquorice, page 425
- Ketoprofen, page 425
- Paracetamol (Acetaminophen), page 425
- Propranolol, page 425
- Quinidine, page 425
- Verapamil, page 426

S

Senna + Corticosteroids

Theoretically, the risk of hypokalaemia might be increased in patients taking corticosteroids, who also regularly use, or abuse, anthraquinone-containing substances such as senna.

Clinical evidence

Chronic diarrhoea as a result of long-term use, or abuse, of stimulant laxatives such as senna can cause excessive water and potassium loss; one paper (cited as an example) describes a number of cases of this.[1] Systemic corticosteroids with mineralocorticoid effects can cause water retention and potassium loss. The effect of senna over-use combined with systemic corticosteroids is not known, but, theoretically at least, the risk of hypokalaemia might be increased. Although this is mentioned in some reviews on herbal interactions[2] there do not appear to be any case reports of such an interaction.

It has also been suggested that senna, by increasing gastrointestinal transit times, might theoretically reduce the absorption of oral corticosteroids.[2] However, there appears to be no published clinical data suggesting that the absorption of corticosteroids is affected by senna or other drugs that alter gastrointestinal transit time, such as metoclopramide or loperamide.

Experimental evidence

No relevant data found.

Mechanism

In theory the additive loss of potassium caused by anthraquinone-containing substances and systemic corticosteroids, may result in hypokalaemia.

Importance and management

The interaction between senna and corticosteroids is theoretical, but be aware of the potential in patients who regularly use, or abuse, anthraquinone-containing substances such as senna. However, note that if anthraquinone laxatives are used as recommended (at a dose producing a comfortable soft-formed motion), then this interaction would not be expected to be clinically relevant.

1. Cummings JH, Sladen GE, James OFW, Sarner M, Misiewicz JJ. Laxative-induced diarrhoea: a continuing clinical problem. *BMJ* (1974) 1, 537–41.
2. Abebe W. An overview of herbal supplement utilization with particular emphasis on possible interactions with dental drugs and oral manifestations. *J Dent Hyg* (2003) 77, 37–46.

Senna + Digitalis glycosides

Theoretically, digitalis toxicity could develop if patients regularly use, or abuse, anthraquinone-containing substances such as senna.

Clinical evidence

For the risk of digitalis toxicity including cardiac arrhythmias because of hypokalaemia induced by abuse of anthraquinone laxatives, see Aloes + Digitalis glycosides, page 28. For mention of a case of **digoxin** toxicity and mild hypokalaemia in a patient taking **digoxin** and furosemide, who started to take a laxative containing *rhubarb* and *liquorice,* see Liquorice + Digitalis glycosides, page 331.

Experimental evidence

The effects of anthraquinones found in senna (rhein 100 micromoles, danthron 100 micromoles, sennidins A and B, sennosides A and B), and senna leaf infusion (senna tea) 10 mg/mL, on the absorption of **digoxin** was examined in human cell lines.[1] Rhein and danthron decreased the absorptive permeability of **digoxin**, whereas the other anthraquinones and the senna leaf infusion had no effect.

Mechanism

Little understood. Digoxin is a substrate of P-glycoprotein, a drug transporter protein, and it is thought that the relatively small molecular size of rhein and danthron alter the fluidity of the apical membrane and interfere with the action of P-glycoprotein.[1]

Importance and management

Determining the clinical relevance of the *in vitro* absorption study results is difficult. The authors suggest that an effect of anthraquinone-containing laxatives on the absorption of poorly permeable drugs such as digoxin cannot be excluded. More study is required before any clinical recommendations can be made.

1. Laitinen L, Takala E, Vuorela H, Vuorela P, Kaukonen AM, Marvola M. Anthranoid laxatives influence the absorption of poorly permeable drugs in human intestinal cell culture model (Caco-2). *Eur J Pharm Biopharm* (2007) 66, 135–45.

Senna + Diuretics; Potassium-depleting

Theoretically, patients taking potassium-depleting diuretics could experience excessive potassium loss if they also regularly use, or abuse, anthraquinone-containing substances such as senna.

Clinical evidence

For information on the additive risk of hypokalaemia with the use of potassium-depleting diuretics and abuse of anthraquinone-containing laxatives. See Aloes + Diuretics; Potassium-depleting, page 28.

Experimental evidence

The effects of the anthraquinones found in senna (rhein, danthron, sennidins A and B, sennosides A and B), and senna leaf infusion (senna tea), on the absorption of **furosemide** 100 micromoles, a poorly permeable drug, was examined in human cell lines.[1] Rhein and danthron increased the absorptive permeability of **furosemide** by about 3.6- and 3-fold, respectively. **Furosemide** permeability was reduced by more than a third by the sennidins and sennosides, but senna leaf infusion had little effect.

Mechanism

Little understood. The changes in furosemide absorptive permeability may be caused by interference with P-glycoprotein or other transporter proteins.[1]

Importance and management

Determining the clinical relevance of the *in vitro* absorption results is difficult. The authors suggest that an effect of anthraquinone-containing laxatives on the absorption of poorly permeable drugs such as furosemide cannot be excluded. More study is required before any clinical recommendations can be made.

1. Laitinen L, Takala E, Vuorela H, Vuorela P, Kaukonen AM, Marvola M. Anthranoid laxatives influence the absorption of poorly permeable drugs in human intestinal cell culture model (Caco-2). *Eur J Pharm Biopharm* (2007) 66, 135–45.

Senna + Estradiol

Senna does not appear to affect the pharmacokinetics of estradiol.

Clinical evidence

In a clinical study in 19 women, the maximum daily tolerated dose of senna tablets (*Senokot*) was taken for 10 to 12 days with a single 1.5-mg dose of estradiol glucuronide given 4 days before the end of the assessment period. Senna had no significant effect on the median AUC of estradiol or estrone.[1]

Experimental evidence

No relevant data found.

Mechanism

It was thought that reducing intestinal transit time with senna might lead to reduced blood levels of estradiol.

Importance and management

Limited evidence suggests that there is unlikely to be a clinically relevant pharmacokinetic interaction between anthraquinone-containing laxatives and estradiol.

1. Lewis SJ, Oakey RE, Heaton KW. Intestinal absorption of oestrogen: the effect of altering transit-time. *Eur J Gastroenterol Hepatol* (1998) 10, 33–9.

Senna + Food

No interactions found.

Senna + Herbal medicines; Liquorice

Consider Liquorice + Laxatives, page 332, for the potential additive effects of anthraquinone-containing laxatives and liquorice.

Senna + Ketoprofen

The interaction between senna and ketoprofen is based on experimental evidence only.

Clinical evidence

No interactions found.

Experimental evidence

The effects of the anthraquinones found in senna (rhein, danthron, sennidins A and B, sennosides A and B), and senna leaf infusion (senna tea), on the absorption of ketoprofen 100 micromoles was examined in human cell lines.[1] Danthron reduced the absorptive permeability of ketoprofen by almost 30% and the senna leaf infusion enhanced ketoprofen permeability by about 1.5-fold.

Mechanism

Little understood. The reduction in absorptive permeability of ketoprofen caused by danthron may be due to reduced ATP production in the cells. The enhanced permeability caused by senna leaf infusion is more difficult to explain because of the many different active compounds contained within the extract.[1]

Importance and management

Evidence is sparse, but what is known suggests that the use of anthraquinone-containing laxatives is unlikely to affect the intestinal permeability of ketoprofen.

1. Laitinen L, Takala E, Vuorela H, Vuorela P, Kaukonen AM, Marvola M. Anthranoid laxatives influence the absorption of poorly permeable drugs in human intestinal cell culture model (Caco-2). *Eur J Pharm Biopharm* (2007) 66, 135–45.

Senna + Paracetamol (Acetaminophen)

The information regarding the use of senna with paracetamol is based on experimental evidence only.

Clinical evidence

No interactions found.

Experimental evidence

The effects of the anthraquinones found in senna (rhein, danthron, sennidins A and B, sennosides A and B), and senna leaf infusion (senna tea), on the absorption of paracetamol 100 micromoles was examined in human cell lines.[1] The *in vitro* absorption of highly permeable drugs such as paracetamol was not significantly altered.

Mechanism

No mechanism expected.

Importance and management

Evidence is sparse, but what is known suggests that the use of anthraquinone-containing laxatives is unlikely to affect the intestinal permeability of paracetamol (acetaminophen).

1. Laitinen L, Takala E, Vuorela H, Vuorela P, Kaukonen AM, Marvola M. Anthranoid laxatives influence the absorption of poorly permeable drugs in human intestinal cell culture model (Caco-2). *Eur J Pharm Biopharm* (2007) 66, 135–45.

Senna + Propranolol

The information regarding the use of senna with propranolol is based on experimental evidence only.

Clinical evidence

No interactions found.

Experimental evidence

The effects of the anthraquinones found in senna (rhein, danthron, sennidins A and B, sennosides A and B), and senna leaf infusion (senna tea), on the absorption of propranolol 100 micromoles was examined in human cell lines.[1] The *in vitro* absorption of highly permeable drugs such as propranolol was not significantly altered.

Mechanism

No mechanism expected.

Importance and management

Evidence is sparse, but what is known suggests that the use of anthraquinone-containing laxatives seems unlikely to affect the intestinal permeability of propranolol.

1. Laitinen L, Takala E, Vuorela H, Vuorela P, Kaukonen AM, Marvola M. Anthranoid laxatives influence the absorption of poorly permeable drugs in human intestinal cell culture model (Caco-2). *Eur J Pharm Biopharm* (2007) 66, 135–45.

Senna + Quinidine

Quinidine plasma levels can be reduced by the anthraquinone-containing laxative senna.

Clinical evidence

In a study in 7 patients with cardiac arrhythmias taking sustained-release quinidine bisulfate 500 mg every 12 hours, senna reduced plasma quinidine levels, measured 12 hours after the last dose of quinidine, by about 25%.[1]

Experimental evidence

No relevant data found.

Mechanism

Not understood.

Importance and management

The modest reduction in quinidine levels might be of clinical importance in patients whose plasma levels are barely adequate to control their arrhythmia.

1. Guckenbiehl W, Gilfrich HJ, Just H. Einfluß von Laxantien und Metoclopramid auf die Chindin-Plasmakonzentration während Langzeittherapie bei Patienten mit Herzrhythmusstörugen. *Med Welt* (1976) 27, 1273–6.

Senna + Verapamil

The information regarding the use of senna with verapamil is based on experimental evidence only.

Clinical evidence

No interactions found.

Experimental evidence

The effects of the anthraquinones found in senna (rhein, danthron, sennidins A and B, sennosides A and B) and senna leaf infusion (senna tea), on the absorption of verapamil 100 micromoles was examined in human cell lines.[1] The *in vitro* absorption of highly permeable drugs such as verapamil was not significantly altered.

Mechanism

No mechanism expected.

Importance and management

Evidence is sparse, but what is known suggests that the use of anthraquinone-containing laxatives seems unlikely to affect the intestinal permeability of verapamil.

1. Laitinen L, Takala E, Vuorela H, Vuorela P, Kaukonen AM, Marvola M. Anthranoid laxatives influence the absorption of poorly permeable drugs in human intestinal cell culture model (Caco-2). *Eur J Pharm Biopharm* (2007) 66, 135–45.

S

Shatavari

Asparagus racemosus Willd. (Asparagaceae)

Synonym(s) and related species

Wild asparagus. Not to be confused with asparagus, page 48, which is *Asparagus officinalis,* the species used as a food.

Constituents

The root and rhizome of shatavari contain a series of steroidal saponins, the shatavarins and others, based on sarsapogenin, diosgenin and arasapogenin. The polycyclic alkaloid asparagamine A; benzofurans such as racemofuran and racemosol; and the **isoflavone** 8-methoxy-5, 6, 4'-trihydroxyisoflavone 7-O-beta-D-glucopyranoside are also present.

Use and indications

Shatavari is widely used in Ayurvedic medicine for dealing with problems related to women's fertility, loss of libido, threatened miscarriage, menopausal problems and to increase the flow of breast milk. It is also reported to be antispasmodic, aphrodisiac, demulcent, diuretic, anti-diarrhoeal, antirheumatic and antidiabetic. Some of these indications are supported by pharmacological (but little clinical) evidence.

Pharmacokinetics

No relevant pharmacokinetic data found.

Interactions overview

Shatavari may have additive effects with conventional antidiabetic drugs, and may alter the absorption of a number of drugs by delaying gastric emptying. Shatavari contains phytoestrogens and therefore has the potential to be antagonistic or synergistic with oestrogens or oestrogen antagonists.

Interactions monographs

- Antidiabetics, page 428
- Food, page 428
- Herbal medicines, page 428
- Miscellaneous, page 428
- Oestrogens or Oestrogen antagonists, page 428

S

Shatavari + Antidiabetics

The interaction between shatavari and antidiabetics is based on experimental evidence only.

Evidence, mechanism, importance and management

In pharmacological studies, shatavari extracts have been shown to lower blood-glucose and stimulate insulin secretion. In one *in vitro* study, the insulin stimulatory effect of various extracts and partition fractions of shatavari was potentiated by **tolbutamide**.[1] This suggests that shatavari might have some antidiabetic effects; this is in line with one of its traditional uses as an antidiabetic. The evidence is too slim to say whether a clinically important effect is likely for usual preparations of the herb, but an additive antidiabetic effect with conventional medicines for diabetes seems possible. Bear this information in mind in the event of an unexpected response to treatment.

1. Hannan JMA, Marenah L, Ali L, Rokeya B, Flatt PR, Abdel-Wahab YH. Insulin secretory actions of extracts of *Asparagus racemosus* root in perfused pancreas, isolated islets and clonal pancreatic β-cells. *J Endocrinol* (2007) 192, 159–68.

Shatavari + Food

No interactions found.

Shatavari + Herbal medicines

No interactions found.

Shatavari + Miscellaneous

Limited evidence suggests that shatavari increases the gastric emptying rate similarly to metoclopramide, which is known to decrease the absorption of atovaquone, digoxin and ketoprofen, and increase the absorption of ciclosporin, dantrolene, morphine and paracetamol (acetaminophen). Shatavari has the potential to interact similarly.

Evidence, mechanism, importance and management

In a crossover study in 8 healthy subjects,[1] powdered root of shatavari 2 g reduced the gastric emptying half-life from a mean baseline of about 160 minutes to 101 minutes after two radio-labelled jam sandwiches were eaten. This was similar to the effect of a single 10-mg dose of oral metoclopramide (85 minutes). If shatavari increases the gastric emptying rate, it has the potential to increase or decrease the absorption of other drugs that are taken concurrently. Metoclopramide is known to have this effect and modestly decreases the absorption of **atovaquone**, **digoxin** and **ketoprofen**, and increases the absorption of **ciclosporin**, **dantrolene**, **morphine** and **paracetamol (acetaminophen)**. Based on the limited evidence presented, it is possible that shatavari might interact similarly. Until more is known, some caution might be appropriate; however, note that, with the exception of **atovaquone**, in most cases the interactions of metoclopramide with these drugs are of limited clinical importance.

1. Dalvi SS, Nadkarni PM, Gupta KC. Effect of Asparagus racemosus (Shatavari) on gastric emptying time in normal healthy volunteers. *J Postgrad Med* (1990) 36, 91–4.

Shatavari + Oestrogens or Oestrogen antagonists

The interaction between shatavari and oestrogens or oestrogen antagonists is based on a prediction only.

Evidence, mechanism, importance and management

Shatavari contains phytoestrogens and has been investigated in a variety of pharmacological and clinical studies for its effect on lactation, dysfunctional uterine bleeding, pre-menstrual syndrome and menopausal symptoms; this has been the subject of a review.[1] Based on these studies, a cautious approach would be to recommend care when combining shatavari with conventional oestrogenic drugs or oestrogen antagonists such as **tamoxifen**, because it is unknown whether the effects might be antagonistic or synergistic (or indeed, not clinically relevant). For further discussion of this subject, see Isoflavones + Tamoxifen, page 304.

1. Bopana N, Saxena S. *Asparagus racemosus* – ethnopharmacological evaluation and conservation needs. *J Ethnopharmacol* (2007) 110, 1–15.

S

Skullcap

Scutellaria lateriflora L. (Lamiaceae)

Synonym(s) and related species

Helmet flower, Hoodwort, Quaker bonnet, Scullcap, Scutellaria.

Constituents

The major active components of skullcap are the **flavonoids** scutellarin, scutellarein, baicalein, baicalin (the glucuronide of baicalein), dihydrobaicalin, apigenin, luteolin, and other methoxyflavones. The iridoid catalpol, and gamma amino benzoic acid (GABA) have also been found and there is a small amount of essential oil present composed of monoterpenes and sesquiterpenes.

Use and indications

Skullcap has been used traditionally as a sedative and to treat nervous disorders. Previous reports about its possible toxicity have been found to be because of contamination with *Teucrium* species; skullcap itself is now considered to be safe to use.

Pharmacokinetics

No relevant pharmacokinetic data found for skullcap, but see flavonoids, page 213, for information on individual flavonoids present in the herb.

Interactions overview

No interactions with skullcap found, but for information on the interactions of individual flavonoids present in skullcap, see under flavonoids, page 213.

S

Soya

Glycine max (L.) Merr. (Fabaceae)

Synonym(s) and related species

Soy.

Glycine soja Siebold and Zucc.

Pharmacopoeias

Hydrogenated Soya Oil (*BP 2012*); Hydrogenated Soy(a-)bean Oil (*PhEur 7.5, USP35–NF30 S1*); Powdered Soy Isoflavones Extract (*USP35–NF30 S1*); Refined Soya Oil (*BP 2012*); Soybean Oil (*USP35–NF30 S1*); Soya-bean Oil, Refined (*PhEur 7.5*); Soy Isoflavones Capsules (*USP35–NF30 S1*); Soy Isoflavones Tablets (*USP35–NF30 S1*).

Constituents

The **isoflavones** in soya beans consist mainly of **genistein** and **daidzein**, with smaller amounts of isoformononetin, ononin, glycetin, desmethyltexasin and others. They are present mainly as glycosides, and the amount varies between the different soya products. Soya beans also contain **coumestans** (mainly in the sprouts) and **phytosterols**. The fixed oil from soya beans contains linoleic and linolenic acids.

Fermented soya products contain variable amounts of tyramine.

Use and indications

Soya is a widely used food, particularly in Japanese and Chinese cuisine. Flour and protein from the beans are used as tofu and as a substitute for meat. Fermented products include soy sauce, natto and miso, and these can contain high concentrations of the isoflavones. Soya milk is used as a substitute for individuals who are allergic to cow's milk, including in infant formula. Edamame beans are soya beans eaten while still green.

There are numerous purported benefits of soya protein, the most well-studied being possible reductions in hyperlipidaemia, menopausal symptoms and osteoporosis, and prevention of some cancers. Epidemiological studies suggest that a diet with a high intake of soya might protect against breast cancer.[1] Numerous randomised clinical studies show a small benefit for soya protein on blood lipids (which is probably independent of isoflavone content),[2,3] and there is also evidence of a modest benefit in patients with diabetes.[4] Soya protein and the isoflavone fraction have also shown some benefits for menopausal symptoms[5] and postmenopausal osteoporosis[6] in some studies. One paper notes that many of the demonstrable actions of isoflavones in soya are attributed to the aglycones genistein and daidzein, however these occur in negligible amounts unless the product has been fermented.[7] For further information on the individual isoflavones present in soya, see isoflavones, page 300. Despite numerous studies and meta-analyses, the health benefits of soya have not been conclusively proven and remain controversial. In a 2006 analysis, the American Heart Advisory Committee concluded that the main benefit of a soya-based diet probably relates to its high content of polyunsaturated fats and fibre and low content of saturated fat.[8]

Pharmacokinetics

In healthy subjects, a soya extract did not induce the cytochrome P450 isoenzyme CYP3A4.[9] *In vitro,* soya bean products and a hydrolysed soya extract, as well as the soya isoflavones daidzein and genistein, inhibited CYP3A4,[9,10] and CYP2C9.[9] However, in one of these studies,[10] St John's wort also inhibited CYP3A4, but clinically this herb is known to be an inducer of CYP3A4. This highlights the problems of extrapolating the findings of *in vitro* studies to clinical situations.[9] Soya-based infant formulas (as well as cow-milk infant formulas) induced CYP1A2 *in vitro* see caffeine, page 432).

The pharmacokinetics of the isoflavone constituents of soya are further discussed under isoflavones, page 300.

Interactions overview

Soya products may increase the metabolism of caffeine and reduce the absorption of levothyroxine. Fermented soya bean products contain high levels of tyramine and vitamin K and may therefore cause hypertensive reactions with MAOIs, and decrease the activity of warfarin and related anticoagulants.

Potential interactions of isoflavone constituents of soya are covered under isoflavones; see antibacterials, page 302, nicotine, page 303, paclitaxel, page 303, tamoxifen, page 304, and theophylline, page 305.

Interactions monographs

- Caffeine, page 432
- Food, page 432
- Herbal medicines, page 432
- Levothyroxine and related drugs, page 432
- MAOIs or RIMAs, page 432
- Warfarin and related drugs, page 433

1. Trock BJ, Hilakivi-Clarke L, Clarke R. Meta-analysis of soy intake and breast cancer risk. *J Natl Cancer Inst* (2006) 98, 459–71.
2. Anderson JW, Johnstone BM, Cook-Newell ME. Meta-analysis of the effects of soy protein intake on serum lipids. *N Engl J Med* (1995) 333, 276–82.

3. Dewell A, Hollenbeck PLW, Hollenbeck CB. Clinical review: a critical evaluation of the role of soy protein and isoflavone supplementation in the control of plasma cholesterol concentrations. *J Clin Endocrinol Metab* (2006) 91, 772–80.
4. Bhathena SJ, Velasquez MT. Beneficial role of dietary phytoestrogens in obesity and diabetes. *Am J Clin Nutr* (2002) 76, 1191–1201.
5. Nelson HD, Vesco KK, Haney E, Fu R, Nedrow A, Miller J, Nicolaidis C, Walker M, Humphrey L. Nonhormonal therapies for menopausal hot flashes: systematic review and meta-analysis. *JAMA* (2006) 295, 2057–71.
6. Cassidy A, Albertazzi P, Lise Nielsen I, Hall W, Williamson G, Tetens I, Atkins S, Cross H, Manios Y, Wolk A, Steiner C, Branca F. Critical review of health effects of soyabean phyto-oestrogens in post-menopausal women. *Proc Nutr Soc* (2006) 65, 76–92.
7. Setchell KDR, Brown NM, Zimmer-Nechemias L, Brashear WT, Wolfe BE, Kirschner AS, Heubi JE. Evidence for lack of absorption of soy isoflavone glycosides in humans, supporting the crucial role of intestinal metabolism for bioavailability. *Am J Clin Nutr* (2002) 76, 447–53.
8. Sacks FM, Lichtenstein A, Van Horn L, Harris W, Kris-Etherton P, Winston M;. Soy protein, isoflavones, and cardiovascular health: an American Heart Association Science Advisory for professionals from the Nutrition Committee. *Circulation* (2006) 113, 1034–44.
9. Anderson GD, Rosito G, Mohustsy MA, Elmer GW. Drug Interaction potential of soy extract and Panax ginseng. *J Clin Pharmacol* (2003) 43, 643–8.
10. Foster BC, Vandenhoek S, Hana J, Krantis A, Akhtar MH, Bryan M, Budzinski JW, Ramputh A, Arnason JT. *In vitro* inhibition of human cytochrome P450-mediated metabolism of marker substrates by natural products. *Phytomedicine* (2003) 10, 334–42.

S

Soya + Antibacterials

No data for soya found. For the theoretical possibility that broad-spectrum antibacterials might reduce the metabolism of the isoflavone constituents of soya, such as daidzein, by colonic bacteria, and so alter their efficacy, see Isoflavones + Antibacterials, page 302.

Soya + Caffeine

Soya products may increase the metabolism of caffeine.

Clinical evidence

Caffeine elimination is low in neonates, but increases faster in those receiving formula feeds (type not specified), than in breast-fed infants.[1] In another study of caffeine for apnoea, formula-fed (type not specified) infants required higher caffeine doses than breast-fed infants (4.4 mg/kg compared with 8.3 mg/kg), but still had lower trough caffeine levels.[2]

Experimental evidence

Both soya-based and cow milk-based infant formulas induced the cytochrome P450 isoenzyme CYP1A2 in *in vitro* studies, whereas breast milk samples from 29 women did not.[3] Conversely, note that high doses of the soya isoflavone daidzein modestly inhibit CYP1A2, see Isoflavones + Theophylline, page 305.

Mechanism

Neonates are less able to metabolise caffeine than adults: hepatic metabolism matures in the first year of life. Infant formula appears to induce the cytochrome P450 isoenzyme CYP1A2, by which caffeine is metabolised. This property is common to both cow's milk and soya, so must be due to a common constituent of both,[3] or the lack of a constituent present in breast milk.[2] The fact that soya isoflavones have some CYP1A2 *inhibitory* activity does not appear to counteract this effect.

Importance and management

Clinical evidence in support of an interaction between soya and caffeine is limited, because the two studies do not state the formula feeds used, although it seems likely that soya feeds are implicated; this suggestion is supported by experimental evidence. In infants, caffeine is dosed individually, but be aware that required doses are likely to increase in those receiving formula feeds, including soya-based formula.

Note that, conversely, in high doses, soya isoflavone supplements might reduce the required dose of CYP1A2 substrates such as Isoflavones + Theophylline, page 305.

1. Blake MJ, Abdel-Rahman SM, Pearce RE, Leeder JS, Kearns GL. Effect of diet on the development of drug metabolism by cytochrome P-450 enzymes in healthy infants. *Pediatr Res* (2006) 60, 717–23.
2. Le Guennec J-C, Billon B. Delay in caffeine elimination in breast-fed infants. *Pediatrics* (1987) 79, 264–8.
3. Xu H, Rajesan R, Harper P, Kim RB, Lonnerdal B, Yang M, Uematsu S, Hutson J, Watson-MacDonell J, Ito S. Induction of cytochrome P450 1A by cow milk-based formula: a comparative study between human milk and formula. *Br J Pharmacol* (2005) 146, 296–305.

Soya + Food

No interactions found.

Soya + Herbal medicines

No interactions found.

Soya + Levothyroxine and related drugs

Soya products or soya isoflavones might increase the dose required of thyroid hormone replacement therapy.

Clinical evidence

A 45-year-old woman who had hypothyroidism after a near-total thyroidectomy and radioactive iodine ablative therapy for papillary carcinoma of the thyroid, required unusually high oral doses of levothyroxine (300 micrograms daily) to achieve clinically effective levels of free thyroxine (T4); suppression of thyroid-stimulating hormone (TSH) was unsatisfactory, even at this dose. She had routinely been taking a 'soya cocktail' protein supplement immediately after her levothyroxine. Taking the soya protein cocktail in the morning, and the levothyroxine in the evening avoided this effect.[1]

A newborn infant with primary hypothyroidism failed to respond to a usual dose of levothyroxine until his soya formula was replaced with cow's milk formula.[2] In another report, three infants with primary hypothyroidism fed soya formula required 18 to 25% decreases in their levothyroxine dose after soya formula was discontinued.[3] In a retrospective study of primary hypothyroidism, TSH values took longer to normalise in 8 infants fed soya formula than in 70 other infants not given soya.[4]

Historical data (from before the 1960s) show that soya formula without iodine supplementation caused goitre, which could be reversed by iodine supplementation.[2]

Experimental evidence

Soya isoflavones inhibited the activity of thyroid peroxidase, an enzyme required for thyroid hormone synthesis, in cell culture and *animal* studies (this has been the subject of a review[5]). However, soya isoflavones do not appear to cause thyroid hormone abnormalities in euthyroid individuals (also reviewed[6]).

Mechanism

Soya isoflavones clearly inhibit thyroid peroxidase; however, hypothyroidism does not usually occur unless iodine deficiency is also present. Soya formula or other similar products might decrease levothyroxine absorption in some individuals.

Importance and management

There is a good body of evidence, which suggests that soya products or soya isoflavones might increase the dose required of thyroid hormone replacement therapy. It would seem prudent to closely monitor the resolution of primary hypothyroidism in infants receiving soya formula, and expect to use higher dose of levothyroxine than anticipated in these individuals. Monitor thyroxine levels and either discontinue the soya formula, or further increase the dose if necessary. Similar precautions would seem prudent if patients receiving levothyroxine wish to take soya supplements; however, remember that the intake of soya supplementation will need to remain relatively constant.

1. Bell DS, Ovalle F. Use of soy protein supplement and resultant need for increased dose of levothyroxine. *Endocr Pract* (2001) 7, 193–4.
2. Chorazy PA, Himelhoch S, Hopwood NJ, Greger NG, Postellon DC. Persistent hypothyroidism in an infant receiving a soy formula: case report and review of the literature. *Pediatrics* (1995) 96, 148–50.
3. Jabbar MA, Larrea J, Shaw RA. Abnormal thyroid function tests in infants with congenital hypothyroidism: the influence of soy-based formula. *J Am Coll Nutr* (1997) 16, 280–282.
4. Conrad SC, Chiu H, Silverman BL. Soy formula complicates management of congenital hypothyroidism. *Arch Dis Child* (2004) 89, 37–40.
5. Doerge DR, Sheehan DM. Goitrogenic and estrogenic activity of soy isoflavones. *Environ Health Perspect* (2002) 110 (Suppl 3), 349–53.
6. Messina M, Redmond G. Effects of soy protein and soybean isoflavones on thyroid function in healthy adults and hypothyroid patients: a review of the relevant literature. *Thyroid* (2006) 16, 249–58.

S

Soya + MAOIs or RIMAs

A potentially fatal hypertensive reaction can occur between the non-selective MAOIs and tyramine-rich foods. Significant amounts of tyramine may be present in fermented or preserved soya products such as soy sauce and tofu, and it may be prudent to avoid these while taking an MAOI. Effects may last for up to two weeks after discontinuation of the MAOI. However, other soya products such as dried textured soya protein and fresh soya beans are unlikely to contain important amounts of tyramine. The risk of a serious hypertensive reaction with moclobemide (or other RIMAs) is very much reduced. Most patients therefore do not need to follow the special dietary restrictions required with the non-selective MAOIs.

Clinical evidence

A 33-year-old woman taking **tranylcypromine** 10 mg four times daily presented to an emergency department with global headache and stiffness of the neck and was found to have a blood pressure of 230/140 mmHg and bradycardia of 55 bpm. Twenty minutes earlier she had eaten chicken teriyaki containing aged soy sauce. She was successfully treated with intravenous labetalol.[1]

Experimental evidence

The tyramine content of a variety of soya products showed marked variability, including clinically significant tyramine levels in tofu when stored for one week and high tyramine content in one of 5 soy sauces (a tyramine level of 6 mg or less was considered safe).[2] In another analysis, high tyramine levels were found in two soy sauces, fermented soya beans, fermented soya bean paste and a soya bean curd condiment.[3] Other non-fermented soya products (tofu, soya bean soup, bean flour, dried bean curd, soya bean drink) had low levels of tyramine, as did one fermented soya bean soup product (miso soup).[3]

Mechanism

Potentiation of the pressor effect of tyramine.[2] Tyramine is formed in foods by the bacterial degradation of proteins, firstly to tyrosine and other amino acids, and the subsequent decarboxylation of the tyrosine to tyramine. This interaction is therefore not associated with fresh foods, but with those which have been allowed to over-ripen or 'mature' in some way,[4] or if spoilage occurs. Tyramine is an indirectly-acting sympathomimetic amine, one of its actions being to release noradrenaline (norepinephrine) from the adrenergic neurones associated with blood vessels, which causes a rise in blood pressure by stimulating their constriction.[4]

Normally any ingested tyramine is rapidly metabolised by the enzyme monoamine oxidase in the gut wall and liver before it reaches the general circulation. However, if the activity of the enzyme at these sites is inhibited (by the presence of an MAOI), any tyramine passes freely into the circulation, causing not just a rise in blood pressure, but a highly exaggerated rise due to the release from the adrenergic neurones of the large amounts of noradrenaline that accumulate there during inhibition of MAO.[4]

RIMAs such as moclobemide and toloxatone selectively inhibit MAO-A, which leaves MAO-B still available to metabolise tyramine. This means that they have less effect on the tyramine pressor response than non-selective MAOIs.

Importance and management

A potentially fatal hypertensive reaction can occur between the non-selective MAOIs and tyramine-rich foods. Significant amounts of tyramine may be present in fermented or preserved soya products such as soy sauce and tofu, and it may be prudent to avoid these while taking an MAOI. Effects may last for up to two weeks after discontinuation of the MAOI. However, other soya products such as dried textured soya protein and fresh soya beans are unlikely to contain important amounts of tyramine.

Moclobemide is safer (in the context of interactions with tyramine-rich foods and drinks) than the non-selective MAOIs, because they it is more readily reversible and selective. Therefore the risk of a serious hypertensive reaction with moclobemide (or other RIMAs) is very much reduced. Most patients therefore do not need to follow the special dietary restrictions required with the non-selective MAOIs.

1. Abrams JH, Schulman P, White WB. Successful treatment of a monoamine oxidase inhibitor-tyramine hypertensive emergency with intravenous labetolol (sic). *N Engl J Med* (1985) 313, 52.
2. Shulman KI, Walker SE. Refining the MAOI diet: tyramine content of pizzas and soy products. *J Clin Psychiatry* (1999) 60, 191–3.
3. Da Prada M, Zürcher G. Tyramine content of preserved and fermented foods or condiments of Far Eastern cuisine. *Psychopharmacology (Berl)* (1992) 106, 32–4.
4. Generali JA, Hogan LC, McFarlane M, Schwab S, Hartman CR. Hypertensive crisis resulting from avocados and a MAO inhibitor. *Drug Intell Clin Pharm* (1981) 15, 904–6.

Soya + Nicotine

For discussion of a study showing that soya isoflavones (daidzein and genistein) caused a minor decrease in the metabolism of nicotine, see Isoflavones + Nicotine, page 303.

Soya + Paclitaxel

No data for soya found. For the possibility that genistein, an isoflavone present in soya, might markedly increase paclitaxel levels, see Isoflavones + Paclitaxel, page 303.

S

Soya + Tamoxifen

The data relating to the use of soya products and isoflavone supplements (containing the isoflavones daidzein and genistein, among others) with tamoxifen are covered under Isoflavones + Tamoxifen, page 304.

Soya + Theophylline

No data for soya found. For the possibility that high doses of daidzein present in soya might modestly increase theophylline levels, see Isoflavones + Theophylline, page 305.

Soya + Warfarin and related drugs

Natto, a Japanese food made from fermented soya bean, can markedly reduce the effects of warfarin and acenocoumarol, because of the high levels of vitamin K_2 substance produced in the fermentation process. In one study, soya bean protein also modestly reduced the effects of warfarin, and a similar case has been reported with soy milk. Two cases of 'warfarin resistance' have been seen in patients given intravenous soya oil emulsions.

Clinical evidence

(a) Fermented soya bean products (natto)

In a controlled study in 12 healthy subjects stabilised on **acenocoumarol**, a single meal containing 100 g of natto decreased the mean INR from 2.1 to 1.5 after 24 hours, and the INR had still not returned to the original level after 7 days (INR 1.75 one week later). The effect was considered clinically important in 6 of the 12 subjects.[1] Similarly, in an earlier retrospective study of 10 patients taking warfarin, eating natto caused the thrombotest values to rise from a range of 12 to 29% up to a range of 33 to 100%. The extent of the rise appeared to be related to the amount of natto eaten. The thrombotest values fell again when the natto was stopped. A healthy subject taking warfarin, with a thrombotest value of 40%, ate 100 g of natto. Five hours later the thrombotest value was unchanged, but 24 hours later it was 86%, and after 48 hours it was 90% (suggesting that the anticoagulant effect was decreased).[2]

(b) Soya milk

In a 70-year-old man stabilised on warfarin 3 mg daily, consumption of soya milk 480 mL daily (240 mL of both *Sun Soy* and *8th Continent* mixed together) decreased the INR from 2.5 to 1.6 after about 4 weeks.[3] One week after stopping the soya milk, his INR was 1.9, and 4 weeks after it was 2.5.

(c) Soya oil

Soya oil is an important source of dietary vitamin K.

In a study in 115 Brazilian patients with vascular disease, consumption of soybean oil (median 11.4 g per day) contributed about 29% of the vitamin K_1 intake, as estimated by 24-hour diet recall. Recent vitamin K_1 consumption was associated with a reduced INR and prothrombin time. The other major contributor to recent vitamin K_1 consumption was kidney beans, which although low in vitamin K themselves, are traditionally prepared in Brazil in soybean oil.[4]

Two cases of 'warfarin resistance' have been seen in patients given intravenous soya oil emulsions.[5,6]

(d) Soya protein

In a study in 10 patients with hypercholesterolaemia who were stabilised on warfarin, substitution of all animal protein for textured soya protein for 4 weeks caused a marked reduction (Quick value approximately doubled) in the anticoagulant effects of warfarin by the second week.[7]

Experimental evidence

Experiments in *animals* to investigate the clinical observations for natto found that natto strongly antagonised the effects of warfarin.[2] In one *in vitro* metabolism study in human liver microsomes,[8] hydrolysed soya extract inhibited all of the cytochrome P450 isoenzymes tested, particularly CYP2C9 and CYP3A4 (which are responsible for the metabolism of warfarin). This suggests an increased warfarin effect might have been expected, but the authors point out there is a lack of concordance between *in vitro* and *in vivo* findings.

Mechanism

Soya beans are a moderate source of vitamin K_1 (19 micrograms per 100 g),[9] and soya oil and products derived from it are an important dietary source of vitamin K. However, the soya milk brand taken in the case report did not contain vitamin K,[3] and another reference source lists soya milk as containing just 7.5 micrograms vitamin K per 250 mL,[9] which would not be expected to cause an interaction. Why this product decreased the effect of warfarin is therefore open to speculation.

The vitamin K content of textured soya protein is unknown. Note that soy sauce made from soya and wheat is reported to contain no vitamin K, and soft tofu made from the curds by coagulating soya milk contains only low levels (2 micrograms per 100 g).[9]

In contrast, fermented soya bean products such as natto contain very high levels of a particular vitamin K_2 substance (MK-7),[10] because of the fermentation process with *Bacillus natto*. In addition, the bacteria might continue to act in the gut to increase the synthesis and subsequent absorption of vitamin K_2.[2] Although the role of vitamin K_2 in anticoagulation is less well established than vitamin K_1, it appears that this also opposes the actions of coumarins and indanediones, which are vitamin K antagonists.

Importance and management

The interaction between warfarin and fermented soya bean products is established, marked, and likely to be clinically relevant in all patients. Patients taking coumarin and probably **indanedione** anticoagulants should be advised to avoid natto, unless they want to consume a regular, constant amount.

Although information is limited, it appears that soya protein might also modestly reduce the effect of warfarin. In particular, complete substitution of animal protein for soya protein appears to reduce the effect of warfarin. A single report suggests that soy milk might also interact, and similarly, case reports suggest that soya milk and soya oil might also interact, and therefore some caution would be prudent with these products. On the basis of known vitamin K-content, whole soya beans could potentially reduce the effect of warfarin, whereas **soy sauce** should not.[9] Note that patients taking coumarins and **indanediones** are advised to have their INR checked if they markedly change their diet. This would seem particularly important if they decide to change their intake of soya-related products.

1. Schurgers LJ, Shearer MJ, Hamulyák K, Stöcklin E, Vermeer C. Effect of vitamin K intake on the stability of oral anticoagulant treatment: dose-response relationships in healthy subjects. *Blood* (2004) 104, 2682–9.
2. Kudo T. Warfarin antagonism of natto and increase in serum vitamin K by intake of natto. *Artery* (1990) 17, 189–201.
3. Cambria-Kiely JA. Effect of soy milk on warfarin efficacy. *Ann Pharmacother* (2002) 36, 1893–6.
4. Custódio das Dôres SM, Booth SL, Martini LA, de Carvalho Gouvêa VH, Padovani CR, de Abreu Maffei FH, Campana ÁO, Rupp de Paiva SA. Relationship between diet and anticoagulant response to warfarin: a factor analysis. *Eur J Nutr* (2007) 46, 147–54.
5. Lutomski DM, Palascak JE, Bower RH. Warfarin resistance associated with intravenous lipid administration. *J Parenter Enteral Nutr* (1987) 11, 316–18.
6. MacLaren R, Wachsman BA, Swift DK, Kuhl DA. Warfarin resistance associated with intravenous lipid administration: discussion of propofol and review of the literature. *Pharmacotherapy* (1997) 17, 1331–7.
7. Gaddi A, Sangiorgi Z, Ciarrocchi A, Braiato A, Descovich GC. Hypocholesterolemic soy protein diet and resistance to warfarin therapy. *Curr Ther Res* (1989) 45, 1006–10.
8. Anderson GD, Rosito G, Mohustsy MA, Elmer GW. Drug Interaction potential of soy extract and Panax ginseng. *J Clin Pharmacol* (2003) 43, 643–8.
9. USDA National Nutrient Database for Standard Reference, Release 17. Vitamin K (phylloquinone) (μg) Content of selected foods per common measure. http://www.nal.usda.gov/fnic/foodcomp/Data/SR17/wtrank/sr17a430.pdf (accessed 17/08/2007).
10. Schurgers LJ, Vermeer C. Determination of phylloquinone and menaquinones in food. Effect of food matrix on circulating vitamin K concentrations. *Haemostasis* (2000) 30, 298–307.

Squill

Drimia maritima (L.) Stearn (Asparagaceae/Hyacinthaceae)

Synonym(s) and related species

Scilla, Sea onion, Sea squill.

Urginea maritima Baker, *Scilla maritima* L., *Urginea scilla* Steinh.

Note that Red squill and White squill are derived from different varieties of the same species, with the name corresponding to the colour of the flowers. Indian squill is *Drimia indica* (Roxb.) Jessop, (*Urginea indica* (Roxb.) Kunth).

Constituents

The bulb contains **cardiac glycosides**, mainly scillaren A and proscillaridin A; flavonoids including apigenin, luteolin, orientin, quercetin, taxifolin, vitexin, and others; and the **phytosterol** stigmasterol.

Red and white squill contain similar compounds, but red squill also contains scilliroside and scillirubroside. Indian squill contains scilliglaucosidin in addition to the constituents described above.

Use and indications

Traditionally, squill has been used as an expectorant for chronic bronchitis, asthma with bronchitis, and whooping cough. It is an ingredient of a variety of proprietary preparations (such as Gee's linctus; Opiate Squill linctus BP) for the relief of the symptoms of coughs and colds. The cardiac glycosides present possess digitalis-like cardiotonic properties, but are poorly absorbed from the gastrointestinal tract and are less potent than digitalis glycosides used therapeutically. Squill is reported to induce vomiting as a result of both a central action and local gastric irritation, but a sub-emetic dose appears to exhibit an expectorant effect, causing an increase in the flow of gastric secretions. As with other cardiotonic drugs, squill is purported to have a diuretic effect. The scilliroside content of red squill is very toxic to rats and has been incorporated into rat poisons.

Pharmacokinetics

No relevant pharmacokinetic data found. For information on the pharmacokinetics of individual flavonoids present in squill, see under flavonoids, page 213.

Interactions overview

Squill contains cardiac glycosides, which could, in theory, have additive effects with digoxin or digitoxin, or interfere with their assays. However, due to the poor oral absorption of cardiac glycosides in squill, it is unlikely through normal therapeutic use that sufficient quantities of cardiac glycosides will be consumed in order to pose a risk. For information on the interactions of individual flavonoids present in squill, see under flavonoids, page 213.

Interactions monographs

- Digitalis glycosides, page 436
- Food, page 436
- Herbal medicines, page 436

S

Squill + Digitalis glycosides   [?✓]

Many herbal medicines contain cardiac glycosides, which could in theory have additive effects with digoxin or digitoxin, or interfere with their assays. However, there appear to be few such interactions reported.

Clinical evidence

No interactions found. However, there are a small number of isolated reports of cardiotoxicity and myopathy after abuse of cough linctuses containing opioids and squill.[1–5] It is therefore theoretically possible that if squill-containing preparations are taken in overdose, levels of digitalis glycosides could be reached that may be additive with digoxin or digitoxin, or interfere with their assays.

Experimental evidence

No relevant data found.

Mechanism

The cardiotoxicities and myopathies seen in the reports[1–3,5,4] were attributed to the cardiac glycoside content of squill present in the formulations.

Importance and management

The theoretical interaction between squill and digitalis glycosides is a prediction that is based on a small number of reports of cardiac glycoside toxicity as a result of abuse of cough linctuses containing squill. A number of proprietary cough preparations still contain squill and the German Commission E monograph for squill contraindicates its use with digitalis glycosides. However, theoretical interactions with herbal medicines are not always translated into practice and it is unlikely through normal therapeutic use that sufficient quantities of the cardiac glycosides present in squill will be consumed to pose a risk. In addition, toxic effects resulting from therapeutic use of these products have not been reported. It would be prudent to exercise caution in patients who are taking digitalis glycosides and who regularly use/abuse squill-containing preparations. However, note that if these products are used as recommended, then this interaction is unlikely to be important.

1. M Kennedy. Cardiac glycoside toxicity: an unusual manifestation of drug addiction. *Med J Aust* (1981) 2, 686–9.
2. Kilpatrick C, Braund W, Burns R . Myopathy with myasthenic features possibly induced by codeine linctus. *Med J Aust* (1982) 2, 41–410.
3. Seow SSW. Abuse of APF linctus codeine and cardiac glycoside toxicity. *Med J Aust* (1984) 140, 54.
4. Smith W, Gould BA, Marshall AJ. Wenckebach's phenomenon induced by cough linctus. *BMJ* (1986) 292, 868.
5. Thurston D, Taylor K. Gee's Linctus *Pharm J* (1984) 233, 63.

Squill + Food

No interactions found.

Squill + Herbal medicines

No interactions found.

S

St John's wort

Hypericum perforatum L. (Clusiaceae)

Synonym(s) and related species

Hypericum, Millepertuis.

Hypericum noeanum Boiss., *Hypericum veronense* Schrank.

Pharmacopoeias

Powdered St. John's Wort (*USP35–NF30 S1*); Powdered St. John's Wort Extract (*USP35–NF30 S1*); St John's Wort (*BP 2012, PhEur 7.5, USP35–NF30 S1*); St John's Wort Dry Extract, Quantified (*BP 2012, PhEur 7.5*).

Constituents

The main groups of active constituents of St John's wort are thought to be the anthraquinones, including **hypericin**, isohypericin, pseudohypericin, protohypericin, protopseudohypericin and cyclopseudohypericin, and the prenylated phloroglucinols, including **hyperforin** and adhyperforin. **Flavonoids**, which include kaempferol, quercetin, luteolin, hyperoside, isoquercitrin, quercitrin and rutin, biflavonoids, which include biapigenin and amentoflavone, and catechins are also present. Other polyphenolic constituents include caffeic and chlorogenic acids, and a volatile oil containing methyl-2-octane.

Most St John's wort products are standardised at least for their **hypericin** content (*BP 2009*), even though **hyperforin** is known to be a more relevant therapeutic constituent, and some preparations are now standardised for both (*USP 32*). It is important to note that there will be some natural variation, and as both hypericin and hyperforin are sensitive to light, they are relatively unstable, so processes used during extraction and formulation, as well as storage conditions, can affect composition of the final product. Therefore different preparations of St John's wort have different chemical profiles and they may not be equivalent in effect.

Use and indications

St John's wort is widely used to treat mild to moderate depression, seasonal affective disorder, low mood, anxiety and insomnia, particularly if associated with menopause. It has also been used topically for its astringent properties.

Pharmacokinetics

St John's wort has been implicated in numerous clinical interactions with conventional drugs and has therefore been extensively studied. Alongside the extensive clinical studies and case reports, there is also a plethora of *in vitro* and *animal* experimental data regarding its interactions and pharmacokinetics. This monograph will discuss the clinical evidence in preference to experimental data, where extensive literature is available and the clinical data are conclusive.

The main constituent found to be responsible for the activity of St John's wort is hyperforin, but other constituents are considered to contribute to its antidepressant activity, such as hypericin and pseudohypericin, the flavonoid quercetin and its glycosides, and rutin. Bioavailability from varying formulations and extracts appears to be low, giving variable steady-state plasma concentrations.[1] For information on the pharmacokinetics of individual flavonoids present in St John's wort, see under flavonoids, page 213.

(a) Cytochrome P450 isoenzymes

St John's wort is known to affect several cytochrome P450 isoenzymes and this accounts for the wide range of drugs with which St John's wort has been reported to interact. It is thought to exert a biphasic effect on these isoenzymes, with inhibition occurring in *in vitro* studies with the initial exposure, and induction following long-term use.[2] Therefore, predicting the overall effect from *in vitro* and *animal* experiments may not always be reliable.

The following is a list of cytochrome P450 isoenzymes that have been assessed with St John's wort in a clinical setting:

- **CYP3A4:** The main clinically relevant effect of St John's wort on cytochrome P450 is the induction of CYP3A4. This has been shown to be related to the constituent, hyperforin. Products vary in their hyperforin content; preparations with a high-hyperforin content, given for a long period of time, will induce CYP3A4 activity, and therefore decrease the levels of drugs metabolised by CYP3A4, by a greater extent than preparations containing low-hyperforin levels taken for a shorter period of time.

  Conventional drugs are often used as probe substrates in order to establish the activity of another drug on specific isoenzyme systems. For CYP3A4 the preferred probe drug is midazolam, because it has no effects of its own on CYP3A4, and is metabolised almost exclusively by CYP3A4, with no known interference from other metabolic processes, such as transporter proteins. See St John's wort + Benzodiazepines, page 442 for an example of the effects of St John's wort on CYP3A4. Studies have assessed the duration of the effects of St John's wort on CYP3A4. One study found that CYP3A4 activity returned to baseline in about one week after St John's wort was taken for 14 days. This may provide an indication of how long to leave between using St John's wort and starting another drug, and therefore avoiding clinically important interactions.[3] However, another study found that the effects of St John's wort lasted for more than 2 weeks in some patients.[4] See the table Drugs and herbs affecting or metabolised by the cytochrome P450 isoenzyme CYP3A4, page 7 for a list of known CYP3A4 substrates.

- **CYP2C19:** There are some clinical reports suggesting that St John's wort induces CYP2C19. See St John's wort + Proton pump inhibitors, page 455, for a clinically relevant example of this.
- **CYP2C8:** St John's wort does not appear to induce CYP2C8 to a clinically relevant extent, see *repaglinide,* under St John's wort + Antidiabetics, page 440.
- **CYP2C9:** St John's wort may induce CYP2C9 (see St John's wort + Warfarin and related drugs, page 459), but the mechanism for these interactions is not conclusive because not all CYP2C9 substrates have been found to interact (see *tolbutamide,* under St John's wort + Antidiabetics, page 440).
- **CYP2E1:** St John's wort may induce CYP2E1 but the general clinical importance of this is unclear, see St John's wort + Chlorzoxazone, page 444.
- **CYP1A2:** St John's wort is also thought to be an inducer of CYP1A2 as levels of caffeine, page 443, and theophylline, page 458, both of which are CYP1A2 substrates, have been reduced by St John's wort. However, the general clinical importance of this is unclear as other studies have found no clinically significant effect on these drugs. This may be because St John's wort only has a minor inducing effect on CYP1A2, which may depend on the level of exposure to hyperforin.
- **CYP2D6:** St John's wort does not appear to affect the activity of CYP2D6 to a clinically relevant extent, see St John's wort + Dextromethorphan, page 446, and St John's wort + Tricyclic antidepressants, page 458.

(b) P-glycoprotein

St John's wort is known to affect P-glycoprotein activity, especially intestinal P-glycoprotein, and it is generally thought that inhibition takes place initially, and briefly, but is followed by a more potent and longer-acting induction. It is the induction that leads to the clinically relevant drug interactions of St John's wort that occur as a result of this mechanism.[5] Hyperforin is implicated as the main constituent responsible for the effect, see St John's wort + Digoxin, page 447.

(c) Serotonin syndrome

St John's wort inhibits the reuptake of 5-hydroxytryptamine (5-HT, serotonin) and this has resulted in a pharmacodynamic interaction, namely the development of serotonin syndrome (see under pharmacodynamics, 8) with conventional drugs that also have serotonergic properties. These include bupropion, page 442, SNRIs, page 455, SSRIs, page 456, and triptans, page 459.

Interactions overview

St John's wort is known to interact with many conventional drugs because of its ability to induce the activity of CYP3A4 and P-glycoprotein, which are involved in the metabolism and distribution of the majority of drugs. CYP2C19 and CYP2E1 may also be induced by St John's wort, although the evidence is not conclusive and further study is needed. In general, CYP2C9, CYP2C8 and CYP1A2 do not appear to be significantly affected by St John's wort, however, isolated reports of an interaction have still occurred. Hyperforin

is the active constituent believed to be central to the inducing effects of St John's wort. As St John's wort preparations and dose regimens are varied, the amount of hyperforin exposure will also vary a great deal, which makes predicting whether an interaction will occur and to what extent, difficult. For more information concerning the pharmacokinetic and pharmacodynamic properties of St John's wort that are relevant to drug interactions, see under *Pharmacokinetics,* above, and for detail on the interactions of St John's wort, see the sections that follow. For information on the interactions of individual flavonoids present in St John's wort, see under flavonoids, page 213.

Interactions monographs

- 5-Aminolevulinic acid, page 440
- Anaesthetics, general, page 440
- Antidiabetics, page 440
- Antiepileptics, page 441
- Benzodiazepines, page 442
- Bupropion, page 442
- Buspirone, page 443
- Caffeine, page 443
- Calcium-channel blockers, page 444
- Chlorzoxazone, page 444
- Ciclosporin, page 445
- Cimetidine, page 445
- Clopidogrel, page 446
- Clozapine, page 446
- Dextromethorphan, page 446
- Digoxin, page 447
- Eplerenone, page 447
- Etoposide, page 448
- Fexofenadine, page 448
- Finasteride, page 448
- Food; Tyramine-rich, page 448
- Herbal medicines, page 449
- HIV-protease inhibitors, page 449
- Hormonal contraceptives, page 449
- Ibuprofen, page 451
- Imatinib, page 451
- Interferons, page 451
- Irinotecan, page 452
- Ivabradine, page 452
- Laboratory tests, page 452
- Lithium, page 453
- Loperamide, page 453
- Methotrexate, page 453
- Methylphenidate, page 453
- Mycophenolate, page 453
- NNRTIs, page 454
- Opioids, page 454
- Prednisone, page 454
- Procainamide, page 455
- Proton pump inhibitors, page 455
- SNRIs, page 455
- SSRIs, page 456

1. Wurglics M, Schubert-Zsilavecz M. Hypericum perforatum: a 'modern' herbal antidepressant: pharmacokinetics of active ingredients. *Clin Pharmacokinet* (2006) 45, 449–68.
2. Xie H-G, Kim RB. St John's wort-associated drug interactions: Short-term inhibition and long-term induction? *Clin Pharmacol Ther* (2005) 78, 19–24.
3. Imai H, Kotegawa T, Tsutsumi K, Morimoto T, Eshima N, Nakano S, Ohashi K. The recovery time-course of CYP3A after induction by St John's wort administration. *Br J Clin Pharmacol* (2008) 65, 701–7.
4. Bauer S, Störmer E, Johne A, Krüger H, Budde K, Neumayer H-H, Roots I, Mai I. Alterations in cyclosporin A pharmacokinetics and metabolism during treatment with St John's wort in renal transplant patients. *Br J Clin Pharmacol* (2003) 55, 203–11.
5. Hennessey M, Kelleher D, Spiers JP, Barry M, Kavanagh P, Back D, Mulcahy F, Feely J. St John's Wort increases expression of P-glycoprotein: Implications for drug interactions. *Br J Clin Pharmacol* (2002) 53, 75–82.

S

St John's wort + 5-aminolevulinic acid

An isolated case report describes a severe phototoxic reaction attributed to a synergistic effect of 5-aminolevulinic acid and St John's wort.

Clinical evidence

A 47-year-old woman who was taking St John's wort (*Hyperiforce,* dose not stated), experienced a phototoxic reaction on skin areas exposed to light 6 hours after receiving 5-aminolevulinic acid 40 mg/kg. She developed a burning erythematous rash and severe swelling of the face, neck and hands. Treatment with oral corticosteroids resulted in complete resolution after skin desquamation.[1]

Experimental evidence

An *in vitro* study using human cell lines found that the combination of 5-aminolevulinic acid and an extract of St John's wort (*Hyperiforce*), increased light-induced toxicity by up to 15%.[1]

Mechanism

It was suggested that there was a synergistic photosensitivity reaction between the two drugs.

Importance and management

This appears to be the only report of such an effect, but bear it in mind in the event of an unexpected adverse reaction to 5-aminolevulinic acid.

1. Ladner DP, Klein SD, Steiner RA, Walt H. Synergistic toxicity of delta-aminolaevulinic acid-induced protoporphyrin IX used for photodiagnosis and hypericum extract, a herbal antidepressant. *Br J Dermatol* (2001) 144, 901–22.

St John's wort + Anaesthetics, general

It has been predicted that St John's wort may prolong the effects of anaesthetics, which is supported by an isolated case. A case of profound hypotension during anaesthesia following the long-term use of St John's wort has also been reported. The American Society of Anesthesiologists recommends that all herbal medicines should be stopped two weeks prior to elective surgery.

Clinical evidence

Prolonged anaesthesia has been reported in a 21-year-old woman who had been taking St John's wort 1 g three times daily for 3 months before general anaesthetics were given for the surgical removal of an abscess. Anaesthesia was induced by intravenous **fentanyl citrate** 1 microgram/kg and **propofol** 3 mg/kg, and maintained throughout the procedure by **sevoflurane** and **nitrous oxide** using a facemask.[1]

Another case report describes a healthy 23-year-old woman who had been taking St John's wort on a daily basis for 6 months, who developed severe hypotension (BP 60/20 mmHg) during general anaesthesia, which responded poorly to ephedrine and phenylephrine (BP increased to 70/40 mmHg).[2]

Experimental evidence

No relevant data found.

Mechanism

It has been suggested that St John's wort may prolong anaesthesia,[3–6] but there are no reports of this occurring. This appears to have been based on the possibility that St John's wort acts as an MAOI,[4,6,7] (although this has been disputed[8]) and the limited evidence that MAOIs may cause hepatic enzyme inhibition and potentiate the effects of barbiturates.[9,10]

However, there is now increasing evidence that St John's wort induces hepatic enzymes, and might therefore increase the metabolism of barbiturates, which suggests that it could increase requirements for **thiopental** anaesthesia. The possible MAOI activity of St John's wort has led to the recommendation that the same considerations apply as for other MAOIs and general anaesthetics.[6,7]

The authors of the second case report suggest that St John's wort might have caused adrenergic desensitisation with decreased responsiveness to the vasopressors.[2]

Importance and management

Not established. The evidence presented suggests that some caution may be warranted in patients using St John's wort if they are given general anaesthetics. Because of the limited information, the American Society of Anesthesiologists have recommended discontinuation of all herbal medicines 2 weeks before an elective anaesthetic[3,5] and if there is any doubt about the safety of a product, this may be a prudent precaution.[4]

1. Crowe S, McKeating K. Delayed emergence and St. John's wort [case reports]. *Anesthesiology* (2002) 96, 1025–7.
2. Irefin S, Sprung J. A possible cause of cardiovascular collapse during anesthesia: long-term use of St John's wort. *J Clin Anesth* (2000) 12, 498–9.
3. Larkin M. Surgery patients at risk for herb-anaesthesia interactions. *Lancet* (1999) 354, 1362.
4. Cheng B, Hung CT, Chiu W. Herbal medicine and anaesthesia. *Hong Kong Med J* (2002) 8, 123–30.
5. Leak JA. Perioperative considerations in the management of the patient taking herbal medicines. *Curr Opin Anaesthesiol* (2000) 13, 321–5.
6. Lyons TR. Herbal medicines and possible anesthesia interactions. *AANA J* (2002) 70, 47–51.
7. Klepser TB, Klepser ME. Unsafe and potentially safe herbal therapies. *Am J Health-Syst Pharm* (1999) 56, 125–38.
8. Miller LG. Herbal medicinals. Selected clinical considerations focusing on known or potential drug-herb interactions. *Arch Intern Med* (1998) 158, 2200–2211.
9. Domino EF, Sullivan TS, Luby ED. Barbiturate intoxication in a patient treated with a MAO inhibitor. *Am J Psychiatry* (1962) 118, 941–3.
10. Buchel L, Lévy J. Mécanisme des phénomènes de synergie du sommeil expérimental. II. Étude des associations iproniazide-hypnotiques, chez le rat et la souris. *Arch Sci Physiol (Paris)* (1965) 19, 161–79.

St John's wort + Antidiabetics

St John's wort slightly decreases the exposure to rosiglitazone, but its effects on pioglitazone are unclear. The pharmacokinetics of repaglinide are unaffected by St John's wort. St John's wort also slightly decreased the exposure to gliclazide, but, in contrast, it did not affect the metabolism of tolbutamide.

Clinical evidence

(a) Meglitinides

In a crossover study in 15 healthy subjects, St John's wort 325 mg three times daily was given for 14 days with a single 1-mg dose of **repaglinide** and 75 g of glucose given on day 15. St John's wort had no statistically significant effect on the pharmacokinetics of **repaglinide**, or on its effects on blood glucose or insulin concentrations.[1]

(b) Sulfonylureas

In a study in 21 healthy subjects, a 300-mg dose of a St John's wort preparation with a high hyperforin content (*LI 160, Lichtwer Pharma*) was given three times daily for 15 days. On the last day of treatment, a single 80-mg dose of **gliclazide** was given, followed 30 minutes later by glucose 75 g. St John's wort reduced the maximum plasma concentration and AUC of **gliclazide** by 22% and 35%, respectively. The clearance was increased by 47%. No statistically significant changes were found in the AUC_{0-4} or blood concentrations of glucose or insulin.[2]

In another study, St John's wort 900 mg had no effect on the metabolism of a single dose of **tolbutamide** either after one day or after 2 weeks of use. The St John's wort product used was from

Sundown Herbals and provided about 33 mg of hyperforin daily.[3] Similarly, in another study, a St John's wort preparation with low hyperforin content (*Esbericum*) at a dose of 240 mg daily (which provided about 3.5 mg of hyperforin daily) had no effect on **tolbutamide** metabolism.[4]

(c) Thiazolidinediones

A preliminary report of a pharmacokinetic study[5] states that St John's wort 900 mg daily decreased the AUC of a single dose of **rosiglitazone** by 26% and increased its clearance by 35%.

Experimental evidence

No relevant data found.

Mechanism

Gliclazide is a substrate of CYP2C9 and the authors suggest that St John's wort induces this isoenzyme, thereby increasing the metabolism of gliclazide and reducing its exposure. The magnitude of this effect was not influenced by CYP2C9 genotype.[2] However, the fact that tolbutamide, commonly used as a probe substrate to assess CYP2C9 activity, was unaffected by St John's wort suggests that other factors could be involved.

Rosiglitazone is known to be metabolised principally by CYP2C8, and it was therefore concluded that St John's wort induces this isoenzyme. The magnitude of the effect of St John's wort does not appear to be influenced by CYP2C8 genotype.[5] However, repaglinide is also principally metabolised by CYP2C8, but was not affected by St John's wort. Note that the subjects in the repaglinide study[1] had been screened for CYP2C8 phenotype and any poor metabolisers (that is, those with low activity of this isoenzyme) were excluded. Note also, that there was some variability in the effects seen according to genotype for the organic anion transporting polypeptide, OATP1B1, but this was not statistically significant. Further study is needed.

Importance and management

The clinical relevance of the slight reduction in rosiglitazone exposure has not been assessed, but it would seem unlikely to be important. However, the authors of the report[5] state that concurrent use of St John's wort should be monitored when patients are also given CYP2C8 substrates. Note that repaglinide is also a CYP2C8 substrate, of CYP2C8, but its pharmacokinetics and effects on blood glucose and insulin concentrations were not affected by St John's wort. No precautions would seem necessary on concurrent use. The likely effect of St John's wort on **pioglitazone**, another CYP2C8 substrate, is unclear. However, large decrease in pioglitazone exposure would not be expected on the basis that rifampicin, a more potent enzyme inducer than St John's wort, only caused a 54% reduction in the AUC of pioglitazone. However, the UK manufacturer[6] recommends caution when prescribing pioglitazone with drugs that induce CYP2C8. All three drugs are also substrates for CYP3A4, of which St John's wort is an established inducer. Further study is needed.

The slight reduction in the exposure to gliclazide does not appear to be clinically important as its blood-glucose-lowering effects were unaffected.

No special precautions appear to be necessary if tolbutamide and St John's wort are used together.

1. Fan L, Zhou G, Guo D, Liu Y-L, Chen W-Q, Liu Z-Q, Tan Z-R, Sheng D, Zhou H-H, Zhang W. The pregnane X receptor agonist St John's wort has no effects on the pharmacokinetics and pharmacodynamics of repaglinide. *Clin Pharmacokinet* (2011) 50, 605–11.
2. Xu H, Williams KM, Liauw WS, Murray M, Day RO, McLachlan AJ. Effects of St John's wort and *CYP2C9* genotype on the pharmacokinetics and pharmacodynamics of gliclazide. *Br J Pharmacol* (2008) 153, 1579–86.
3. Wang Z, Gorski JC, Hamman MA, Huang S-M, Lesko LJ, Hall SD. The effects of St John's wort (*Hypericum perforatum*) on human cytochrome P450 activity. *Clin Pharmacol Ther* (2001) 70, 317–26.
4. Arold G, Donath F, Maurer A, Diefenbach K, Bauer S, Henneicke von Zepelin H-H, Friede M, Roots I. No relevant interaction with alprazolam, caffeine, tolbutamide, and digoxin by treatment with a low-hyperforin St John's wort extract. *Planta Med* (2005) 71, 331–7.
5. Hruska MW, Cheong JA, Langaee TY, Frye RF. Effect of St John's wort administration on CYP2C8 mediated rosiglitazone metabolism. *Clin Pharmacol Ther* (2005) 77, P35.
6. Actos (Pioglitazone hydrochloride). Takeda UK Ltd. UK Summary of product characteristics, December 2011.

St John's wort + Antiepileptics

St John's wort modestly increased the clearance of single-dose carbamazepine, but had no effect on multiple-dose carbamazepine pharmacokinetics. Carbamazepine does not appear to significantly affect the pharmacokinetics of hypericin or pseudohypericin (constituents of St John's wort). St John's wort increased the clearance of mephenytoin by about 3-fold and is predicted to reduce the blood levels of phenytoin and phenobarbital, but this awaits clinical confirmation.

Clinical evidence

In a multiple-dose study in 8 healthy subjects, St John's wort had no effect on the pharmacokinetics of **carbamazepine** or its metabolite (carbamazepine-10,11-epoxide). In this study, subjects took **carbamazepine** 200 mg increased to 400 mg daily alone for 20 days, then with St John's wort 300 mg (standardised to hypericin 0.3%) three times daily for a further 14 days.[1] In contrast, the AUC of a single 400-mg dose of **carbamazepine** was reduced by 21% after St John's wort 300 mg was given three times daily for 14 days, and the AUC of the 10,11-epoxide metabolite was increased by 26%.[2]

A double-blind, placebo-controlled study in healthy subjects found that, apart from a modest 29% decrease in the AUC of pseudohypericin, **carbamazepine** did not significantly affect the pharmacokinetics of either hypericin or pseudohypericin, which are both constituents of St John's wort.[3]

In another placebo-controlled study in 6 extensive metabolisers of CYP2C19, St John's wort 300 mg three times daily for 14 days increased the clearance of a single oral dose of **mephenytoin** 100 mg given on day 15, by about 3-fold. There were no significant effects when **mephenytoin** was given to 6 poor metabolisers of CYP2C19. Each St John's wort tablet contained 0.3% hypericin and 4% hyperforin.[4]

Experimental evidence

Because of the quality of the clinical evidence (controlled pharmacokinetic studies), experimental data have not been sought.

Mechanism

St John's wort is a known inducer of CYP3A4, and the results with single-dose carbamazepine are as predicted. However, carbamazepine is also an inducer of CYP3A4, and induces its own metabolism (autoinduction). It is suggested that St John's wort is not sufficiently potent an inducer to further induce carbamazepine metabolism when autoinduction has occurred,[1] and therefore a small interaction is seen with single doses but no interaction is seen with multiple doses. However, the lack of effect seen in some of these studies may also be due to the different preparations used, and therefore differing levels of hyperforin.

Mephenytoin is a substrate of CYP2C19 and St John's wort appears to induce this isoenzyme.

Importance and management

The available evidence suggests that a clinically significant interaction between carbamazepine and St John's wort is unlikely. Before the publication of the above reports, the CSM in the UK had advised that patients taking a number of drugs including the antiepileptics carbamazepine, **phenytoin** and **phenobarbital** should not take St John's wort.[5] This advice was based on predicted pharmacokinetic interactions. In the light of the above studies, this advice may no longer apply to carbamazepine, although further study is needed. Until more is known, it would probably be prudent to avoid concurrent use in patients taking mephenytoin, **phenytoin** and **phenobarbital** (and therefore **primidone**), especially as **phenytoin** is also a substrate of CYP2C19, which St John's wort also appears to induce. The situation with carbamazepine is less clear. As the pharmacokinetic effects reported were modest, it may not be necessary to avoid St John's wort, however concurrent use should probably still be monitored to ensure adequate carbamazepine levels and efficacy.

S

Note that St John's wort does not appear to interfere with laboratory assays for carbamazepine, **phenytoin**, **phenobarbital** or **valproate**. See St John's wort + Laboratory tests, page 452.

1. Burstein AH, Horton RL, Dunn T, Alfaro RM, Piscitelli SC, Theodore W. Lack of effect of St John's wort on carbamazepine pharmacokinetics in healthy volunteers. *Clin Pharmacol Ther* (2000) 68, 605–12.
2. Burstein AH, Piscitelli SC, Alfaro RM, Theodore W. Effect of St John's wort on carbamazepine single-dose pharmacokinetics. *Epilepsia* (2001) 42 (Suppl 7), 253.
3. Johne A, Perloff ES, Bauer S, Schmider J, Mai I, Brockmöller J, Roots I. Impact of cytochrome P-450 inhibition by cimetidine and induction by carbamazepine on the kinetics of hypericin and pseudohypericin in healthy volunteers. *Eur J Clin Pharmacol* (2004) 60, 617–22.
4. Wang L-S, Zhu B, El-Aty AMA, Zhou G, Li Z, Wu J, Chen G-L, Liu J, Tang ZR, An W, Li Q, Wang D, Zhou H-H. The influence of St. John's wort on CYP2C19 activity with respect to genotype. *J Clin Pharmacol* (2004) 44, 577–81.
5. Committee on the Safety of Medicines (UK). Message from Professor A Breckenridge (Chairman of CSM) and Fact Sheet for Health Care Professionals. Important interactions between St John's wort (*Hypericum perforatum*) preparations and prescribed medicines. February 2000 http://www.mhra.gov.uk/home/groups/comms-ic/documents/websiteresources/con019563.pdf (accessed 27/11/2008).

St John's wort + Benzodiazepines

Long-term use of St John's wort decreases the plasma levels of alprazolam, midazolam and quazepam. St John's wort preparations taken as a single dose, or containing low-hyperforin levels, appear to have less of an effect.

Clinical evidence

(a) Alprazolam

In a study in 12 healthy subjects, St John's wort (*LI 160, Lichtwer Pharma,* 0.12 to 0.3% hypericin) 300 mg three times daily for 16 days with a single 2-mg dose of alprazolam on day 14. The AUC of alprazolam was halved by St John's wort and the clearance was increased by about twofold.[1]

In another study, alprazolam 1 or 2 mg was given to 7 healthy subjects on the third day of a 3-day treatment period with St John's wort (*Solaray*; hypericin content standardised at 0.3%) 300 mg three times daily. The pharmacokinetics of alprazolam were unchanged by St John's wort, but the authors note that 3 days may have been an insufficient time for St John's wort to fully induce cytochrome P450 isoenzymes.[2] In another study, 16 healthy subjects were given St John's wort extract 120 mg (*Esbericum* capsules; corresponding to 0.5 mg total hypericins and 1.76 mg hyperforin) twice daily for 10 days. A single 1-mg dose of alprazolam was given on the day before treatment with St John's wort and on the last day of treatment. St John's wort extract at this low dosage and low hyperforin content had no clinically relevant effects on the pharmacokinetics of alprazolam, when compared with 12 subjects given placebo.[3]

(b) Midazolam

An open-label study in 12 healthy subjects found that a single 900-mg dose of St John's wort had no significant effect on the pharmacokinetics of single doses of either *oral* midazolam 5 mg or *intravenous* midazolam 0.05 mg/kg, although there was a trend for increased oral clearance. However, St John's wort 300 mg three times daily for 14 or 15 days decreased the AUC and maximum plasma concentration of *oral* midazolam by about 50% and 40%, respectively. Intravenous midazolam was not significantly affected. Similar results were found in another six studies.[4–9] In one of the studies, although no serious adverse events occurred, 3 subjects reported that the sedative effects of midazolam were less noticeable when St John's wort was taken at the same time.[6]

(c) Quazepam

In a placebo-controlled study, 13 healthy subjects were given St John's wort (*TruNature*; hypericin content standardised at 0.3%) 300 mg three times daily for 14 days with a single 15-mg dose of quazepam on day 14. St John's wort modestly decreased the AUC and maximum plasma levels of quazepam by 26% and 29%, respectively, but the pharmacodynamic effects of quazepam were not affected.[10]

Experimental evidence

No relevant data found.

Mechanism

Alprazolam, midazolam and quazepam are substrates of the cytochrome P450 isoenzyme CYP3A4. St John's wort appears to induce CYP3A4 thus increasing the metabolism of *oral* midazolam,[5–9,11] alprazolam,[1] and quazepam,[10] and reducing the bioavailability of these benzodiazepines.

Hyperforin appears to be the main active constituent that induces CYP3A4, because high-hyperforin extracts have more of an inducing effect than low-hyperforin extracts.[6–9]

Importance and management

Although not all the studies found an interaction between St John's wort and alprazolam or midazolam, those that did found a reduction in levels, which is in line with the known CYP3A4 inducing effects of St John's wort. The variable findings reported in the studies (some found no interaction) could be due to the preparation of St John's wort used and the duration of treatment.[2,9] Until more is known about the interacting constituents of St John's wort, and the amount necessary to provoke an interaction it would seem prudent to monitor patients receiving alprazolam and oral midazolam concurrently for any signs of reduced efficacy. Single doses of *intravenous* midazolam do not appear to be significantly affected. Note that **triazolam** is also a substrate of CYP3A4 and is likely to be affected in the same way as alprazolam and midazolam.

The modest reduction in quazepam levels did not reduce its efficacy; however, it may be prudent to bear the potential for an interaction in mind should a patient taking St John's wort have a reduced response to quazepam.

Those benzodiazepines that undergo glucuronidation, such as **lorazepam**, **oxazepam** and **temazepam**, would not be expected to be affected by St John's wort, and may be useful alternatives.

1. Markowitz JS, Donovan JL, DeVane CL, Taylor RM, Ruan Y, Wang J-S, Chavin KD. Effect of St John's wort on drug metabolism by induction of cytochrome P450 3A4 enzyme. *JAMA* (2003) 290, 1500–1504.
2. Markowitz JS, DeVane CL, Boulton DW, Carson SW, Nahas Z, Risch SC. Effect of St John's wort (*Hypericum perforatum*) on cytochrome P-450 2D6 and 3A4 activity in healthy volunteers. *Life Sci* (2000) 66, 133–9.
3. Arold G, Donath F, Maurer A, Diefenbach K, Bauer S, Henneike von Zepelin H-H, Friede M, Roots I. No relevant interaction with alprazolam, caffeine, tolbutamide, and digoxin by treatment with a low hyperforin St John's wort extract. *Planta Med* (2005) 71, 331–7.
4. Dresser GK, Schwarz UI, Wilkinson GR, Kim RB. Coordinate induction of both cytochrome P4503A and MDR1 by St John's wort in healthy subjects. *Clin Pharmacol Ther* (2003) 73, 41–50.
5. Xie R, Tan LH, Polasek EC, Hong C, Teillol-Foo M, Gordi T, Sharma A, Nickens DJ, Arakawa T, Knuth DW, Antal EJ. CYP3A and P-glycoprotein activity induction with St. John's wort in healthy volunteers from 6 ethnic populations. *J Clin Pharmacol* (2005) 45, 352–6.
6. Gurley BJ, Gardner SF, Hubbard MA, Williams DK, Gentry WB, Cui Y, Ang CYW. Cytochrome P450 phenotypic ratios for predicting herb-drug interactions in humans. *Clin Pharmacol Ther* (2002) 72, 276–87.
7. Gurley BJ, Gardner SF, Hubbard MA, Williams DK, Gentry WB, Cui Y, Ang CYW. Clinical assessment of botanical supplementation on cytochrome P450 phenotypes in the elderly: St John's wort, garlic oil, *Panax ginseng*, and *Ginkgo biloba*. *Drugs Aging* (2005) 22, 525–39.
8. Imai H, Kotegawa T, Tsutsumi K, Morimoto T, Eshima N, Nakano S, Ohashi K. The recovery time-course of CYP3A after induction by St John's wort administration. *Br J Clin Pharmacol* (2008) 65, 701–7.
9. Mueller SC, Majcher-Peszynska J, Uehleke B, Klammt S, Mundkowski RG, Miekisch W, Sievers H, Bauer S, Frank B, Kundt G, Drewelow B. The extent of induction of CYP3A by St. John's wort varies among products and is linked to hyperforin dose. *Eur J Clin Pharmacol* (2006) 62, 29–36.
10. Kawaguchi A, Ohmori M, Tsuruoka S, Harada K, Miyamori I, Yano R, Nakamura T, Masada M, Fujimura A. Drug interaction between St John's wort and quazepam. *Br J Clin Pharmacol* (2004) 58, 403–10.
11. Wang Z, Gorski JC, Hamman MA, Huang S-M, Lesko LJ, Hall SD. The effects of St John's wort (*Hypericum perforatum*) on human cytochrome P450 activity. *Clin Pharmacol Ther* (2001) 70, 317–26.

St John's wort + Bupropion

St John's wort negligibly reduces the exposure to bupropion. A single case describes dystonia when bupropion was started in a patient taking HRT and St John's wort. A case of mania was attributed to the use of St John's wort in a patient taking bupropion.

Clinical evidence

(a) Pharmacokinetic effects

In an open, two-phase pharmacokinetic study in 18 healthy subjects, St John's wort 325 mg three times daily for 14 days, decreased the AUC of a single 150-mg dose of bupropion by about 16% and increased its clearance by about 20%. The AUC and clearance of the active metabolite, hydroxybupropion, were unaffected, but its half-life was reduced by about 18%.[1]

(b) Other effects

1. Dystonia   A 58-year-old woman taking St John's wort 300 mg daily and menopausal HRT (oestradiol and medroxyprogesterone), developed acute facial dystonia 4 days after starting bupropion 150 mg daily for smoking cessation. She was treated with a variety of drugs, and over a couple of weeks the spasm-free interval lengthened, and by 5 months the dystonia resolved completely and all medications were withdrawn without recurrence of the dystonia.[2]

2. Mania   A brief report describes the development of mania in one patient, which was associated with the concurrent use of St John's wort and bupropion.[3]

Experimental evidence

No relevant data found.

Mechanism

The reason for the increased clearance of St John's wort in the pharmacokinetic study[1] is unclear, as bupropion is principally metabolised by CYP2B6, which is not known to be affected by St John's wort.

Dystonia is a rare adverse effect of bupropion alone, and the authors suggested that the combination of bupropion with St John's wort led to additive effects on serotonin reuptake inhibition, making dopaminergic adverse effects such as dystonia more likely.[2] Note also that one HRT preparation has been shown to inhibit the metabolism of bupropion to hydroxybupropion, so it could be hypothesised that there might also be a pharmacokinetic element to this case.

Importance and management

Information on a pharmacodynamic or pharmacokinetic interaction between bupropion and St John's wort appears to be limited to two reports and one study. Nevertheless because of the potential severity of the reactions it would seem prudent to monitor concurrent use closely for an increased incidence of adverse reactions.

1. Lei H-P, Yu X-Y, Xie H-T, Li H-H, Fan L, Dai L-L, Chen Y, Zhou H-H. Effect of St. John's wort supplementation on the pharmacokinetics of bupropion in healthy male Chinese volunteers *Xenobiotica* (2010) 40, 275–81.
2. Milton JC, Abdulla A. Prolonged oro-facial dystonia in a 58 year old female following therapy with bupropion and St John's Wort. *Br J Clin Pharmacol* (2007) 64, 717–18.
3. Griffiths J, Jordan S, Pilan K. Natural health products and adverse reactions. *Can Adverse React News* (2004) 14, 2–3.

St John's wort + Buspirone

Two patients taking buspirone developed marked CNS effects after starting to take herbal medicines including St John's wort.

Clinical evidence

A 27-year-old woman who had been taking buspirone 30 mg daily for over one month started to take St John's wort (*Hypericum 2000 Plus,* Herb Valley, Australia) three tablets daily. After 2 months she complained of nervousness, aggression, hyperactivity, insomnia, confusion and disorientation, which was attributed to serotonin syndrome. The St John's wort was stopped, the buspirone was increased to 50 mg daily and her symptoms resolved over a week.[1] A 42-year-old woman who was taking fluoxetine 20 mg twice daily and buspirone 15 mg twice daily started to develop symptoms of anxiety, with episodes of over-sleeping and memory deficits. It

was discovered that she had been self-medicating with St John's wort, **ginkgo biloba** and **melatonin**. She was asked to stop the non-prescribed medication and her symptoms resolved.[2]

Experimental evidence

No relevant data found.

Mechanism

The exact mechanism of these interactions are not clear, but it is possible they were due to the additive effects of the buspirone and the herbal medicines, either through their effects on elevating mood or through excess effects on serotonin. Fluoxetine may have had a part to play in one of the cases. See St John's wort + SSRIs, page 456. Note that St John's wort, a moderate CYP3A4 inducer, might theoretically reduce the efficacy of buspirone, a CYP3A4 substrate.

Importance and management

The clinical relevance of these cases describing an interaction between buspirone and St John's wort is unclear, but they highlight the importance of considering adverse effects from herbal medicines when they are used with conventional medicines. Bear in mind the possibility that St John's wort preparations might reduce buspirone efficacy.

1. Dannawi M. Possible serotonin syndrome after combination of buspirone and St John's wort. *J Psychopharmacol* (2002) 16, 401.
2. Spinella M, Eaton LA. Hypomania induced by herbal and pharmaceutical psychotropic medicines following mild traumatic brain injury. *Brain Inj* (2002) 16, 359–67.

St John's wort + Caffeine

Two studies suggest that St John's wort increases the metabolism of caffeine. However, four other studies using preparations of varying hyperforin content suggest that the metabolism of caffeine is not affected by St John's wort.

Clinical evidence

A study in 16 healthy subjects given a single 200-mg dose of caffeine before and after St John's wort 300 mg (containing 900 micrograms of hypericin) three times daily for 14 days, found no overall change in the pharmacokinetics of caffeine. However, when the subset of 8 female patients was considered, it was found that there was an induction of CYP1A2 in this group of patients resulting in an increase in the production of caffeine metabolites.[1]

In another study, St John's wort 300 mg given to 12 healthy subjects three times daily for 28 days, modestly increased the metabolism of caffeine 100 mg (a CYP1A2 probe substrate) to paraxanthine by about 26%, although no serious adverse events occurred. The St John's wort preparation used was standardised to 0.3% hypericin and provided each subject with about 12.2 mg of hyperforin daily.[2] However, a later study using the same criteria in 12 elderly healthy subjects found that St John's wort 300 mg three times daily for 28 days (standardised to hypericin 0.3%) generally had no statistically significant effect on the metabolism of a single 100-mg dose of caffeine to paraxanthine taken on day 28, although some individuals showed moderate changes.[3]

Similarly, another study in 28 healthy subjects found no significant change in caffeine pharmacokinetics when a low-hyperforin (about 3.5 mg daily) St John's wort extract (*Esbericum*) 120 mg was given twice daily for 11 days to patients who had received a single caffeine dose of 100 mg before St John's wort was started, and on the last day of the study.[4] These findings were also reported in two other studies using caffeine as a probe drug for CYP1A2 activity and a St John's wort regimen that provided a high-hyperforin dose. One study gave hyperforin 33 mg and hypericin 2.5 mg daily, and the other gave a minimum of hyperforin 36 mg and hypericin 2.7 mg daily.[5,6]

Experimental evidence

No relevant data found.

Mechanism

These studies investigated whether St John's wort had any effect on the cytochrome P450 isoenzyme CYP1A2 by which caffeine is metabolised.

Importance and management

The extent of any interaction with caffeine may depend on the St John's wort preparation involved and dose used and may be correlated with the dose of hyperforin.[4] However, these studies generally suggest that an interaction between St John's wort and caffeine is unlikely to be clinically important. Caffeine is often used as a probe drug for CYP1A2 activity, and therefore these results also suggest that a significant pharmacokinetic interaction as a result of this mechanism between St John's wort and other CYP1A2 substrates is unlikely. Note that St John's wort has only minimal effects on the metabolism of theophylline, which is also a CYP1A2 substrate, consider also St John's wort + Theophylline, page 458.

1. Wenk M, Todesco L, Krähenbühl S. Effect of St John's wort on the activities of CYP1A2, CYP3A4, CYP2D6, N-acetyltransferase 2, and xanthine oxidase in healthy males and females. *Br J Clin Pharmacol* (2004) 57, 494–9.
2. Gurley BJ, Gardner SF, Hubbard MA, Williams DK, Gentry WB, Cui Y, Ang CYW. Cytochrome P450 phenotypic ratios for predicting herb-drug interactions in humans. *Clin Pharmacol Ther* (2002) 72, 276–87.
3. Gurley BJ, Gardner SF, Hubbard MA, Williams DK, Gentry WB, Cui Y, Ang CYW. Clinical assessment of botanical supplementation on cytochrome P450 phenotypes in the elderly: St John's wort, garlic oil, *Panax ginseng*, and *Ginkgo biloba*. *Drugs Aging* (2005) 22, 525–39.
4. Arold G, Donath F, Maurer A, Diefenbach K, Bauer S, Henneicke von Zepelin HH, Friede M, Roots I. No relevant interaction with alprazolam, caffeine, tolbutamide and digoxin by treatment with a low-hyperforin St John's wort extract. *Planta Med* (2005) 71, 331–7.
5. Wang Z, Gorski JC, Hamman MA, Huang S-M, Lesko LJ, Hall SD. The effects of St John's wort (*Hypericum perforatum*) on human cytochrome P450 activity. *Clin Pharmacol Ther* (2001) 70, 317–26.
6. Wang L-S, Zhu B, El-Aty AMA, Zhou G, Li Z, Wu J, Chen G-L, Liu J, Tang ZR, An W, Li Q, Wang D, Zhou H-H. The influence of St. John's wort on CYP2C19 activity with respect to genotype. *J Clin Pharmacol* (2004) 44, 577–81.

St John's wort + Calcium-channel blockers

St John's wort significantly reduces the bioavailability of nifedipine and verapamil. Other calcium-channel blockers would be expected to interact similarly.

Clinical evidence

(a) Nifedipine

In a study in 10 healthy subjects, St John's wort 900 mg daily for 14 days decreased the maximum levels and AUC of a single oral dose of nifedipine 10 mg by about 38% and 45%, respectively. The maximum levels and AUC of the active metabolite of nifedipine, dehydronifedipine, were raised by about 45% and 26%, respectively. The St John's wort preparation used was standardised to contain hypericin 0.3% and hyperforin 5%.[1]

(b) Verapamil

In a study in 8 healthy subjects, verapamil 24 mg was given as a jejunal perfusion over 100 minutes both before and after treatment with St John's wort tablets (*Movina*; containing 3 to 6% hyperforin) 300 mg three times daily for 14 days. St John's wort did not affect jejunal permeability or the absorption of either *R*- or *S*-verapamil. The AUCs of *R*- and *S*-verapamil were decreased by 78% and 80%, respectively, and the peak plasma levels were decreased by 76% and 78%, respectively. The terminal half-life was not changed significantly. The AUC for *R*-verapamil was sixfold higher than that of *S*-verapamil and St John's wort did not change this ratio.[2]

Experimental evidence

No relevant data found.

Mechanism

It appears that St John's wort decreased the bioavailability of both nifedipine and verapamil by inducing their metabolism by the cytochrome P450 isoenzyme CYP3A4 in the gut. An effect on P-glycoprotein-mediated transport is not likely, as intestinal permeability was not significantly altered.[2]

Importance and management

The general importance of this interaction is unclear, as neither study reported on the clinical outcome of these reductions in calcium-channel blocker levels. Patients taking St John's wort with nifedipine or verapamil should have their blood pressure and heart rate monitored to ensure they are still effective, and the dose should be adjusted if needed. There appears to be no information about other calcium-channel blockers, but as they are all metabolised by CYP3A4, to a greater or lesser extent, it would seem prudent to monitor concurrent use carefully.

1. Wang X-D, Li J-L, Lu Y, Chen X, Huang M, Chowbay B, Zhou S-F. Rapid and simultaneous determination of nifedipine and dehydronifedipine in human plasma by liquid chromatography-tandem mass spectrometry: Application to a clinical herb-drug interaction study. *J Chromatogr B Analyt Technol Biomed Life Sci* (2007) 852, 534.
2. Tannergren C, Engman H, Knutson L, Hedeland M, Bondesson U, Lennernäs H. St John's wort decreases the bioavailability of *R*- and *S*-verapamil through induction of first-pass metabolism. *Clin Pharmacol Ther* (2004) 75, 298–309.

St John's wort + Chlorzoxazone

St John's wort increases the clearance of chlorzoxazone.

Clinical evidence

In a study in 12 healthy subjects, St John's wort 300 mg three times daily for 28 days more than doubled the clearance of chlorzoxazone 500 mg (a CYP2E1 probe substrate). The St John's wort preparation used was standardised to a concentration of hypericin 0.3% and provided each subject with about 12.2 mg of hyperforin daily.[1] A later study using the same criteria in 12 healthy subjects (aged between 60 and 76 years old) found that St John's wort 300 mg three times daily for 28 days increased the metabolism of a single 500-mg dose of chlorzoxazone to hydroxychlorzoxazone by only 26%. The St John's wort preparation used in this study provided a daily dose of 4.8 mg of hyperforin.[2]

Experimental evidence

No relevant data found.

Mechanism

It appears that St John's wort increases the clearance of chlorzoxazone by inducing its metabolism by the cytochrome P450 isoenzyme CYP2E1.

Importance and management

The clinical relevance of this interaction is unclear but as no adverse events were reported in the studies, it is unlikely to be of general importance. The authors of the second study suggested that the lower induction of CYP2E1 may have occurred because of inter-individual variability or because there is an age-related reduction in CYP2E1 activity.[2] However, the dose of hyperforin was only about one-third of the dose used in the first study, and this may also account for the difference in degree of induction seen. Nevertheless, because only a single dose of chlorzoxazone was used in these studies, if a patient is taking St John's wort, it may be prudent to monitor for any signs of reduced chlorzoxazone efficacy. As chlorzoxazone is used as a probe drug for CYP2E1 activity, be aware that St John's wort may induce the metabolism of other CYP2E1 substrates.

1. Gurley BJ, Gardner SF, Hubbard MA, Williams DK, Gentry WB, Cui Y, Ang CYW. Cytochrome P450 phenotypic ratios for predicting herb-drug interactions in humans. *Clin Pharmacol Ther* (2002) 72, 276–87.
2. Gurley BJ, Gardner SF, Hubbard MA, Williams DK, Gentry WB, Cui Y, Ang CYW. Clinical assessment of botanical supplementation on cytochrome P450 phenotypes in the elderly: St John's wort, garlic oil, *Panax ginseng*, and *Ginkgo biloba*. *Drugs Aging* (2005) 22, 525–39.

S

St John's wort + Ciclosporin

Marked reductions in ciclosporin blood levels and transplant rejection can occur within a few weeks of starting St John's wort.

Clinical evidence

A marked drop in ciclosporin blood levels was identified in one kidney transplant patient as being due to the addition of St John's wort extract 300 mg three times daily. When the St John's wort was stopped the ciclosporin levels rose. The authors of this report identified another 35 kidney and 10 liver transplant patients whose ciclosporin levels had dropped by an average of 49% (range 30 to 64%) after starting St John's wort. Two of them had rejection episodes.[1,2] In addition, subtherapeutic ciclosporin levels in 7 kidney transplant patients,[3–7] one liver transplant patient,[8] and 6 heart transplant patients[9–11] have been attributed to self-medication with St John's wort. Acute graft rejection episodes occurred in 7 cases,[3,5,7–9,11] and one patient subsequently developed chronic rejection, requiring a return to dialysis.[5] Another case of subtherapeutic ciclosporin levels occurred in a kidney transplant patient during the concurrent use of a herbal tea containing St John's wort. The patient's levels remained subtherapeutic despite a ciclosporin dose increase from 150 to 250 mg daily. The levels recovered within 5 days of stopping the herbal tea and the ciclosporin dose was reduced to 175 mg daily.[12]

These case reports are supported by a small study in which 11 renal transplant patients, with stable dose requirements for ciclosporin, were given St John's wort extract (*Jarsin 300*) 600 mg daily for 14 days. Pharmacokinetic changes were noted 3 days after the St John's wort was added. By day 10 the ciclosporin dose had to be increased from an average of 2.7 to 4.2 mg/kg daily in an attempt to keep ciclosporin levels within the therapeutic range. Two weeks after the St John's wort was stopped, only 3 patients had been successfully re-stabilised on their baseline ciclosporin dose. Additionally, the pharmacokinetics of various ciclosporin metabolites were substantially altered.[13]

Another study in 10 kidney transplant patients stable taking ciclosporin found that the content of hyperforin in the St John's wort affected the extent of the interaction with ciclosporin. In patients taking St John's wort with a high hyperforin content (hyperforin 7 mg; hypericin 0.45 mg) the reduction in the AUC_{0-12} of ciclosporin was 45% greater than that in patients taking St John's wort with a low hyperforin content (hyperforin 0.1 mg; hypericin 0.45 mg). The maximum blood ciclosporin level and the trough ciclosporin level were also reduced by 36% and 45%, respectively, in the patients taking the higher hyperforin-containing St John's wort preparation, when compared with the patients taking the preparation with a lower hyperforin content. The patients taking the high-hyperforin preparation required a mean ciclosporin dose increase of 65% whereas the patients taking the low-hyperforin preparation did not require any ciclosporin dose alterations.[14]

Experimental evidence

Because of the extensive clinical evidence available, experimental data have not been sought.

Mechanism

St John's wort is a known inducer of the cytochrome P450 isoenzyme CYP3A4 by which ciclosporin is metabolised. Concurrent use therefore reduces ciclosporin levels. It has also been suggested that St John's wort affects ciclosporin reabsorption by inducing the drug transporter protein, P-glycoprotein, in the intestine.[9,13]

Importance and management

An established and clinically important interaction. The incidence is not known, but all patients taking ciclosporin should avoid St John's wort because of the potential severity of this interaction.

Transplant rejection can develop within 3 to 4 weeks. It is possible to accommodate this interaction by increasing the ciclosporin dosage[11] (possibly about doubled) but this raises the costs of an already expensive drug. Also, the varying content of natural products would make this hard to monitor. The advice of the CSM in the UK is that patients receiving ciclosporin should avoid or stop taking St John's wort. In the latter situation, the ciclosporin blood levels should be well monitored and the dosage adjusted as necessary.[15] The study described above suggests that increased monitoring will be needed for at least 2 weeks after the St John's wort is stopped.[13]

Note that St John's wort does not appear to interfere with laboratory assays for ciclosporin, see St John's wort + Laboratory tests, page 452.

1. Breidenbach T, Hoffmann MW, Becker T, Schlitt H, Klempnauer J. Drug interaction of St John's wort with ciclosporin. *Lancet* (2000) 355, 1912.
2. Breidenbach T, Kliem V, Burg M, Radermacher J, Hoffmann MW, Klempnauer J. Profound drop of cyclosporin A whole blood trough levels caused by St John's wort (Hypericum perforatum). *Transplantation* (2000) 69, 2229–30.
3. Barone GW, Gurley BJ, Ketel BL, Abul-Ezz SR. Herbal supplements: a potential for drug interactions in transplant recipients. *Transplantation* (2001) 71, 239–41.
4. Mai I, Kreuger H, Budde K, Johne A, Brockmoeller J, Neumayer H-H, Roots I. Hazardous pharmacokinetic interaction of Saint John's wort (Hypericum perforatum) with the immunosuppressant cyclosporin. *Int J Clin Pharmacol Ther* (2000) 38, 500–502.
5. Barone GW, Gurley BJ, Ketel BL, Lightfoot ML, Abul-Ezz SR. Drug interaction between St John's wort and cyclosporine. *Ann Pharmacother* (2000) 34, 1013–16.
6. Moschella PA-C, Jaber BL. Interaction between cyclosporine and Hypericum perforatum (St John's wort) after organ transplantation. *Am J Kidney Dis* (2001) 38, 1105–7.
7. Turton-Weeks SM, Barone GW, Gurley BJ, Ketel BL, Lightfoot ML, Abul-Ezz SR. St John's wort: a hidden risk for transplant patients. *Prog Transplant* (2001) 11, 116–20.
8. Karliova M, Treichel U, Malagò M, Frilling A, Gerken G, Broelsch CE. Interaction of *hypericum perforatum* (St John's wort) with cyclosporin A metabolism in a patient after liver transplantation. *J Hepatol* (2000) 33, 853–5.
9. Ruschitzka F, Meier PJ, Turina M, Lüscher TF, Noll G. Acute heart transplant rejection due to Saint John's wort. *Lancet* (2000) 355, 548–9.
10. Ahmed SM, Banner NR, Dubrey SW. Low cyclosporin-A level due to Saint-John's-wort in heart-transplant patients. *J Heart Lung Transplant* (2001) 20, 795.
11. Bon S, Hartmann K, Kuhn M. Johanniskraut: ein enzyminductor? *Schweiz Apothekerzeitung* (1999) 16, 535–6.
12. Alscher DM, Klotz U. Drug interaction of herbal tea containing St. John's wort with cyclosporine. *Transpl Int* (2003) 16, 543–4.
13. Bauer S, Störmer E, Johne A, Krüger H, Budde K, Neumayer H-H, Roots I, Mai I. Alterations in cyclosporin A pharmacokinetics and metabolism during treatment with St John's wort in renal transplant patients. *Br J Clin Pharmacol* (2003) 55, 203–11.
14. Mai I, Bauer S, Perloff ES, Johne A, Uehleke B, Frank B, Budde K, Roots I. Hyperforin content determines the magnitude of the St John's wort-cyclosporine drug interaction. *Clin Pharmacol Ther* (2004) 76, 330–340.
15. Committee on the Safety of Medicines (UK). Message from Professor A Breckenridge (Chairman of CSM) and Fact Sheet for Health Care Professionals. Important interactions between St John's wort (*Hypericum perforatum*) preparations and prescribed medicines. February 2000 http://www.mhra.gov.uk/home/groups/comms-ic/documents/websiteresources/con019563.pdf (accessed 27/11/2008).

St John's wort + Cimetidine

Cimetidine does not significantly alter the metabolism of the constituents of St John's wort, hypericin and pseudohypericin.

Clinical evidence

A placebo-controlled study in healthy subjects taking St John's wort (*LI 160, Lichtwer Pharma*) 300 mg three times daily found that, apart from a modest 25% increase in the AUC of pseudohypericin, cimetidine 1 g daily (in divided doses) did not significantly affect the pharmacokinetics of either the hypericin or pseudohypericin constituents of St John's wort.[1]

Experimental evidence

No relevant data found.

Mechanism

Cimetidine is an inhibitor of the cytochrome P450 isoenzymes CYP3A4, CYP1A2 and CYP2D6. This study suggests that St John's wort is not significantly metabolised by these isoenzymes.

Importance and management

The available evidence suggests that cimetidine is unlikely to affect the dose requirements of St John's wort.

1. Johne A, Perloff ES, Bauer S, Schmider J, Mai I, Brockmöller J, Roots I. Impact of cytochrome P-450 inhibition by cimetidine and induction by carbamazepine on the kinetics of hypericin and pseudohypericin in healthy volunteers. *Eur J Clin Pharmacol* (2004) 60, 617–22.

S

St John's wort + Clopidogrel

St John's wort caused a small increase in the antiplatelet effect of clopidogrel in one study in hyporesponsive patients, and a small decrease in platelet reactivity in another.

Clinical evidence

In an open-label study, 10 healthy subjects who had been classified as hyporesponsive to clopidogrel after administration of a single 300-mg dose, were given St John's wort 300 mg (containing 1.7% hyperforin) three times daily for 14 days (after a 7-day washout period) followed by another single 300-mg dose of clopidogrel. Platelet aggregation was decreased by about 30% by St John's wort.[1] Similarly, in a randomised, double-blind study, 20 post-coronary stent patients taking clopidogrel 75 mg daily and aspirin 81 mg to 325 mg daily, and classified as hyporesponsive to clopidogrel, were given St John's wort, 300 mg three times daily for 14 days, or placebo. Platelet reactivity was decreased by 18%, and platelet inhibition was increased by 78% by St John's wort.[1]

Experimental evidence

No relevant data found.

Mechanism

Clopidogrel is a prodrug and is metabolised to its active thiol metabolite by CYP3A4 and CYP2C19, as well as by CYP1A2 and CYP2B6. St John's wort is a known inducer of CYP3A4 and CYP2C19, and might also have some effects on CYP1A2 and CYP2B6. Metabolism of clopidogrel to its active metabolite might therefore be expected to be increased by St John's wort.

Importance and management

Evidence for an interaction between clopidogrel and St John's wort is limited to these studies. The clinical importance of the increased antiplatelet effect and decreased platelet reactivity seen is unclear, particularly because platelet reactivity studies might not be directly relevant to clinical outcomes, and whether this results in an increase in beneficial cardiovascular effects and/or an increase in the bleeding risk with clopidogrel requires further study. The authors of the studies[1] suggest that St John's wort might offer a therapeutic option for increasing the antiplatelet effects of clopidogrel in hyporesponders, but this also requires further study. Until further data are available on the clinical outcomes of this interaction, caution is advised on the concurrent use of clopidogrel and St John's wort. Bear this interaction in mind should any otherwise unexplained bleeding occur in a patient taking both drugs.

1. Lau WC, Welch TD, Shields T, Rubenfire M, Tantry US, Gurbel PA. The effect of St John's wort on the pharmacodynamic response of clopidogrel in hyporesponsive volunteers and patients: increased platelet inhibition by enhancement of CYP3A4 activity. *J Cardiovasc Pharmacol* (2011) 57, 86–93.

St John's wort + Clozapine

An isolated report describes reduced clozapine concentrations in a patient stabilised on clozapine, shortly after St John's wort was started.

Clinical evidence

A case report describes a 41-year-old patient with disorganised schizophrenia who had been stable on clozapine for 6 months and had a minimum plasma clozapine concentration of 0.46 to 0.57 mg/L at a dose of 500 mg daily. Shortly after starting St John's wort 300 mg three times daily (with each tablet containing hypericin 0.36 to 0.8 mg and hyperforin 9 mg), her clozapine plasma concentration decreased to 0.19 mg/L and she showed signs of increased disorganisation. Three weeks later, her clozapine plasma concentration was found to be 0.16 mg/L. One month after stopping St John's wort her clozapine plasma concentration

had increased to 0.32 mg/L and after another month it had further increased to 0.41 mg/L, and her psychiatric condition improved.[1]

Experimental evidence

No relevant data found.

Mechanism

Not established. Clozapine is principally metabolised by CYP1A2, with some involvement of other isoenzymes, such as CYP3A4. St John's wort is known to induce CYP3A4, and possibly affects CYP1A2, although evidence of clinically important interactions with St John's wort via CYP1A2 is lacking (see St John's wort + Theophylline, page 458). It is therefore possible that induction of CYP3A4 led to the decreased clozapine plasma concentrations seen.

Importance and management

The report of reduced clozapine concentrations in a patient taking St John's wort is isolated and as such its general clinical importance is not known. Nevertheless, it is consistent with the way St John's wort interacts with other drugs, and it would seem prudent to monitor clozapine concentrations in patients taking St John's wort, or consider this as a possible cause in cases of otherwise unexplained reductions in clozapine concentrations.

1. Van Strater ACP, Bogers JPAM. Interaction of St John's wort (*Hypericum perforatum*) with clozapine. *Int Clin Psychopharmacol* (2012) 27, 121–3.

St John's wort + Dextromethorphan

St John's wort does not affect the pharmacokinetics of dextromethorphan or debrisoquine.

Clinical evidence

In a study in 12 healthy subjects, St John's wort (*LI 160, Lichtwer Pharma*, 0.12 to 0.3% hypericin) 300 mg three times daily was taken for 16 days with a single 30-mg dose of dextromethorphan on day 14. There was no consistent change in the urinary dextromethorphan to dextrorphan metabolic ratio: 6 subjects had an increase in the production of dextrorphan while the other 6 subjects had a reduction in dextrorphan production. This finding was within the normal inter-patient variation in dextromethorphan metabolism.[1] Similar findings were reported in another study in 16 healthy subjects given a single 25-mg dose of dextromethorphan on the last day of a 14-day course of St John's wort (*Jarsin*; 900 micrograms of hypericin) 300 mg three times daily.[2] Similarly, the metabolism of dextromethorphan was not significantly affected by St John's wort when 12 healthy subjects were given a single 30-mg dose of dextromethorphan after 14 days of St John's wort (*Jarsin, Lichtwer Pharma*) 300 mg three times daily.[3] In yet another study in 12 healthy subjects, St John's wort 300 mg three times daily for 14 days had no significant effect on the urinary excretion of a single 30-mg oral dose of dextromethorphan either after one day or after 2 weeks of use. The St John's wort product used was from *Sundown Herbals* and provided about 33 mg of hyperforin daily.[4]

Three further studies found that St John's wort 300 mg three times daily (containing up to 24 mg of hyperforin) for 14 or 28 days had no clinically relevant effect on the pharmacokinetics of a single 5-mg dose of debrisoquine.[5–7]

Experimental evidence

An *in vitro* study[8] found that a St John's wort extract (*Hypericum Stada*) inhibited the metabolism of dextromethorphan when used as a probe substrate for cytochrome P450 isoenzyme CYP2D6.

Mechanism

St John's wort taken as a multiple-dose regimen does not appear to have a clinically relevant effect on the metabolism of dextromethorphan or debrisoquine, both of which are used as substrates to assess the activity of the cytochrome P450 isoenzyme CYP2D6. Inhibition of CYP2D6, seen in the single dose *in vitro* study is therefore not expected to be clinically relevant.

Importance and management

St John's wort is unlikely to interact with dextromethorphan to a clinically relevant extent. Dextromethorphan and debrisoquine are used as a probe drugs for CYP2D6 activity, and therefore these results also suggest that a pharmacokinetic interaction as a result of this mechanism between St John's wort and other CYP2D6 substrates is unlikely.

1. Markowitz JS, Donovan JL, DeVane CL, Taylor RM, Ruan Y, Wang J-S, Chavin KD. Effect of St John's wort on drug metabolism by induction of cytochrome P450 3A4 enzyme. *JAMA* (2003) 290, 1500–1504.
2. Wenk M, Todesco L, Krähenbühl S. Effect of St John's wort on the activities of CYP1A2, CYP3A4, CYP2D6, N-acetyltransferase 2, and xanthine oxidase in healthy males and females. *Br J Clin Pharmacol* (2004) 57, 494–9.
3. Roby CA, Dryer DA, Burstein AH. St. John's wort: effect on CYP2D6 activity using dextromethorphan-dextrorphan ratios. *J Clin Psychopharmacol* (2001) 21, 530–532.
4. Wang Z, Gorski JC, Hamman MA, Huang S-M, Lesko LJ, Hall SD. The effects of St John's wort (*Hypericum perforatum*) on human cytochrome P450 activity. *Clin Pharmacol Ther* (2001) 70, 317–26.
5. Gurley BJ, Gardner SF, Hubbard MA, Williams DK, Gentry WB, Cui Y, Ang CYW. Cytochrome P450 phenotypic ratios for predicting herb-drug interactions in humans. *Clin Pharmacol Ther* (2002) 72, 276–87.
6. Gurley BJ, Gardner SF, Hubbard MA, Williams DK, Gentry WB, Cui Y, Ang CYW. Clinical assessment of botanical supplementation on cytochrome P450 phenotypes in the elderly: St John's wort, garlic oil, *Panax ginseng*, and *Ginkgo biloba*. *Drugs Aging* (2005) 22, 525–39.
7. Gurley BJ, Swain A, Hubbard MA, Williams DK, Barone G, Hartsfield F, Tong Y, Carrier DJ, Cheboyina S, Battu SK. Clinical assessment of CYP2D6-mediated herb-drug interactions in humans: effects of milk thistle, black cohosh, goldenseal, kava kava, St. Johns wort, and *Echinacea*. *Mol Nutr Food Res* (2008) 52, 755–64.
8. Hellum BH, Nilsen OG. The *in vitro* inhibitory potential of trade herbal products on human CYP2D6-mediated metabolism and the influence of ethanol. *Basic Clin Pharmacol Toxicol* (2007) 101, 350–358.

St John's wort + Digoxin

Digoxin toxicity occurred in a patient taking digoxin when he stopped taking St John's wort. There is good evidence that some preparations of St John's wort can reduce the levels of digoxin by about one-quarter to one-third.

Clinical evidence

An 80-year-old man taking long-term digoxin and St John's wort herbal tea (2 litres daily) developed symptoms of digoxin toxicity (nodal bradycardia of 36 bpm and bigeminy) when he stopped taking the herbal tea.[1]

In a study 13 healthy subjects were given digoxin for 5 days until steady-state had been achieved, and then St John's wort extract (*LI 160, Lichtwer Pharma*) 300 mg three times daily for a further 10 days. The AUC and trough level of digoxin decreased by 28% and 37%, respectively. When compared with a parallel group of 12 subjects taking digoxin and placebo, the St John's wort group had 26.3% lower maximum plasma digoxin levels, 33.3% lower trough digoxin levels and a 25% lower AUC.[2]

In another study, 8 healthy subjects pretreated with St John's wort 300 mg 3 times daily for 14 days were given a single 500-microgram dose of digoxin. St John's wort decreased the AUC_{0-7} of digoxin by 18%.[3]

Another study in 18 healthy subjects found that St John's wort 300 mg 3 times daily (*Nature's Way,* containing a daily dose of 24 mg of hyperforin) for 14 days reduced the maximum levels and AUC_{0-24} of a single 250-microgram dose of digoxin by 36% and 23%, respectively. These findings were comparable to rifampicin (an established P-glycoprotein inducer) 600 mg daily for 7 days. No significant adverse effects were reported.[4]

In a further randomised placebo-controlled study, 93 healthy subjects were given digoxin alone for 7 days and then with one of ten St John's wort preparations for 14 days. The extract used in the earlier study (*LI 160, Jarsin 300, Lichtwer Pharma*) 300 mg three times daily similarly reduced the digoxin AUC, peak and trough plasma levels by 25%, 37%, and 19%, respectively. Comparable results were found with hypericum powder containing similar

amounts of hyperforin (about 21 mg daily), while hypericum powder with half the hyperforin content (about 10 mg daily) reduced the AUC, peak and trough plasma levels by about 18%, 21%, and 13%, respectively. Some St John's wort products, including tea, juice, oil extract, and powder with low-dose hyperforin (all 5 mg daily or less), did not significantly affect the pharmacokinetics of digoxin.[5] Similarly, a further study in 28 healthy subjects found no statistically significant change in digoxin pharmacokinetics when another low-hyperforin (about 3.5 mg daily) St John's wort extract (*Esbericum*) 120 mg was given twice daily for 11 days to patients who had received a digoxin loading dose of 750 micrograms daily for 2 days before starting St John's wort, and then received digoxin 250 micrograms daily each day during the study.[6]

Experimental evidence

In a study using human cell lines, St John's wort and hyperforin, a major active constituent, were found to induce P-glycoprotein transport of digoxin out of the cells in a reversible manner, which was comparable to rifampicin, a known inducer of P-glycoprotein. When treated with hypericin, another active constituent of St John's wort, the transport of digoxin out of the cells was not increased.[7]

Mechanism

St John's wort, and specifically hyperforin, a major active constituent, has been shown to increase the activity of the P-glycoprotein drug transporter protein in the intestines, which reduces the absorption of digoxin.[2-4,7]

Importance and management

Information seems to be limited to these reports, but the interaction would appear to be established. The extent of the interaction may depend on the St John's wort preparation involved and dose used and seems to be correlated with the dose of hyperforin.[4-7] Reductions in serum digoxin levels of the size seen with *LI 160* could diminish the control of arrhythmias or heart failure. Digoxin serum levels should therefore be closely monitored if St John's wort is either started or stopped, and appropriate dosage adjustments made if necessary. The recommendation of the CSM in the UK is that St John's wort should not be used by patients taking digoxin.[8]

Note that St John's wort does not appear to interfere with various immunoassays used for therapeutic drug monitoring of digoxin, see St John's wort + Laboratory tests, page 452.

1. Anđelić S. Bigeminija - rezultat interakcije digoksina i kantariona. *Vojnosanit Pregl* (2003) 60, 361–4.
2. Johne A, Brockmöller J, Bauer S, Maurer A, Langheinrich M, Roots I. Pharmacokinetic interaction of digoxin with an herbal extract from St John's wort (*Hypericum perforatum*). *Clin Pharmacol Ther* (1999) 66, 338–45.
3. Dürr D, Stieger B, Kullak-Ublick GA, Rentsch KM, Steinert HC, Meier PJ, Fattinger K. St John's wort induces intestinal P-glycoprotein/MDR1 and intestinal and hepatic CYP3A4. *Clin Pharmacol Ther* (2000) 68, 598–604.
4. Gurley BJ, Swain A, Williams DK, Barone G, Battu SK. Gauging the clinical significance of P-glycoprotein-mediated herb-drug interactions: Comparative effects of St John's wort, Echinacea, clarithromycin, and rifampin on digoxin pharmacokinetics. *Mol Nutr Food Res* (2008) 52, 772–9.
5. Mueller SC, Uehleke B, Woehling H, Petzsch M, Majcher-Peszynska J, Hehl E-M, Sievers H, Frank B, Riethling A-K, Drewelow B. Effect of St John's wort dose and preparations on the pharmacokinetics of digoxin. *Clin Pharmacol Ther* (2004) 75, 546–57.
6. Arold G, Donath F, Maurer A, Diefenbach K, Bauer S, Henneicke von Zepelin HH, Friede M, Roots I. No relevant interaction with alprazolam, caffeine, tolbutamide and digoxin by treatment with a low-hyperforin St John's wort extract. *Planta Med* (2005) 71, 331–7.
7. Tian R, Koyabu N, Morimoto S, Shoyama Y, Ohtani H, Sawada Y. Functional induction and de-induction of P-glycoprotein by St. John's wort and its ingredients in a human colon adenocarcinoma cell line. *Drug Metab Dispos* (2005) 33, 547–54.
8. Committee on the Safety of Medicines (UK). Message from Professor A Breckenridge (Chairman of CSM) and Fact Sheet for Health Care Professionals. Important interactions between St John's wort (*Hypericum perforatum*) preparations and prescribed medicines. February 2000 http://www.mhra.gov.uk/home/groups/comms-ic/documents/websiteresources/con019563.pdf (accessed 26/11/2008).

St John's wort + Eplerenone

St John's wort slightly decreases the AUC of eplerenone.

Clinical evidence

St John's wort caused a small 30% decrease in the AUC of a single 100-mg dose of eplerenone.[1,2]

Experimental evidence

No relevant data found.

Mechanism

Eplerenone is metabolised by the cytochrome P450 isoenzyme CYP3A4, and therefore inducers of this isoenzyme, such as St John's wort, would be expected to decrease its levels.

Importance and management

Because of the possibility of decreased efficacy of eplerenone, the UK manufacturers do not recommend the concurrent use of potent CYP3A4 inducers with eplerenone and they specifically name St John's wort.[1] However, it is unlikely that the decrease seen with St John's wort is clinically relevant. Further study is needed to demonstrate the clinical significance.

1. Inspra (Eplerenone). Pfizer Ltd. UK Summary of product characteristics, April 2007.
2. Inspra (Eplerenone). Pfizer Inc. US Prescribing information, April 2008.

St John's wort + Etoposide

The interaction between St John's wort and etoposide is based on experimental evidence only.

Clinical evidence

No interactions found.

Experimental evidence

In vitro studies suggest that hypericin, a component of St John's wort may antagonise the effects of etoposide. It may also stimulate the hepatic metabolism of etoposide by the cytochrome P450 isoenzyme CYP3A4.[1]

Mechanism

Etoposide is metabolised by the cytochrome P450 isoenzyme CYP3A4, and therefore inducers of this isoenzyme, such as St John's wort, would be expected to decrease its levels.

Importance and management

Information is very limited but it seems that it would be prudent to avoid St John's wort in patients taking etoposide or related drugs. More study is needed.

1. Peebles KA, Baker RK, Kurz EU, Schneider BJ, Kroll DJ. Catalytic inhibition of human DNA topoisomerase IIα by hypericin, a naphthodianthrone from St. John's wort (*Hypericum perforatum*). *Biochem Pharmacol* (2001) 62, 1059–70.

St John's wort + Fexofenadine

Pretreatment with St John's wort had no clinically relevant effect on the plasma levels of single-dose fexofenadine in one study, but markedly reduced fexofenadine levels in two others.

Clinical evidence

In a study in 12 healthy subjects, a single 900-mg dose of St John's wort (*Hypericum perforatum*) increased the maximum plasma level and AUC of a single 60-mg dose of fexofenadine by 45% and 31%, respectively.

Conversely, St John's wort 300 mg three times daily for 14 days caused a slight 5 to 10% decrease in the maximum level and AUC of a single dose of fexofenadine 60 mg in the same subjects.[1] In contrast, in another study, 12 days of pretreatment with St John's wort increased the oral clearance of a single dose of fexofenadine by about 1.6-fold in healthy subjects.[2] Similarly, a study in 30 healthy

subjects found that 10 days of pretreatment with St John's wort 300 mg 3 times daily, almost doubled the oral clearance of a single 60-mg dose of fexofenadine.[3]

Experimental evidence

No relevant data found.

Mechanism

In these studies St John's wort was thought to be interacting via its effects on P-glycoprotein.

Importance and management

The findings from these multiple-dose studies suggest that St John's wort either has no clinically relevant effect on fexofenadine, or that a decrease occurs that is possibly clinically important. It may be prudent to monitor closely for signs of reduced fexofenadine efficacy in a patient taking regular St John's wort, and if this is the case, consider St John's wort as a possible cause. Further study is needed.

1. Wang Z, Hamman MA, Huang S-M, Lesko LJ, Hall SD. Effect of St John's wort on the pharmacokinetics of fexofenadine. *Clin Pharmacol Ther* (2002) 71, 414–20.
2. Dresser GK, Schwarz UI, Wilkinson GR, Kim RB. Coordinate induction of both cytochrome P4503A and MDR1 by St John's wort in healthy subjects. *Clin Pharmacol Ther* (2003) 73, 41–50.
3. Xie R, Tan LH, Polasek EC, Hong C, Teillol-Foo M, Gordi T, Sharma A, Nickens DJ, Arakawa T, Knuth DW, Antal EJ. CYP3A and P-glycoprotein activity induction with St. John's wort in healthy volunteers from 6 ethnic populations. *J Clin Pharmacol* (2005) 45, 352–6.

St John's wort + Finasteride

St John's wort moderately reduces the exposure to finasteride.

Clinical evidence

An open study in 12 healthy men given 5 mg finasteride directly into the intestine via a catheter, found that St. John's wort (*Movina*) 300 mg twice daily (equivalent to hyperforin 4%) for 14 days reduced the maximum plasma concentration and AUC of finasteride by 34% and 58%, respectively. The clearance of finasteride was increased almost 2.5-fold. The AUC of the finasteride metabolite, carboxy-finasteride, remained largely unaffected but the maximum plasma concentration was increased by 62%.[1]

A patient with BPH controlled with finasteride had an increase in his serum prostate-specific antigen (PSA) concentration when St John's wort 900 mg (containing 4% hyperforin) daily was started. St John's wort was stopped and PSA concentrations gradually returned to baseline. Urological tests showed no changes in disease status.[2,3]

Experimental evidence

No relevant data found.

Mechanism

Finasteride is primarily metabolised by CYP3A4 in the liver, which is known to be induced by St. John's wort, and this most likely leads to the reduction in exposure seen.

Importance and management

The study and case report seem to be the only clinical evidence of the effects of St John's wort on finasteride. However, the moderate reduction in finasteride exposure seen in the study suggests that it is possible that finasteride will be less effective in those taking St John's wort. There is insufficient evidence to suggest that St John's wort should be avoided in patients taking finasteride. Nevertheless, it would seem prudent to bear the potential for reduced efficacy in mind, especially in patients taking finasteride for BPH.

1. Lundahl A, Hedeland M, Bondesson U, Knutson L, Lennernäs H. The effect of St. John's wort on the pharmacokinetics, metabolism and biliary excretion of finasteride and its metabolites in healthy men. *Eur J Pharm Sci* (2009) 36, 433–43.
2. Lochner S. Interaktionen zwischen Johanniskrautextrakt und Finasterid? *Med Monatsschr Pharm* (2010) 33, 307.
3. Lochner S 07 2012.

St John's wort + Food; Tyramine-rich

An isolated report describes a patient taking St John's wort who experienced a hypertensive crisis after consuming tyramine-rich food and drink.

Clinical evidence

A man who had taken a St John's wort supplement for 7 days (preparation and dose not stated) was admitted to hospital with confusion and disorientation. He was unable to recall events after eating aged cheeses and pouring a glass of red wine 8 hours earlier. On examination he had a pulse rate of 115 bpm, a respiratory rate of 16 breaths per minute and his blood pressure was 210/140 mmHg. He was treated with intravenous phentolamine and oral labetalol and his blood pressure decreased to 160/100 mmHg after 2 hours and the delirium also resolved. Extensive laboratory investigations did not find any cause for the hypertension and delirium.[1]

Experimental evidence

No relevant data found.

Mechanism

It was suggested that the time scale of starting to regularly take St John's wort and the onset of delirium and hypertension after the consumption of tyramine-rich food and drink was suggestive of hypertension associated with MAOIs. Normally any ingested tyramine is rapidly metabolised by the enzyme monoamine oxidase in the gut wall and liver before it reaches the general circulation. However, if the activity of the enzyme at these sites is inhibited (by the presence of an MAOI), any tyramine passes freely into the circulation, causing not just a rise in blood pressure, but a highly exaggerated rise due to the release from the adrenergic neurones of the large amounts of noradrenaline that accumulate there during inhibition of MAO.[2] Although St John's wort is a potent inhibitor of monoamine oxidase, this effect has not been demonstrated at recommended doses. It was concluded that the hypertensive crisis in this patient may have been mediated by monoamine oxidase inhibition, but there was also a possibility of another, as yet unknown, pharmacological action of St John's wort being involved.[1]

Importance and management

Given the widespread use of St John's wort, this case would seem to be unusual, and there is currently little grounds for suggesting any dietary restriction in those taking St John's wort.

1. Patel S, Robinson R, Burk M. Hypertensive crisis associated with St. John's wort. *Am J Med* (2002) 112, 507–8.
2. Generali JA, Hogan LC, McFarlane M, Schwab S, Hartman CR. Hypertensive crisis resulting from avocados and a MAO inhibitor. *Drug Intell Clin Pharm* (1981) 15, 904–6.

St John's wort + Herbal medicines

For a case report describing delirium following the use of St John's wort, valerian and loperamide, see under St John's wort + Loperamide, page 453.

St John's wort + HIV-protease inhibitors

St John's wort causes a marked reduction in the serum levels of indinavir, which may result in HIV treatment failure. Other HIV-protease inhibitors, whether used alone or boosted by ritonavir, are predicted to interact similarly.

Clinical evidence

In a single-drug pharmacokinetic study, 8 healthy subjects were given three 800-mg doses of **indinavir** on day 1 of to achieve steady-state serum levels, and then an 800-mg dose on day 2. For the next 14 days they were given St John's wort extract 300 mg three times daily. Starting on day 16, the **indinavir** dosing was repeated. It was found that the St John's wort reduced the mean AUC of **indinavir** by 54% and decreased the 8-hour **indinavir** trough serum level by 81%.[1]

Experimental evidence

No relevant data found.

Mechanism

Not fully understood, but it seems highly likely that St John's wort induces the activity of the cytochrome P450 isoenzyme CYP3A4, thereby increasing the metabolism of indinavir and therefore reducing its levels.

Importance and management

Direct information seems to be limited to this study, but the interaction would appear to be established. Such a large reduction in the serum levels of indinavir is likely to result in treatment failures and the development of viral resistance. Therefore St John's wort should be avoided. There seems to be no direct information about other HIV-protease inhibitors, but since they are also metabolised by CYP3A4 it is reasonable to expect that they will be similarly affected by St John's wort. The FDA in the US has suggested that concurrent use of St John's wort and HIV-protease inhibitors is not recommended.[2] Similarly, the CSM in the UK has advised that patients taking HIV-protease inhibitors should avoid St John's wort and that anyone already taking both should stop the St John's wort and have their HIV RNA viral load measured.[3] The levels of the HIV-protease inhibitors are likely to increase as the induction effects of St John's wort diminish, usually over one to two weeks.[4,5] Therefore the dose of the HIV-protease inhibitor will probably need adjusting. The US and UK manufacturers of all HIV-protease inhibitors (**amprenavir, atazanavir, darunavir, fosamprenavir, lopinavir/ritonavir, nelfinavir, ritonavir, saquinavir, tipranavir**) either contraindicate or advise against the use of St John's wort.

1. Piscitelli SC, Burstein AH, Chaitt D, Alfaro RM, Falloon J. Indinavir concentrations and St John's wort. *Lancet* (2000) 355, 547–8.
2. Lumpkin MM, Alpert S. FDA Public Healthy Advisory. Risk of drug interactions with St John's wort and indinavir and other drugs. February 2000 http://www.fda.gov/cder/drug/advisory/stjwort.htm (accessed 21/08/2007).
3. Committee on the Safety of Medicines (UK). Message from Professor A Breckenridge (Chairman of CSM) and Fact Sheet for Health Care Professionals. Important interactions between St John's wort (*Hypericum perforatum*) preparations and prescribed medicines. February 2000 http://www.mhra.gov.uk/home/groups/comms-ic/documents/websiteresources/con019563.pdf (accessed 26/11/2008).
4. Imai H, Kotegawa T, Tsutsumi K, Morimoto T, Eshima N, Nakano S, Ohashi K. The recovery time-course of CYP3A after induction by St John's wort administration. *Br J Clin Pharmacol* (2008) 65, 701–7.
5. Bauer S, Störmer E, Johne A, Krüger H, Budde K, Neumayer H-H, Roots I, Mai I. Alterations in cyclosporin A pharmacokinetics and metabolism during treatment with St John's wort in renal transplant patients. *Br J Clin Pharmacol* (2003) 55, 203–11.

St John's wort + Hormonal contraceptives

St John's wort may affect the pharmacokinetics of desogestrel, ethinylestradiol, and norethisterone. Both breakthrough bleeding and, more rarely, combined oral contraceptive failure has been reported in women taking St John's wort. Two cases describe the failure of emergency hormonal contraception, which was attributed to the use of St John's wort.

Clinical evidence

(a) Combined hormonal contraceptives

A study in 17 healthy women taking **ethinylestradiol/desogestrel** 20/150 micrograms daily found that St John's wort (300 mg twice

S

or three times daily) did not affect the AUC or maximum levels of **ethinylestradiol**. However, the AUC and maximum levels of the active metabolite of **desogestrel** were significantly decreased by about 40% and 20%, respectively. There was no evidence that ovulation occurred. However, the frequency of breakthrough bleeding increased significantly from 35% to around 80%, which may affect compliance.[1] Another study in 12 healthy women taking **ethinylestradiol/norethisterone** 35 micrograms/1 mg (*Ortho-Novum*) found that St John's wort 300 mg three times daily for 8 weeks increased the oral clearance of **norethisterone** and reduced the half-life of **ethinylestradiol,** but the serum levels of LH, FSH and progesterone were unaffected. However, of more importance, was the increase in breakthrough bleeding, which the authors state as a major cause of patients stopping hormonal contraceptives.[2] A further study in 16 subjects also found reductions in the levels of low-dose **ethinylestradiol/norethisterone** 20 micrograms/1 mg. Furthermore, they found increased progesterone levels of more than 3 nanograms/mL (an indication that ovulation occurred) in 3 patients who also took St John's wort compared with one subject who took placebo. Breakthrough bleeding was also increased.[3] In a secondary analysis of this study,[4] the anti-androgenic effects of **ethinylestradiol/norethisterone**, utilised in the treatment of hirsutism and acne, were not significantly affected by St John's wort.

The Adverse Drug Reactions Database of the Swedish Medical Products Agency has on record 2 cases of pregnancy due to the failure of a combined oral contraceptive, which was attributed to the use of products containing St John's wort (*Esberikum* and *Kira*). One woman was taking **ethinylestradiol** and **norethisterone** and the other was taking **ethinylestradiol** and **levonorgestrel**.[5] This follows an earlier report from the Swedish Medical Products Agency of 8 cases of breakthrough bleeding in women aged 23 to 31 taking long-term oral contraceptives and St John's wort. Breakthrough bleeding occurred within about a week of starting St John's wort in 5 of the cases, and was known to have resolved in 3 cases when the St John's wort was stopped.[6] The CSM in the UK has on record a further 7 cases of pregnancy in women taking St John's wort and oral contraceptives in the two-year period from February 2000 to February 2002.[7] Another earlier brief report describes 3 women taking a combined oral contraceptive (**ethinylestradiol/desogestrel** 30/150 micrograms) who developed breakthrough bleeding one week (2 cases) and 3 months (1 case) after starting to take St John's wort.[8] A single case of pregnancy has also been reported in a patient taking St John's wort with **ethinylestradiol/dienogest** (*Valette*).[9] The German Federal Institute for Drugs and Medical Devices has received a total of 8 case reports of ineffective contraception with St John's wort.[10]

In contrast, in a study, 16 healthy women took **ethinylestradiol/desogestrel** 20/150 micrograms daily on days 1 to 21 of a 28 day cycle, and an extract of St John's wort with a low hyperforin content of 650 micrograms, (Ze117, standardised to 0.2% hypericin), 250 mg twice daily on days 7 to 21. The plasma levels of **ethinylestradiol** and the active metabolite of **desogestrel** were not significantly altered by St John's wort. None of the women experienced any breakthrough bleeding or spotting, and measurements of plasma hormone levels indicated that the contraceptive efficacy was unchanged.[11]

(b) Emergency hormonal contraceptives

The CSM in the UK has received reports of 2 women taking St John's wort who became pregnant despite taking **emergency hormonal contraception**. One of them was also taking an oral contraceptive.[7]

Experimental evidence

No relevant data found.

Mechanism

It is believed that St John's wort can induce the metabolism of the contraceptive steroids by the cytochrome P450 isoenzyme CYP3A4, thereby reducing their serum levels and their effects.[6,8,12] This can lead to breakthrough bleeding and, in some

cases, contraceptive failure. This is consistent with the way St John's wort appears to lower the serum levels of some other drugs. Note that although hyperforin is the most likely constituent responsible for enzyme induction (supported by the study that found no interaction with a low-hyperforin preparation), others may contribute and the levels of individual constituents can vary between different preparations of the herb.

Importance and management

Information appears to be limited to these reports but the interaction between hormonal contraceptives and St John's wort appears to be established. Its incidence is not known but the evidence so far suggests that breakthrough bleeding may be a problem, although pregnancy resulting from this interaction appears to be uncommon. Only two cases of emergency hormonal contraceptive failure attributed to an interaction with St John's wort have so far been reported, but the effects of any interaction here would be very difficult to assess. Since it is not known who is particularly likely to be at risk, the recommendation of the CSM/MCA and the Faculty of Family Planning and Reproductive Health Care (FFPRHC) in the UK[12,13] is that women taking **oral contraceptives** (both **combined** and **progestogen-only pills**) should either avoid St John's wort or they should use an additional form of contraception. The FFPRHC Clinical Effectiveness Unit is in agreement with the CSM advice but recommends that, if St John's wort must be continued, the following general guidelines[13] for the use of liver enzyme inducers with hormonal contraceptives should be followed:

- Women taking **combined oral contraceptives** should use an ethinylestradiol dose of at least 50 micrograms daily. The dose may be increased further above 50 micrograms if breakthrough bleeding occurs. Omitting or reducing the pill-free interval has not been shown to reduce the risk of ovulation with liver enzyme inducers. Additional non-hormonal methods of contraception, such as condoms, should also be used by patients using combined hormonal contraceptives, both when taking the liver enzyme inducers and for at least 4 weeks after stopping the drug. Alternatives to all forms of combined hormonal contraceptives should be considered with long-term use of liver enzyme inducers.
- The **combined contraceptive patch** may be continued in the usual manner. Additional, non-hormonal methods of contraception, such as condoms, should also be used by patients using the combined contraceptive patch, both when taking the liver enzyme inducers and for at least 4 weeks after stopping the drug. Using more than one patch is not recommended.
- The **progestogen-only oral contraceptive** is not recommended for use with liver enzyme inducers. Alternative methods of contraception are advised.
- The **progestogen-only implant** may be continued with short courses of enzyme inducers. Additional non-hormonal methods of contraception, such as condoms, should also be used by patients using the progestogen-only implant, both when taking the liver enzyme inducers and for at least 4 weeks after stopping the drug. Alternatives to the progestogen-only implant should be considered with long-term use of liver enzyme inducers.
- The effectiveness of both **combined** and the **progestogen-only emergency hormonal contraceptive** will be reduced in women taking liver enzyme inducers. The FFPRHC Clinical Effectiveness Unit states that there appears to be no good evidence on how to manage the interaction between emergency hormonal contraception and enzyme inducers such as St John's wort, but current clinical practice is to increase the contraceptive dose by approximately 50%.[13] The British National Formulary recommends giving a single 3-mg dose of **levonorgestrel**, although this is unlicensed.[14] A copper IUD may also be used as an effective alternative.[13] In the UK it is possible to buy the progestogen-only emergency hormonal contraception without a prescription; however, it has been advised that patients taking enzyme inducers should not be supplied the emergency hormonal contraceptive but should be referred to a doctor or family planning service.[13,15] Given the

potential consequences of an unwanted pregnancy, these seem sensible precautions.

- The depot **progestogen-only injection**, **copper** and **levonorgestrel-releasing intrauterine devices** (**IUD**) do not appear to be affected by enzyme-inducing drugs, such as St John's wort, and may be used as alternative contraceptive methods, particularly for women requiring hormonal contraception who are likely to be taking the enzyme inducer in the long-term, as these are unaffected by liver enzyme inducers.

Although the considerable worldwide popularity of St John's wort is fairly recent, it is currently the most widely used antidepressant in Germany and has been used for very many years in both Germany and Austria. Yet, there seems to be no published evidence that oral contraceptive failure in those countries is more frequent than anywhere else. This would seem to confirm that contraceptive failure leading to pregnancy occurring as a result of this interaction is very uncommon, or perhaps that it has failed to be identified as a possible cause.

The anti-androgenic effects of ethinylestradiol/norethisterone, utilised in the treatment of hirsutism and acne, do not appear to be significantly affected by St John's wort. However, as this was a small study, it may be prudent to still monitor the effectiveness of the combined hormonal contraceptive for this indication until further evidence is available.

1. Pfrunder A, Schiesser M, Gerber S, Haschke M, Bitzer J, Drewe J. Interaction of St John's wort with low-dose oral contraceptive therapy: a randomized controlled trial. *Br J Clin Pharmacol* (2003) 56, 683–90.
2. Hall SD, Wang Z, Huang S-M, Hamman MA, Vasavada N, Adigun AQ, Hilligoss JK, Miller M, Gorski JC. The interaction between St John's wort and an oral contraceptive. *Clin Pharmacol Ther* (2003) 74, 525–35.
3. Murphy PA, Kern SE, Stanczyk FZ, Westhoff CL. Interaction of St John's wort with oral contraceptives: effects on the pharmacokinetics of norethindrone and ethinyl estradiol, ovarian activity and breakthrough bleeding. *Contraception* (2005) 71, 402–8.
4. Fogle RH, Murphy PA, Westhoff CL, Stanczyk FZ. Does St. John's Wort interfere with the antiandrogenic effect of oral contraceptive pills? *Contraception* (2006) 74, 245–8.
5. Swedish Medical Products Agency. St John's wort may influence other medication. Data on file. 2002.
6. Yue Q-Y, Bergquist C, Gerdén B. Safety of St John's wort (Hypericum perforatum). *Lancet* (2000) 355, 576–7.
7. Committee on Safety of Medicines. Personal communication. February 2002.
8. Bon S, Hartmann K, Kuhn M. Johanniskraut: Ein Enzyminduktor? *Schweiz Apothekerzeitung* (1999) 16, 535–6.
9. Schwarz UI, Büschel B, Kirch W. Unwanted pregnancy on self-medication with St John's wort despite hormonal contraception. *Br J Clin Pharmacol* (2003) 55, 112–13.
10. Bundesinstitut für Arzneimittel und Medizinprodukte. March 2007.
11. Will-Shahab L, Bauer S, Kunter U, Roots I, Brattström A. St John's wort extract (Ze 117) does not alter the pharmacokinetics of a low-dose oral contraceptive. *Eur J Clin Pharmacol* (2009) 65, 287–94.
12. Committee on the Safety of Medicines (UK). Message from Professor A Breckenridge (Chairman of CSM) and Fact Sheet for Health Care Professionals. Important interactions between St John's wort (*Hypericum perforatum*) preparations and prescribed medicines. February 2000 http://www.mhra.gov.uk/home/groups/comms-ic/documents/websiteresources/con019563.pdf (accessed 26/11/2008).
13. Faculty of Family Planning and Reproductive Health Care Clinical Effectiveness Unit. FFPRHC Guidance: Drug interactions with hormonal contraception. April 2005 http://www.ffprhc.org.uk/admin/uploads/DrugInteractionsFinal.pdf (accessed 27/11/2008).
14. British National Formulary 57th ed. London: The British Medical Association and The Pharmaceutical Press; 2009. p. 448.
15. Royal Pharmaceutical Society of Great Britain. Practice guidance on the supply of emergency hormonal contraception as a pharmacy medicine. September 2004 http://www.rpsgb.org/pdfs/ehcguid.pdf (accessed 27/11/2008).

St John's wort + Ibuprofen

St John's wort does not affect the pharmacokinetics of ibuprofen.

Clinical evidence

Eight healthy male subjects were given an oral dose of ibuprofen 400 mg before, and at the end of, a 21 day course of St John's wort 300 mg three times daily. The pharmacokinetics of ibuprofen were unaffected by St John's wort. The St John's wort extract was standardised to contain hypericin (probably 0.3%) and a minimum of 4% hyperforin.[1]

Experimental evidence

No relevant data found.

Mechanism

As ibuprofen is a substrate for the cytochrome P450 isoenzymes CYP2C9 and CYP2C8, the authors of the study suggest that the lack of interaction is evidence that St John's wort has no significant effects on these isoenzymes.[1] Minor or no significant effects on pharmacokinetics have similarly been reported for rosiglitazone, a substrate for CYP2C8, and gliclazide, and tolbutamide both of which are substrates for CYP2C9. See St John's wort + Antidiabetics, page 440.

Importance and management

St John's wort does not appear to interact with ibuprofen and therefore no special precautions seem necessary on concurrent use.

1. Bell EC, Ravis WR, Lloyd KB, Stokes TJ. Effects of St. John's wort supplementation on ibuprofen pharmacokinetics. *Ann Pharmacother* (2007) 41, 229–34.

St John's wort + Imatinib

St John's wort lowers serum imatinib levels.

Clinical evidence

In a study in 12 healthy subjects, the pharmacokinetics of a single dose of imatinib was determined before, and on day 12, of two weeks of treatment with St John's wort extract (Kira [*LI 160*], Lichtwer Pharma) 300 mg three times daily. The AUC and maximum plasma level of imatinib was decreased by 30% and 15%, respectively. Imatinib clearance was increased by 43% and its half-life was decreased from 12.8 to 9 hours.[1] Similar results were found in another study.[2]

Experimental evidence

No relevant data found.

Mechanism

St John's wort induces intestinal CYP3A4 and it therefore also reduces imatinib levels.

Importance and management

This study suggests that St John's wort may modestly reduce the exposure to imatinib, which could result in a reduction in its efficacy. The manufacturers suggest that concurrent use of imatinib and potent enzyme-inducing drugs should be avoided.[3,4] St John's wort has smaller effects than other known CYP3A4 inducers, but nevertheless, some suggested that concurrent use should also be avoided.[1] However, if this is not possible it would be prudent to monitor the outcome of concurrent use closely, and increase the imatinib dose as necessary.

1. Frye RF, Fitzgerald SM, Lagattuta TF, Hruska MW, Egorin MJ. Effect of St John's wort on imatinib mesylate pharmacokinetics. *Clin Pharmacol Ther* (2004) 76, 323–9.
2. Smith P. The influence of St John's wort on the pharmacokinetics and protein binding of imatinib mesylate. *Pharmacotherapy* (2004) 24, 1508–14.
3. Glivec (Imatinib mesilate). Novartis Pharmaceuticals UK Ltd. UK Summary of product characteristics, November 2007.
4. Gleevec (Imatinib mesylate). Novartis Pharmaceuticals Corporation. US Prescribing information, September 2008.

St John's wort + Interferons

An isolated report describes acute hepatotoxicity in a patient taking peginterferon alfa and St John's wort.

Evidence, mechanism, importance and management

A case report describes a 61-year-old woman with chronic hepatitis C receiving peginterferon alfa-2a 180 micrograms weekly, who developed acute hepatitis while taking St John's wort. The patient had undetectable hepatitis C virus RNA after 8 weeks of peginterferon, but at week 8 her ALT and AST concentrations were

S

grossly elevated (at 700 units/L and 1200 units/L respectively) and treatment with peginterferon alfa-2a was stopped. Three weeks later, her ALT and AST concentrations continued to increase, intense jaundice developed, and her prothrombin time became prolonged. On further questioning, the patient revealed she had been taking St John's wort, 2 capsules daily (exact dose not stated), for 6 weeks. Due to the worsening liver failure, the patient was admitted to hospital for treatment and was discharged 4 weeks later. The authors concluded that while the initial hepatotoxicity might have been caused by peginterferon alfa-2a, the continuation of St John's wort (including after the peginterferon was stopped) might have contributed to the severity of the reaction.[1] This is an isolated report and as such its general clinical importance is not known.

1. Piccolo P, Gentile S, Alegiani F, Angelico M. Severe drug induced acute hepatitis associated with use of St John's wort (*Hypericum perforatum*) during treatment with pegylated interferon α. *BMJ Case Rep* (2009) Epub, .

St John's wort + Irinotecan

St John's wort increases the metabolism of irinotecan, which may decrease its efficacy.

Clinical evidence

In a randomised, crossover study St John's wort decreased the AUC of the active metabolite of irinotecan, SN-38, by 42%, but had no statistically significant effect on the AUC of the inactive metabolite, APC. Myelosuppression was also reduced; with irinotecan alone the leucocyte and neutrophil counts decreased by 56% and 63%, respectively, but in the presence of St John's wort the decreases were only 8.6% and 4.3%, respectively. In this study, irinotecan was given as a single 350-mg/m² intravenous dose every 3 weeks, and during one cycle a St John's wort preparation was given three times daily, beginning 14 days before and stopping 4 days after the irinotecan.[1]

Experimental evidence

In an experimental study in *rats,* St John's wort 400 mg/kg given daily for 14 days reduced the maximum levels of irinotecan and its active metabolite, SN-38, by 39.5% and 38.9%, respectively. The AUC of SN-38 was also reduced by 26.3%.[2]

Mechanism

St John's wort induces CYP3A4 and P-glycoprotein, which are both involved in the metabolism of irinotecan. The evidence suggests that St John's wort increases the metabolism of irinotecan to an unknown inactive metabolite (other than APC), rather than the active metabolite, SN-38, thereby reducing its effects.[1]

Importance and management

Evidence for an interaction between irinotecan and St John's wort appears to be limited. Irinotecan has a narrow therapeutic range, and as it is a prodrug that is metabolised to its active metabolite SN-38, the lower levels of SN-38 suggest that its efficacy will be reduced in the presence of St John's wort. It would therefore seem sensible to warn patients who are about to receive irinotecan to avoid St John's wort. Note that the manufacturers state that the use of St John's wort with irinotecan is contraindicated,[3,4] and that St John's wort should be stopped at least 2 weeks before irinotecan is given.[4] It seems likely that **topotecan**, a related drug that is also a substrate for CYP3A4, will be similarly affected by St John's wort, but evidence for this is lacking.

1. Mathijssen RHJ, Verweij J, de Bruijn P, Loos WJ, Sparreboom A. Effects of St John's wort on irinotecan metabolism. *J Natl Cancer Inst* (2002) 94, 1247–9.
2. Hu Z-P, Yang X-X, Chen X, Cao J, Chan E, Duan W, Huang M, Yu X-Q, Wen J-Y, Zhou S-F. A mechanistic study on altered pharmacokinetics of irinotecan by St. John's wort. *Curr Drug Metab* (2007) 8, 157–71.
3. Campto (Irinotecan hydrochloride trihydrate). Pfizer Ltd. UK Summary of product characteristics, May 2009.
4. Camptosar (Irinotecan hydrochloride). Pfizer Inc. US Prescribing information, August 2010.

St John's wort + Ivabradine

The metabolism of ivabradine is increased by St John's wort.

Clinical evidence

Twelve healthy subjects were given a single oral dose of ivabradine 10 mg 24 hours before St John's wort (*Jarsin* tablets) 300 mg three times daily was given for 14 days. On day 16, they were given a further dose of ivabradine 10 mg with a single 300-mg dose of St John's wort. The maximum levels and AUC of ivabradine were reduced by more than half by St John's wort. The maximum levels and AUC of its active metabolite were reduced by 25% and 32%, respectively. No adverse effects were reported, and the heart rate and blood pressure remained unchanged.[1] Similar findings are also reported by the manufacturers of ivabradine.[2]

Experimental evidence

No relevant data found.

Mechanism

St John's wort is a known inducer of the cytochrome P450 isoenzyme CYP3A4, by which ivabradine is metabolised. Concurrent use therefore increases the metabolism of ivabradine, which results in a reduction in its plasma levels, and a potential reduction in effects.

Importance and management

Evidence is limited to the study above, and despite the lack of change in pharmacodynamic effects seen in this study, the pharmacokinetic changes may be significant to affect individual patients. Monitor concurrent use for ivabradine efficacy and adjust the dose as necessary. Remember to re-adjust the dose of ivabradine if concurrent use of these drugs is stopped. The UK manufacturer suggests that the use of St John's wort should be restricted in patients taking ivabradine.[2]

1. Portolés A, Terleira A, Calvo A, Martrnez I, Resplandy G. Effects of Hypericum perforatum on ivabradine pharmacokinetics in healthy volunteers: an open-label, pharmacokinetic interaction clinical trial. *J Clin Pharmacol* (2006) 46, 1188–94.
2. Procoralan (Ivabradine hydrochloride). Servier Laboratories Ltd. UK Summary of product characteristics, March 2007.

St John's wort + Laboratory tests

St John's wort does not interfere with *in vitro* assays for carbamazepine, ciclosporin, digoxin, phenobarbital, phenytoin, procainamide, quinidine, tacrolimus, theophylline, tricyclic antidepressants, and valproate.

Clinical evidence

No interactions found.

Experimental evidence

In *in vitro* experiments, St John's wort added to serum samples did not interfere with a fluorescence polarization immunoassay (FPIA, Abbott Laboratories) for **carbamazepine**, **digoxin**, **phenytoin**, **quinidine**, **theophylline**, **tricyclic antidepressants**, and **valproate**. It also did not interfere with a serum sample microparticle enzyme immunoassay (MEIA, Abbott Laboratories) for **digoxin**, or other assays (exact assays not specified, Roche Diagnostics/Hitachi) for **phenobarbital** or **procainamide**. Whole-blood FPIA analysis of **ciclosporin** levels and whole-blood MEIA analysis of **tacrolimus** levels were also not affected by the addition of St John's wort.[1]

Mechanism

No mechanism expected.

Importance and management

St John's wort does not appear to interfere with various immuno-assays used for therapeutic drug monitoring of carbamazepine, ciclosporin, digoxin, phenobarbital, phenytoin, procainamide, quinidine, tacrolimus, theophylline, tricyclics, and valproate.

1. Dasgupta A, Tso G, Szelei-Stevens K. St. John's wort does not interfere with thera-peutic drug monitoring of 12 commonly monitored drugs using immunoassays. *J Clin Lab Anal* (2006) 20, 62–7.

St John's wort + Lithium

A brief report describes mania in a patient taking lithium who also took St John's wort.

Evidence, mechanism, importance and management

A search of Health Canada's database of spontaneous adverse reac-tions identified one case in which St John's wort was suspected of inducing mania in a patient also taking lithium.[1] The reasons for this effect are unknown, although it seems likely that the symptoms could be due to the effects of both lithium and St John's wort on serotonin. No further details were given of this case.

1. Griffiths J, Jordan S, Pilan K. Natural health products and adverse reactions. *Can Adverse React News* (2004) 14, 2–3.

St John's wort + Loperamide

A case report describes delirium in a woman taking St John's wort and valerian root who also took loperamide.

Clinical evidence

A 39-year-old woman who had been taking two tablets of St John's wort with **valerian** root daily for 6 months (exact products and doses not specified), was hospitalised after becoming disorientated, agitated and confused. The patient had also recently started lop-eramide for diarrhoea prior to admission. The delirium subsided within two days of stopping these drugs.[1]

Experimental evidence

No relevant data found.

Mechanism

Unclear. A MAOI-induced reaction caused by the combination of St John's wort and loperamide was suggested as a possible cause for the delirium. However, an interaction between St John's wort and valerian, or valerian and loperamide, cannot not be ruled out.[1]

Importance and management

This appears to be the only report of delirium associated with the combination of St John's wort, valerian and loperamide. Its general relevance is therefore unclear.

1. Khawaja IS, Marotta RF, Lippmann S. Herbal medicines as a factor in delirium. *Psy-chiatr Serv* (1999) 50, 969–70.

St John's wort + Methotrexate

The interaction between St John's wort and methotrexate is based on experimental evidence only.

Clinical evidence

No interactions found.

Experimental evidence

In a study in rats given oral methotrexate 5 mg/kg, the AUC of methotrexate was 55% higher in those also given oral St John's wort 150 mg/kg (standardised to contain 0.3% hypericin) when compared with those given methotrexate alone. A larger 300 mg/kg dose of St John's wort had a greater effect, with the AUC and maximum con-centration of methotrexate 163% and 60% higher, respectively, than with methotrexate alone. At both St John's wort doses, the increased exposure to methotrexate was associated with greater mortality than with methotrexate alone.[1]

Mechanism

St John's wort metabolites inhibited multi-drug resistance protein 2 (MRP 2) *in vitro* and it was suggested that methotrexate transport was affected by this mechanism.

Importance and management

Evidence for an interaction between St John's wort and methotrex-ate appears to be limited to this study, which found greater methotrexate exposure and mortality in the presence of St John's wort. Although the findings of *animal* studies cannot always be reliably extrapolated to clinical practice, they do suggest that St John's wort might increase methotrexate toxicity. In this study, **diclofenac**, which is known to have a clinically relevant interaction with methotrexate, was used as a positive control and its effects on methotrexate exposure were of a similar order of magnitude to those of St John's wort. Therefore, until more is known, if concurrent use cannot be avoided, it might be prudent to increase the frequency of monitoring of full blood counts, and renal and liver function. Patients should be told to report any sign or symptom suggestive of infection, particularly sore throat (which might possibly indicate that white cell counts have fallen) or dyspnoea or cough (suggestive of pulmonary toxicity).

1. Yang S-H, Juang S-H, Tsai S-Y, Chao P-DL, Hou Y-C. St John's wort significantly increased the systemic exposure and toxicity of methotrexate in rats. *Toxicol Appl Pharmacol* (2012) 263, 39–43.

St John's wort + Methylphenidate

St John's wort may decrease the efficacy of methylphenidate in the treatment of attention deficit hyperactivity disorder.

Evidence, mechanism, importance and management

A 22-year-old man who had been successfully treated with methylphenidate 20 mg daily for attention deficit hyperactiv-ity disorder (ADHD) for 6 months started to take St John's wort 600 mg daily. Over the next 4 months the efficacy of methylphenidate decreased, but 3 weeks after St John's wort was stopped, methylphenidate became more effective. No adverse effects were seen during the concurrent use of the herbal medicine and the drug.[1]

This is an isolated case report and therefore no general recommendations can be made. However, if the efficacy of methylphenidate becomes reduced, it may be worth questioning the patient about St John's wort use, and giving consideration to stopping the herb.

1. Niederhofer H. St John's wort may diminish methylphenidate's efficacy in treating patients suffering from attention deficit hyperactivity disorder. *Med Hypotheses* (2007) 68, 1189.

St John's wort + Mycophenolate

St John's wort does not appear to alter the pharmacokinetics of mycophenolate.

Clinical evidence

In a pharmacokinetic study, 8 stable kidney transplant patients tak-ing mycophenolate 1 g to 2 g daily and **tacrolimus** were given 600 mg of St John's wort extract (*Jarsin 300*) daily for 14 days.

S

The levels of mycophenolic acid, the main metabolite of mycophenolate, were measured before St John's wort was started, on day 14, and two weeks after St John's wort was stopped. The pharmacokinetics of mycophenolic acid were unchanged throughout the study, and no dosage adjustments were needed in any of the 8 patients.[1]

Experimental evidence

No relevant data found.

Mechanism

No mechanism. St John's wort is an inducer of the cytochrome P450 isoenzyme CYP3A4 and P-glycoprotein. As mycophenolate is not significantly metabolised or transported by these routes, an interaction would not be expected.

Importance and management

St John's wort does not appear to affect the pharmacokinetics of mycophenolate and therefore no additional precautions seem necessary on concurrent use.

1. Mai I, Störmer E, Bauer S, Krüger H, Budde K, Roots I. Impact of St John's wort treatment on the pharmacokinetics of tacrolimus and mycophenolic acid in renal transplant patients. *Nephrol Dial Transplant* (2003) 18, 819–22.

St John's wort + NNRTIs

There is some evidence to suggest that St John's wort may decrease the levels of nevirapine. Delavirdine and efavirenz would be expected to be similarly affected.

Clinical evidence

Nevirapine levels, obtained by routine monitoring, were noted to be lower in 5 men who were also taking St John's wort. Based on a pharmacokinetic modelling analysis, it was estimated that St John's wort increased the oral clearance of **nevirapine** by about 35%.[1]

Experimental evidence

No relevant data found.

Mechanism

This finding supports predictions based on the known metabolism of the NNRTIs **delavirdine**, **efavirenz** and nevirapine by the cytochrome P450 isoenzyme CYP3A4, of which St John's wort is a known inducer.

Importance and management

The interaction between St John's wort and nevirapine confirms advice issued by the CSM in the UK,[2] that St John's wort may decrease blood levels of the NNRTIs with possible loss of HIV suppression. Therefore concurrent use should be avoided.

1. de Maat MMR, Hoetelmans RMW, Mathôt RAA, van Gorp ECM, Meenhorst PL, Mulder JW, Beijnen JH. Drug interaction between St John's wort and nevirapine. *AIDS* (2001) 15, 420–421.
2. Committee on the Safety of Medicines (UK). Message from Professor A Breckenridge (Chairman of CSM) and Fact Sheet for Health Care Professionals. Important interactions between St John's wort (*Hypericum perforatum*) preparations and prescribed medicines. February 2000 http://www.mhra.gov.uk/home/groups/comms-ic/documents/websiteresources/con019563.pdf (accessed 26/11/2008).

St John's wort + Opioids

St John's wort reduces the plasma concentrations of methadone. Exposure to oxycodone was halved in one study. St John's wort is predicted to induce the metabolism of tapentadol.

Clinical evidence

(a) Methadone

In a study in 4 patients taking **methadone**, St John's wort (*Jarsin*) 900 mg daily for 14 to 47 days decreased **methadone** plasma concentration-to-dose ratios (indicating decreased **methadone** levels) by 19 to 60%. Two patients reported symptoms that suggested a withdrawal syndrome.[1]

(b) Oxycodone

In a crossover study in 12 healthy subjects, St John's wort (*Jarsin* containing hyperforin 2 to 6%) 300 mg three times daily was given for 15 days, with a single 15-mg oral dose of oxycodone on day 14. The AUC and maximum plasma concentration of oxycodone were reduced by 50% and 29%, respectively, and the AUC and maximum plasma concentration of the oxycodone metabolite, noroxycodone, were increased by 13% and 50%, respectively. The AUC of another metabolite, oxymorphone, was reduced by 52%, but its maximum plasma concentration was not notably affected. St John's wort reduced the self-reported analgesic effect of oxycodone (using visual analogue scales), but had no effect on cold pain intensity and threshold, as assessed using the cold pressor test. All but two of the subjects were extensive CYP2D6 metabolisers (that is, they had normal CYP2D6 activity).[2]

Experimental evidence

No relevant data found.

Mechanism

St John's wort is a known inducer of CYP3A4, and so can affect plasma concentrations of drugs metabolised by this isoenzyme, such as methadone.[1] Oxycodone is metabolised to noroxycodone by CYP3A4, and to oxymorphone by CYP2D6. St John's wort therefore increases the metabolism of oxycodone to noroxycodone, increasing its exposure. The mechanism of the proposed interaction with tapentadol is unclear, as tapentadol is principally metabolised by a number of glucuronidases. *In vitro* and *animal* studies suggest that some constituents of St. John's wort can alter the activity of glucuronidases, but the *in vivo* consequences of this effect are unknown.[3] Further study is needed.

Importance and management

St John's wort appears to reduce the plasma concentrations of methadone causing withdrawal symptoms in some patients. Therefore, concurrent use should be avoided. It might be prudent to follow the same advice for other opioids[4] that are mainly metabolised by CYP3A4, such as **buprenorphine**, **fentanyl** or **alfentanil**. Exposure to oxycodone is halved by St John's wort, but its analgesic effects do not appear to be notably altered. Concurrent use need not be avoided, but consider this interaction in the case of any unexpected reduction in analgesic effect, and adjust the oxycodone dose accordingly.

The UK manufacturer of **tapentadol** states that caution is necessary if a strong enzyme inducer (they name St John's wort) is started or stopped in a patient taking tapentadol, as this might lead to decreased efficacy or an increased risk of adverse effects.[5] The clinical importance of this prediction is unclear, but until more is known, be aware that the dose of tapentadol might need to be adjusted on concurrent use.

1. Eic-Höchli D, Oppliger R, Powell Golay K, Baumann P, Eap CB. Methadone maintenance treatment and St John's wort. *Pharmacopsychiatry* (2003) 36, 35–7.
2. Nieminen TH, Hagelberg NM, Saari TI, Neuvonen M, Laine K, Neuvonen PJ, Olkkola KT. St John's wort greatly reduces the concentrations of oral oxycodone. *Eur J Pain* (2010) 14, 854–9.
3. Mohamed M-EF, Frye RF. Effects of herbal supplements on drug glucuronidation. Review of clinical, animal, and in vitro studies. *Planta Med* (2011) 77, 311–21.
4. Kumar NB, Allen K, Bel H. Perioperative herbal supplement use in cancer patients: potential implications and recommendations for presurgical screening. *Cancer Control* (2005) 12, 149–57.
5. Palexia Tapentadol hydrochloride. Grünenthal Ltd UK Summary of product characteristics, February 2011.

St John's wort + Prednisone

St John's wort does not appear to affect the pharmacokinetics of prednisone.

Clinical evidence

Eight healthy male subjects were given a single oral dose of prednisone 20 mg before, and at the end, of a 28 day course of St John's wort 300 mg three times daily. The pharmacokinetics of prednisone, and its metabolite prednisolone, were not significantly affected by St John's wort. The St John's wort extract was standardised to contain hypericin 0.3% and a minimum of 4% hyperforin.[1]

Experimental evidence

No relevant data found.

Mechanism

It was thought that St John's wort, a known inducer of the cytochrome P450 isoenzyme CYP3A4, would increase the metabolism of prednisone and prednisolone and reduce their levels. While prednisone and prednisolone are substrates of CYP3A4, it is not a major metabolic pathway as they have been shown to be relatively unaffected by potent CYP3A4 inhibitors in healthy subjects.

Importance and management

St John's wort does not appear to induce the metabolism of a single dose of prednisone, or its metabolite prednisolone, in healthy male subjects; however, further study is needed to clarify significance of this in patients receiving long-term prednisone.

1. Bell EC, Ravis WR, Chan HM, Lin Y-J. Lack of pharmacokinetic interaction between St. John's wort and prednisone. *Ann Pharmacother* (2007) 41, 1819–24.

St John's wort + Procainamide

The interaction between St John's wort and procainamide is based on experimental evidence only.

Clinical evidence

No interactions found.

Experimental evidence

In a study in *mice,* a single dose of St John's wort extract significantly raised the bioavailability of procainamide 100 mg/kg for a period of up to 4 hours. A trend towards an increase in procainamide levels was seen in the *mice* given St John's wort for 2 weeks, with the procainamide dose given the day after St John's wort stopped, however this was not statistically significant. Other pharmacokinetic parameters remained unaffected by both single-dose and long-term use of St John's wort.[1]

Mechanism

Not understood.

Importance and management

The evidence for any significant effect of St John's wort on the pharmacokinetics of procainamide is extremely limited and although the bioavailability of procainamide may have been raised slightly in *mice,* its metabolism was unchanged. The clinical significance of this in humans is unknown and further study is needed.

St John's wort also does not interfere with laboratory assays for procainamide, see St John's wort + Laboratory tests, page 452.

1. Dasgupta A, Hovanetz M, Olsen M, Wells A, Actor JK. Drug-herb interaction. Effect of St John's wort on bioavailability and metabolism of procainamide in mice. *Arch Pathol Lab Med* (2007) 131, 1094–8.

St John's wort + Proton pump inhibitors

St John's wort induces the metabolism of omeprazole, and this might result in reduced efficacy. Other proton pump inhibitors are likely to be similarly affected.

Clinical evidence

In a crossover study, 12 healthy subjects (6 of the extensive CYP2C19 metaboliser phenotype and 6 of the poor CYP2C19 metaboliser phenotype) were given St John's wort 300 mg three times daily or placebo for 14 days, followed by a single 20-mg dose of **omeprazole** on day 15. St John's wort modestly decreased the AUC of **omeprazole** in all subjects (by 49% in extensive metabolisers and 41% in poor metabolisers), and also increased the plasma levels of **hydroxyomeprazole** by 35% in those who were extensive metabolisers. It also markedly increased the levels of the inactive CYP3A4 sulfone metabolite of **omeprazole** in both extensive and poor metabolisers (by 148% and 132%, respectively).[1]

Experimental evidence

No relevant data found.

Mechanism

St John's wort increases the metabolism of omeprazole by inducing both CYP2C19 and CYP3A4.[1]

Importance and management

This appears to be the only study examining the effects of St John's wort on proton pump inhibitors. However, the reduction seen in the AUC of omeprazole (about 40%) suggest that there is a possibility that omeprazole will be less effective in patients taking St John's wort. As all PPIs are metabolised by CYP2C19 to varying extents, it is likely that the effects of St John's wort seen in these studies will be similar with other PPIs, although note that **rabeprazole** is much less dependent on this route of metabolism than other PPIs.

There is insufficient evidence to suggest that St John's wort should be avoided in patients taking PPIs. However, the potential reduction in the efficacy of the PPI should be borne in mind, particular where the consequences may be serious, such as in patients with healing ulcers.

1. Wang LS, Zhou G, Zhu B, Wu J, Wang JG, Abd El-Aty AM, Li T, Liu J, Yang TL, Wang D, Zhong XY, Zhou HH. St John's wort induces both cytochrome P450 3A4-catalyzed sulfoxidation and 2C19-dependent hydroxylation of omeprazole. *Clin Pharmacol Ther* (2004) 75, 191–7.

St John's wort + SNRIs

Serotonin syndrome has been reported in one patient taking venlafaxine and St John's wort.

Clinical evidence

An interaction between **venlafaxine** and St John's wort was reported to the Centre Régional de Pharmacovigilance de Marseille involving a 32-year-old man who had been taking **venlafaxine** 250 mg daily for several months. He started taking St John's wort at a dose of 200 drops 3 times daily (usual dose up to 160 drops daily) and on the third day felt faint and anxious, and had symptoms of diaphoresis, shivering and tachycardia. St John's wort was stopped and his symptoms resolved in 3 days without altering the dose of **venlafaxine**.[1] A search of Health Canada's database of spontaneous adverse reactions for the period 1998 to 2003 also found one case of suspected serotonin syndrome as a result of an interaction between **venlafaxine** and St John's wort.[2]

Experimental evidence

No relevant data found.

Mechanism

A pharmacodynamic interaction may occur between St John's wort and venlafaxine because they can both inhibit the reuptake of 5-hydroxytryptamine (serotonin). Serotonin syndrome has been seen with St John's wort alone,[3] and so additive serotonergic effects appear to be the explanation for what occurred in the cases described here.

Importance and management

Information appears to be limited to these reports. **Duloxetine** would be expected to interact similarly and the manufacturers of both **duloxetine** and venlafaxine generally advise caution if they are given with drugs that affect the serotonergic neurotransmitter systems,[4–6] a similar caution with St John's wort would be prudent.

1. Prost N, Tichadou L, Rodor F, Nguyen N, David JM, Jean-Pastor MJ. Interaction millepertuis-venlafaxine. *Presse Med* (2000) 29, 1285–6.
2. Griffiths J, Jordan S, Pilan K. Natural health products and adverse reactions. *Can Adverse React News* (2004) 14, 2–3.
3. Demott K. St. John's wort tied to serotonin syndrome. *Clin Psychiatry News* (1998) 26, 28.
4. Efexor (Venlafaxine hydrochloride). Wyeth Pharmaceuticals. UK Summary of product characteristics, March 2008.
5. Effexor (Venlafaxine hydrochloride). Wyeth Pharmaceuticals Inc. US Prescribing information, November 2008.
6. Cymbalta (Duloxetine hydrochloride). Eli Lilly and Company Ltd. UK Summary of product characteristics, July 2008.

St John's wort + SSRIs

Cases of severe sedation, mania and serotonin syndrome have been reported in patients taking St John's wort with SSRIs.

Clinical evidence

(a) Citalopram

A brief case report describes serotonin syndrome in a woman who had been taking citalopram 20 mg daily for 2 months, three weeks after she also started taking St John's wort. She presented to hospital extremely agitated with unusual behaviour and was expressing suicidal thoughts. On admission, she was perspiring and complained of nausea and abdominal discomfort, with a tachycardia of 120 beats per minute and fluctuating blood pressure.[1] No further details are given.

(b) Fluoxetine

For a report of hypomania that occurred when St John's wort, **ginkgo biloba** and **melatonin** were added to treatment with fluoxetine and buspirone, see St John's wort + Buspirone, page 443.

For a report of serotonin syndrome when **eletriptan**, fluoxetine and St John's wort were used together, see St John's wort + Triptans, page 459.

(c) Paroxetine

In one report, a woman stopped taking paroxetine 40 mg daily after 8 months, and 10 days later started to take 600 mg of St John's wort powder daily. No problems occurred until the next night when she took a single 20-mg dose of paroxetine because she thought it might help her sleep. The following day at noon she was found still to be in bed, rousable but incoherent, groggy and slow moving and almost unable to get out of bed. Two hours later she still complained of nausea, weakness and fatigue, but her vital signs and mental status were normal. Within 24 hours all symptoms had resolved.[2]

(d) Sertraline

Four elderly patients taking sertraline developed symptoms characteristic of serotonin syndrome within 2 to 4 days of also taking St John's wort 300 mg, either two or three times daily. The symptoms included dizziness, nausea, vomiting, headache, anxiety, confusion, restlessness, and irritability. Two of them were treated with oral cyproheptadine 4 mg either two or three times daily, and the symptoms of all of them resolved within a week. They later resumed treatment with sertraline without problems.[3] A search of Health Canada's database of spontaneous adverse reactions from 1998 to

2003 found 2 cases of suspected serotonin syndrome as a result of an interaction between sertraline and St John's wort.[4]

Mania developed in a 28-year-old man, who continued to take St John's wort against medical advice whilst also receiving sertraline 50 mg daily for depression; he was also receiving testosterone replacement post-orchidectomy.[5]

Experimental evidence

No relevant data found.

Mechanism

A pharmacodynamic interaction might occur between St John's wort and SSRIs because they can both inhibit the reuptake of 5-hydroxytryptamine (serotonin).[6] Serotonin syndrome has been seen with St John's wort alone,[7] and so additive serotonergic effects appear to be the explanation for what occurred in the cases described here.

Importance and management

Information appears to be limited to these reports, but interactions between SSRIs and St John's wort would seem to be established. The incidence is not known but it is probably small, nevertheless because of the potential severity of the reaction it would seem prudent to avoid concurrent use. The advice of the CSM in the UK is that St John's wort should be stopped if patients are taking any SSRI because of the risk of increased serotonergic effects and an increased incidence of adverse reactions.[8]

1. Witharana S, Pollard A, Vaughan J. Continuing awareness of serotonin syndrome needed. *Pharm J* (2007) 278, 487.
2. Gordon JB. SSRIs and St. John's wort: possible toxicity? *Am Fam Physician* (1998) 57, 950–953.
3. Lantz MS, Buchalter E, Giambanco V. St. John's wort and antidepressant drug interactions in the elderly. *J Geriatr Psychiatry Neurol* (1999) 12, 7–10.
4. Griffiths J, Jordan S, Pilan K. Natural health products and adverse reactions. *Can Adverse React News* (2004) 14, 2–3.
5. Barbenel DM, Yusufi B, O'Shea D, Bench CJ. Mania in a patient receiving testosterone replacement post-orchidectomy taking St John's wort and sertraline. *J Psychopharmacol* (2000) 14, 84–6.
6. Izzo AA. Drug interactions with St. John's wort (Hypericum perforatum): a review of the clinical evidence. *Int J Clin Pharmacol Ther* (2004) 42, 139–48.
7. Demott K. St. John's wort tied to serotonin syndrome. *Clin Psychiatry News* (1998) 26, 28.
8. Committee on the Safety of Medicines (UK). Message from Professor A Breckenridge (Chairman of CSM) and Fact Sheet for Health Care Professionals. Important interactions between St John's wort (Hypericum perforatum) preparations and prescribed medicines. February 2000 http://www.mhra.gov.uk/home/groups/comms-ic/documents/websiteresources/con019563.pdf (accessed 26/11/2008).

St John's wort + Statins

St John's wort moderately decreases the exposure to simvastatin and reduces its lipid-lowering effect. Similarly, St John's wort reduces the lipid-lowering effect of atorvastatin. An isolated report unexpectedly describes reduced rosuvastatin efficacy during the use of St John's wort. St John's wort does not alter the pharmacokinetics of pravastatin.

Clinical evidence

In a placebo-controlled, crossover study, 16 healthy subjects took St John's wort 300 mg three times daily for 14 days. On day 14 **simvastatin** 10 mg was given to 8 subjects and **pravastatin** 20 mg was given to the other 8 subjects. St John's wort did not affect the plasma concentration of **pravastatin**, but it tended to reduce the AUC of **simvastatin** and moderately reduce the AUC of its active metabolite, simvastatin acid, by 62%.[1]

In a crossover study in 24 patients with hypercholesterolemia taking long-term **simvastatin** 10 to 40 mg daily (an average dose of 20.8 mg daily), St John's wort (*Movina*) 300 mg twice daily for 4 weeks, raised the levels of total cholesterol from 4.56 mmol/L (pre-treatment) to 5.08 mmol/L and LDL-cholesterol from 2.30 mmol/L to 2.72 mmol/L. The authors equate the magnitude of the increased LDL-cholesterol levels to a halving of the effects of **simvastatin**.[2]

In a similar study by the same authors, 16 patients with hypercholesterolemia taking long-term **atorvastatin** 10 to 40 mg daily (an average dose of 14.4 mg daily), were given St John's wort (*Movina*) 300 mg twice daily for 4 weeks. St John's wort raised the levels of total cholesterol from 4.76 mmol/L (pre-treatment) to 5.1 mmol/L and LDL-cholesterol from 2.39 mmol/L to 2.66 mmol/L. The levels of **atorvastatin** were not measured in this study. The authors equate the magnitude of the increased LDL-cholesterol levels to a loss of one-third of the effects of **atorvastatin**. No adverse effects were reported.[3]

A case report describes a 59-year-old man who was taking rosuvastatin 10 mg daily with satisfactory lipid levels. Six months later, a routine blood test indicated that his total cholesterol had risen from 4.27 mmol/L to 6.1 mmol/L. On questioning he said that he had been taking a supplement containing St John's wort 600 mg daily. He stopped taking the supplement, and 4 months later his cholesterol levels had reduced to about the former level.[4]

Experimental evidence

No relevant data found.

Mechanism

St John's wort is a weak inducer of CYP3A4, by which simvastatin, and to a lesser extent atorvastatin, are metabolised; however, this on its own does not seem sufficient to explain the reduction in statin efficacy seen. Rosuvastatin is less than 10% metabolised, so a reduction in its metabolism seems unlikely, and the case report is therefore unexplained. A lack of a pharmacokinetic interaction with pravastatin is as expected.

Importance and management

Although the evidence is limited, it appears that St John's wort can reduce the efficacy of atorvastatin and simvastatin, which appears to result in a clinically relevant increase in total cholesterol and LDL-cholesterol levels, depending on the patients baseline result and medical history. It might be prudent to consider an interaction if lipid-lowering targets are not met, and advise the patient to stop taking St John's wort or adjust the dose of the statin, as needed.

No pharmacokinetic interaction would be expected with pravastatin as it is not metabolised by CYP3A4, and this was demonstrated in the study above. Similarly, no pharmacokinetic interaction would be expected with **rosuvastatin**, but the case report adds a note of caution. Bear it in mind in the event of an unexpected response to treatment.

1. Sugimoto K, Ohmori M, Tsuruoka S, Nishiki K, Kawaguchi A, Harada K, Arakawa M, Sakomoto K, Masada M, Miyamori I, Fujimura A. Different effects of St John's wort on the pharmacokinetics of simvastatin and pravastatin. *Clin Pharmacol Ther* (2001) 70, 518–24.
2. Eggertsen R, Andreasson Å, Andrén L. Effects of treatment with a commercially available St John's Wort product (Movina®) on cholesterol levels in patients with hypercholesterolemia treated with simvastatin. *Scand J Prim Health Care* (2007) 25, 154–9.
3. Andrén L, Andreasson Å, Eggertsen R. Interaction between a commercially available St. John's wort product (Movina) and atorvastatin in patients with hypercholesterolemia. *Eur J Clin Pharmacol* (2007) 63, 913–16.
4. Gordon RY, Becker DJ, Rader DJ. Reduced efficacy of rosuvastatin by St John's wort. *Am J Med* (2009) 122, e1–e2.

St John's wort + Tacrolimus

St John's wort decreases tacrolimus levels.

Clinical evidence

In a clinical study, 10 healthy subjects were given a single 100-microgram/kg dose of tacrolimus alone, or after they took St John's wort 300 mg three times daily for 14 days. On average St John's wort decreased the maximum blood level of tacrolimus by 65% and its AUC by 32%. However, the decrease in AUC ranged from 15% to 64%, with one patient having a 31% *increase* in AUC.[1] Similar results have been found in a study in 10 kidney transplant patients given St John's wort (*Jarsin 300*) 600 mg daily for 2 weeks. In order to achieve target levels, the tacrolimus dose was increased in all patients, from a median of 4.5 mg daily to 8 mg daily. Two weeks after stopping St John's wort, tacrolimus

doses were reduced to a median of 6.5 mg daily, and then to the original dose of 4.5 mg daily after about 4 weeks.[2]

A case report describes a 65-year-old patient taking tacrolimus following a kidney transplant. The patient started to take St John's wort (*Neuroplant*) 600 mg daily, and after one month the tacrolimus trough blood levels had dropped from a range of 6 to 10 nanograms/mL down to 1.6 nanograms/mL, with an unexpected improvement in creatinine levels. When the St John's wort was stopped, tacrolimus levels and creatinine returned to the previous range. Subsequently a lower target range of tacrolimus was set.[3]

Experimental evidence

No relevant data found.

Mechanism

St John's wort induces the cytochrome P450 isoenzyme CYP3A4 and affects the transporter protein P-glycoprotein. CYP3A4 and P-glycoprotein are involved in the metabolism and clearance of tacrolimus, so an increase in their effects would be expected to result in a decrease in tacrolimus levels.[1,3]

Importance and management

Although the evidence currently seems limited to these reports, the interaction between tacrolimus and St John's wort has been predicted from the pharmacokinetics of these two drugs. Given the unpredictability of the interaction (and the variability in content of St John's wort products) it would seem prudent to avoid St John's wort in transplant patients, and possibly other types of patient taking tacrolimus. If St John's wort is started or stopped, monitor tacrolimus levels closely and adjust the dose accordingly.

St John's wort also does not interfere with laboratory assays for tacrolimus, see St John's wort + Laboratory tests, page 452.

1. Hebert MF, Park JM, Chen Y-L, Akhtar S, Larson AM. Effects of St John's wort (Hypericum perforatum) on tacrolimus pharmacokinetics in healthy volunteers. *J Clin Pharmacol* (2004) 44, 89–94.
2. Mai I, Störmer E, Bauer S, Krüger H, Budde K, Roots I. Impact of St John's wort treatment on the pharmacokinetics of tacrolimus and mycophenolic acid in renal transplant patients. *Nephrol Dial Transplant* (2003) 18, 819–22.
3. Bolley R, Zülke C, Kammerl M, Fischereder M, Krämer BK. Tacrolimus-induced nephrotoxicity unmasked by induction of the CYP3A4 system with St John's wort. *Transplantation* (2002) 73, 1009.

St John's wort + Talinolol

St John's wort modestly decreases the plasma levels of talinolol.

Clinical evidence

In a pharmacokinetic study, a single dose of talinolol (50 mg orally or 30 mg intravenously) was given to 9 healthy subjects alone and after St John's wort (*Jarsin, Lichtwer Pharma*) 900 mg daily for 12 days. St John's wort was found to reduce the AUC and oral bioavailability of talinolol by about 31% and 25%, respectively. The non-renal clearance of talinolol 30 mg given as a 30 minute infusion was increased by about 26%. Other pharmacokinetic parameters of both oral and intravenous talinolol were not significantly affected.[1]

Experimental evidence

No relevant data found.

Mechanism

Talinolol is a known substrate for P-glycoprotein. This study found that the levels of intestinal P-glycoprotein in the duodenal biopsy samples of 9 subjects were raised by St John's wort, leading to a reduction in the absorption of talinolol.

Importance and management

Information about an interaction between St John's wort and talinolol appears to be limited to this study but it is in line with the known effects of St John's wort on substrates of P-glycoprotein, such as digoxin. Consider St John's wort + Digoxin, page 447. The modest decrease in talinolol levels suggests that, in most patients, this interaction is unlikely to be clinically significant. Nevertheless, consider this interaction if blood pressure is difficult to control.

1. Schwarz UI, Hanso H, Oertel R, Miehlke S, Kuhlisch E, Glaeser H, Hitzl M, Dresser GK, Kim RB, Kirch W. Induction of intestinal P-glycoprotein by St John's wort reduces the oral bioavailability of talinolol. *Clin Pharmacol Ther* (2007) 81, 669–78.

St John's wort + Theophylline

A patient needed a large increase in the dose of theophylline while taking St John's wort. In contrast, no pharmacokinetic interaction was found in a two-week study in healthy subjects.

Clinical evidence

A study in 12 healthy subjects found that a standardised preparation of St John's wort 300 mg (hypericin 0.27%) three times daily for 15 days had no significant effects on the plasma level of a single 400-mg oral dose of theophylline.[1]

However, an isolated case has been reported of a woman, previously stable for several months taking theophylline 300 mg twice daily, who was found to need a large increase in her theophylline dose (to 800 mg twice daily) to achieve serum levels of 9.2 mg/L. Two months previously she had started to take 300 mg of a St John's wort supplement (hypericin 0.3%) each day. When she stopped taking the St John's wort, her serum theophylline levels doubled within a week to 19.6 mg/L and her theophylline dose was consequently reduced. This patient was also taking a whole spectrum of other drugs (amitriptyline, furosemide, ibuprofen, inhaled triamcinolone, morphine, potassium, prednisone, salbutamol (albuterol), valproic acid, zolpidem and zafirlukast) and was also a smoker. No changes in the use of these drugs or altered compliance were identified that might have offered an alternative explanation for the changed theophylline requirements.[2]

Experimental evidence

In vitro data suggest hypericin can act as an inducer of the cytochrome P450 isoenzyme CYP1A2.[2]

Mechanism

Uncertain. It has been suggested that treatment with St John's wort for 15 days was unlikely to induce the isoenzymes sufficiently to cause changes in plasma theophylline.[1] This is supported by studies in which the use of St John's wort for 4 weeks,[3] but not 2 weeks,[4] modestly increased the paraxanthine/caffeine ratio, used as a measure of CYP1A2 activity. The patient in the case report had been taking St John's wort for 2 months, although at a lower dose, therefore differences in duration of treatment may account for the discrepancy.

Importance and management

Direct information about this apparent interaction between theophylline and St John's wort appears to be limited. Despite the isolated case report describing a large decrease in theophylline levels, no pharmacokinetic interaction was noted in healthy subjects, and mechanistic studies suggest a modest interaction at most. Furthermore most clinically significant interactions with St John's wort are mediated by CYP3A4. Until further evidence is available to confirm the absence of an interaction, it would be prudent to be aware of the possibility if theophylline adverse effects (headache, nausea, tremor) develop. In 2000, the CSM in the UK recommended that patients taking theophylline should not take St John's wort. In those patients already taking the combination, the St John's wort should be stopped and the theophylline dose monitored and adjusted if necessary.[5,6] However, this guidance was issued before the pharmacokinetic study that suggests that an interaction is generally unlikely. There appears to be no direct evidence regarding aminophylline, but as it is metabolised to theophylline, no clinically relevant interaction would generally be expected with St John's wort.

Note that St John's wort does not appear to interfere with laboratory assays for theophylline, see St John's wort + Laboratory tests, page 452.

1. Morimoto T, Kotegawa T, Tsutsumi K, Ohtani Y, Imai H, Nakano S. Effect of St John's wort on the pharmacokinetics of theophylline in healthy volunteers. *J Clin Pharmacol* (2004) 44, 95–101.
2. Nebel A, Schneider BJ, Baker RK, Kroll DJ. Potential metabolic interaction between St John's wort and theophylline. *Ann Pharmacother* (1999) 33, 502.
3. Gurley BJ, Gardner SF, Hubbard MA, Williams DK, Gentry WB, Cui Y, Ang CYW. Cytochrome P450 phenotypic ratios for predicting herb-drug interactions in humans. *Clin Pharmacol Ther* (2002) 72, 276–87.
4. Wang Z, Gorski JC, Hamman MA, Huang S-M, Lesko LJ, Hall SD. The effects of St John's wort (*Hypericum perforatum*) on human cytochrome P450 activity. *Clin Pharmacol Ther* (2001) 70, 317–26.
5. Committee on the Safety of Medicines (UK). Message from Professor A Breckenridge (Chairman of CSM) and Fact Sheet for Health Care Professionals. Important interactions between St John's wort (*Hypericum perforatum*) preparations and prescribed medicines. February 2000 http://www.mhra.gov.uk/home/groups/comms-ic/documents/websiteresources/con019563.pdf (accessed 16/12/2011).
6. Committee on Safety of Medicines/Medicines Control Agency. Reminder: St John's Wort (*Hypericum perforatum*) interactions. *Current Problems* (2000) 26, 6–7.

St John's wort + Tibolone

An isolated case describes liver damage in a woman taking tibolone and St John's wort.

Clinical evidence

A 57-year-old woman who had been taking tibolone 2.5 mg daily for the past two years for postmenopausal symptoms, and hydroxychloroquine sulfate 200 mg daily for the past 7 years for rheumatoid arthritis, without complaint, was hospitalised for liver damage after taking a 2-g infusion of St John's wort daily for 10 weeks for mild depression. The patient was suffering from fatigue, reduced appetite and jaundice. Her liver function normalised after about one year of taking ursodesoxycholic acid 250 mg twice daily.[1]

Experimental evidence

No relevant data found.

Mechanism

Unknown.

Importance and management

The general clinical importance of this isolated report is uncertain. Both tibolone and hydroxychloroquine sulfate have been associated with liver toxicity alone but cases with hydroxychloroquine sulfate are quite rare. Therefore the authors of the report suggest that an interaction between tibolone and St John's wort was to blame for the liver damage in this case; however, both drugs may cause liver damage alone. Both tibolone and St John's wort are widely used long-term, which suggests that this interaction is not common. Nevertheless, it may be prudent to be aware of a possible interaction if symptoms of liver toxicity (fatigue, reduced appetite, dark urine) become apparent.

1. Etogo-Asse F, Boemer F, Sempoux C, Geubel A. Acute hepatitis with prolonged cholestasis and disappearance of interlobular bile ducts following tibolone and Hypericum perforatum (St. John's wort). Case of drug interaction? *Acta Gastroenterol Belg* (2008) 71, 36–8.

St John's wort + Tricyclic antidepressants

The plasma levels of amitriptyline and its active metabolite, nortriptyline, are modestly reduced by St John's wort.

Clinical evidence

Twelve depressed patients were given **amitriptyline** 75 mg twice daily and St John's wort extract (*Jarsin, Lichtwer Pharma*) 900 mg daily for at least 14 days. The AUC_{0-12} of **amitriptyline**

S

was reduced by about 22% and the AUC of nortriptyline (its metabolite) was reduced by about 41%.[1]

Experimental evidence

No relevant data found.

Mechanism

Not fully understood. St John's wort is known to induce the activity of the cytochrome P450 isoenzyme CYP3A4, which is a minor route of metabolism of the tricyclic antidepressants. However, the tricyclics are predominantly metabolised by CYP2D6, so an effect on CYP3A4 is unlikely to lead to a clinically relevant reduction in their levels. Induction of P-glycoprotein by St John's wort may also contribute; however, the extent of its involvement in the transport of the tricyclics is unclear.

Importance and management

The evidence for an interaction is limited to this study, and based on the minor reduction in amitriptyline levels seen, it seems unlikely that a clinically significant reduction in efficacy would occur. Other tricyclics would be expected to interact similarly.

Both the tricyclics and St John's wort are antidepressants, but whether concurrent use is beneficial or safe is not known, and it was not assessed in this study.[1] Further study is needed.

Note that St John's wort does not appear to interfere with laboratory assays for tricyclics, see St John's wort + Laboratory tests, page 452.

1. Johne A, Schmider J, Brockmöller J, Stadelmann AM, Störmer E, Bauer S, Scholler G, Langheinrich M, Roots I. Decreased plasma levels of amitriptyline and its metabolites on comedication with an extract from St. John's wort (*Hypericum perforatum*). *J Clin Psychopharmacol* (2002) 22, 46–54.

St John's wort + Triptans

Serotonin syndrome has been reported in a patient taking eletriptan and St John's wort.

Clinical evidence

A 28-year-old woman who had been taking **fluoxetine** 60 mg daily for one year for an eating disorder, and St John's wort (dose and frequency not stated) for one month, suffered a loss of consciousness, convulsions, and mental confusion after **eletriptan** 40 mg daily was started 3 days earlier for a recurrent migraine. Previous use of **eletriptan** and **fluoxetine** had not resulted in any reported adverse effects. After admission to hospital, the patient developed acute rhabdomyolysis and transient mild acute renal failure. Serotonin syndrome was diagnosed, all medications were stopped and the symptoms gradually resolved over 10 days.[1]

Experimental evidence

No relevant data found.

Mechanism

Both the triptans and St John's wort have been implicated in cases of serotonin syndrome when they were given with other serotonergic drugs. Additive serotonergic effects are the likely explanation for the case report above.

Importance and management

Published evidence for an interaction between St John's wort and the triptans appears to be limited to the case report cited. Most UK manufacturers of triptans warn about the potential increase in undesirable effects. The possible concern is that concurrent use might result in the development of serotonin syndrome.

1. Bonetto N, Santelli L, Battistin L, Cagnin A. Serotonin syndrome and rhabdomyolysis induced by concomitant use of triptans, fluoxetine and hypericum. *Cephalalgia* (2007) 27, 1421–3.

St John's wort + Voriconazole

St John's wort, taken for two weeks, more than halved the AUC of a single dose of voriconazole.

Clinical evidence

In a study in 17 healthy subjects, a single 400-mg dose of oral voriconazole was given alone and on the first and last day of a 15-day course of St John's wort (*Jarsin, Lichtwer Pharma*), given at a dose of 300 mg three times daily. Taking St John's wort for one day had no effect on the voriconazole $AUC_{0-\infty}$, but increased the maximum plasma concentration and AUC_{0-10} by 22%. However, when voriconazole was given on day 15 of treatment with St John's wort, the AUC of voriconazole was decreased by 59% and there was a 2.4-fold increase in oral clearance.[1]

Experimental evidence

No relevant data found.

Mechanism

These results suggest that the short-term effect of St John's wort is to enhance the absorption of voriconazole, whereas the longer-term effect is to induce absorption-limiting transport proteins and intestinal metabolism by cytochrome P450 isoenzymes.[1]

Importance and management

The increase in voriconazole absorption with a single dose of St John's wort is small and therefore not clinically relevant. However, the reduction in the plasma concentration and AUC of voriconazole after 15 days of St John's wort could reduce clinical efficacy. For this reason, the UK and US manufacturers contraindicate the concurrent use of St John's wort and voriconazole.[2,3] Patients already taking voriconazole should be advised not to take St John's wort. Patients requiring voriconazole should be asked about current or recent use of St John's wort, as this might indicate the need to use an increased voriconazole dose, at least initially, while the metabolic effects of the herb decline.

1. Rengelshausen J, Banfield M, Riedel KD, Burhenne J, Weiss J, Thomsen T, Walter-Sack I, Haefeli WE, Mikus G. Opposite effects of short-term and long-term St John's wort on voriconazole pharmacokinetics. *Clin Pharmacol Ther* (2005) 78, 25–33.
2. VFEND (Voriconazole). Pfizer Ltd. UK Summary of product characteristics, April 2012.
3. VFEND (Voriconazole). Pfizer Inc. US Prescribing information, November 2011.

St John's wort + Warfarin and related drugs

St John's wort can reduce in the anticoagulant effects of phenprocoumon and warfarin. An isolated report described an increased anticoagulant effect in response to warfarin on the concurrent use of St John's Wort.

Clinical evidence

(a) Phenprocoumon

In a randomised, placebo-controlled crossover study in 10 healthy men,[1] St John's wort extract (*LI 160, Lichtwer Pharma*) 900 mg daily for 11 days negligibly reduced the AUC of a single 12-mg dose of phenprocoumon by 17%.

A case report describes a 75-year-old woman taking phenprocoumon who had a reduced anticoagulant response (a rise in the Quick value) 2 months after starting to take St John's wort.[2]

(b) Warfarin

In a randomised, crossover study in 12 healthy subjects, one tablet of St John's wort three times daily for 3 weeks modestly decreased the AUC of both *R*- and *S*-warfarin by about 25%. In this study, the brand of St John's wort used was *Bioglan* tablets, each tablet containing an extract equivalent to 1 g of *Hypericum perforatum* flowering herb top containing 825 micrograms of hypericin and 12.5 mg of hyperforin, and warfarin was given as a single 25-mg dose on day 14.[3]

Over the 1998 to 1999 period, the Swedish Medical Products Agency received 7 case reports of patients stabilised on warfarin whose INRs decreased when St John's wort was started. Their INRs fell from the normal therapeutic range of about 2 to 4 to about 1.5. Two patients needed warfarin dose increases of 6.6% and 15%, respectively, when St John's wort was added. The INRs of 4 patients returned to their former values when St John's wort was stopped.[4] A retrospective study[5] similarly found that the concurrent use of enzyme inducers (including St John's wort) greatly influenced the total weekly warfarin dose; further analysis found that an average additional amount of warfarin of 17.2 mg weekly was required in patients taking these drugs.

In contrast, a case report describes an 85-year-old patient taking warfarin 5 mg daily for almost a year without problems, who developed upper gastrointestinal bleeding, requiring hospitalisation, one month after starting St John's wort. On admission his haemoglobin was 7.9 g/dL and his INR was 6.2. After supportive treatment, the bleeding ceased and endoscopy before discharge revealed no clinically important pathology.[6]

Experimental evidence

No relevant data found.

Mechanism

Uncertain, but it is suggested that St John's wort increases the metabolism and clearance of the coumarins[1,3,4] possibly by induction of CYP3A4, and CYP2C9, as both *R*- and *S*-warfarin were affected.[3] However, note that St John's wort had no effect on the metabolism of tolbutamide, which is commonly used as a probe substrate for CYP2C9 activity. See St John's wort + Antidiabetics, page 440. Note also that St John's wort does not generally *inhibit* cytochrome P450 isoenzymes *in vivo*, as was suggested by the authors of the case report showing increased warfarin effects.[6]

Importance and management

Information seems to be limited to these reports, but a modest pharmacokinetic interaction between the coumarins and St John's wort would seem established, which might be clinically important in some patients. It would be prudent to monitor the INRs of patients taking phenprocoumon, warfarin or any other coumarin if they start taking St John's wort, being alert for the need to increase the anticoagulant dose accordingly. This interaction should also be borne in mind as a possible cause in cases where an otherwise unexplained decrease in INR occurs, and scrutiny of the patients other medications, particularly self medications, should be undertaken for the presence of St John's wort. Note that the CSM in the UK advise that St John's wort should not be used with warfarin. They state that the degree of induction of warfarin metabolism is likely to vary because levels of active ingredients can vary between St John's wort preparations. If a patient is already taking warfarin and St John's wort, they advise checking the INR, stopping the St John's wort, and then monitoring the INR closely and adjusting the anticoagulant dosage as necessary.[7]

Note that the case report of increased effect of warfarin,[6] is in stark contrast to the other evidence and is not in line with how St John's wort is understood to affect drug metabolism. It is therefore unlikely to be of any general importance.

1. Maurer A, Johne A, Bauer S, Brockmöller J, Donath F, Roots I, Langheinrich M, Hübner W-D. Interaction of St John's wort extract with phenprocoumon. *Eur J Clin Pharmacol* (1999) 55, 22.
2. Bon S, Hartmann K, Kuhn M. Johanniskraut. Ein Enzyminduktor? *Schweiz Apothekerzeitung* (1999) 16, 535–6.
3. Jiang X, Williams KM, Liauw WS, Ammit AJ, Roufogalis BD, Duke CC, Day RO, McLachlan AJ. Effect of St John's wort and ginseng on the pharmacokinetics and pharmacodynamics of warfarin in healthy subjects. *Br J Clin Pharmacol* (2004) 57, 592–9.
4. Yue Q-Y, Bergquist C, Gerdén B. Safety of St John's wort (*Hypericum perforatum*). *Lancet* (2000) 355, 576–7.
5. Whitley HP, Fermo JD, Chumney ECG, Brzezinski WA. Effect of patient-specific factors on weekly warfarin dose. *Ther Clin Risk Manag* (2007) 3, 499–504.
6. Uygur Bayramiçli O, Kalkay MN, Oskay Bozkaya E, Doğan Köse E, Iyigün O, Görük M, Sezgin G. St. John's wort (Hypericum perforatum) and warfarin: Dangerous liaisons. *Turk J Gastroenterol* (2011) 22, 115.
7. Committee on the Safety of Medicines (UK). Message from Professor A Breckenridge (Chairman of CSM) and Fact Sheet for Health Care Professionals. Important interactions between St John's wort (*Hypericum perforatum*) preparations and prescribed medicines. February 2000 http://www.mhra.gov.uk/Safetyinformation/Safetywarningsalertsandrecalls/Safetywarningsandmessagesformedicines/CON2015756 (accessed 03/02/2011).

S

Starflower oil

Borago officinalis L. (Boraginaceae)

Synonym(s) and related species

Beebread, Bee plant, Borage, Borage oil, Burrage.

Pharmacopoeias

Refined Borage Oil (*BP 2012*); Borage (Starflower) Oil, Refined (*PhEur 7.5*).

Constituents

The oil from starflower seeds contains the essential fatty acids of the omega-6 series, **linoleic acid** (about 30 to 41%) and **gamolenic acid** (gamma-linolenic acid, about 17 to 27%). Other fatty acids include oleic acid, alpha-linolenic acid, palmitic acid and stearic acid.

Starflower leaves contain potentially hepatotoxic pyrrolizidine alkaloids including lycopsamine, intermedine and their derivatives.

Use and indications

Starflower is thought to possess diuretic, expectorant and anti-inflammatory properties. The main use of starflower comes from its seed oil, which contains none of the hepatotoxic pyrrolizidine alkaloids found in the leaves. The oil is used as an alternative to evening primrose oil, page 206 as a source of gamolenic acid.

Infusions of the leaves have traditionally been used for fevers and coughs but it is not recommended that starflower leaves are taken internally, especially if fresh, because they contain small amounts of the hepatotoxic pyrrolizidine alkaloids. The leaves have also been used as an emollient poultice.

Pharmacokinetics

No relevant pharmacokinetic data found, but see evening primrose oil, page 206 for information on the pharmacokinetics of *cis*-linoleic acid.

Interactions overview

Evening primrose oil contains linoleic acid and gamolenic acid, which are the main active constituents implicated in its interactions. Starflower oil also contains these constituents, and is therefore expected to interact in the same way. See evening primrose oil, page 206.

S

Sweet wormwood

Artemisia annua L. (Asteraceae)

Synonym(s) and related species

Annual wormwood, Sweet Annie.

Not to be confused with Wormwood (*Artemisia absinthium*).

Constituents

The major active constituent of the herb is the sesquiterpene endoperoxide **artemisinin** (qinghaosu or qinghao). Related compounds including artemisinic acid, artemisia ketone, artemisinic alcohol, arteannuin B and others are also present, along with **flavonoids** such as casticin, artemetin, chrysoplenetin, cirsilineol, eupatin and chrysosplenol-D. Some of these constituents are also present in the **volatile oil**, which also contains borneol, farnesene, sabinene, germacrene D, β-caryophyllene, and others.

Use and indications

Sweet wormwood has traditionally been used in Chinese medicine to treat fever and malaria. The main active constituent, artemisinin, is a potent and rapidly acting antiplasmodial agent, but has poor pharmaceutical properties, which has led to the development of a number of derivatives that are used clinically for the treatment of malaria. The herb is still taken in the form of a tea by rural populations of Asia and Africa for the treatment of malaria, although this use is controversial, due to high recrudescence rates (the reappearance of a disease after a period of inactivity) and concerns about the development of resistance if used alone. There is some evidence that the presence of other constituents in extracts of sweet wormwood (possibly flavonoids) contribute to its antimalarial activity.

Pharmacokinetics

A study in healthy subjects given freshly prepared sweet wormwood tea, showed that artemisinin is rapidly absorbed and may have similar bioavailability to artemisinin taken in a capsule formulation (based on a comparison to historical data).[1] For information on the pharmacokinetics of flavonoids, see under flavonoids, page 213.

Interactions overview

No interactions with sweet wormwood found. Note that, as the amount of artemisinin obtained from usual doses of traditionally prepared herbal tea is considerably less than the doses used therapeutically, it would seem highly unlikely that the drug interactions seen with pharmaceutical preparations of artemisinin would occur if sweet wormwood is taken with conventional medicines. However, while use of pure artemisinin as a supplement is outside the scope of this monograph (which concerns the use of the herb), it should be noted that the amount of artemisinin present in such preparations could be similar to the doses used therapeutically and the possibility of interactions cannot be ruled out, such as increased exposure to caffeine and other CYP1A2 substrates.

Artemisinin derivatives used therapeutically also have a high risk of causing QT prolongation. The concurrent use of more than one drug that prolongs the QT interval increases the risk of torsade de pointes, which may lead to life-threatening ventricular arrhythmias.

Sweet wormwood needs much more research before any firm recommendations can be made about its potential to interact with CYP1A2 substrates and drugs that prolong the QT interval; however, until more is known some caution is warranted.

1. Rath K, Taxis K, Walz G, Gleiter CH, Li S-M, Heide L. Pharmacokinetic study of artemisinin after oral intake of a traditional preparation of *Artemisia annua* L. (Annual wormwood). *Am J Trop Med Hyg* (2004) 70, 128–32.

Tea

Camellia sinensis (L.) Kuntze (Theaceae)

Synonym(s) and related species

Camellia thea Link, *Thea sinensis* L.

Note that Green tea (predominantly produced in China and Japan) is produced from steam-treated tea leaves. Black tea or Red tea (predominantly produced in India, Sri Lanka and Kenya) is processed by fermentation and heating, whereas Oolong tea is partially fermented.

Pharmacopoeias

Powdered Decaffeinated Green Tea Extract (*USP35–NF30 S1*).

Constituents

Tea contains **caffeine** (around 1 to 5%), with minor amounts of other xanthines such as theophylline and theobromine. Tea also contains **flavonoids**, the content of which varies between green (unfermented) and black (fermented) tea. Green tea appears to contain greater quantities of the flavonol-type of **flavonoids** than black tea. Black tea also contains theaflavins, which are produced during the fermentation process. Other flavonols present include quercetin and kaempferol. Oolong tea contains some unique flavones known as oolonghomobisflavins. Tea also contains up to 24% tannins.

Use and indications

The leaf buds and very young leaves of tea are used as a stimulant and diuretic, actions which can be attributed to the caffeine content. They are also used as an astringent for gastrointestinal disorders, which may be attributed to the polyphenols and tannins. Tea is very widely used to make a beverage. Green tea extracts, which are rich in polyphenolics, are available as supplements. There is also a prescription-only ointment containing green tea extract (sinecatechins), which is used for the treatment of genital warts.[1]

Pharmacokinetics

The pharmacokinetics of caffeine are discussed under caffeine, page 106. Black tea does not appear to affect the cytochrome P450 isoenzyme CYP2C9, as shown by the lack of effect on the pharmacokinetics of flurbiprofen, page 466. Similarly green tea catechins do not appear to affect the metabolism of caffeine, page 465, losartan, page 468, dextromethorphan, page 466, or alprazolam, page 464, suggesting a lack of effect on the isoenzymes CYP1A2, CYP2C9, CYP2D6, and CYP3A4, respectively.

For information on the pharmacokinetics of individual flavonoids present in tea, see flavonoids, page 213.

Interactions overview

Tea can contain significant amounts of caffeine, therefore the interactions of caffeine, page 106, are relevant to tea, unless the product is stated as decaffeinated. Black tea appears to reduce the absorption of iron, whereas green tea appears to have much smaller, if any, effects. Both black and green tea may cause a modest increase in blood pressure, which may be detrimental to the treatment of hypertension. Tea, particularly green tea catechins, may have some antiplatelet effects, which may be additive with those of conventional antiplatelet drugs. Case reports suggest that tea may reduce the INR in response to warfarin.

Green tea extracts do not appear to affect the pharmacokinetics of alprazolam, caffeine, ciclosporin, dextromethorphan, irinotecan, losartan, and have only modest effects on the pharmacokinetics of buspirone, but some of this data needs confirming in patients. Black tea does not appear to have a clinically relevant effect on the pharmacokinetics of flurbiprofen.

Milk does not appear to affect the absorption of flavonoids or catechins from tea, suggesting that the addition of milk does not impair the antioxidant effects of tea.

For information on the interactions of individual flavonoids present in tea, see under flavonoids, page 213.

Interactions monographs

- Alprazolam, page 464
- Antihypertensives, page 464
- Antiplatelet drugs, page 465
- Buspirone, page 465
- Caffeine, page 465
- Ciclosporin or Tacrolimus, page 466
- Dextromethorphan, page 466
- Flurbiprofen, page 466
- Food, page 467
- Herbal medicines; Pepper, page 467
- Irinotecan, page 467
- Iron compounds, page 467
- Losartan, page 468
- Warfarin and related drugs, page 468

1. Veregen (Sinecatechins). Doak Dermatologics. US Prescribing information, December 2007.

T

Tea + Alprazolam

Green tea extract does not affect the pharmacokinetics of alprazolam.

Clinical evidence

In a pharmacokinetic study, 10 healthy subjects were given a single 2-mg dose of alprazolam before and after *Decaffeinated Super Green Tea Extract* 2 capsules twice daily for 14 days. The **green tea extract** did not affect the pharmacokinetics of alprazolam.[1]

Experimental evidence

Because of the quality of the clinical evidence available, experimental data have not been sought.

Mechanism

These studies provide evidence that green tea catechins, at similar[1] doses to the amount provided by average green tea consumption are unlikely to affect the metabolism of drugs by the cytochrome P450 isoenzyme CYP3A4.

Importance and management

The available data suggests that no clinically relevant pharmacokinetic interaction would be expected between green tea and alprazolam. Alprazolam is used as a probe drug for CYP3A4 activity, and therefore these results also suggest that a pharmacokinetic interaction as a result of this mechanism between green tea and other CYP3A4 substrates is unlikely.

For the possible pharmacodynamic interaction between caffeine (a constituent of tea) and benzodiazepines, see Caffeine + Benzodiazepines and related drugs, page 109. Tea can contain significant amounts of caffeine, and this interaction should be applied to tea, unless the product is stated to be decaffeinated.

1. Donovan JL, Chavin KD, Devane CL, Taylor RM, Wang JS, Ruan Y, Markowitz JS. Green tea (Camellia sinensis) extract does not alter cytochrome p450 3A4 or 2D6 activity in healthy volunteers. *Drug Metab Dispos* (2004) 32, 906–8.

Tea + Antihypertensives

Both black and green tea may cause a modest increase in blood pressure, which may be detrimental to the treatment of hypertension.

Clinical evidence

There is a possibility that the effect of tea on blood pressure might differ from that of pure caffeine. There are few data on the effect of tea on blood pressure in patients treated with antihypertensives. One study in stable hypertensive patients taking beta blockers, calcium-channel blockers, nitrates and ACE inhibitors reported that 450 mL of **black tea** (containing approximately 190 mg of caffeine) increased systolic blood pressure by 5 mmHg two hours after consumption. This effect was similar to the increase seen with a single dose of 200-mg of caffeine. Drinking 900 mL of **black tea** daily for 4 weeks had no significant effect on blood pressure. However, the acute effects of tea remained: systolic blood pressure was still increased by 5 mmHg two hours after the patients drank 450 mL of **black tea**.[1] There are a number of short-term intervention studies on the effect of tea on blood pressure, mainly in healthy subjects or patients with untreated mild hypertension. In one meta-analysis of 5 randomised studies of the effect of tea consumption for at least 7 days (median 4 weeks) on blood pressure, tea consumption was associated with no change in blood pressure, when compared with the control group (although this group took caffeine in two of the studies).[2] In one of the studies in this review, the acute increase in blood pressure seen with both **green tea** and **black (fermented)** tea 30 minutes after consumption was actually higher than that from an equivalent dose of caffeine. However, the increases seen in ambulatory blood pressure after 7 days of regular consumption of **green** or **black tea** were small and not different to that of caffeine.[3] In another study by the same research group, the acute effects of **black (fermented)** tea on blood pressure were not apparent when the tea was taken with a meal (high fat).[4]

The only long-term studies are of epidemiological type. In the Nurses Health prospective cohort study I, tea consumption was not associated with an increased risk of developing hypertension, whereas in the cohort study II, there was a slight trend for increased risk of hypertension with increased caffeinated tea intake.[5] However, in a cohort study in Taiwan, the risk of developing hypertension was reduced by regular tea (**green** or **oolong**) consumption.[6] Similarly, in a cross-sectional study, tea intake (mostly **black (fermented)** tea with added milk) was related to lower blood pressure in older women.[7]

There appears to be very little data on the effect of supplements containing tea extracts on blood pressure. In one study, which compared the addition of **green tea extract** or placebo to a low-energy diet, the **green tea extract** had no additional benefit on blood pressure over that achieved by modest weight loss.[8] In a single-dose study, a supplement containing **black tea extract** (polyphenols and caffeine), **guarana extract** (caffeine), ginger extract, dill weed extract, rutin and vitamin C (*TeaLean*), there was an average 3.7 mmHg increase in systolic blood pressure in the 2 hours after ingestion, but no increase in diastolic blood pressure.[9]

Experimental evidence

Because of the extensive clinical evidence available, experimental data has not been sought.

Mechanism

Acute intake of caffeine raises blood pressure, but some tolerance to this effect might possibly develop with regular consumption. See also Caffeine + Antihypertensives, page 108. Polyphenolics in tea might improve endothelial function, and might therefore lower blood pressure.

Importance and management

The evidence presented here is conflicting, and it is not possible to be conclusive about the long-term effect of tea intake (green or black) on blood pressure. However, any adverse effect appears to be modest. On acute intake, both green and black (fermented) teas and some herbal supplements (particularly if they contain caffeine) might increase blood pressure, although from the limited information above, these increases appear to be small and not necessarily sustained during long-term intake. Bear this in mind in patients with poorly controlled hypertension who frequently consume tea, particularly in large quantities. Further study on the effects of tea on antihypertensives is needed. However, note that similar effects are known to occur with caffeine alone, see Caffeine + Antihypertensives, page 108.

1. Duffy SJ, Keaney JF, Holbrook M, Gokce N, Swerdloff PL, Frei B, Vita JA. Short- and long-term black tea consumption reverses endothelial dysfunction in patients with coronary artery disease. *Circulation* (2001) 104, 151–6.
2. Taubert D, Roesen R, Schömig E. Effect of cocoa and tea intake on blood pressure: a meta-analysis. *Arch Intern Med* (2007) 167, 626–34.
3. Hodgson JM, Puddey IB, Burke V, Beilin LJ, Jordan N. Effects on blood pressure of drinking green and black tea. *J Hypertens* (1999) 17, 457–63.
4. Hodgson JM, Burke V, Puddey IB. Acute effects of tea on fasting and postprandial vascular function and blood pressure in humans. *J Hypertens* (2005) 23, 47–54.
5. Winkelmayer WC, Stampfer MJ, Willett WC, Curhan GC. Habitual caffeine intake and the risk of hypertension in women. *JAMA* (2005) 294, 233–5.
6. Yang YC, Lu FH, Wu JS, Wu CH, Chang CJ. The protective effect of habitual tea consumption on hypertension. *Arch Intern Med* (2004) 164, 1534–40.
7. Hodgson JM, Devine A, Puddey IB, Chan SY, Beilin LJ, Prince RL. Tea intake is inversely related to blood pressure in older women. *J Nutr* (2003) 133, 2883–6.
8. Diepvens K, Kovacs EM, Vogels N, Westerterp-Plantenga MS. Metabolic effects of green tea and of phases of weight loss. *Physiol Behav* (2006) 87, 185–91.
9. Roberts AT, de Jonge-Levitan L, Parker CC, Greenway F. The effect of an herbal supplement containing black tea and caffeine on metabolic parameters in humans. *Altern Med Rev* (2005) 10, 321–5.

Tea + Antiplatelet drugs

Tea, particularly green tea catechins, may have some antiplatelet effects, which may be additive with those of conventional antiplatelet drugs.

Clinical evidence

(a) Pharmacodynamic effects

In studies in healthy medication-free subjects, neither acute[1,2] nor chronic[3] tea consumption of **black (fermented) tea**, (with or without added milk) affected platelet aggregation, whereas two studies did report a reduction in platelet activation with chronic tea intake.[2,4] Another study, in 49 patients with known coronary artery disease taking **aspirin** 325 mg daily, found no evidence that acute or chronic ingestion of **black (fermented) tea** affected ADP-induced platelet aggregation.[5] There appears to be just one clinical study of **green tea**, which did not find any significant effect on platelet aggregation.[6]

(b) Pharmacokinetic effects

A study in 5 healthy subjects found that 200 mL of tea (at a temperature of 50°C) increased the rate of absorption of salicylate from a single 500-mg dose of **aspirin**, when compared with water, but the maximum concentration of salicylate was not significantly affected. The authors note that this result may have been influenced by the high temperature of the tea and an alkaline pH, both of which can increase the dissolution rate of **aspirin**.[7] Note that caffeine is known to have a modest effect on the absorption of **aspirin**, see Caffeine + Aspirin or Diclofenac, page 108.

Experimental evidence

Green tea catechins have been reported to inhibit platelet aggregation in *mice* and *in vitro,* in a dose-dependent manner. Bleeding time was also prolonged in *mice,* but aPTT, prothrombin time and thrombin time were not affected by **green tea catechins** added to human plasma. This suggested an antiplatelet rather than an antithrombotic effect.[8] Another *animal* study by the same research group found that oral **green tea catechins** 25 and 50 mg/kg inhibited arachidonic acid-induced platelet aggregation and the production of thromboxane A_2 and prostaglandin D_2.[9]

Mechanism

There is *in vitro* evidence that flavonoids, and flavanols and procyanidin oligomers in particular, inhibit platelet aggregation,[10] and this has been suggested as a mechanism to explain why some epidemiological studies show that a diet high in these substances is associated with a reduced risk of cardiovascular disease (see also Flavonoids + Anticoagulant or Antiplatelet drugs, page 215).

Importance and management

In general the evidence appears to suggest that black (fermented) tea does not have a clinically relevant effect on platelet aggregation. However, experimental studies using green tea catechins have found an antiplatelet effect, and this effect may, in theory, be additive with those of conventional antiplatelet drugs. Concurrent use need not be avoided (indeed combinations of antiplatelet drugs are often prescribed together) but it may be prudent to be aware of the potential for increased bleeding if green tea extracts, particularly in high doses, are given with other antiplatelet drugs such as aspirin and **clopidogrel**. Patients should discuss any episode of prolonged bleeding with a healthcare professional. Modest consumption is unlikely to cause any problems.

1. Hodgson JM, Puddey IB, Burke V, Beilin LJ, Mori TA, Chan SY. Acute effects of ingestion of black tea on postprandial platelet aggregation in human subjects. *Br J Nutr* (2002) 87, 141–5.
2. Wolfram RM, Oguogho A, Efthimiou Y, Budinsky AC, Sinzinger H. Effect of black tea on (iso-)prostaglandins and platelet aggregation in healthy volunteers. *Prostaglandins Leukot Essent Fatty Acids* (2002) 66, 529–33.
3. Hodgson JM, Puddey IB, Mori TA, Burke V, Baker RI, Beilin LJ. Effects of regular ingestion of black tea on haemostasis and cell adhesion molecules in humans. *Eur J Clin Nutr* (2001) 55, 881–6.
4. Steptoe A, Gibson EL, Vuononvirta R, Hamer M, Wardle J, Rycroft JA, Martin JF, Erusalimsky JD. The effects of chronic tea intake on platelet activation and inflammation: a double-blind placebo controlled trial. *Atherosclerosis* (2007) 193, 277–82.
5. Duffy SJ, Vita JA, Holbrook M, Swerdloff PL, Keaney JF. Effect of acute and chronic tea consumption on platelet aggregation in patients with coronary artery disease. *Arterioscler Thromb Vasc Biol* (2001) 21, 1084–9.
6. Hirano-Ohmori R, Takahashi R, Momiyama Y, Taniguchi H, Yonemura A, Tamai S, Umegaki K, Nakamura H, Kondo K, Ohsuzu F. Green tea consumption and serum malondialdehyde-modified LDL concentrations in healthy subjects. *J Am Coll Nutr* (2005) 24, 342–6.
7. Odou P, Barthélémy C, Robert H. Influence of seven beverages on salicylate disposition in humans. *J Clin Pharm Ther* (2001) 26, 187–93.
8. Kang W-S, Lim I-H, Yuk D-Y, Chung K-H, Park J-B, Yoo H-S, Yun Y-P. Antithrombotic activities of green tea catechins and (-)-epigallocatechin gallate. *Thromb Res* (1999) 96, 229–37.
9. Son D-J, Cho M-R, Jin Y-R, Kim S-Y, Park Y-H, Lee S-H, Akiba S, Sato T, Yun Y-P. Antiplatelet effect of green tea catechins: a possible mechanism through arachidonic acid pathway. *Prostaglandins Leukot Essent Fatty Acids* (2004) 71, 25–31.
10. Nardini M, Natella F, Scaccini C. Role of dietary polyphenols in platelet aggregation. A review of the supplementation studies. *Platelets* (2007) 18, 224–43.

Tea + Buspirone

Green tea catechins have only modest effects on the pharmacokinetics of buspirone.

Clinical evidence

In a study in 41 healthy subjects, **green tea catechin extract** 4 capsules daily for 4 weeks caused a minor 21% increase in the AUC of a single 10-mg dose of buspirone. The **green tea catechin extract** used in this study, *Polyphenon E,* contained 80 to 98% total catechins, of which 50 to 75% (200 mg) was epigallocatechin gallate. It was essentially decaffeinated (0.5% w/w caffeine).[1]

Experimental evidence

Because of the quality of the clinical evidence available, experimental data have not been sought.

Mechanism

These studies provide evidence that green tea catechins (at higher doses than the amount provided by average green tea consumption[1]) are unlikely to affect the metabolism of drugs principally metabolised via cytochrome P450 isoenzyme CYP3A4.

Importance and management

No clinically relevant pharmacokinetic interaction is expected between *decaffeinated* green tea and buspirone. However, there is a possible pharmacodynamic interaction between caffeine (a constituent of tea) and benzodiazepines, see Caffeine + Benzodiazepines and related drugs, page 109. Tea can contain significant amounts of caffeine, and therefore this interaction is relevant to tea, unless the product is stated to be decaffeinated.

1. Chow HH, Hakim IA, Vining DR, Crowell JA, Cordova CA, Chew WM, Xu MJ, Hsu CH, Ranger-Moore J, Alberts DS. Effects of repeated green tea catechin administration on human cytochrome P450 activity. *Cancer Epidemiol Biomarkers Prev* (2006) 15, 2473–6.

Tea + Caffeine

Green tea catechins do not appear to affect the pharmacokinetics of caffeine.

Clinical evidence

In a study in 41 healthy subjects, 4 capsules of a **green tea catechin extract** taken daily for 4 weeks had no effect on the metabolism of caffeine to paraxanthine after a single 100-mg dose of caffeine. The **green tea catechin extract** used in this study, *Polyphenon E,* contained 80 to 98% total catechins, of which 50 to 75% (200 mg) was

T

epigallocatechin gallate per capsule. It was essentially decaffeinated (0.5% w/w caffeine).[1]

Experimental evidence

Because of the quality of the clinical evidence available, experimental data have not been sought.

Mechanism

This study provides evidence that green tea catechins (at higher[1] doses than the amount provided by average green tea consumption) are unlikely to affect the metabolism of drugs principally metabolised by the cytochrome P450 isoenzyme CYP1A2.

Importance and management

No pharmacokinetic interaction is expected between *decaffeinated* green tea and caffeine or other CYP1A2 substrates.

Note that tea usually contains caffeine, and therefore the interactions of caffeine, page 106, (including caffeine found in other medicines, supplements or foods) are relevant. Excess caffeine consumption can cause adverse effects, including headache, jitteriness, restlessness, and insomnia. Reduce caffeine intake if problems develop.

1. Chow HH, Hakim IA, Vining DR, Crowell JA, Cordova CA, Chew WM, Xu MJ, Hsu CH, Ranger-Moore J, Alberts DS. Effects of repeated green tea catechin administration on human cytochrome P450 activity. *Cancer Epidemiol Biomarkers Prev* (2006) 15, 2473–6.

Tea + Ciclosporin or Tacrolimus

Green tea catechins do not appear to affect ciclosporin levels, and may protect against the adverse renal effects of ciclosporin and tacrolimus.

Evidence, mechanism, importance and management

In a study in *rats,* epigallocatechin gallate (a **green tea catechin**) had no significant effect on ciclosporin levels and also appeared to protect against ciclosporin-induced renal damage.[1] In another *animal* study, pre-treatment with **green tea polyphenolic extract**, followed by the addition of ciclosporin or tacrolimus blunted the decrease in glomerular filtration rates seen with these drugs.[2] Similar findings were reported in another *animal* study with ciclosporin.[3]

These findings in *animals* provide limited evidence that green tea supplements are unlikely to interact adversely with ciclosporin or tacrolimus, and might actually be beneficial. However, until clinical data are available, it would be unwise for transplant patients taking these immunosuppressants to take tea supplements. Usual consumption of tea beverages does not appear to be a problem.

1. Mun KC. Effect of epigallocatechin gallate on renal function in cyclosporine-induced nephrotoxicity. *Transplant Proc* (2004) 36, 2133–4.
2. Zhong Z, Connor HD, Li X, Mason RP, Forman DT, Lemasters JJ, Thurman RG. Reduction of ciclosporin and tacrolimus nephrotoxicity by plant polyphenols. *J Pharm Pharmacol* (2006) 58, 1533–43.
3. Shi S, Zheng S, Zhu Y, Jia C, Xie H. Inhibitory effect of tea polyphenols on renal cell apoptosis in rat test subjects suffering from cyclosporine-induced chronic nephrotoxicity. *Chin Med J (Engl)* (2003) 116, 1345–50.

Tea + Dextromethorphan

Green tea catechins do not appear to affect the pharmacokinetics of dextromethorphan.

Clinical evidence

In a study in 32 healthy subjects, 4 capsules of a **green tea catechin extract** taken daily for 4 weeks had no effect on the metabolism of dextromethorphan to dextrorphan after a single 30-mg dose of dextromethorphan. The **green tea catechin extract** used in this

study, *Polyphenon E,* contained 80 to 98% total catechins, of which 50 to 75% (200 mg per capsule) was epigallocatechin gallate. It was essentially decaffeinated (0.5% w/w caffeine).[1] Similar findings (a lack of a pharmacokinetic interaction with dextromethorphan) were reported in another study in which 7 subjects received a single 30-mg dose of dextromethorphan before and after *Decaffeinated Super Green Tea Extract* 2 capsules twice daily for 14 days.[2]

Experimental evidence

Because of the quality of the clinical evidence (controlled pharmacokinetic studies), experimental data have not been sought.

Mechanism

These studies provide evidence that green tea catechins (at similar[2] or higher[1] doses than the amount provided by average green tea consumption) are unlikely to affect the metabolism of dextromethorphan.

Importance and management

Evidence from two well-designed clinical studies suggests that green tea does not affect the pharmacokinetics of dextromethorphan. Dextromethorphan is used as a probe drug for CYP2D6 activity, and therefore these results also suggest that a pharmacokinetic interaction as a result of this mechanism between green tea and other CYP2D6 substrates is unlikely.

1. Chow HH, Hakim IA, Vining DR, Crowell JA, Cordova CA, Chew WM, Xu MJ, Hsu CH, Ranger-Moore J, Alberts DS. Effects of repeated green tea catechin administration on human cytochrome P450 activity. *Cancer Epidemiol Biomarkers Prev* (2006) 15, 2473–6.
2. Donovan JL, Chavin KD, Devane CL, Taylor RM, Wang JS, Ruan Y, Markowitz JS. Green tea (Camellia sinensis) extract does not alter cytochrome p450 3A4 or 2D6 activity in healthy volunteers. *Drug Metab Dispos* (2004) 32, 906–8.

Tea + Flurbiprofen

Black tea does not appear to have a clinically relevant effect on the pharmacokinetics of flurbiprofen.

Clinical evidence

In a single-dose study in healthy subjects, brewed **black tea** (*Lipton Brisk* tea) had no effect on the clearance of elimination half-life of flurbiprofen.[1]

Experimental evidence

An *in vitro* study reported that a sample containing brewed **black tea** 2.5% inhibited the hydroxylation of flurbiprofen by CYP2C9 by 89%.[1]

Mechanism

These studies provide evidence that black (fermented) tea is unlikely to affect the metabolism of flurbiprofen.

Importance and management

Although experimental studies[1] suggested that black tea may inhibit the metabolism of flurbiprofen, the study in healthy subjects suggests that any effects is not clinically relevant. No pharmacokinetic interaction is therefore expected between black (fermented) tea and flurbiprofen. Flurbiprofen can be used as a probe drug for CYP2C9 activity, and therefore these results also suggest that a pharmacokinetic interaction as a result of this mechanism between black tea and other CYP2C9 substrates is unlikely.

1. Greenblatt DJ, von Moltke LL, Perloff ES, Luo Y, Harmatz JS, Zinny MA. Interaction of flurbiprofen with cranberry juice, grape juice, tea, and fluconazole: in vitro and clinical studies. *Clin Pharmacol Ther* (2006) 79, 125–33.

Tea + Food

Milk does not appear to affect the absorption of flavonoids or catechins from tea, suggesting that the addition of milk does not impair the antioxidant effects of tea.

Clinical evidence

In a study in 12 healthy subjects, blood levels of catechins did not differ when **black (fermented) tea** was taken with the addition of milk (100 mL semi-skimmed plus water 500 mL with 3 g of instant tea) compared with no milk (3 g instant tea with water 600 mL).[1] Similarly, in another study, plasma levels of the flavonoids quercetin and kaempferol did not differ when **black (fermented) tea** was drunk alone or with the addition of 15 mL of milk to 135 mL of tea.[2] Another study showed similar findings (no difference in increase in total phenols, catechins, quercetin and kaempferol).[3] Conversely, a slight 17% decrease in the AUC of catechins when **black tea** was taken with the addition of 70 mL milk was reported in another study.[4] As regards the plasma antioxidant effect of tea, three studies[3–5] found that the addition of milk to **black (fermented) tea** did not alter the increase in antioxidant potential, whereas one study found that the addition of milk to **black tea** (3 measures consumed between 9 am and 12 noon) markedly reduced the increase in antioxidant effect at 12 noon, but it was only slightly reduced at 3 pm.[6] The addition of milk also had no effect on the antioxidant effect of **green tea** in one study.[5]

In another study in 16 healthy women, the addition of milk (to a final concentration of 10%) to **black tea** completely prevented the increase in endothelial-dependent flow-mediated dilation seen with black tea alone. However, the increase in endothelial-independent vasodilation was not affected by the addition of milk to tea.[7]

Experimental evidence

Because of the extensive clinical evidence available, experimental data have not been sought.

Mechanism

It has been suggested that substances in milk (such as casein[7]) might reduce the absorption of catechins and flavonoids from tea, but this has not been demonstrated in many of the studies.

Importance and management

Although the evidence is not entirely conclusive, there appears to be no important interaction between milk and black (fermented) tea suggesting that the addition of milk does not reduce the antioxidant effects of tea. Similar levels of potentially active catechins and flavonoids can be expected however the tea is taken. This suggests that milk is also unlikely to alter the absorption of catechins from green tea supplements.

1. van het Hof KH, Kivits GA, Weststrate JA, Tijburg LB. Bioavailability of catechins from tea: the effect of milk. *Eur J Clin Nutr* (1998) 52, 356–9.
2. Hollman PC, Van Het, Hof KH, Tijburg LB, Katan MB. Addition of milk does not affect the absorption of flavonols from tea in man. *Free Radic Res* (2001) 34, 297–300.
3. Kyle JA, Morrice PC, McNeill G, Duthie GG. Effects of infusion time and addition of milk on content and absorption of polyphenols from black tea. *J Agric Food Chem* (2007) 55, 4889–94.
4. Reddy VC, Vidya Sagar GV, Sreeramulu D, Venu L, Raghunath M. Addition of milk does not alter the antioxidant activity of black tea. *Ann Nutr Metab* (2005) 49, 189–95.
5. Leenen R, Roodenburg AJ, Tijburg LB, Wiseman SA. A single dose of tea with or without milk increases plasma antioxidant activity in humans. *Eur J Clin Nutr* (2000) 54, 87–92.
6. Langley-Evans SC. Consumption of black tea elicits an increase in plasma antioxidant potential in humans. *Int J Food Sci Nutr* (2000) 51, 309–15.
7. Lorenz M, Jochmann N, von Krosigk A, Martus P, Baumann G, Stangl K, Stangl V. Addition of milk prevents vascular protective effects of tea. *Eur Heart J* (2007) 28, 219–23.

Tea + Herbal medicines; Pepper

The interaction between green tea and pepper is based on experimental evidence only.

Clinical evidence

No interactions found.

Experimental evidence

In a study in *mice*, **piperine** modestly increased the bioavailability of epigallocatechin-3-gallate (EGCG) from **green tea**, with a 30% increase in the AUC_{1-5} and maximum plasma levels.[1]

In vitro, **piperine** inhibited the intestinal glucuronidation of epigallocatechin-3-gallate by up to 60% when used at a concentration of 500 micromol/L.[1]

Mechanism

Piperine appeared to increase EGCG bioavailability by inhibiting glucuronidation and gastrointestinal transit.[1]

Importance and management

The available evidence is from experimental studies only, but it does provide some evidence that piperine (an alkaloid derived from black pepper, page 372) can modestly increase bioavailability of the green tea catechin studied. However, the increases seen are probably unlikely to be clinically important, even if they were to be replicated in a clinical study. Evidence regarding the interactions of other herbal medicines with tea is limited, but the caffeine content of tea suggests that it may interact with other herbal medicines in the same way as caffeine, see Caffeine + Herbal medicines; Bitter orange, page 111, and Ephedra + Caffeine, page 202.

1. Lambert JD, Hong J, Kim DH, Mishin VM, Yang CS. Piperine enhances the bioavailability of the tea polyphenol (-)-epigallocatechin-3-gallate in mice. *J Nutr* (2004) 134, 1948–52.

Tea + Irinotecan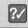

The information regarding the use of green tea with irinotecan is based on experimental evidence only.

Evidence, mechanism, importance and management

Based on the results of *in vitro* studies, it was considered that usual pharmacological doses of **green tea catechins** were unlikely to inhibit the formation of active metabolites of irinotecan. There was no induction of CYP3A4 metabolism, and just modest and variable induction of glucuronidation (UGT1A1). However, the authors did conclude that these effects require confirmation in patients.[1]

1. Mirkov S, Komoroski BJ, Ramırez J, Graber AY, Ratain MJ, Strom SC, Innocenti F. Effects of green tea compounds on irinotecan metabolism. *Drug Metab Dispos* (2007) 35, 228–33.

Tea + Iron compounds

Black tea appears to reduce the absorption of iron and may contribute to iron-deficiency anaemia. Green tea appears to have much smaller, if any, effects.

Clinical evidence

(a) Black tea

There is little data on the effect of tea on the absorption of iron from supplements. One case report describes an impaired response to iron, given to correct iron-deficiency anaemia, in a patient drinking

T

2 litres of black tea daily. The patient recovered when the black tea was stopped. This report did not specify whether the black tea was tea without milk, or black (fermented) tea.[1]

Some short-term controlled studies show a marked reduction in the absorption of *dietary* non-haem iron with black (fermented) tea beverage, some of which are cited for information.[2-5] In one of these, in a series of studies in healthy subjects, a 275 mL serving of black (fermented, Assam) tea reduced the absorption of radiolabelled iron from a 50 g bread roll by 79 to 94%. The tea was prepared by adding 300 mL of boiling water to 3 g of Assam tea, then infusing for 10 minutes before straining and serving. Milk added to the tea had very little effect on the reduction in iron absorption.[5] A study found that 150 mL of black tea reduced the absorption of radiolabelled iron from a test meal by 59% in 10 women with iron deficiency anaemia and by 49% in 10 control subjects without anaemia. When the quantity of tea was increased to 300 mL iron absorption was reduced by about 66% in both groups.[6]

Whether these reductions in iron absorption are important in the development of iron deficiency anaemia is less clear. Various epidemiological studies have looked at the correlation between tea consumption and iron deficiency in different populations. In one review of 16 of these studies, tea consumption did not influence iron status in people with adequate iron stores (as is common in the West), but there seemed to be a negative association between tea consumption and iron status in people with marginal iron status.[7] Another report describes no change in the absorption of a single dose of iron (2 to 15.8 mg/kg) in 10 iron-deficient children when the iron was given with 150 mL of tea (type unspecified) instead of water.[8]

(b) Green tea

A study found that green tea extract (37 mg catechins) showed a modest 26% reduction in iron absorption,[9] and another study, of pure epigallocatechin gallate 150 mg and 300 mg, found only a 14% and 27% reduction in iron absorption, respectively.[10] A study in 4 elderly patients with iron deficiency anaemia and 11 control patients found no evidence that green tea inhibited the absorption of iron from sodium ferrous citrate.[11] Another study in pregnant women with iron deficiency anaemia reported a slightly higher resolution rate for anaemia in patients taking green tea.[12]

Note that tea has been used with some success in reducing iron accumulation and the frequency of phlebotomy in patients with iron overload syndromes.[13]

Experimental evidence

Because of the extensive clinical evidence available, experimental data have not been sought.

Mechanism

Tannins found in tea are thought to form insoluble complexes with non-haem iron and thus reduce its absorption.[2,3] Other polyphenolic compounds found in tea may also reduce the bioavailability of non-haem iron. One study reported that beverages containing 100 to 400 g of polyphenols may reduce iron absorption by 60 to 90%.[5]

Importance and management

The general importance of these findings is uncertain, but be aware that black tea consumption may contribute to iron-deficiency anaemia. However, it has been suggested that no restrictions are required in healthy patients not at risk of iron deficiency.[14] Conversely, the suggestion is that patients at risk of iron deficiency (which would include those requiring iron supplements) should be advised to avoid tea with meals and for one hour after eating.[14] Note that tea is not generally considered to be a suitable drink for babies and children, because of its effects on iron absorption. Milk does not attenuate the effect of black (fermented) teas on iron absorption.

The available data suggest that green tea extracts rich in catechins have less effect on iron absorption than tea beverages from black (fermented) teas. Furthermore, a reduction in absorption of about 20% would not generally be considered to be clinically relevant. No general restrictions are therefore required.

1. Mahlknecht U, Weidmann E, Seipelt G. Black tea delays recovery from iron-deficiency anaemia. *Haematologica* (2001) 86, 559.
2. Disler PB, Lynch SR, Charlton RW, Torrance JD, Bothwell TH, Walker RB, Mayet F. The effect of tea on iron absorption. *Gut* (1975) 16, 193–200.
3. Morck TA, Lynch SR, Cook JD. Inhibition of food iron absorption by coffee. *Am J Clin Nutr* (1983) 37, 416–20.
4. Rossander L, Hallberg L, Björn-Rasmussen E. Absorption of iron from breakfast meals. *Am J Clin Nutr* (1979) 32, 2484–9.
5. Hurrell RF, Reddy M, Cook JD. Inhibition of non-haem iron absorption in man by polyphenolic-containing beverages. *Br J Nutr* (1999) 81, 289–95.
6. Thankachan P, Walczyk T, Muthayya S, Kurpad AV, Hurrell RF. Iron absorption in young Indian women: the interaction of iron status with the influence of tea and ascorbic acid. *Am J Clin Nutr* (2008) 87, 881–6.
7. Temme EHM, Van Hoydonck PGA. Tea consumption and iron status. *Eur J Clin Nutr* (2002) 56, 379–86.
8. Koren G, Boichis H, Keren G. Effects of tea on the absorption of pharmacological doses of an oral iron preparation. *Isr J Med Sci* (1982) 18, 547.
9. Samman S, Sandström B, Bjørndal Toft M, Bukhave K, Jensen M, Sørensen SS, Hansen M. Green tea or rosemary extract added to foods reduces nonheme-iron absorption. *Am J Clin Nutr* (2001) 73, 607–12.
10. Ullmann U, Haller J, Bakker GCM, Brink EJ, Weber P. Epigallocatechin gallate (EGCG) (TEAVIGO) does not impair non-haem-iron absorption in man. *Phytomedicine* (2005) 12, 410–415.
11. Kubota K, Sakuri T, Nakazato K, Shirakura T. Effect of green tea on iron absorption in elderly patients with iron deficiency anaemia [in Japanese]. *Nippon Ronen Igakkai Zasshi* (1990) 27, 555–8.
12. Mitamura T, Kitazono M, Yoshimura O, Yakushiji M. The influence of green tea upon the improvement of iron deficiency anemia with pregnancy treated by sodium ferrous citrate [in Japanese]. *Nippon Sanka Fujinka Gakkai Zasshi* (1989) 41, 688–94.
13. Kaltwasser JP, Werner E, Schalk K, Hansen C, Gottschalk R, Seidl C. Clinical trial on the effect of regular tea drinking on iron accumulation in genetic haemochromatosis. *Gut* (1998) 43, 699–704.
14. Nelson M, Poulter J. Impact of tea drinking on iron status in the UK: a review. *J Hum Nutr Diet* (2004) 17, 43–54.

Tea + Losartan

Green tea extracts do not appear to affect the pharmacokinetics of losartan.

Clinical evidence

In a study in 42 healthy subjects, **green tea extract** four capsules daily for 4 weeks had no effect on the metabolism of a single 25-mg dose of losartan to the metabolite E3174. The **green tea catechin extract** used in this study, *Polyphenon E,* contained 80 to 98% total catechins, of which 50 to 75% (200 mg per capsule) was epigallocatechin gallate. It was essentially decaffeinated (0.5% w/w caffeine).[1]

Experimental evidence

Because of the quality of the clinical evidence (controlled pharmacokinetic studies), experimental data have not been sought.

Mechanism

This study suggests that green tea catechins do not affect the metabolism of losartan.

Importance and management

Evidence is limited to this one study, which suggests that no pharmacokinetic interaction is expected between decaffeinated green tea extract and losartan. Losartan can be used as a probe drug for CYP2C9 activity, and therefore these results also suggest that a pharmacokinetic interaction as a result of this mechanism between green tea extracts and other CYP2C9 substrates is unlikely.

1. Chow HH, Hakim IA, Vining DR, Crowell JA, Cordova CA, Chew WM, Xu MJ, Hsu CH, Ranger-Moore J, Alberts DS. Effects of repeated green tea catechin administration on human cytochrome P450 activity. *Cancer Epidemiol Biomarkers Prev* (2006) 15, 2473–6.

Tea + Warfarin and related drugs

Case reports suggest that tea may reduce the INR in response to warfarin.

Clinical evidence

A patient taking warfarin had a reduction in his INR from a range of 3.2 to 3.79 down to 1.37, which was attributed to the ingestion of very large quantities of **green tea** (about 2 to 4 litres each day for one week). This interaction was attributed to the vitamin-K content of the tea.[1] However, although dried tea, including **green tea**, is very high in vitamin-K$_1$, the brewed liquid made from the tea contains negligible amounts of vitamin K$_1$,[2] and is therefore not considered to contribute any vitamin K$_1$ to the diet.[2] The reason for this interaction is therefore unclear, unless the patient was eating some of the brewed tea leaves.

Another man stabilised on warfarin was found to have an INR of 4.43 at a routine clinic visit, which was increased from 3.07 six weeks previously. The patient had stopped taking a herbal product *Nature's Life Greens* that month because he did not have enough money to buy it. He had been taking it for the past 7 years as a vitamin supplement because he had previously been instructed to limit his intake of green leafy vegetables. He was eventually restabilised on warfarin and the same nutritional product.[3] The product label listed 25 vegetables without stating the amounts or concentrations,[3] but at least 5 of the listed ingredients are known to contain high levels of vitamin K$_1$ including parsley, **green tea leaves**, spinach, broccoli, and cabbage. It is therefore likely it contained sufficient vitamin to antagonise the effect of the warfarin so that when it was stopped the warfarin requirements fell, and without an appropriate adjustment in dose, this resulted in an increased INR.

A further case report describes a 67-year-old woman who had an increase in her INR from a range of 1.7 to 2.7 up to 5, one week after she stopped drinking black tea (brewed from tea bags). The warfarin was temporarily withheld and then restarted at a reduced dose of 26 mg/week (previous dose had been 32 mg/week) and her INR remained between 1.7 and 3.3 over the following 2 months.[4]

Experimental evidence

Because of the clinical evidence available, experimental data have not been sought.

Mechanism

Unknown. Green and black (fermented) tea do not alter the pharmacokinetics of some CYP2C9 substrates. See losartan, page 468, and flurbiprofen, page 466. Therefore it is unlikely that a pharmacokinetic interaction occurs with warfarin, which is principally metabolised by this isoenzyme.

Importance and management

Evidence for an interaction between tea and warfarin appears to be limited to two case reports with green tea and one with black tea. Vitamin K$_1$ antagonises the effect of warfarin and similar anticoagulants, and this is present in high levels in tea leaves. However, vitamin K$_1$ is a fat soluble vitamin, and is therefore not present in brewed tea or water extracts of green tea. In general, a reduction in warfarin effects via this mechanism would be unexpected with tea or tea supplements. Nevertheless, some consider that increased monitoring of INR is advisable when patients taking warfarin want to stop or start any herbal medicine or nutritional supplement. Because of the many other factors influencing anticoagulant control, it is not possible to reliably ascribe a change in INR specifically to a drug interaction in a single case report without other supporting evidence. It may be better to advise patients to discuss the use of any herbal products they wish to try, and to increase monitoring if this is thought advisable. Cases of uneventful use should be reported, as they are as useful as possible cases of adverse effects.

However, note that it has been suggested that tea, particularly green tea, may have antiplatelet effects. See Tea + Antiplatelet drugs, page 465. There is a well-established small increased risk of bleeding when aspirin at antiplatelet doses is combined with the anticoagulant drug warfarin. Theoretically, very high intake of green tea catechins may be sufficient to increase the risk of bleeding with anticoagulant drugs; however, firm evidence for this is lacking. Modest consumption is unlikely to cause any problems.

1. Taylor JR, Wilt VM. Probable antagonism of warfarin by green tea. *Ann Pharmacother* (1999) 33, 426–8.
2. Booth SL, Madabushi HT, Davidson KW, Sadowski JA. Tea and coffee brews are not dietary sources of vitamin K-1 (phylloquinone). *J Am Diet Assoc* (1995) 95, 82–3.
3. Bransgrove LL. Interaction between warfarin and a vitamin K-containing nutritional supplement: a case report. *J Herb Pharmacother* (2001) 1, 85–9.
4. Parker DL, Hoffmann TK, Tucker MA, Meier DJ. Interaction between warfarin and black tea *Ann Pharmacother* (2009) 43, 150–151.

T

Thyme

Thymus vulgaris L. (Lamiaceae)

Synonym(s) and related species

Common thyme, French thyme, Garden thyme, Rubbed thyme.

Thymus aestivus Reut. ex Willk., *Thymus ilerdensis* Gonz. Frag. ex Costa., *Thymus × valentinus* Rouy., *Thymus webbianus* Rouy, *Thymus welwitschii* Boiss. subsp *ilerdensis* (Gonz. Frag. ex Costa) Nyman, and *Thymus zygis* L. are also used.

Not to be confused with wild thyme, which is *Thymus serpyllum* L.

Pharmacopoeias

Thyme (*BP 2012, PhEur 7.5*); Thyme Oil (*BP 2012*); Thyme Oil, Thymol Type (*PhEur 7.5*); Thymol (*BP 2012, PhEur 7.5*).

Constituents

The major non-volatile constituents of thyme are the **flavonoids** including apigenin, eriodictyol, luteolin, naringenin, and others. Other non-volatile constituents include caffeic acid, rosmarinic acid, saponins and tannins. The oil contains up to 70% **thymol**, with carvacrol, *p*-cymene, linalool, α-terpineol and thujan-4-ol. Other species contain similar constituents, although some varieties contain less thymol and more of the other components.

Use and indications

Thyme is used traditionally as a carminative, spasmolytic and antimicrobial, particularly for the respiratory system.

Thymol is widely used in dentistry as a mouthwash, but it is toxic in high doses and should not be taken internally or applied externally in large amounts. Thyme is commonly used as a flavouring ingredient in foods.

Pharmacokinetics

An aqueous extract of thyme has been identified as a potent inhibitor of several cytochrome P450 isoenzymes, namely CYP2C9, CYP2C19, CYP2D6 and CYP3A4, in an *in vitro* study.[1] However, these findings should be interpreted with caution, as the study also found St John's wort to be a CYP3A4 inhibitor, whereas clinically, it is a CYP3A4 inducer.

For information on the pharmacokinetics of individual flavonoids present in thyme, see under flavonoids, page 213.

Interactions overview

No interactions with thyme found. Note that thyme is commonly used as a flavouring ingredient in foods.

For information on the interactions of individual flavonoids present in thyme, see under flavonoids, page 213.

1. Foster BC, Vandenhoek S, Hana J, Krantis A, Akhtar MH, Bryan M, Budzinski JW, Ramputh A, Arnason JT. *In vitro* inhibition of human cytochrome P450-mediated metabolism of marker substrates by natural products. *Phytomedicine* (2003) 10, 334–42.

T

Tolu balsam

Myroxylon balsamum (L.) Harms (Fabaceae)

Synonym(s) and related species

Balsam tolu, Balsamum tolutanum, *Myroxylon balsamum* (L.) var. *balsamum, Myroxylon toluiferum* Kunth, *Toluifera balsamum* L.

Note that Peru balsam is a similar resin obtained from *Myroxylon balsamum* var *pereirae*.

Pharmacopoeias

Tolu Balsam (*BP 2012, PhEur 7.5, USP35–NF30 S1*); Tolu Balsam Syrup (*USP35–NF30 S1*); Tolu Balsam Tincture (*USP35–NF30 S1*).

Constituents

The major constituents of the resin (or balsam), which is collected from incisions in the bark and sapwood, are **cinnamic acid** (to which it may be standardised) and **benzoic acid** and their esters such as cinnamyl cinnamate and benzyl benzoate, and also **resin alcohols** such as coniferyl benzoate and hydroconiferyl benzoate. Vanillin, ferulic acid, and triterpenoids such as oleanolic acid and sumaresinolic acid are also present.

Use and indications

Tolu balsam is considered to have mild expectorant and antiseptic properties. It may be taken orally as a constituent of cough medicines and lozenges. It may also be an ingredient of topical preparations used for the treatment of minor skin abrasions. Compound benzoin tincture can contain tolu balsam, and may be known as Friars' balsam. Tolu balsam is a cause of contact allergy.

Pharmacokinetics

No relevant pharmacokinetic data found.

Interactions overview

No interactions with tolu balsam found.

T

Tribulus

Tribulus terrestris L. (Zygophyllaceae)

Synonym(s) and related species

Caltrops, Gokhru, Puncture vine, *Tribulus lanuginosus* L.

Constituents

The fruits contain a wide range of **saponins** such as gitonin, protodioscin, tribulosaponins A and B, tribulosin, various terrestrosins, and others; lignans known as tribulusamides A and B; and **flavonoids**, such as kaempferol, quercetin and rutin. The flowers contain saponins based on ruscogenin, hecogenin and diosgenin.

Use and indications

The fruit, flowers and root of tribulus are used. Traditionally tribulus has been used for the treatment of inflammation, digestive disorders, cough, headache, mastitis, kidney and bladder stones, and as an aphrodisiac. It is also used as a general tonic, but is now widely used as an anabolic agent. There is some supporting experimental evidence that it has androgenic effects.

Pharmacokinetics

No relevant pharmacokinetic information found. For information about the pharmacokinetics of individual flavonoids present in tribulus, see under flavonoids, page 213.

Interactions overview

No interactions with tribulus found. For information on the interactions of individual flavonoids present in tribulus, see under flavonoids, page 213.

T

Turmeric

Curcuma longa L. (Zingiberaceae)

Synonym(s) and related species

Indian saffron.

Curcuma domestica Valeton is generally accepted to be the same species as *Curcuma longa*.

The related species *Curcuma aromatica* Salisb., is known as wild or aromatic turmeric and *Curcuma xanthorrhiza* D. Dietr., is known as Javanese turmeric.

Not to be confused with *Curcuma zedoaria* (Christmann) Roscoe, which is zedoary.

Pharmacopoeias

Turmeric (*USP35–NF30 S1*); Powdered Turmeric (*USP35–NF30 S1*); Powdered Turmeric Extract (*USP35–NF30 S1*).

Constituents

The active constituents are **curcuminoids**, and include a mixture known as **curcumin** which contains diferuloyl-methane, (sometimes referred to as curcumin or curcumin I), desmethoxycurcumin (curcumin II), bisdesmethoxy-curcumin (curcumin III), and cyclocurcumin (curcumin IV). Most commercially available preparations of 'curcumin' are not pure, but also contain desmethoxycurcumin and bisdesmethoxycurcumin. The related species *Curcuma aromatica* and *Curcuma xanthorrhiza* also contain curcuminoids.

The essential oil contains mainly turmerones, including zingiberene.

Use and indications

Turmeric has many biological activities, which are mainly attributed to the curcuminoids it contains. It is widely used as an anti-inflammatory and liver protecting agent, and its chemopreventive effects for cancer (inhibition of tumour formation, promotion, progression and dissemination in many *animal* models) are the subject of much research. Turmeric is also used for disorders related to the ageing process. Curcumin has an anti-oxidant and anti-inflammatory activity, and has been proposed as a treatment for many degenerative diseases with an inflammatory or oxidative basis, such as cardiovascular diseases, type 2 diabetes, arthrosis and arthritis, among others.

Turmeric is also used as a spice in food.

Pharmacokinetics

An *in vitro* study suggested that curcumin-containing extracts from *Curcuma longa* may inhibit intestinal CYP3A4;[1] this finding is supported by a study in *rats,* see midazolam, page 475. A study in *rats* fed curcumin, found that even large amounts of curcumin (5 g/kg) did not alter the activity of hepatic cytochrome P450 isoenzymes.[2]

Several *in vitro* studies have suggested that curcumin inhibits or alters the effects of P-glycoprotein.[3–5] See also beta blockers, page 474. Further study using individual curcumin constituents extracted from turmeric powder found that curcumin I has a greater inhibitory action on P-glycoprotein than curcumin II or curcurmin III,[6] although curcumin III has been shown to have a greater influence on the multidrug resistance gene (of which P-glycoprotein is a product).[7]

Interactions overview

Turmeric or its constituent curcumin affects the absorption of some beta blockers, increases the absorption of midazolam, but does not affect the absorption of iron. Piperine, from pepper, enhances the bioavailability of curcumin.

Interactions monographs

- Beta blockers, page 474
- Food, page 474
- Herbal medicines; Pepper, page 474
- Iron compounds, page 474
- Midazolam, page 475

1. Hou XL, Takahashi K, Kinoshita N, Qiu F, Tanaka K, Komatsu K, Takahashi K, Azuma J. Possible inhibitory mechanism of Curcuma drugs on CYP3A4 in 1alpha,25 dihydroxyvitamin D3 treated Caco-2 cells. *Int J Pharm* (2007) 337, 169–77.
2. Sugiyama T, Nagata J, Yamagishi A, Endoh K, Saito M, Yamada K, Yamada S, Umegaki K. Selective protection of curcumin against carbon tetrachloride-induced inactivation of hepatic cytochrome P450 isozymes in rats. *Life Sci* (2006) 78, 2188–93.
3. Anuchapreeda S, Leechanachai P, Smith MM, Ambudkar SV, Limtrakul PN. Modulation of P-glycoprotein expression and function by curcumin in multidrug-resistant human KB cells. *Biochem Pharmacol* (2002) 64, 573–82.
4. Zhang W, Lim LY. Effects of spice constituents in P-glycoprotein-mediated transport and CYP3A4-mediated metabolism *in vitro*. *Drug Metab Dispos* (2008) 36, 1283–90.
5. Junyaprasert VB, Soonthornchareonnon N, Thongpraditchote S, Murakami T, Takano M. Inhibitory effect of Thai plant extracts on P-glycoprotein mediated efflux. *Phytother Res* (2006) 20, 79–81.
6. Chearwae W, Anuchapreeda S, Nandigama K, Ambudkar SV, Limtrakul P. Biochemical mechanism of modulation of human P-glycoprotein (ABCB1) by curcumin I, II, and III purified from Turmeric powder. *Biochem Pharmacol* (2004) 68, 2043–52.
7. Limtrakul P, Anuchapreeda S, Buddhasukh D. Modulation of human multidrug-resistance MDR-1 gene by natural curcuminoids. *BMC Cancer* (2004) 4, 13.

T

Turmeric + Beta blockers

In a clinical study, curcumin, a major constituent of turmeric, *decreased* the absorption of talinolol, a P-glycoprotein substrate. Curcumin *increased* the absorption of celiprolol, another P-glycoprotein substrate, in *rats*.

Clinical evidence

In a randomised study, 12 healthy subjects were given a single 50-mg dose of **talinolol** after taking **curcumin**, a major constituent of turmeric, 300 mg daily for 6 days. **Curcumin** was found to reduce the AUC and maximum plasma level of **talinolol** by 33% and 28%, respectively, but no clinically significant changes in heart rate or blood pressure occurred.[1]

Experimental evidence

In a study, *rats* were given curcumin 60 mg/kg daily for 5 days. Thirty minutes after the last dose of **curcumin**, a single 30-mg/kg dose of **celiprolol** was given. **Curcumin** increased the AUC and maximum plasma concentration of **celiprolol** by 30% and 90%, respectively. In a parallel single-dose study in *rats* **curcumin** 60 mg/kg, given 30 minutes before a single 30-mg/kg dose of **celiprolol** had no effect on the pharmacokinetics of **celiprolol**.[2]

Mechanism

It was thought that curcumin inhibits P-glycoprotein and therefore increases the absorption of P-glycoprotein substrates such as talinolol. This appears to be the case in a *rat* study, where curcumin had effects similar to (but weaker than) other known, clinically relevant P-glycoprotein inhibitors, that is, it increased the absorption of celiprolol, another P-glycoprotein substrate. However, in a clinical study the absorption of talinolol was unexpectedly *decreased* by curcumin; however, clinically, the known P-glycoprotein inhibitor verapamil also decreases talinolol absorption. This suggests that there may be other mechanisms involved in talinolol absorption. Differential effects on hepatic and intestinal P-glycoprotein may also be of relevance.

Importance and management

Evidence for an interaction between curcumin (a major constituent of turmeric) and beta blockers is sparse, but the available evidence does suggest that curcumin can modify the absorption of beta blockers that are P-glycoprotein substrates. The findings with talinolol were similar to the effects seen clinically with other P-glycoprotein inhibitors (see *Mechanism*). However, the effects on absorption were modest, and beta blockers are generally accepted to have a wide therapeutic margin, so these findings would not be expected to be clinically relevant. It is unclear whether the effects of curcumin on celiprolol in *rats* will be replicated in humans. However, as with talinolol the effects were modest and are therefore unlikely to be clinically relevant.

1. Juan H, Terhaag B, Cong Z, Bi-Kui Z, Rong-Hua Z, Feng W, Fen-Li S, Juan S, Jung T, Wen-Xing P. Unexpected effect of concomitantly administered curcumin on the pharmacokinetics of talinolol in healthy Chinese volunteers. *Eur J Clin Pharmacol* (2007) 63, 663–8.
2. Zhang W, Tan TMC, Lim L-Y. Impact of curcumin-induced changes in P-glycoprotein and CYP3A expression on the pharmacokinetics of peroral celiprolol and midazolam in rats. *Drug Metab Dispos* (2007) 35, 110–115.

Turmeric + Food

Consider Turmeric + Herbal medicines; Pepper, below. Turmeric is used as a spice in food.

Turmeric + Herbal medicines; Pepper

Piperine, a major constituent of pepper, increases the bioavailability of curcumin, a major constituent of turmeric.

Clinical evidence

In a crossover study, 8 healthy subjects were given a single 2-g dose of **curcumin**, a major constituent of turmeric, powder alone, or with **piperine**, a major constituent of pepper, powder 20 mg. When **curcumin** was given alone, its serum levels were either very low, or undetectable. The addition of **piperine** increased **curcumin** levels 30-fold over the first 45 minutes, and the relative bioavailability of **curcumin** was increased 20-fold. Concurrent use was well tolerated.[1]

Experimental evidence

In an experimental study, *rats* were given a single 2-g/kg dose of curcumin alone, or with piperine 20 mg/kg. Although piperine modestly increased the maximum levels and AUC of curcumin, these changes were not statistically significant. Note that curcumin was reasonably well absorbed in *rats,* in contrast to humans, where absorption is poor, but this may have been due to the much greater doses given.[1]

Mechanism

Unknown. It was suggested that piperine may inhibit the metabolism of curcumin.

Importance and management

In general the evidence supports the suggestion that piperine (a constituent of pepper) increases the bioavailability of curcumin (a major constituent of turmeric). This interaction may be beneficial because the effects of curcumin may be increased; however, it may also increase the potential for curcumin to interact with other medicines. The effect of piperine on the absorption of curcumin from turmeric extracts does not appear to have been studied, but it seems reasonable to expect a similar increase in bioavailability.

1. Shoba G, Joy D, Joseph T, Majeed M, Rajendran R, Srinivas PSSR. Influence of piperine on the pharmacokinetics of curcumin in animals and human volunteers. *Planta Med* (1998) 64, 353–6.

Turmeric + Iron compounds

Turmeric does not appear to affect the bioavailability of dietary levels of iron.

Clinical evidence

In a randomised, crossover study, 30 healthy women were given a standard Thai meal (fortified with about 4 mg of isotopically labelled ferrous sulfate), with rice, to which 500 mg of ground turmeric had been added. Turmeric was found to have no effect on the absorption of iron.[1]

Experimental evidence

No relevant data found.

Mechanism

It was thought that polyphenols in turmeric may inhibit iron absorption.

Importance and management

The study cited suggests that turmeric does not inhibit the absorption of dietary levels of iron. However, the authors note that the amount of turmeric used was relatively low, when compared with the intake from some Asian diets. Furthermore, the effects of turmeric on iron supplementation (e.g. ferrous sulfate in doses of 200 mg) does not appear to have been studied, so it is difficult to predict the effect of the use of turmeric as a herbal medicine on iron replacement therapy. However, what is known suggests that an interaction would not be expected.

1. Tuntipopipat S, Judprasong K, Zeder C, Wasantwisut E, Winichagoon P, Charoenki-atkul S, Hurrell R, Walczyk T. Chili, but not turmeric, inhibits iron absorption in young women from an iron-fortified composite meal. *J Nutr* (2006) 136, 2970–2974.

Turmeric + Midazolam

The interaction between curcumin, a major constituent of turmeric, and midazolam is based on experimental evidence only.

Clinical evidence
No interactions found.

Experimental evidence
In a study, *rats* were given **curcumin**, a major constituent of turmeric, 60 mg/kg daily for 5 days. Thirty minutes after the last dose of **curcumin**, a single 20-mg/kg dose of midazolam was given. **Curcumin** increased the AUC of midazolam 3.8-fold, and although the maximum plasma level was approximately doubled, this was not statistically significant.[1]

Mechanism
Midazolam is a substrate of the cytochrome P450 subfamily CYP3A (specifically the isoenzyme CYP3A4). The authors of the study suggest that curcumin inhibited intestinal CYP3A, resulting in a decrease in the metabolism of midazolam by this route, which led to an increase in its bioavailability.

Importance and management
Evidence appears to be limited to this study in *rats,* which demonstrated a large increase in the bioavailability of midazolam. These findings are difficult to reliably extrapolate to humans, but as the effect was so large, it would seem reasonable to assume that curcumin could cause a clinically relevant increase in the bioavailability of midazolam, which may lead to an increase in the sedative effects of midazolam. It is not clear whether turmeric, of which curcumin is a major constituent, would have similar effects, but if large doses are given an effect seems possible. It would seem prudent to warn patients taking curcumin, and turmeric, about the possible increase in sedative effects.

Midazolam is used as a probe drug for CYP3A4 activity, and therefore these results also suggest that a pharmacokinetic interaction between curcumin (and therefore possibly turmeric) and other CYP3A4 substrates is possible. See the table Drugs and herbs affecting or metabolised by the cytochrome P450 isoenzyme CYP3A4, page 7, for a list of known CYP3A4 substrates.

1. Zhang W, Tan TMC, Lim L-Y. Impact of curcumin-induced changes in P-glycoprotein and CYP3A expression on the pharmacokinetics of peroral celiprolol and midazolam in rats. *Drug Metab Dispos* (2007) 35, 110–115.

No interactions have been included for herbal medicines or dietary supplements beginning with the letter U

Valerian

Valeriana officinalis L. (Valerianaceae)

Synonym(s) and related species

All-heal, Belgian valerian, Common valerian, Fragrant valerian, Garden valerian.

Many other *Valerian* species are used in different parts of the world.

Pharmacopoeias

Cut Valerian (*BP 2012*); Powdered Valerian (*USP35−NF30 S1*); Powdered Valerian Extract (*USP35−NF30 S1*);Valerian (*BP 2012, USP35−NF30 S1*); Valerian Dry Aqueous Extract (*BP 2012, PhEur 7.5*); Valerian Dry Hydroalcoholic Extract (*BP 2012, PhEur 7.5*); Valerian Root (*PhEur 7.5*); Valerian Root, Cut (*PhEur 7.5*); Valerian Tablets (*USP35−NF30 S1*); Valerian Tincture (*BP 2012, PhEur 7.5*).

Constituents

Valerian root and rhizome contains a large number of constituents which vary considerably according to the source of the plant material and the method of processing and storage. Many are known to contribute to the activity, and even those that are known to be unstable may produce active decomposition products. The valepotriates include the valtrates, which are active constituents, but decompose on storage to form other actives including baldrinal, and volatile constituents. The volatile oil is composed of valerenic acids and their esters, and other derivatives including isovaleric acid (which is responsible for the odour of valerian), and others. Other constituents present include the free amino acids gamma-aminobutyric acid (GABA); the **flavonoids** flavone 6-methylapigenin, hesperidin and linarin; alkaloids of the pyridine type including valerianine and valerine, and sterols including β-sitosterol.

Valerian dry hydroalcoholic extract is an extract produced from valerian root and contains a minimum of 0.25% sesquiterpenic acids, expressed as valerenic acid.

Use and indications

Valerian is used particularly for stress and insomnia. It has long been used as a hypnotic, sedative, anxiolytic, antispasmodic, carminative and antihypertensive, and for hypochondriasis, migraine, cramp, intestinal colic, rheumatic pains and dysmenorrhoea. Despite many pharmacological studies showing sedative and anxiolytic effects, and binding or modulation of constituents to GABA and other neurotransmitter receptors, the clinical efficacy is not conclusively proven. A recent study suggested it is safe, but not necessarily effective; however many analytical reports also show that extracts and products of valerian vary greatly in both chemical composition and biological activity, and it may be that only certain preparations have any therapeutic benefit. Many commercial products use valerian in combination with hops, passiflora, and other herbal extracts and there is some evidence that these may be more efficacious, although again this is not clinically proven. The use of valerian as an aid to benzodiazepine withdrawal has been suggested on the basis of GABA-receptor binding effects, and there is a small study in *mice* which suggests it may be useful to a limited extent; again this has not been shown clinically.

Pharmacokinetics

An *in vitro* study using a number of different valerian root preparations (capsules or tablets of the powdered extract, and teas) found that the products tested inhibited the cytochrome P450 isoenzyme CYP3A4.[1] Other *in vitro* studies have found no effects,[2] or an inductive effect at levels unlikely to be obtained clinically.[3] Generally, studies suggest that any effect on CYP3A4 is unlikely to be of clinical importance, see benzodiazepines, page 479.

A further *in vitro* study[2] suggests that valerian has no effect, or weak effects, on CYP1A2 (see also caffeine, page 480), CYP2C9, or CYP2C19. This study also suggests that valerian does not affect CYP2D6, although another *in vitro* study suggests that valerian may cause induction of CYP2D6, but this was at concentrations that are unlikely to be attained *in vivo*.[3] These effects are unlikely to be clinically relevant because a study in 12 healthy subjects found that valerian root extract had no significant effects on the metabolism of debrisoquine, a probe substrate for CYP2D6,[4] as did another clinical study using dextromethorphan, page 480). A further clinical study suggests that valerian also has no clinically relevant effect on CYP2E1, see chlorzoxazone, page 480.

In vitro investigations have suggested that valerian may inhibit P-glycoprotein,[1,5] although the authors of one study concluded that this is unlikely to be clinically relevant, because the concentration at which this occurred is unlikely to be attained *in vivo*,[5] and the findings of another study suggested that the effects were much weaker than those of verapamil, a known, clinically relevant P-glycoprotein inhibitor.[1]

For information on the pharmacokinetics of individual flavonoids present in valerian, see under flavonoids, page 213.

Interactions overview

Valerian does not appear to affect the metabolism of alprazolam, caffeine, chlorzoxazone, dextromethorphan, or midazolam to a clinically relevant extent. Valerian may increase the sleeping time in *mice* in response to alcohol and barbiturates. Case reports describe possible interactions with ginkgo, see Ginkgo + Herbal medicines; Valerian, page 246 and St John's wort and/or loperamide, see St John's wort + Loperamide, page 453. For information on the interactions of individual flavonoids present in valerian, see under flavonoids, page 213.

Interactions monographs

1. Lefebvre T, Foster BC, Drouin CE, Krantis A, Arnason JT, Livesey JF, Jordan SA. *In vitro* activity of commercial valerian root extracts against human cytochrome P450 3A4. *J Pharm Pharm Sci* (2004) 7, 265–73.
2. Zou L, Harkey MR, Henderson GL. Effects of herbal components on cDNA-expressed cytochrome P450 enzyme catalytic activity. *Life Sci* (2002) 71, 1579–89.
3. Hellum BH, Hu Z, Nilsen OG. The induction of CYP1A2, CYP2D6 and CYP3A4 by six trade herbal products in cultured primary human hepatocytes. *Basic Clin Pharmacol Toxicol* (2007) 100, 23–30.
4. Gurley BJ, Gardner SF, Hubbard MA, Williams DK, Gentry WB, Khan IA, Shah A. *In vivo* effects of goldenseal, kava kava, black cohosh, and valerian on human cytochrome P450 1A2, 2D6, 2E1, and 3A4/5 phenotypes. *Clin Pharmacol Ther* (2005) 77, 415–26.
5. Hellum BH, Nilsen OG. In vitro inhibition of CYP3A4 metabolism and P-glycoprotein-mediated transport by trade herbal products. *Basic Clin Pharmacol Toxicol* (2008) 102, 466–75.

Valerian + Alcohol

The interaction between valerian and alcohol is based on experimental evidence only.

Clinical evidence

No interactions found.

Experimental evidence

In a study in *mice,* a valepotriates extract of valerian, given in high doses, almost doubled the sleeping time in response to alcohol. In contrast, in a separate experiment, the extract appeared to antagonise the effects of alcohol on motor activity.[1]

Mechanism

Additive CNS depressant effects.

Importance and management

The evidence of an interaction between valerian and alcohol appears to be limited to a study in *mice.* However, valerian is said to have sedative effects, and is used for insomnia, and so additive effects on sedation seem possible. The manufacturers[2,3] of two herbal products containing valerian that are registered by the MHRA in the UK, advise against excessive alcohol intake while taking valerian because the sedative effect of valerian may be potentiated by alcohol. It seems reasonable to suggest that additive sedative effects are possible. It would be prudent to warn patients that they may be more sedated if they drink alcohol while taking valerian, and if this occurs, to avoid undertaking skilled tasks. Note that in the study in *mice,* the sedative effects of valepotriates, even in large doses were more modest than those of diazepam and chlordiazepoxide. Remember that not all the indications of valerian are as an anxiolytic/hypnotic.

1. von Eickstedt K-W. Die Beeinflussung der Alkohol-Wirkung durch valepotriate. *Arzneimittelforschung* (1969) 19, 995–7.
2. Niteherb Tablets (Dry extract of valerian root). MH Pharma (UK) Ltd. UK Summary of product characteristics, December 2007.
3. Valdrian Capsules (Valerian root). Bio-Health Ltd. UK Summary of product characteristics, July 2008.

Valerian + Barbiturates

The interaction between valerian and barbiturates is based on experimental evidence only.

Clinical evidence

No interactions found.

Experimental evidence

In a study in *mice,* **valerenic acid** (an active constituent of valerian) 50 or 100 mg/kg was found to increase sedation (measured by balance tests), but only at the highest doses. The effect was strongest 10 to 15 minutes after administration. **Pentobarbital** 60 mg/kg also sedated the *mice,* but the effects were more pronounced than those with **valerenic acid**. When both substances were given together, **valerenic acid** prolonged the sleeping time in response to **pentobarbital**. The effect was dose-dependent, with the higher **valerenic acid** dose approximately doubling the **pentobarbital** sleeping time.[1]

Mechanism

Valerenic acid has non-specific central nervous depressant properties, which appear to enhance the effects of pentobarbital.[1]

Importance and management

Evidence for an interaction between valerenic acid and pentobarbital appears to be limited to this study in *mice*; however, the effects are in line with the known activities of both substances. It is unclear whether the use of valerian would result in an effect of similar magnitude, but some additive sedation seems likely. Other barbiturates do not appear to have been studied, but it seems likely that they will interact similarly. It may therefore be prudent to consider the potential additive sedative effects in any patient taking barbiturates with valerian. This seems most likely to be of importance with the use of **phenobarbital** (or other barbiturates) for epilepsy, when sedative effects are less desirable. It would be prudent to warn patients that they may be more sedated, and if this occurs, to avoid undertaking skilled tasks. Remember that not all the indications of valerian are as an anxiolytic/hypnotic.

1. Hendriks H, Bos R, Woerdenbag HJ, Koster AS. Central nervous depressant activity of valerenic acid in the mouse. *Planta Med* (1985) 51, 28–31.

Valerian + Benzodiazepines

Valerian does not affect the pharmacokinetics of alprazolam or midazolam to a clinically relevant extent. However, additive sedative effects are a possibility.

Clinical evidence

In a crossover study, 12 healthy subjects were given valerian root extract 1 g each night for 14 days, with a single 2-mg dose of **alprazolam** on the morning of day 15. Valerian increased the maximum plasma concentration of **alprazolam** by 20%, but there were no other statistically significant changes in the pharmacokinetics of **alprazolam**.[1] The valerian extract used in this study contained 11 mg of valerenic acid per gram.

In another study, 12 healthy subjects were given valerian root extract 125 mg three times daily for 28 days before receiving a single dose of **midazolam**. Valerian root extract caused no significant changes in the metabolism of **midazolam**.[2]

Experimental evidence

No relevant data found.

Mechanism

Valerian has been found in some *in vitro* studies to be an inhibitor of the cytochrome P450 isoenzyme CYP3A4. See pharmacokinetics, page 477. Alprazolam and midazolam are metabolised by this isoenzyme. The minor pharmacokinetic changes reported therefore suggest that clinically, valerian has only slight effects on CYP3A4.

Importance and management

Evidence from two well-designed clinical studies suggest that valerian does not have a clinically relevant effect on the pharmacokinetics of either alprazolam or midazolam (the 20% rise in alprazolam levels seen in one study would not be expected to be clinically relevant). Therefore no dosage adjustment of either benzodiazepine would appear to be needed if valerian is also given. However, note that valerian is said to have sedative effects, and is used for insomnia, and so additive effects on sedation seem possible. There seems to be no reason to avoid the concurrent use of valerian with alprazolam or midazolam, but as with any combination of CNS depressant drugs, warn patients that they be more drowsy, and caution against undertaking skilled tasks if this occurs.

Midazolam is used as a probe drug for CYP3A4 activity, and therefore these results also suggest that a pharmacokinetic interaction between valerian and other CYP3A4 substrates is unlikely.

1. Donovan JL, DeVane CL, Chavin KD, Wang J-S, Gibson BB, Gefroh HA, Markowitz JS. Multiple night-time doses of valerian (*Valeriana officinalis*) had minimal effects on CYP3A4 activity and no effect on CYP2D6 activity in healthy volunteers. *Drug Metab Dispos* (2004) 32, 1333–6.
2. Gurley BJ, Gardner SF, Hubbard MA, Williams DK, Gentry WB, Khan IA, Shah A. In vivo effects of goldenseal, kava kava, black cohosh, and valerian on human cytochrome P450 1A2, 2D6, 2E1, and 3A4/5 phenotypes. *Clin Pharmacol Ther* (2005) 77, 415–26.

Valerian + Caffeine

Valerian does not affect the pharmacokinetics of caffeine to a clinically relevant extent. However, the stimulant effects of caffeine may oppose the hypnotic effects of valerian.

Clinical evidence

In a study, 12 non-smoking healthy subjects were given valerian root extract 125 mg three times daily for 28 days with a single 100-mg dose of oral caffeine at the end of supplementation. Valerian root extract caused no significant changes in the metabolism of caffeine.[1]

Experimental evidence

No relevant data found.

Mechanism

Opposing pharmacological effects.

Importance and management

Although the evidence is limited to one study, it was a well-designed study in healthy subjects. It suggests that the use of valerian will not alter the pharmacokinetics of caffeine. However, the effects of caffeine (a stimulant) are likely to be in direct opposition to the effects of valerian (a hypnotic), and although this does not appear to have been studied, caffeine has been shown to diminish the effects of other known hypnotic drugs. Therefore patients requiring valerian for its hypnotic properties should probably also consider their caffeine intake.

Caffeine is used as a probe drug for CYP1A2 activity, and therefore these results also suggest that a pharmacokinetic interaction between valerian and other CYP1A2 substrates is unlikely.

1. Gurley BJ, Gardner SF, Hubbard MA, Williams DK, Gentry WB, Khan IA, Shah A. In vivo effects of goldenseal, kava kava, black cohosh, and valerian on human cytochrome P450 1A2, 2D6, 2E1, and 3A4/5 phenotypes. Clin Pharmacol Ther (2005) 77, 415–26.

Valerian + Chlorzoxazone

Valerian does not affect the pharmacokinetics of chlorzoxazone to a clinically relevant extent. However, additive sedative effects are a possibility.

Clinical evidence

In a study, 12 healthy subjects were given valerian root extract 125 mg three times daily for 28 days with a single 250-mg dose of oral chlorzoxazone at the end of supplementation. Valerian root extract caused no significant changes in the metabolism of chlorzoxazone.[1]

Experimental evidence

No relevant data found.

Mechanism

Additive pharmacological effects.

Importance and management

Although the evidence is limited to one study, it was a well-designed study in healthy subjects. It suggests that the use of valerian will not alter the pharmacokinetics of chlorzoxazone. However, note that chlorzoxazone has sedative effects, and although this was not studied, it may be prudent to consider the possibility of additive sedation when valerian is also given.

Chlorzoxazone is used as a probe drug for CYP2E1 activity, and therefore these results also suggest that a pharmacokinetic interaction between valerian and other CYP2E1 substrates is unlikely.

1. Gurley BJ, Gardner SF, Hubbard MA, Williams DK, Gentry WB, Khan IA, Shah A. In vivo effects of goldenseal, kava kava, black cohosh, and valerian on human cytochrome P450 1A2, 2D6, 2E1, and 3A4/5 phenotypes. Clin Pharmacol Ther (2005) 77, 415–26.

Valerian + Dextromethorphan

Valerian does not affect the pharmacokinetics of dextromethorphan to a clinically relevant extent.

Clinical evidence

In a crossover study, 12 healthy subjects were given valerian root extract 1 g each night for 14 days, with a single 30-mg dose of dextromethorphan on the morning of day 15. Valerian extract caused no significant changes in the pharmacokinetics of dextromethorphan. The valerian extract used in this study contained 11 mg of valerenic acid per gram.[1]

Experimental evidence

See pharmacokinetics, page 477, for in vitro studies of the possible inducing effects of valerian on the cytochrome P450 isoenzyme CYP2D6.

Mechanism

Although in vitro study suggests that valerian may induce the cytochrome P450 isoenzyme CYP2D6, this effect only occurred at high dose, and the clinical study suggests that this effect does not occur in humans.

Importance and management

Although the evidence is limited to one study, it was a well-designed study in healthy subjects. It suggests that the use of valerian will not alter the pharmacokinetics of dextromethorphan.

Dextromethorphan is used as a probe drug for CYP2D6 activity, and therefore these results also suggest that a pharmacokinetic interaction between valerian and other CYP2D6 substrates is unlikely.

1. Donovan JL, DeVane CL, Chavin KD, Wang J-S, Gibson BB, Gefroh HA, Markowitz JS. Multiple night-time doses of valerian (Valeriana officinalis) had minimal effects on CYP3A4 activity and no effect on CYP2D6 activity in healthy volunteers. Drug Metab Dispos (2004) 32, 1333–6.

Valerian + Food

No interactions found.

Valerian + Herbal medicines

For a report of a possible interaction between valerian and ginkgo, see Ginkgo + Herbal medicines; Valerian, page 246. For a case describing delirium in a patient taking St John's wort, valerian and loperamide, see St John's wort + Loperamide, page 453.

Valerian + Loperamide

For a case of delirium, involving the use of loperamide, St John's wort and valerian, see under St John's wort + Loperamide, page 453.

Vervain

Verbena officinalis L. (Verbenaceae)

Synonym(s) and related species

Verbena, *Verbena setosa* M. Martens & Galeotti.

Not to be confused with Lemon verbena, which is unrelated.

Pharmacopoeias

Verbena Herb (*BP 2012, PhEur 7.5*).

Constituents

Vervain contains **iridoid glycosides** including verbenalin (verbanaloside), to which it may be standardised, verbenin (aucubin) and hastatoside; **phenylpropanoid glycosides** including acteoside (verbascoside) and eukovoside; **flavonoids** such as luteolin; and an **essential oil**, the main components of which are citral, geraniol, limonene and verbenone.

Use and indications

Vervain has been used to treat a wide variety of disorders, and has purported bitter, secretolytic and sedative properties. It is used as a tonic to aid convalescence, for mild nervous system disorders such as anxiety and depression, and for jaundice, nasal congestion and sinusitis, and digestive disorders, often in combination with other herbs. However, clinical trial evidence is generally lacking for any of these uses.

Pharmacokinetics

No relevant pharmacokinetic data found. For information on the pharmacokinetics of individual flavonoids present in vervain, see under flavonoids, page 213.

Interactions overview

Vervain may reduce the absorption of iron compounds. For information on the interactions of individual flavonoids present in vervain, see under flavonoids, page 213.

Interactions monographs

- Food, page 482
- Herbal medicines, page 482
- Iron compounds, page 482

V

Vervain + Food

No interactions found.

Vervain + Herbal medicines

No interactions found.

Vervain + Iron compounds

Vervain tea caused a modest reduction in iron absorption in one study.

Clinical evidence

In a study in 10 healthy subjects, a 275 mL serving of vervain tea reduced the absorption of iron from a 50 g bread roll by about 59%. The tea was prepared by adding 300 mL of boiling water to 3 g of the herbal tea, then infusing for 10 minutes before straining and serving. In this study, the inhibitory effect of vervain tea on iron absorption was modestly less than that of black tea (Assam tea, *Camellia sinensis* L.), which is known to inhibit iron absorption,[1] see also, Tea + Iron compounds, page 467.

Experimental evidence

No relevant data found.

Mechanism

The polyphenols in vervain may bind to iron in the intestine and reduce its absorption.

Importance and management

The clinical relevance of this interaction is unclear, as the effect on absorption was smaller than that of black tea (Assam tea, *Camellia sinensis* L.), which is known to inhibit iron absorption (see Tea + Iron compounds, page 467). Until more is known it may be prudent to consider intake of herbal teas such as vervain in patients requiring iron supplementation and in patients that are particularly unresponsive to iron replacement therapy.

1. Hurrell RF, Reddy M, Cook JD. Inhibition of non-haem iron absorption in man by polyphenolic-containing beverages. *Br J Nutr* (1999) 81, 289–95.

White horehound

Marrubium vulgare L. (Lamiaceae)

Synonym(s) and related species

Common hoarhound, Hoarhound, Horehound, Marrubium, *Marrubium hamatum* L.

Not to be confused with Black horehound (*Ballota nigra*).

Pharmacopoeias

White Horehound (*BP 2012, PhEur 7.5*)

Constituents

White horehound contains **diterpenes**, mainly **marrubiin**, to which it may be standardised, and various alcohols including marrubenol, marrubiol, peregrinol and vulgarol. Marrubiin may be an artefact formed from premarrubiin during extraction. **Flavonoids** are also present and include apigenin, luteolin, quercetin and their glycosides, and there is also a small amount of **volatile oil** containing bisabolol, camphene, *p*-cymene, limonene, β-pinene, sabinene and others.

Use and indications

White horehound has been used mainly for its supposed expectorant and antispasmodic properties for conditions such as acute or chronic bronchitis and whooping cough, and for loss of appetite and dyspepsia. Marrubiin is thought to be responsible for the expectorant properties.

Pharmacokinetics

No relevant pharmacokinetic data found. For information on the pharmacokinetics of individual flavonoids present in white horehound, see under flavonoids, page 213.

Interactions overview

No interactions with white horehound found. For information on the interactions of individual flavonoids present in white horehound see under flavonoids, page 213.

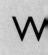

Wild yam

Dioscorea villosa L. (Dioscoreaceae)

Synonym(s) and related species

Colic root, Rheumatism root.

Constituents

The major constituents of the root and rhizome are saponins based mainly on diosgenin and other sapogenins; they include dioscin and dioscorin.

Use and indications

Traditionally, wild yam was used to treat rheumatism and intestinal colic. However, more recently wild yam extract has found favour as a form of topical hormone replacement therapy for women. It is often claimed that wild yam is a source of 'natural progesterone', but this is not the case – it is a source of diosgenin, which is used by the pharmaceutical industry as a chemical precursor for the production of progesterone.

Pharmacokinetics

No relevant pharmacokinetic data found.

Interactions overview

No interactions with wild yam found.

Willow

Salix species (Salicaceae)

Synonym(s) and related species

European willow, Salix, White willow,

Salix alba L., *Salix cinerea* L., *Salix daphnoides*, *Salix fragilis* L., *Salix pentandra* L., *Salix purpurea* L.

Pharmacopoeias

Willow Bark (*BP 2012, PhEur 7.5*); Willow Bark Dry Extract (*BP 2012, PhEur 7.5*).

Constituents

The bark of willow contains the phenolic glycosides **salicin** (up to 10%), acetylsalicin, salicortin, salireposide, picein, triandrin. Esters of salicylic acid, salicyl alcohol, and **flavonoids** and tannins are also present. Extracts are sometimes standardised to a minimum of 1.5% of total salicylic derivatives, expressed as **salicin** (*BP 2012, PhEur 7.5*).

Use and indications

The bark of willow is reported to have analgesic, anti-inflammatory, antipyretic and astringent properties. It has long been used for treating all kinds or fevers, headache, influenza, rheumatism, gout and arthritis.

Pharmacokinetics

In a pharmacokinetic study, 10 healthy subjects were given two oral doses of *Salix purpurea* bark extract, each standardised to contain 120 mg of salicin, 3 hours apart and 30 minutes before meals. Salicylic acid was the most prominent metabolite detected in the serum, with peak levels achieved approximately 1 hour after the dose. The AUC of salicylic acid from the willow bark extract was equivalent to the AUC of salicylic acid from an 87-mg dose of aspirin (given to healthy subjects in another study).[1] However, it is not clear if this amount of salicylic acid has the same antiplatelet effects as aspirin: one study found that taking an extract of the bark of *Salix purpurea* and *Salix daph-*

noides, to achieve a salicin dose of 240 mg daily, had a much smaller effect on platelet aggregation than aspirin.[2]

Interactions overview

No interactions with willow found. It has been suggested that willow bark is likely to interact with antiplatelet drugs and NSAIDs (which have antiplatelet effects), and increase the risk of bleeding with anticoagulants. This is because one constituent, **salicin**, is metabolised to salicylic acid, a substance that is also derived from aspirin. Given that pharmacokinetic studies (see above) suggest that doses of willow bark extracts can achieve levels of salicylic acid that are equivalent to an 87-mg dose of aspirin, this seems reasonable. However, other studies suggest that the antiplatelet effects of aspirin are much greater than those of willow bark, which suggests that willow bark extracts may be less likely to interact than aspirin. The antiplatelet effects of willow bark need much more research before any firm recommendations can be made about its potential to interact with antiplatelet drugs, NSAIDs, and anticoagulants; however, until more is known some caution is warranted.

The concurrent use of willow bark and antiplatelet drugs (such as aspirin or clopidogrel) need not be avoided: indeed combinations of antiplatelet drugs are often prescribed together, but it may be prudent to be aware of the potential for increased bleeding. Patients should discuss any episode of prolonged bleeding with a healthcare professional.

Clinically, the use of an antiplatelet drug with an anti-coagulant should generally be avoided in the absence of a specific indication. It may therefore be prudent to advise against concurrent use with willow bark. However, if concurrent use is felt desirable it would seem sensible to warn patients to be alert for any signs of bruising or bleeding, and report these immediately, should they occur.

This advice is probably applicable to any herb with known antiplatelet effects.

1. Schmid B, Kötter I, Heide L. Pharmacokinetics of salicin after oral administration of a standardised willow bark extract. *Eur J Clin Pharmacol* (2001) 7, 387–91.
2. Krivoy N, Pavlotzky E, Chrubasik S, Eisenberg E, Brook G. Effect of Salicis cortex extract on human platelet aggregation. *Planta Med* (2001) 67, 209–12.

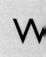

No interactions have been included for herbal medicines or dietary supplements beginning with the letter X

Yarrow

Achillea millefolium L. (Asteraceae)

Synonym(s) and related species

Achillea, Milfoil, Nosebleed.

Achillea collina Becker and *Achillea lanulosa* Nutt. are closely related and are also frequently used.

Pharmacopoeias

Yarrow (*BP 2012, PhEur 7.5*).

Constituents

Yarrow contains a volatile oil composed of various monoterpenes (including limonene and α-thujone), and sesquiterpene lactones (including achillicin, achillin, millefin and millefolide). Azulene is the major component in the closely related *Achillea collina* and *Achillea lanulosa* but it is reported to be absent in *Achillea millefolium*. Yarrow also contains pyrrolidine and pyridine alkaloids, **flavonoids** (including apigenin, quercetin and rutin), tannins and sugars.

Use and indications

Yarrow has been used in the treatment of bruises, swellings and strains, and for fevers and colds. It has also been used for essential hypertension, amenorrhoea, dysentery, diarrhoea, and specifically for thrombotic conditions. There is little, if any, clinical evidence to support these uses, but extracts and many of the constituents have reported anti-inflammatory and antiplatelet activity.

Pharmacokinetics

An *in vitro* study suggests that ethanol extracts of yarrow leaves and flowers markedly inhibit the cytochrome P450 isoenzyme CYP2C19 but have only weak inhibitory effects on CYP3A4. The clinical significance of the effects on CYP2C19 is unknown.[1] For information on the pharmacokinetics of individual flavonoids present in yarrow, see under flavonoids, page 213.

Interactions overview

No interactions with yarrow found. For information on the interactions of individual flavonoids present in yarrow, see under flavonoids, page 213.

1. Scott IM, Leduc RI, Burt AJ, Marles RJ, Arnason JT, Foster BC. The inhibition of human cytochrome P450 by ethanol extracts of North American botanicals. *Pharm Biol* (2006) 44, 315–27.

No interactions have been included for herbal medicines or dietary supplements beginning with the letter Z

Z

Index

All of the herbal medicines, dietary supplements, nutraceuticals and drugs included in this book, whether interacting or not, are listed in this index. Drugs may also be listed under the group names if the interaction is thought to apply to the group as a whole, or if several members of the group have been shown to interact. Note that in some circumstances, broad terms (e.g. analgesics) have been used, where the information is in sufficient to allow more specific indexing. It is therefore advisable to look up both the individual drug

and its group to ensure that all the relevant information is obtained. It may also be advisable to look up both interactants if you don't initally find what you are looking for as synonyms are also included as lead-ins. You can possibly get a lead on the way unlisted drugs behave if you look up those that are related, but bear in mind that none of them is identical and any conclusions reached should only be tentative.